CLINICAL
NEUROSURGERY

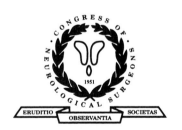

LIPPINCOTT
WILLIAMS
& WILKINS

Copyright ©2002
THE CONGRESS OF NEUROLOGICAL SURGEONS

Accurate indications, adverse reactions, and dosage schedules for drugs are provided in this book, but it is possible that they may have changed. The reader is urged to review the package information data of the manufacturer of the medications mentioned.

Printed in the United States of America
(ISBN 0-7817-4236-6)

CLINICAL NEUROSURGERY

Volume 49

Proceedings

OF THE
CONGRESS OF NEUROLOGICAL SURGEONS

San Diego, California
2001

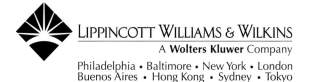
LIPPINCOTT WILLIAMS & WILKINS
A **Wolters Kluwer** Company
Philadelphia • Baltimore • New York • London
Buenos Aires • Hong Kong • Sydney • Tokyo

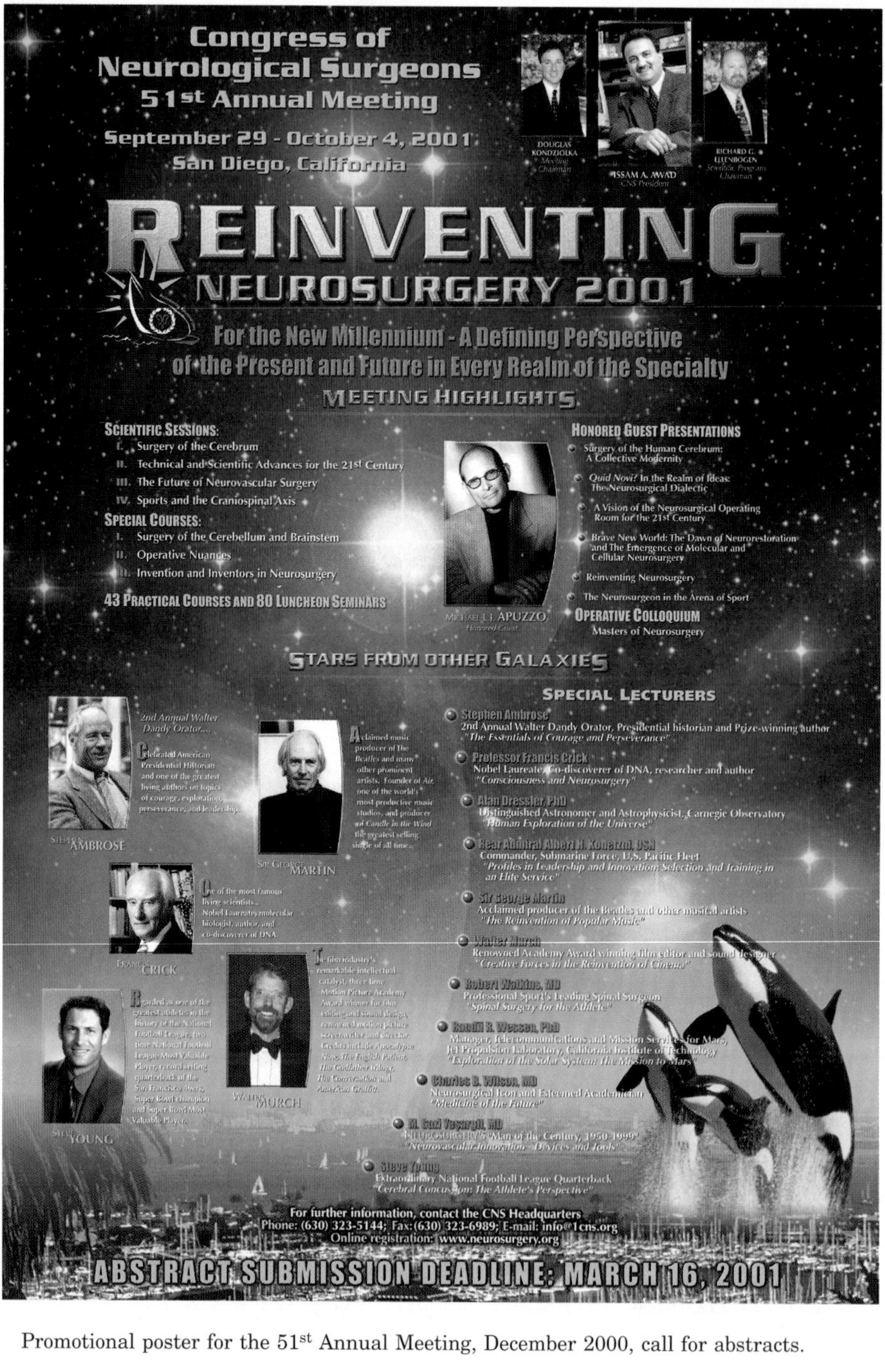

Promotional poster for the 51st Annual Meeting, December 2000, call for abstracts.

Preface

REINVENTING NEUROSURGERY: 9/11: THE MIRACLE OF SAN DIEGO, 2001

The formulation of the fall 2001 Annual Meeting of the Congress of Neurological Surgeons began in February 2000 as the principals met on site. At that time, it was decided that the general theme would be *Reinventing Neurosurgery*, reflecting the dramatic changes in the discipline that had taken place in the previous generation and the ongoing rapid metamorphosis of the field during the past decade.

According to tradition, the scientific program's fabric and design was to be fashioned according to the career and interests of the honored guest and, therefore, themes of cerebral surgery, advanced technology, futurism, molecular biology, minimalism, and the neurosurgeon in sport were established. These elements were to be rendered on a backdrop of international collegiality and mutual contribution. In addition, it was decided that a number of innovations would be added to the program. The most significant of these was an expanded array of individuals and topics presented in a special lecture mode designed to stimulate not only the scientific, but also other intellectual interests and facets of those in attendance. These included discussions related to reinvention themes in astronomy, space-exploration, popular music, film, history, sports, and military leadership.

Program Chair—Richard Ellenbogen—along with his committee, Meeting Chair—Doug Kondziolka, and President Issam Awad worked creatively and harmoniously to establish what was a new benchmark in educational meeting design and presentation. The list of special lecturers was unusually stellar and included Nobel Laureate Frances Crick; prize-winning historian Stephen Ambrose; the noted musical producer Sir George Martin; Academy Award winning filmmaker Walter Murch; Carnegie Observatory astronomer Allan Dressler; Jet Propulsion Laboratory scientist and Mars Mission Director Randii Wesson; Chief of Staff of the United States, Atlantic Fleet Vice Admiral Albert H. Konetzni; the exceptional athlete, National Football League and Super Bowl Most Valuable Player Steve Young; former Honored Guests, Gazi Yasagil and Charles Wilson; and other neurosurgical icons. By late August 2001, advance registration and projected meeting attendance were at record high levels.

With the tragic and horrific attack on New York's World Trade Center on Tuesday, September 11, 2001, the nation and world entered a surrealistic period, which virtually paralyzed our country for days. Generalized cancellation of events and a disruption of travel that would be evident in various stages for months to come peaked as all were largely overcome by the event and its practical ramifications. I was in Denver with Issam Awad and his family, completing a visitorship and attending to the New York Football Giants in their season opening Monday night game against the Denver Broncos. I was preparing to travel to Los Angeles on that Tuesday morning, but was delayed, as were many, for five days because the airport closures and surface travel congestion.

During that period, with considerable uncertainty but maximum resolve, the Congress Leadership and Laurie Behncke, the Executive Director, made the decision to go forward with the San Diego Meeting— an action that required both courage and confidence in the ability of the nation and world to sufficiently restore itself after the calamity.

From September 11 until September 26, San Diego was in complete dormancy. All hotels were closed, with only security and a single staff person on hand to answer telephones. All restaurants were closed, meetings were canceled, and every hosting function was inoperative. Such a situation was evident not only in San Diego but also nationally as the country struggled to recover. During this period, a number of cancellations of attendees and speakers occurred.

But as the time of the meeting approached, it became apparent that as the world struggled to recover, the focal point of the Annual Meeting in San Diego was to be a special and restorative event in every sense of the word. With an attendance of over six thousand, the meeting was held in a uniquely celebratory air—the participants rejoiced in neurosurgery, progress, and all of the best elements of the human spirit. A sense of resolve and hope, as well as an unusual bonding, occurred among all in the massive international attendance body. It was a remarkable atmosphere, a truly unique event in the history of neurosurgery and the stream of human history in general. Considering the global air and the truly unique circumstances it could be considered "the miracle of San Diego 2001"—*it was a time like no other!*

This volume represents the essence of the scientific fabric of the invited topical speakers during the general sessions. It has been compiled by Matthew Howard of the University of Iowa and his remote staff of Associate Editors—Charles S. Cobbs, M.D., J. Paul Elliott, M.D.; Guy M. McKhann II, M.D.—with Brenda Gropman deserving special praise for her efforts. The work of Christine M. Arnold of Lippincott Williams & Wilkins and Laura Horowitz of Hearthside Publishing Services has likewise been particularly noteworthy in making this volume a reality.

Michael L.J. Apuzzo, M.D.
Honored Guest 2001
Los Angeles, California

Honored Guests

1952—Professor Herbert Olivecrona, Stockholm, Sweden
1953—Sir Geoffrey Jefferson, Manchester, England
1954—Dr. Kenneth G. McKenzie, Toronto, Canada
1955—Dr. Carl W. Rand, Los Angeles, California
1956—Dr. Wilder G. Penfield, Montreal, Canada
1957—Dr. Francis C. Grant, Philadelphia, Pennsylvania
1958—Dr. A. Earl Walker, Baltimore, Maryland
1959—Dr. William J. German, New Haven, Connecticut
1960—Dr. Paul C. Bucy, Chicago, Illinois
1961—Professor Eduard A. V. Busch, Copenhagen, Denmark
1962—Dr. Bronson S. Ray, New York, New York
1963—Dr. James L. Poppen, Boston, Massachusetts
1964—Dr. Edgar A. Kahn, Ann Arbor, Michigan
1965—Dr. James C. White, Boston, Massachusetts
1966—Dr. Hugh A. Kravenbühl, Zurich, Switzerland
1967—Dr. W. James Gardner, Cleveland, Ohio
1968—Professor Normal M. Dott, Edinburgh, Scotland
1969—Dr. Wallace B. Hamby, Cleveland, Ohio
1970—Dr. Barnes Woodhall, Durham, North Carolina
1971—Dr. Elisha S. Gurdjian, Detroit, Michigan
1972—Dr. Francis Murphey, Memphis, Tennessee
1973—Dr. Henry G. Schwartz, St. Louis, Missouri
1974—Dr. Guy L. Odom, Durham, North Carolina
1975—Dr. William A. Sweet, Boston, Massachusetts
1976—Dr. Lyle A. French, Minneapolis, Minnesota
1977—Dr. Richard C. Schneider, Ann Arbor, Michigan
1978—Dr. Charles G. Drake, London, Ontario, Canada
1979—Dr. Frank H. Mayfield, Cincinnati, Ohio
1980—Dr. Eben Alexander, Jr., Winston-Salem, North Carolina
1981—Dr. J. Garber Galbraith, Birmingham, Alabama
1982—Dr. Keiji Sano, Tokyo, Japan
1983—Dr. C. Miller Fisher, Boston, Massachusetts
1984—Dr. Hugo V. Rizzoli, Washington, DC
   Dr. Walter E. Dandy (posthumously), Baltimore, Maryland
1985—Dr. Sidney Goldring, St. Louis, Missouri
1986—Dr. M. Gazi Yasargil, Zurich, Switzerland
1987—Dr. Thomas W. Langiftt, Philadelphia, Pennsylvania
1988—Professor Lindsay Symon, London, England
1989—Dr. Thoralf M. Sundt, Jr., Rochester, Minnesota

1990—Dr. Charles Byron Wilson, San Francisco, California
1991—Dr. Bennett M. Stein, New York, New York
1992—Dr. Robert G. Ojemann, Boston, Massachusetts
1993—Dr. Albert L. Rhoton, Jr., Gainesville, Florida
1994—Dr. Robert F. Spetzler, Phoenix, Arizona
1995—Dr. John A. Jane, Charlottesville, Virginia
1996—Dr. Peter J. Jannetta, Pittsburgh, Pennsylvania
1997—Dr. Nicholas T. Zervas, Boston, Massachusetts
1998—Dr. John M. Tew, Cincinnati, Ohio
1999—Dr. Duke S. Samson, Dallas, Texas
2000—Dr. Edward R. Laws, Charlottesville, Virginia
2001—Dr. Michael L. J. Apuzzo, Los Angeles, California

Officers of the Congress
of
Neurological Surgeons
2001

ISSAM A. AWAD, M.D.,
President

STEPHEN M. PAPADOPOULOS, M.D.,
President-Elect

MARK N. HADLEY, M.D., F.A.S.C.   GERALD E. RODTS, JR. M.D.,
Vice President   *Secretary*

PAUL J. CAMARATA, M.D.,
Treasurer

DANIEL L. BARROW, M.D.,
Past President

EXECUTIVE COMMITTEE

JOEL D. MACDONALD, M.D.   RICHARD G. ELLENBOGEN, M.D.
P. DAVID ADELSON, M.D.   MICHAEL L. LEVY, M.D.
CHRISTOPHER C. GETCH, M.D.   DAVID F. JIMENEZ, M.D.
CHRISTOPHER E. WOLFLA, M.D.   DOUGLAS KONDZIOLKA, M.D.
DANIEL K. RESNICK, M.D.   ANTHONY L. ASHER, M.D.
B. GREGORY THOMPSON, JR., M.D.   ISABELLE M. GERMANO, M.D.
NELSON M. OYESIKU, M.D.   BEVERLY C. WALTERS, M.D.

Editors-in-Chief
Clinical Neurosurgery

Volume	Date	Editor-in-Chief
1	1953	Raymond K. Thompson, M.D.
2	1954	Raymond K. Thompson, M.D. & Ira J. Jackson, M.D.
3	1955	Raymond K. Thomspon, M.D. & Ira J. Jackson, M.D.
4	1956	Ira J. Jackson, M.D.
5	1957	Robert G. Fisher, M.D.
6	1958	Robert G. Fisher, M.D.
7	1959	Robert G. Fisher, M.D.
8	1960	William H. Mosberg, Jr., M.D.
9	1961	William H. Mosberg, Jr., M.D.
10	1962	William H. Mosberg, Jr., M.D.
11	1963	John Shillito, Jr., M.D., & William H. Mosberg, Jr., M.D.
12	1964	John Shillito, Jr., M.D.
13	1965	John Shillito, Jr., M.D.
14	1966	Robert G. Ojemann, M.D. & John Shillito, Jr., M.D.
15	1967	Robert G. Ojemann, M.D.
16	1968	Robert G. Ojemann, M.D.
17	1969	Robert G. Ojemann, M.D.
18	1970	George T. Tindall, M.D.
19	1971	George T. Tindall, M.D.
20	1972	Robert H. Wilkins, M.D.
21	1973	Robert H. Wilkins, M.D.
22	1974	Robert H. Wilkins, M.D.
23	1975	Ellis B. Keener, M.D.
24	1976	Ellis B. Keener, M.D.
25	1977	Ellis B. Keener, M.D.
26	1978	Peter W. Carmel, M.D.
27	1979	Peter W. Carmel, M.D.
28	1980	Peter W. Carmel, M.D.
29	1981	Martin H. Weiss, M.D.
30	1982	Martin H. Weiss, M.D.
31	1983	Martin H. Weiss, M.D.
32	1984	John R. Little, M.D.
33	1985	John R. Little, M.D.
34	1986	John R. Little, M.D.
35	1987	Peter McL. Black, M.D., Ph.D.
36	1988	Peter McL. Black, M.D., Ph.D.

37   1989   Peter McL. Black, M.D., Ph.D.
38   1990   Warren R. Selman, M.D.
39   1991   Warren R. Selman, M.D.
40   1992   Warren R. Selman, M.D.
41   1993   Christopher M. Loftus, M.D.
42   1994   Christopher M. Loftus, M.D.
43   1995   Christopher M. Loftus, M.D.
44   1996   M. Sean Grady, M.D.
45   1997   M. Sean Grady, M.D.
46   1998   M. Sean Grady, M.D.
47   1999   Matthew A. Howard III, M.D.
48   2000   Matthew A. Howard III, M.D.
49   2001   Matthew A. Howard III, M.D.

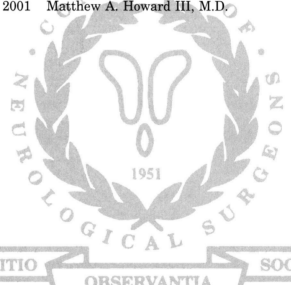

Contributors

P. David Adelson, M.D., F.A.C.S., F.A.A.P.
University of Pittsburgh School of Medicine and Children's
  Hospital of Pittsburgh
Pittsburgh, Pennsylvania

John R. Adler, Jr., M.D.
Departments of Neurosurgery and Radiation Oncology
Stanford University Medical Center
Stanford, California

Arun Paul Amar, M.D.
Clinical Instructor
Neurological Surgery
Keck School of Medicine
University of Southern California
Los Angeles, California

Michael L.J. Apuzzo, M.D.
Edwin M. Todd, M.D./Trent H. Wells Jr. Professor of Neurological
  Surgery
And Radiation Oncology, Biology and Physics
Department of Neurological Surgery
Keck School of Medicine, University of Southern California
Los Angeles, California
and
Principle Neurosurgical Consultant
Department of Athletics
University of Southern California
and
Principle Neurosurgical Consultant
New York Giants Football Club
East Rutherford, New Jersey

Issam A. Awad, M.D.
Department of Neurosurgery
University of Colorado Health Sciences Center
Denver, Colorado

Julian E. Bailes, M.D.
West Virginia University
School of Medicine
Department of Neurosurgery
Morgantown, West Virginia

Daniel L. Barrow, M.D.
MBNA/Bowman Professor and Chairman
Department of Neurosurgery
Emory University School of Medicine
Atlanta, Georgia

Bernard R. Bendok, M.D.
Department of Neurosurgery and Toshiba Stroke Research Center
School of Medicine and Biomedical Sciences
University at Buffalo
State University of New York
Buffalo, New York

Edward C. Benzel, M.D.
Director, Spinal Disorders
The Cleveland Clinic Foundation
Cleveland, Ohio

Cherisse Berry, B.S.
Keck School of Medicine, University of Southern California
Los Angeles, California

Peter Black, M.D., Ph.D.
Neurosurgeon-in-Chief
Department of Neurosurgery
Brigham and Women's Hospital
Boston, Massachusetts

Jeffrey Bost, P.A.-C
Department of Neurological Surgery
University of Pittsburgh Medical Center
Pittsburgh, Pennsylvania

Alan S. Boulos, M.D.
Department of Neurosurgery and Toshiba Stroke Research Center
School of Medicine and Biomedical Sciences
University at Buffalo
State University of New York
Buffalo, New York

Alexandra Chabrerie M.S.
Department of Neurosurgery
Brigham and Women's Hospital
Boston, Massachusetts

Michael Collins, Ph.D.
UPMC Sports Medicine Concussion Program
UPMC Sports Medicine Performance Complex
Pittsburgh, Pennsylvania

Joseph Eskridge, M.D.
Departments of Radiology and Neurological Surgery
University of Washington
Seattle, Washington

Rodrick A. Faccio, B.S.
Staff Editor for Design
Neurosurgery
Los Angeles, California

Lisa A. Ferrara, M.S.
Director, Spine Research Laboratory
Department of Neurosurgery
Department of Orthopaedic Surgery
The Cleveland Clinic Foundation
Cleveland, Ohio

Mauro A. T. Ferreira, M.D.
Neuroscience Research Department
Barrow Neurological Institute
St. Joseph's Hospital and Medical Center
Phoenix, Arizona

Mel Field, M.D.
Department of Neurological Surgery
University of Pittsburgh Medical Center
Presbyterian Hospital
Pittsburgh, Pennsylvania

Amory Fiore, M.D.
The Department of Neurosurgery and the Neurospine Institute
Emory University
Atlanta, Georgia

Aaron J. Fleischman, Ph.D.
Co-Director, BioMEMS Laboratory
Department of Biomedical Engineering
The Cleveland Clinic Foundation
Cleveland, Ohio

John C. Flickinger, M.D.
Departments of Neurological Surgery and Radiation Oncology
University of Pittsburgh Medical Center
Pittsburgh, Pennsylvania

Kevin T. Foley, M.D.
Image-Guided Surgery Research Center and Department of
   Neurosurgery
College of Medicine
University of Tennessee Health Science Center
Memphis, Tennessee

Alexandra Golby, M.D.
Department of Neurosurgery
Brigham and Women's Hospital
Boston, Massachusetts

M. Sean Grady, M.D.
Department of Neurological Surgery
University of Pennsylvania
Philadelphia, Pennsylvania

Laverne Gugino, M.D.
Department of Anesthesia
Brigham and Women's Hospital
Boston, Massachusetts

Lee R. Guterman, Ph.D., M.D.
Department of Neurosurgery and Toshiba Stroke Research Center
School of Medicine and Biomedical Sciences
University at Buffalo
State University of New York
Buffalo, New York

Paul A. Grabb, M.D.
University of Alabama/Neurosurgery
Birmingham, Alabama

Mark N. Hadley, M.D., F.A.C.S.
University of Alabama/Neurosurgery
Birmingham, Alabama

Regis W. Haid, Jr., M.D.
The Department of Neurosurgery and the Neurospine Institute
Emory University
Atlanta, Georgia

Byron Hansen, M.S., ATC
Athletic Trainer
New York Giants Football Club
East Rutherford, New Jersey

Jeffrey S. Henn, M.D.
Division of Neurological Surgery
Barrow Neurological Institute
St. Joseph's Hospital and Medical Center
Phoenix, Arizona

L. Nelson Hopkins, M.D.
Department of Neurosurgery and Toshiba Stroke Research Center
School of Medicine and Biomedical Sciences
University at Buffalo
State University of New York
Buffalo, New York

Juha Jaaskelainen, M.D.
Department of Neurosurgery
Brigham and Women's Hospital
Boston, Massachusetts

Patrick J. Kelly, M.D., F.A.C.S.
Professor and Chairman
Department of Neurosurgery
New York University School of Medicine
New York, New York

Douglas Kondziolka, M.D.,M.Sc., F.R.C.S.C., F.A.C.S.
Professor of Neurological Surgery and Radiation Oncology
Department of Neurological Surgery
Pittsburgh, Pennsylvania

Michael A. Lefkowitz, M.D.
Image-Guided Surgery Research Center and Department of
  Neurosurgery
College of Medicine
University of Tennessee Health Science Center
Memphis, Tennessee

G. Michael Lemole, Jr., M.D.
Division of Neurological Surgery
Barrow Neurological Institute
St. Joseph's Hospital and Medical Center
Phoenix, Arizona

Elad I. Levy, M.D.
Department of Neurosurgery and Toshiba Stroke Research Center
School of Medicine and Biomedical Sciences
University at Buffalo
State University of New York
Buffalo, New York

Michael L. Levy, M.D., Ph.D.
Associate Professor of Neurological Surgery
Division of Neurological Surgery
Children's Hospital of Los Angeles
Los Angeles, California
and
Neurosurgical Consultant
Department of Athletics
University of Southern California

Mark A. Liker, M.D.
Clinical Instructor
Neurological Surgery
Keck School of Medicine
University of Southern California
Los Angeles, California

Charles Y. Liu, M.D., Ph.D.
Clinical Instructor of Neurosurgery
Department of Neurological Surgery
Keck School of Medicine, University of Southern California
Los Angeles, California
and

Visiting Researcher
Division of Chemistry and Chemical Engineering
California Institute of Technology
Pasadena, California

Mark Lovell, Ph.D., A.B.P.N.
Director, UPMC Sports Medicine Concussion Program
UPMC Sports Medicine Performance Complex
Pittsburgh, Pennsylvania

David A. Lundin, M.D.
Department of Neurological Surgery
University of Washington
Seattle, Washington

L. Dade Lunsford, M.D.
Departments of Neurological Surgery and Radiation Oncology
University of Pittsburgh Medical Center
Pittsburgh, Pennsylvania

Joseph C. Maroon, M.D.
Heindl Scholar and Professor
Department of Neurological Surgery
University of Pittsburgh Medical Center
Presbyterian Hospital
Pittsburgh, Pennsylvania

Marc R. Mayberg, M.D.
The Cleveland Clinic
Cleveland, Ohio

Vincent J. Miele M.D.
West Virginia University
School of Medicine
Department of Neurosurgery
Morgantown, West Virginia

Debbie H. Mielke
University of Alabama/Neurosurgery
Birmingham, Alabama

Praveen Mummaneni, M.D
The Department of Neurosurgery and the Neurospine Institute
Emory University
Atlanta, Georgia

David W. Newell, M.D.
Department of Neurological Surgery
University of Washington
Seattle, Washington

Nelson M. Oyesiku, M.D.,
University of Alabama/Neurosurgery
Birmingham, Alabama

Carmen A. Petraglia, B.S.
The Duquesne University
Pittsburgh, Pennsylvania

Mark Preul, M.D.
Neuroscience Research Department
Barrow Neurological Institute
St. Joseph's Hospital and Medical Center
Phoenix, Arizona

Gregory J. Przybylski, M.D.
University of Alabama/Neurosurgery
Birmingham, Alabama

Adnan I. Qureshi, M.D.
Department of Neurosurgery and Toshiba Stroke Research Center
School of Medicine and Biomedical Sciences
University at Buffalo
State University of New York
Buffalo, New York

Daniel K. Resnick, M.D.
University of Alabama/Neurosurgery
Birmingham, Alabama

Gerald E. Rodts, Jr., M.D.
The Department of Neurosurgery and the Neurospine Institute
Emory University
Atlanta, Georgia

Robert H. Rosenwasser, M.D.
Division of Cerebrovascular Surgery
and Interventional Neuroradiology
Thomas Jefferson University Hospital
Philadelphia, Pennsylvania

Shuvo Roy, Ph.D.
Co-Director, BioMEMS Laboratory
Department of Biomedical Engineering
The Cleveland Clinic Foundation
Cleveland, Ohio

Timothy C. Ryken, M.D.
University of Alabama/Neurosurgery
Birmingham, Alabama

Mark Schornak, M.S.
Divisions of Neurological Surgery
Barrow Neurological Institute
St. Joseph's Hospital and Medical Center
Phoenix, Arizona

Christopher I. Shaffrey, M.D.
Department of Neurological Surgery
University of Washington
Seattle, Washington

Joseph Skiba
Assistant Equipment Manager
New York Giants Football Club
East Rutherford, New Jersey

Volker K.H. Sonntag, M.D.
Division of Neurological Surgery
Barrow Neurological Institute
St. Joseph's Hospital and Medical Center
Phoenix, Arizona

Robert F. Spetzler, M.D.
Divisions of Neurological Surgery
Barrow Neurological Institute
St. Joseph's Hospital and Medical Center
Phoenix, Arizona

Jayashree Srinivasan, M.D.
Swedish Medical Center
Seattle, Washington

Kevin L. Stevenson, M.D.
University of Pittsburgh School of Medicine
and Children's Hospital of Pittsburgh
Pittsburgh, Pennsylvania

Brian R. Subach, M.D.
Assistant Professor
Department of Neurosurgery and the Neurospine Institute
Emory University
Atlanta, Georgia

Daniel Sullivan, M.Div.
Managing Editor
Neurosurgery
Los Angeles, California

Joseph L. Voelker, M.D.
West Virginia University
School of Medicine
Department of Neurosurgery
Morgantown, West Virginia

Beverly C. Walters, M.D.
University of Alabama/Neurosurgery
Birmingham, Alabama

Michael Y. Wang, M.D.
Clinical Instructor Department of Neurological Surgery
Keck School of Medicine
University of Southern California
Los Angeles, California

H. Richard Winn, M.D.
Department of Neurological Surgery
University of Washington
Seattle, Washington

Diana B. Wiseman, M.D.
Department of Neurological Surgery
University of Washington
Seattle, Washington

Geoffrey P. Zubay, M.D.
Division of Neurological Surgery
Barrow Neurological Institute
St. Joseph's Hospital and Medical Center
Phoenix, Arizona

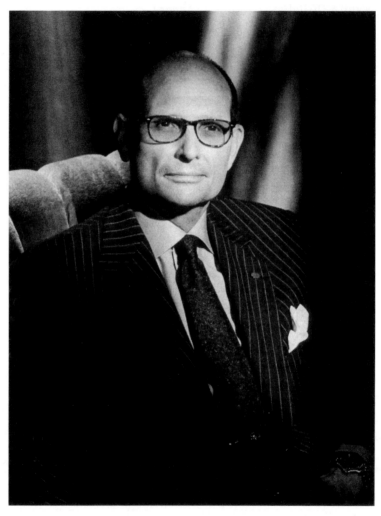

Michael L. J. Apuzzo, M.D.

Biography

Michael L.J. Apuzzo was born in New Haven Connecticut, the son of a fine craftsman/precision machinist and an operating room nurse. The Apuzzo family had a long maritime heritage with roots in Amalfi on the southern Italian coast. The maternal Lorenz family was Austrian with ties to the Art department at the University of Vienna. From an early age he was influenced by family interests in music, art, and sports as well as significant cultural influences created by the Yale University environments working at the Yale Bowl and campus for various athletic and cultural events. As a child he acquired an admiration for refined craftsmanship while watching his father create exquisite wooden yachts and sailboats in a boatyard on the Quinnipiac River and later worked on commercial boats bearthed in this area harvesting at the oyster beds in Long Island Sound.

He received his secondary education at the Hopkins Grammar School. Founded in 1660 with yearly classes of 40 or fewer students, the highly intense and disciplined environment was singularly influential in developing his academic style and interests. Within that setting, the appreciation of classicism, art, history, literature, physical and biological science and particularly competitive sport were further developed and fostered.

He entered Yale College with a primary interest in architecture, but as a work study student was serendipitously assigned to catalogue books at the Harvey Cushing Library under the direction of Madeline Stanton, Cushing's former secretary. This experience helped to redirect his goals. He ultimately graduated with a major focus in psychology and zoology with active participation in varsity-level intercollegiate sports and enjoying highly stimulating experiences at the Bingham Oceanographic Laboratories at the University that included biological research activities and performing hypophysectomies on various fish species.

After entering the Boston University School of Medicine, he was particularly influenced by noted neuroanatomist Arthur Lassek, gastroenterologist Franz Inglefinger (Editor, *New England of Medicine*), renologist Arnold Relman (later to become Editor of the *New England Journal of Medicine*), the esteemed neurologist and physiologist Derek Denny-Brown at the Boston City Hospital and the academic surgeons Reginald Smithwick, Richard Egdahl, John Mannick and Francis Moore, who were instrumental in initiating his concept of the surgeon as a physiologist and innovator. His senior thesis under Denny-

Brown's direction was entitled, "The Enigma of Parkinsonism" and dealt with basal ganglia pathophysiological states.

At Egdahl's urging, he entered a period of general surgical training at McGill's Royal Victoria Hospital under the direction of the brilliant and ebullient Lloyd B. MacLean. At that time he was influenced in his development channels by his contact with the famous cardiac surgeon and innovator Arthur Vineberg and the faculty of the Montreal Neurological Institute, particularly Theodore Rassmussen and William Feindel, who helped to arrange a residency opportunity within the Yale Medical School setting. There he was encouraged by William German (a former Cushing fellow and long-time Yale chairman), the flamboyant and creative William B. Scoville, and Benjamin B. Whitcomb. Finally, William F. Collins, Jr. (later Editor of the *Journal of Neurosurgery*), who came to Yale in a chair transition, was highly supportive but, more importantly, became powerfully influential as a quintessential academic role model who solidified his perception of career surgical objectives and fundamental standards. Under Collins' direction, he undertook complex electrophysiological studies of thalamic and dorsal horn lamina mapping over an eighteen month period.

With Scoville he was introduced to the concept of minimally invasive techniques and the power of creativity and progressive thinking in the operative setting.

Apuzzo went on to enter the United States Navy Nuclear Powered Submarine Service where, after special training in submarine operations, deep sea diving, and nuclear, submarine, and diving medicine, he was assigned to hazardous duty on extended submarine patrols to Polar regions, the Mediterranean and Black Seas. During the course of service on the U.S.S. Robert E. Lee (SSBN-601), he earned Submarine Dolphins qualifying in submarines and deep sea diving. His thesis entitled *The Management of Acute Head Injuries on Polaris Submarines* was selected by Admiral Hyman Rickover and his advisors for inclusion within the medical resources throughout the nuclear submarine fleet. Subsequently, he was awarded and given special commendations by the United States Surgeon General and the Commander of the Atlantic Submarine Fleet for unusual actions and achievements in connection with patrol duties. This experience and scientific background proved to be singularly important in the development of his career and focus toward introduction and transfer of complex technology to hospital and patient care settings. Additionally he became more appreciative of the potential for the use of methods of employing ionizing radiation in the nervous system.

In 1973 Apuzzo joined the faculty of the department of Neurological Surgery at the University of Southern California School of Medicine, where his associations with Theodore Kurze in the early developmental refinement of microsurgery and its applications, particularly in deep cerebral microsurgery, and Martin Weiss as an academic role model and supporter were highly influential in establishing both directional substance, focus and motivation. During this early and later periods he focused intensely on detailed aspects of microsurgical, instrumentation, methodology, its application in both the head and spine as well as aspects of operating room design. The environment proved to be exceptionally fertile.

In 1976 he established an amalgam with the Jet Propulsion Laboratory in association with the California Institute of Technology working at the time with scientists at Cape Kennedy/Cape Canaveral in conjunction with the Mars Viking project. This interaction fostered a twenty five year relationship that refocused on the development and transfer of complex technology to the operating room and other areas of patient care from the aerospace and defense industries. This included, in part, work on complex imaging utilization in intracranial surgery, robotics, the introduction of biosensors and the biological applications of the free electron laser.

In 1978, through the intercession of Edwin Todd, he established a working relationship with the genius biomechanical engineer Trent H. Wells, Jr. and over a 12 year period working with Wells in his machine shop/laboratory helped to develop and refine the initial and then developing novel imaging directed stereotactic systems for point and volume stereotaxy, and later, early units of linear accelerator developed radiosurgery. Over time he refined, applied, championed and popularized these concepts in the operating room and clinical settings. Importantly, he established dialogue and mutual projects with USC Schools of Engineering and Cinema-Television, developing programs with film industries computer graphics resources. The computer became a neurosurgical tool.

In 1976, at the urging of Harold Young and Stephen Mahaley, he established one of the nation's first central nervous system tumor-immunology laboratories. He introduced the concept and terms "cellular and molecular neurosurgery," eventually performing the first reported series of stereotactically bilaterally implanted adrenal medullary autograft for Parkinson's disease in movement toward the concept of neurorestoration. During a prolonged period of study he focused on tumor immune relations and their therapeutic implications, developing many clinical protocols for application to cerebral malignant neoplasms. Subsequently he initiated studies of auto-immune responses in head injury.

Beginning in 1977, he moved to reintroduce neuroendoscopy as an adjuvant in cerebral surgery performing some of the initial third ventricular surgeries employing the endoscope and stereotactic methodology to facilitate these procedures.

In all of these developments Apuzzo pioneered and championed the concept of minimally invasive neurosurgery as a paradigm shift in the field. During this time he published more than 500 contributions to the scientific literature, including 36 published volumes on the topics of the future of neurosurgery, microsurgery, neuro-oncology, stereotaxy, head injury, epilepsy, benign cerebral gliomas, malignant cerebral gliomas, cerebral surgery, general intracranial neurosurgery and the neurosurgical operating room. His principal atlas texts, *Surgery of the Third Ventricle* and *Brain Surgery: Complication Avoidance and Management*, are universally considered modern classics.

During his career he has been an ardent advocate for internationalism, education and facilitated global communication in neurosurgery. He has presented more than 50 keynote, named, or commemorative lectures. These have included the prestigious Richard C. Schneider (AANS), Herbert Olivecrona (Karolinska Institute), and Sixto Obrador (Her Majesty Queen Sophia of Spain) Academic Lectureships. In addition he has conducted 130 invited professorships worldwide while holding principal leadership and innovative roles in publication, program and educational committees of all major national and international organizations.

Apuzzo has served on more than 25 editorial review boards. Since 1992 as Editor of *NEUROSURGERY*, he has instituted and fostered innovations in scientific publishing, internet activities and the scope of organized neurosurgery in global unification in education.

With a lifetime interest in recreational and competitive sport, for 23 years he has served as the primary neurosurgical consultant for the University of Southern California Athletic Department, caring for a wide range of neurosurgical problems and ultimately serving as an important resource for Olympic and professional level athletics and sports organizations. In particular, he has served as special consultant to the National Football League, currently holding the position as Principal Neurosurgical Consultant for the New York Football Giants.

His professional activities have been influenced by and continue to reflect his avid personal interests in architecture, fine painting, classical musicology, history, mythology, athletics and historical elements of American cinema.

He is the Edwin M. Todd/Trent H. Wells, Jr. Professor of Neurological Surgery, Radiation Oncology, Biology, and Physics at the Keck School of Medicine at the University of Southern California in Los Angeles where he continues to persistently and vigorously pursue progress in multiple focused clinical and more global aspects of the neurosurgical discipline.

He is indebted to his senior neurosurgical colleagues at the University of Southern California, Martin H. Weiss, J. Gordon McComb and Steven L. Giannotta, for their stimulation and for setting an atmosphere of unusual standards, and a long line of remarkable residents who have continued to translate their vitality, ideas and freshness of thought to maintain a nearly daily intellectual renaissance.

His son, filmmaker Jason, has been a source of new perspective, ideas and inspiration.

Bibliography

SELECTED PUBLICATIONS OF
MICHAEL L.J. APUZZO FROM
A CURRENT BIBLIOGRAPHY OF 507
OCTOBER 2001

PEER REVIEW

SCIENTIFIC CONTRIBUTIONS

1. Apuzzo, M.L.J.: The Management of Acute Head Injuries on Polaris Submarines. *Naval Bul. Med.*, 1969.
2. Heiden, J.S., Weiss, M.H., Rosenberg, A.W., Kurze, T., Apuzzo, M.L.J.: Penetrating gunshot wounds of the cervical spine in civilians Review of 38 cases. *J. Neurosurg.* 42:575–579, 1975.
3. Heiden, J.S., Weiss, M.H., Rosenberg, A.W., Apuzzo, M.L.J.: A Conspectus of Management of Cervical Spine Cord Trauma in Southern California. *J. Neurosurg.* 43:732–736, 1975.
4. Kurze, T., Apuzzo, M.L.J., Weiss, M.H., Heiden, J.S.: Collagen Sponge: An Improved Mode of Surface Brain Protection. *J. Neurosurg.* 43:637–638, 1975.
5. Apuzzo, M.L.J., Davey, L.J., Manueledis, E.E.: Pineal Apoplexy Associated with Anticoagulant Therapy. Case Report. *J. Neurosurg.* 45:223–226, 1976.
6. Apuzzo, M.L.J., Heiden, J.S., Weiss, M.H., Ackerson, T.T., Harvey, J.P., Kurze, T.: Acute Fracture of the Odontoid Process: An Analysis of 45 Cases. *J. Neurosurg.* 47:861–863, 1976.
7. Apuzzo, M.L.J., Weiss, M.H., Petersons, V., Small, R.B., Kurze, T., Heiden, J.S.: The Effect of Positive End Expiratory Pressure (PEEP) Ventilation on Intracranial Pressurein Man. *J. Neurosurg.* 46:227–232, 1977.
8. Apuzzo, M.L.J., Heifetz, M.D., Weiss, M.H., Kurze, T.: Neurosurgical Endoscopy Using the Side Viewing Telescope. *J. Neurosurg.* 46:398–400, 1977.
9. Apuzzo, M.L.J., Sheikh, K.M., Kochsiek, K.R., Weiss, M.H.: Malignant Glial Neoplasms: Definition of a Humoral Host Response to Tumor-Associated Antigen(s). *Yale J. Bio. Med.* 50:397–403, 1977.
10. Weiss, M.H., Spence, J., Apuzzo, M.L.J., Heiden, J.S., McComb, J.G., Kurze, T.: The Influence of Nitroprusside on Pressure Cerebral Autoregulations. *Neurosurgery* 4:56–59, 1979.

11. Gott, P.S., Weiss, M.H., Apuzzo, M.L.J., Van Der Meulen, J.: The Checkerboard Visual Evoked Response in Evaluation and Management of Pituitary Tumors. *Neurosurgery* 553–558, 1979.
12. Apuzzo, M.L.J., Mitchell, M.: Immunological Aspects of Intrinsic Glial Tumors. *J. Neurosurg.* 55:1–18, 1981.
13. Apuzzo, M.L.J., Sheikh, K.M.A., Weiss, M.H., Heiden, J.S., Kurze, T.: The Utilization of Native Glioma Antigens in the Assessment of Specific Cellular and Humoral Immune Responses in Malignant Glioma Patients. *Acta Neurochirurgica* 55:181–200, 1981.
14. Iacono, R., Apuzzo, M.L.J., Davis, R., Tsai, F.: Multiple Meningiomas Following Radiation for Medulloblastoma. *J. Neurosurg.* 55:282–286, 1981.
15. Apuzzo, M.L.J., Chikovani, O.K., Gott, M.S., Teng, E.L., Zee, C.S., Giannotta, S.L., Weiss, M.H.: Transcallosal, Interfornicial Approaches for Lesions Affecting the Third Ventricle: Surgical Considerations and Consequences. *Neurosurgery* 10:547–554, 1982.
16. Apuzzo, M.L.J.: Newly Designed Sterilization System for the Operating Microscope: A Technical Note. *Neurosurgery* 12:106–107, 1983.
17. Weiss, M.H., Teal, J., Gott, P., Wycoff, R., Yadley, R., Apuzzo, M.L.J., Giannotta, S.L., Kletsky, O., March, C.: Natural History of Microprolactinomas: Six Year Follow-up. *Neurosurgery* 12:180–183, 1983.
18. Apuzzo, M.L.J., Sabshin, J.K.: Computed Tomographic Guidance Stereotaxis in the Management of Intracranial Mass Lesions. *Neurosurgery* 12:277–285, 1983.
19. Heilbrun, M. Peter, Roberts, Theodore, S., Apuzzo, M.L.J., Wells, Trent H., Jr., Sabshin, James K.: Preliminary Experience With Brown-Roberts-Wells (BRW) Computerized Tomography Stereotaxic Guidance System. *J. Neurosurg.* 59:217–222, 1983.
20. Sabshin, J.K., Apuzzo, M.L.J., Ahmadi, J.: Cervical IntraExtradural Hematoma Secondary to Radicular Artery Injury: A Case Report. *Spine* 8:807–811, 1983.
21. Apuzzo, M.L.J., Zelman, V., Jepson, J., Chandrasoma, P.: Observations with the Utilization of the Brown-Roberts-Wells Stereotactic System in the Management of Intracranial Mass Lesions. *Acta Neruochirurgica, Suplementum* 33:193–195, 1984.
22. Apuzzo, M.L.J., Dobkin, W.R., Zee, C., James C. Chan, M.D. Giannotta, S.L.., Weiss, M.H.: Surgical Considerations in the Treatment of Intraventricular Cysticercosis: An Analysis of 45 Cases. *J. Neurosurgery* 60:400–407, 1984.
23. Giannotta, Steven L., Weiss, Martin H., Apuzzo, M.L.J., Martin Evangeline: High Dose Glucocorticoids in the Management of Severe Head Injury. *Neurosurgery* 15:497–501, 1984.
24. Apuzzo, M.L.J., Chandrasoma, Parakrama T., Zelman, V., Gian-

notta, Steven L., Weiss, Martin H.: Computerized Tomographic Guidance Stereotaxis in the Management of Lesions of the Third Ventricular Region. *Neurosurgery* 15:502–508, 1984.

25. von Hanwehr, R, Hoffman, F., Taylor, C.R., Apuzzo, M.L.J.: Mononuclear Cell Populations Infiltrating the Microenvironment of CNS Tumors: Definition of Phenotype Expression Utilizing Monoclonal Antibodies. *J. Neurosurgery* 60:1138–1147, 1984.

26. Apuzzo, M.L.J.: C.T. Guidance Stereotaxis of the Brain. *Western J. Med.* 140:773–774, 1984.

27. Apuzzo, M.L.J.: Effects of Photoradiation Therapy on Normal Rat Brain. *Neurosurgery* 15:809–810, 1984.

28. Little, F.M., Gomer, C.J., Hyman, S., Apuzzo, M.L.J.: Observations in studies of quantitative kinetics of tritium labelled hematoporphyrin derivatives (H_pD_I and H_pD_{II}) in the normal and neoplastic rat brain model. *J. Neuro-Oncology* 2:361–370, 1984.

29. Apuzzo, M.L.J.: Uptake and Retention of Hemotroporphyrin Derivative in an In Vivo/In Vitro Model of Cerebral Glioma. *Neurosurgery* 17:889, 1985.

30. Erlich, Stephanie S., Apuzzo, M.L.J.: The Pineal Gland: Anatomy, Physiology, and Clinic Significance. *J. Neurosurgery*, 63:321–341, 1985.

31. Apuzzo, M.L.J., Chandrasoma, P.T., Cohen, D., Zee, C.S., Zelman, V.: Computed Imaging Stereotaxy: Experience and Perspective Related to 500 Procedures Applied to Brain Masses. *Neurosurgery*, 20:930–937, 1987.

32. Apuzzo, M.L.J., Petrovich, Z., Luxton, G., J.H. Jepson, D. Cohen, R.E. Breeze: Interstitial Brachytherapy of Malignant Cerebral Neoplasms: Rationale, Methodology and Prospects. *Neurological Research*, 9:91–100, 1987.

33. Kaye, Andrew H., Morstyn, George, M.L.J. Apuzzo: Photoradiation Therapy and Its Potential in the Management of Neurological Tumors. *J. Neurosurgery*, 69:1–14, 1988.

34. Apuzzo, M.L.J.: Magnetic Resonance Imaging Stereotactic Thalamotomy: Report of a Case with Comparison to Computed Tomography. *Neurosurgery*, 23:363–367, 1988.

35. Fitzgibbons, P.L., Appley, A., Turner, R., Bishop, P., Parker, J., Breeze, R., Weiss, M.H., Apuzzo, M.L.J.: Flow Cytometric Analysis of Pituitary Tumors. Correlation of Nuclear Antigen p105 and DNA Content with Clinical Behavior. *Cancer* 62:1556–1560, 1988.

36. Chandrasoma, Parakrama T., Smith, Maurice, M., Apuzzo, M.L.J.: Stereotaxic Biopsy in the Diagnosis of Brain Masses: Comparison of Results of Biopsy and Resected Surgical Specimen. *Neurosurgery* 24:160–165, 1989.

37. Couldwell, William T., Apuzzo, Michael L.J.: Initial Experience

Related to the Cosman-Roberts-Wells Stereotactic Instrument. *J. Neurosurgery* 72:145–148, 1990.

38. Apuzzo, Michael L.J., Neal, John H., Waters, Cheryl H., Appley, Alan J., et al: Utilization of Unilateral and Bilateral Stereotactically Placed Adrenomedullary-Striatal Autografts in Parkinsonian Humans: Rationale, Techniques and Observations. *Neurosurgery*, 26:746–757, 1990.

39. Waters, C., Itabashi, H.H., Apuzzo, M.L.J., Weiner, L.P.: Adrenal Caudate Transplatation-Postmortem Study. *J. Movement Disorders* 5(3):248–250, 1990.

40. Appley, Alan J., Fitzgibbons, Patrick L., Chandrasoma, Parakrama, T., Hinton, David R. Apuzzo, Michael L.J.: Multiparameter Flow Cytometric Analysis of Central Nervous System Neoplasms. Correlation of Nuclear Antigen P105 and DNA Content with Clinical Behavior. *Neurosurgery* 27:83–96, 1990.

41. Breeze, R.E., Nichols, P.W., Apuzzo, M.L.J.: Craniocervical Junction Neuroenteric Cysts. *J.Neurosurgery* 73:788–791, 1990.

42. Apuzzo, M.L.J., Levy, M.L., Tung. H.: Surgical Strategies and Technical Methodologies in Optimal Management of Craniopharyngioma and Masses Affecting the Third Ventricular Chamber. *Acta Neurochirurgica, Suppl.* 53:77–88,1991.

43. Lucas, G.L., Luxton, G., Cohen, D., Petrovich, Z., Langholz, B., Apuzzo, M.L., Sapozink, M.D.: Treatment Results of Stereotactic Interstitial Brachytherapy for Primary and Metastatic Brain Tumors. Nervous System Malignancies—Diagnosis, Treatment. *Int. J. Radiat. Oncol. Biol. Phys.*; 21(3):715–721, l991.

44. Oppenheimer, J.H., Levy, M.L.,Sinha, U., El-Kadi, H., Apuzzo, M.L.J., Luxton, G., Petrovich, Z., Zee, C., Miller, C.A.: Radio-necrosis Secondary to Interstitial Brachytherapy: Correlation of Magnetic Resonance Imaging and Histopathology. *Neurosurgery*, 31 (2):336–343, 1992.

45. Schneider, J., Hofman, F.M., Apuzzo, M.L.J., Hinton, D.R.: Cytokines and Immunoregulatory Molecules in Malignant Glial Neoplasms. *J of Neurosurgery*, 77(2):265–273, 1992.

46. Chen, T.C., Hinton, D.R., Apuzzo, M.L.J., Hoffman, F.M.: Differential Effects of Tumor Necrosis Factor-Alpha on Proliferation, Cell Surface Antigen Expression, and Cytokine Interactions in Malignant Gliomas. *Neurosurgery*,. 32(1):85–94, 1993.

47. Luxton, G., Petrovich, Z., Jozsef, G., Nedzi, L.A., Apuzzo, M.L.J.: Stereotactic Radiosurgery: Principles and Comparison of Treatment Methods. *Neurosurgery*, 32(2):241–259, 1993.

48. Couldwell, W.T., Weiss, M.H., DeGiorgio, C.M., Weiner, L.P., Hinton, D.R., Ehresmann, G.R., Conti, P.S., Apuzzo, M.L.J.: Clinical

and Radiographic Response in a Minority of Patients with Recurrent Malignant Gliomas Treated with High-Dose Tamoxifen. *Neurosurgery*, 32(3):485–490, 1993.

49. Levy, M.L., Rezai, A., Masri, L.S., Litofsky, S.N., Giannotta, S.L., Apuzzo, M.L.J., Weiss, M.H.: The Significance of Subarachnoid Hemorrhage after Penetrating Craniocerebral Injury: Correlations with Angiography and Outcome in a Civilian Population. *Neurosurgery*, 32(4):532–540, 1993.

50. Chin, L.S., Rabb, C.H., Hinton, D.R., Apuzzo, M.L.J.: Hemangiopericytoma of the Temporal Bone Presenting as a Retroauricular Mass. *Neurosurgery*, 33(4): pp. 728–731, 1993.

51. Apuzzo, M.L.J., Weinberg, R.A.: The Architecture and Functional Design of Advanced Neurosurgical Operating Environments, *Neurosurgery*, 33(4): pp. 663–673, 1993.

52. Levy, M.L., Masri, L.S., Levy, K.M., Martin-Thomson, E., Couldwell, W.T., Johnson, F.L., McComb, J.G. and Apuzzo, M.L.J.: Penetrating Craniocerebral Injury Resultant From Gunshot Wounds: Gang-related Injury in Children and Adolescents. *Neurosurgery*, 33(6):1993.

53. Levy, M.L., Masri, L.S., Lavine, S. and Apuzzo, M.L.J.: Outcome Prediction After Penetrating Craniocerebral Injury in a Civilian Population: Agressive Surgical Management in Patients with Admission Glasgow Coma Scale Scores of 3, 4, or 5. *Neurosurgery*, 35(1):77–85, 1994.

54. Ahmadi, J., Savabi, F., Apuzzo, M.L.J., Segall, H.D. and Hinton, D: Magnetic Resonance Imaging and Quantitative Analysis of Intracranial Cystic Lesions: Surgical Implication. *Neurosurgery*, 35(2): 199–207, 1994.

55. Kureshi, S.A., Hofman, F.M., Schneider, J.H., Chin, L.S., Apuzzo, M.L.J. and Hinton, D.R.: Cytokine Expression in Radiation-induced Delayed Cerebral Injury. *Neurosurgery*, 35(5):822–830, 1994.

56. Zee, C.S., Chen, T., Hinton, D.R., Tan, M., Segall, H.D. and Apuzzo, M.L.J.: Magnetic Resonance Imaging of Cystic Meningiomas and Its Surgical Implications. *Neurosurgery*, 36(3):482–488, 1995.

58. Sutton, J.P., Couldwell, W., Lew, M.F., Mallory, L., Grafton, S., DeGiorgio, C., Welsh, M., Apuzzo, M.L.J., Ahmadi, J. and Waters, C.H.: Ventroposterior Medial Pallidotomy in Patients with Advanced Parkinson's Disease. *Neurosurgery*, 36(6):1112–1117, 1995.

60. Apuzzo, M.L.J.: SCHNEIDER LECTURE—New Dimensions of Neurosurgery in the Realm of High Technology: Possibilities, Practicalities, Realities. *Neurosurgery*, 38(4):625–639, 1996.

61. Ko, D., Heck, C., Grafton, S., Apuzzo, M.L.J., Couldwell, W.T., Chen, T., Day, J.D., Zelman, V., Smith, T., DeGiorgio, C.M.: Vagus Nerve Stimulation Activates Central Nervous System Structures in Epileptic Patients During PET $H_2{}^{15}O$ Blood Flow Imaging. *Neurosurgery*, 39(2):426–431, 1996.
62. LeMay, D.R., Chen, T.C., Petrovich, Z., Luxton, G., Zelman, V., Zee, C., Green, J., Apuzzo, M.L.J.: Gamma Unit Facility: Concept Genesis, Architectural Design and Practical Realization. *Stereotactic and Functional Neurosurgery* (Proceedings of the Meeting of the American Society for Stereotactic and Functional Neurosurgery, Calif.), Part II, 66(1–3):41–49, 1996.
63. Apuzzo, M.L.J., Stieg, P.E., Starr, P., Schwartz, R.B., Folkerth, R.D.: Surgery of the Soul's Cistern. *Neurosurgery*, 39(5):1022–1029, 1996.
64. Zlokovic, B.V., Apuzzo, M.L.J.: Cellular and Molecular Neurosurgery: Pathways from Concept to Reality-Part I: Target Disorders and Concept Approaches to Gene Therapy of the Central Nervous System. *Neurosurgery*, 40.(4):.789–804, 1997.
65. Zlokovic, B.V., Apuzzo, M.L.J.: Cellular and Molecular Neurosurgery: Pathways from concept to Reality—Part II: Vector Systems and Delivery Methodologies for Gene Therapy of the Central Nervous System. *Neurosurgery*, 40(4):805–813, 1997.
66. Cheng, Y., Luxton, G., Apuzzo, M.L.J., MacPherson, Zbigniew, P.: Extracranial Radiation Doses in Patients Undergoing Gamma Knife Radiosurgery. *Neurosurgery*, 41(3):553–560, 1997.
67. Amar, P.A., Heck, C.N., Levy, M.L., Smith, T., DeGiorgio, C.M., Oviedo, S. & Apuzzo, M.L.J.: An Institutional Experience with Cervical Vagus Nerve Trunk Stimulation for Medically Refractory Epilepsy: Rationale, Technique, and Outcome: *Neurosurgery*, 43 (6):1265–1280, 1998.
68. Lavine, S.D., Petrovich, Z., Cohen-Gadol, A.A., Masri, L.S., Morton, D.L., O'Day, S.J., Essner, R., Zelman, V., Yu, C., Luxton, G., Apuzzo, M.L.J.: Gamma Knife Radiosurgery for Metastatic Melanoma: An Analysis of Survival, Outcome, and Complications: *Neurosurgery*, 44(1):59–66, 1999.
69. Apuzzo, M.L.J.; Chen, J.C.T. Stereotaxy, Navigation and The Temporal Concatenation. *Stereotactic and Functional Neurosurgery*, 72 (2):82–88, 1999.
70. Cheng, Y., Luxton, G., Jozsef, G., Apuzzo, M.L.J. and Petrovich, Z.: "Posimetric Comparison of Three Photon Radiosurgery Techniques for an Elongated Ellipsoid Target". *Int. J. Radiation Oncology Biol. Phys.*, 45(2):817–826, 1999.
71. Sullivan, D., Langmoen, I., Adams, C.B.T., Sainte-Rose, C. and Apuzzo, M.L.J.: The Bayeux Tapestry: A Charter of a People and

a Unique Testimony of Creative Imagery in Communication: *Neurosurgery* 45(3):663–669, 1999.

72. Yu, C., Luxton, G., Apuzzo, M.L.J. and Petrovich, Z.: TLD Measurements of the Relative Output Factors for the Leksell Gamma Knife: *Stereotactic and Functional Neurosurgery*, 72:150–158,1999.

73. Chen, J.C.T., Amar, A.P., Levy, M.L. and Apuzzo, M.L.J.: The Development of Anatomic Art and Sciences: The Ceroplastica Anatomic Models of La Specola: *Neurosurgery*, 45:883–892, 1999.

74. Yu, H., Wang, Y., Eton, D, Stins, M., Wang, L., Apuzzo, M.L.J., Weaver, F.A., McComb, J. G., Weiss, M.H. and Zlokovic B.V.: Retroviral Vector-Mediated Transfer and Expression of Human Tissue Plasminogen Activator cDNA in Bovine Brain Endothelial Cells: *Neurosurgery*, 45(4):962–970, 1999.

75. Amar, A.R., DeGiorgio, C., Apuzzo, M.L.J. and EO5 Study Group: Long-term Multicenter Experience with Vagus Nerve Stimulation for Intractable Partial Seizures. Proceedings of Quadrennial Meeting of the American Society for Stereotactic and Functional Neurosurgery; Snowbird, Utah; July 7–10, 1999. *Stereotactic and Functional Neurosurgery*, Issue 73:104–108, 1999

76. Apuzzo, M.L.J. and Chen, J.C.T.: "Stereotaxy, Navigation and the Temporal Concatenation" Proceedings of Quadrennial Meeting of the American Society for Stereotactic and Functional Neurosurgery; Snowbird, Utah; July 7–10, 1999. *Stereotactic and Functional Neurosurgery*, Issue 72:82–88, 1999.

77. Apuzzo, M.L.J. & Hodge, Jr., C.J.: The Metamorphosis of Communication, the Knowledge Revolution and the Maintenance of a Contemporary Perspective During the 21st Century. *Neurosurgery*, 46(1):7–15, 2000.

78. Apuzzo, M.L.J.: "Modernity and the Emerging Futurism in Neurosurgery",tempora mutantur nos et mutamur in illis *Journal of Clincal Neuroscience* 7(2):85–87, 2000.

79. Apuzzo, M.L.J., Joseph C.T. Chen, M.D., Ph.D., Zbigniew Petrovich, M.D., Steven Giannotta, M.D., Cheng Yu, Ph.D.,: Radiosurgical Salvage Therapy for Patients Presenting with Recurrence of Metastatic Disease to the Brain, *Neurosurgery*, 46(4):860–867, 2000.

80. Chen JCT, Petrovich Z, O'Day S, Morton D, Essner R, Giannotta SL, Yu C, Apuzzo, M.L.J.:Stereotactic Radiosurgery in the Treatment of Metastatic Disease to the Brain. *Neurosurgery*, 47(2): 268–281, 2000.

81. Chen JCT, Giannotta SL, Yu C, Petrovich Z, Levy ML, Apuzzo MLJ: Radiosurgical management of benign cavernous sinus tumors: Dose profiles and acute complications. *Neurosurgery* 48: 1022–1032, 2001.

82. Yu C, Apuzzo MLJ, Zee C-S, Petrovich Z: A phantom study of the geometric accuracy of computed tomographic and magnetic resonance imaging sterotactic localization with the Leksell stereotactic system. *Neurosurgery* 48:1092–1099, 2001.
83. Long DM, Apuzzo MLJ: Sine qua non: The formulation of a theory of neurosurgery. *Neurosurgery* 49:56 7–574, 2001.
84. Apuzzo MLJ, Liu CY: 2001: Things to come. *Neurosurgery* 49:765–778, 2001.

EDITORIALS

1. Apuzzo, M.L.J.: NEUROSURGERY'S Presence on the Internet: A Work in Progress. *Neurosurgery*, 39(1), 1996.
2. Wilkins, R.H., Watts, C., Laws, Jr., E.R., Apuzzo, M.L.J.: NEUROSURGERY: A Two Decade Metamorphosis—the Editors' Perspective. *Neurosurgery*, 40(6):,1997.
3. Apuzzo, M.L.J.: Exploration of the Solar System and the Introduction of Advanced Technology to Neurosurgery: Pegasus or Pandemonium. *Neurosurgery*, 41(6):1438–1439, 1997.
4. Apuzzo, M.L.J.: Summa Cum Laude: *Neurosurgery*, 45(5): 975, 1999.
5. Apuzzo, M.L.J.: Reinventing Neurosurgery: Entering the Third Millennium, *Neurosurgery*, . 46(1): 1–2, January, 2000.
6. Apuzzo, M.L.J.: Brave New World: Reaching for Utopia, *Neurosurgery*, 46 (5):1033, 2000.
7. Apuzzo, M.L.J., The Legacy of Galen of Pergamon: *Neurosurgery*, 47(3):545, 2000.
8. Apuzzo MLJ: Cadenza. *Neurosurgery* 48:1, 2001.
9. Apuzzo MLJ: Ad astra per aspera: Audacity and reinvention. *Neurosurgery* 49:239, 2001.
10. Apuzzo MLJ: When worlds collide. *Neurosurgery* 49:553, 2001.
11. Apuzzo MLJ: Divina machina versus machina. *Neurosurgery* 49:590–591, 2001.

EDITORIAL VOLUMES

NEUROSURGERY, VOL. 31–49, 1992–2001
Stereotactic and Functional Neurosurgery, Vol. 65, No. 1–3, 1995.
Stereotactic and Functional Neurosurgery, Vol. 66, No. 1–4, 1996.

BOOKS AND CHAPTERS
BOOKS EDITED

1. Apuzzo, M.L.J.: **Surgery of the Third Ventricle.** Apuzzo, M.L.J. (ed), Williams and Wilkins, Baltimore, 1987.

2. Apuzzo, M.L.J.: *Neuroscience and Neurosurgery of the Twenty-First Century.* Hanley and Belfus Medical Publishers, Philadelphia, PA 1988.
3. Apuzzo, M.L.J, Chandrasoma, P: *Sterotactic Brain Biospsy.* Igaku-Shoin Medical Publishers, New York, NY, 1989.
4. Apuzzo, M.L.J.: *Malignant Cerebral Glioma*, AANS Publishers, Chicago, IL, 1990.
5. Apuzzo, M.L.J.: *Surgical Aspects of Epilepsy*, AANS Publishers, Chicago, IL, 1991.
6. Apuzzo, M.L.J.: **Surgery of the Supratentorial Space, Vol. I;** *Brain Surgery: Complication Avoidance and Management*, Churchill Livingstone, New York, NY, November, 1992.
7. Apuzzo, M.L.J.: **Surgery of the Infratentorial Space, Vol. II;** *Brain Surgery, Complication Avoidance and Management*, Churchill Livingstone, New York, NY, November, 1992.
8. Apuzzo, M.L.J.: *Neurosurgery for the Third Millinneum*; American Association of Neurological Surgeons Neurosurgical Topics, November, 1992.
9. Apuzzo, M.L.J.: *Benign Cerebral Glioma, Vol. I*; American Association of Neurological Surgeons Neurosurgical Topics, 1995.
10. Apuzzo, M.L.J. : *Benign Cerebral Glioma, Vol. II*; American Association of Neurological Surgeons Neurosurgical Topics, 1995.
11. Levy, M.L.J, Apuzzo, M.L.J. (Editors): **Penetrating Craniocerebral Injuries: Spectrum of Methods and Salvageability.** *The Neurosurgery Clinics of North America*, W. B. Saunders Co., Philadelphia, PA, 1995.
12. Apuzzo, M.L.J. : *Surgery of the Third Ventricle, Second Edition*, Williams and Wilkins, Baltimore, MD, 1998.
13. Apuzzo, M.L.J.: *Combined Modality Therapy of Central Nervous System Tumors.* Z. Petrovich, L.W. Brady, M.L.J. Apuzzo and M. Bamberg (Editors), Springer , 2000.

CHAPTERS

1. Apuzzo, M.L.J.: Lumbar Laminotomy, Foraminotomy, Root Decompression and Discectomy In the Lateral Position. In Watkins, R.G. (ed): *Surgical Approaches to the Spine.* Springer Verlag, New York, 1982.
2. Apuzzo, M.L.J.: Transcallosal Interfornicial Exposure of Lesions of the Third Ventricle. In Schmidek H.H. (ed): *Operative Neurological Techniques: Indications and Methods.* Grune and Stratton, New York, 1982.
3. Kril, M.P., Apuzzo, M.L.J.: Observations in the Study of T Lymphocyte Subsets by Monoclonal Antibodies and Flow Cytometric

Analysis in Intracranial Neoplastic Disorders. *Clinical Neurosurgery*, 30:125–136, 1983.

4. Apuzzo, M.L.J., Jepson, J.H., Luxton, G., Little, F.M.: Ionizing and Nonionizing Radiation Treatment of Malignant Cerebral Gliomas: Specialized Approaches. *Clinical Neurosurgery*, 31:470–496, 1984.
5. Apuzzo, M.L.J.: Immunology of Brain Tumors. *In* Wilkins, R.H. and Rengachary, S.S. (eds): *Neurosurgery.* McGraw-Hill Book Co., pp. 538–541, 1985.
6. Apuzzo, M.L.J.: Immunotherapy of Human Gliomas. *In* Wilkins, R.H. and Rengachary, SS (eds): *Neurosurgery.* McGraw-Hill Book Co. pp 1139–1142, 1985.
7. Apuzzo, M.L.J.: Computed Tomographic Guidance Stereotaxis in the Management of Ninety-Four Lesions of the Third Ventricular Region. In: Samii, M. (ed) *Surgery in and Around the Brain Stem and the Third Ventricle.* Springer-Verlag, 1985.
8. Apuzzo, M.L.J.: Interforniceal Exposure of the Third Ventricular Chamber. *In*: Samii, M (ed). *Surgery in and Around the Brain Stem and the Third Ventricle.* Springer-Verlag, Berlin Heidelberg, 1985.
9. Apuzzo, M.L.J.: CT Guidance Stereotaxis in the Management of 94 Lesions of the Third Ventricular Region, in Samii, M (ed). *Surgery in and Around the Brain Stem and the Third Ventricle.* Springer-Verlag, Berlin, Heidelberg, 1985.
10. Apuzzo, M.L.J., Watkins, Robert G., Dobkin, William R.: Therapeutic Considerations in the Surgical Management of Lesions Affecting the Mid-Thoracic Spine. *In*: Dunsker, S.B., Schmidek, H.H. (eds) *Focus on Spinal Surgery: The Unstable Spine.* Grune and Stratton, N.Y., pp. 107–126, 1986.
11. Apuzzo, M.L.J., Watkins, Robert, G., Dobkin, William, R.: Biomechanics of the Neural Axis. *In*: Dunsker, S.B., Schmidek, H.H., *Focus on Spinal Surgery: The Unstable Spine.* Grune and Stratton, N.Y., pp. 17–23, 1986.
12. Zee, C.S., Segall, H.D., Apuzzo, M.L.J., Giannotta, S.L.: Computerized Tomographic Assessment of Head Trauma. *In* Wilkins, R.H. and Rengachary, S.S. (eds): *Neurosurgery.* McGraw-Hill Book Co., pp. 1578–1586, 1986.
13. Koos, W., Pendl, G., Apuzzo, M.L.J.: Transcallosal Interfornicial Exposure of Lesions Involving the Third Ventricle. *In*: *Technical Aspects of Pediatric Neurosurgery.* Springer Verlag 1986.
14. Apuzzo, M.L.J.: Techniques of Lumbar Dorsal Decompression Procedures in the Lateral Position. *In*: Watkins, Robert G. (ed): *Principles and Techniques of Spinal Surgery.* Aspen Systems, Rockville, MD, 1986.

15. Apuzzo, M.L.J.: Surgery of Masses Affecting the Third Ventricular Chamber: Techniques and Strategies. *Clinical Neurosurgery*, 34: 499–522, 1987.
16. Apuzzo, M.L.J.: The Brown-Roberts-Wells System. *In*: L. Dade Lundsford (ed) *Modern Neurosurgery*, Martinus Nijhoff Publishing, Boston, pp. 10–12, 1987.
17. Apuzzo, M.L.J.: Interstitial Radiation. *In*: Paul L. Kornblith and Michael L. Walker (eds), *Advances in Neurooncology*, Futura Publishing Company, Mt. Kisco, NY, 1987.
18. Apuzzo, M.L.J.: Lasers in Surgery (Argon, YAG CO_2). *In*: Jon Robertson and W. Craig Clark (eds) *Lasers in Neurosurgery*, Martinus Nijhoff Publishing, Boston, 1987.
19. Apuzzo, M.L.J.: Transcallosal Interfornicial Exposure of Lesions of the Third Ventricle. In Schmidek H.H. (ed): *Operative Neurological Techniques: Indications and Methods*. Second Edition. Grune and Stratton, New York, 1987.
20. Apuzzo, M.L.J.: Interforniceal Approach. *In*: Apuzzo, M.L.J. (ed): *Surgery of the Third Ventricle*. Williams and Wilkins, Baltimore, pp. 354–580, 1987.
21. Apuzzo, M.L.J.: Anterior and Mid Ventricular Lesions: Surgical Overview. *In*: Apuzzo, M.L.J. (ed) *Surgery of the Third Ventricle*. Williams and Wilkins, Baltimore, pp. 495–541, 1987.
22. McComb, J. Gordon, Apuzzo, Michael L.J.: Posterior Interhemispheric Retrocallosal and Transcallosal Approaches to the Pineal Region. *In*: Apuzzo, M.L.J. (ed) *Surgery of the Third Ventricle*. Williams and Wilkins, Baltimore, pp. 611–640, 1987.
23. McComb, J. Gordon, Apuzzo, M.L.J.: Operative Management of Malformations of the Vein of Galen. *In*: Apuzzo, M.L.J. (ed) *Surgery of the Third Ventricle*. Williams and Wilkins, Baltimore, pp. 641–648, 1987.
24. Apuzzo, M.L.J.: Applications of Computerized Tomographic Guidance Stereotaxis. *In*: Apuzzo, M.L.J. (ed) *Surgery of the Third Ventricle*. Williams and Wilkins, Baltimore pp. 751–792, 1987.
25. Apuzzo, M.L.J.: Image-Directed Stereotactic Neurosurgery Biopsy: Methods, Utilization, and Strategies. In: R. Tasker (ed): *Stereotactic Surgery*: State of the Art Reviews. Hanley and Belfus, Inc. Publishers, Philadelphia, PA, 2: 287–308, 1987.
26. Apuzzo, M.L.J.: Applications of Image Directed Stereotaxy in the Management of Intracranial Neoplasms. *In*: Peter M. Heilbrun (ed), *Stereotactic Neurosurgery*, Williams and Wilkins, Baltimore, 1988.
27. Apuzzo, M.L.J., Neal, John H., Fredericks, Craig A., Cohen, Deirdra, Chandrasoma, Parakrama, Breeze, Robert E.: Image Di-

rected Stereotaxy: Instrumentation for Contemporary Assessment and Management of Structural Intracranial Disorders. *In*: Chandler, William F. (ed) *Practice of Surgery*, Ltd., Woodbury, CT, Chapter 21, pp. 1–26, 1988.

28. Apuzzo, M.L.J.: Application of Futuristic Concepts and Technology to the Neurosurgical Operating Room Environments. *Neuroscience and Neurosurgery of the Twenty-First Century.* Apuzzo, M.L.J. (ed.) Hanley and Belfus Medical Publishers, Philadelphia, PA, pp. 223–244, 1988.

29. Valencia, P., Apuzzo, M.L.J.: Computer Development and Applications. In: Apuzzo, M.L.J. (ed.) *Neuroscience and Neurosurgery of the Twenty-First Century.* Hanley and Belfus Medical Publishers, Philadelphia, PA, pp. 245–250, 1988.

30. Apuzzo, M.L.J.: Surgery of Intracranial Tumors: Aspects of Operating Room Design with Integration and Use of Technical Adjuvants. *Clinical Neurosurgery* 35:185–214, 1989.

31. Apuzzo, M.L.J.: Superior Surgical Approaches to the Diencephalic and Paradiencephalic Regions. *In*: Stein, Bennett, M. and Holtzman, Robert, N.N. (eds), *Surgery of the Diencephalon*, Plenum Publishing Corp., New York, NY, 1989.

32. Apuzzo, M.L.J., Chandrasoma, P.: Atlas of Tissue Smear Stereotactically Assayed Cerebral Lesions. In: Apuzzo, M.L.J., Chandrasoma, P. (eds) *Stereotactic Brain Biopsy*. Igaku-Shoin Medical Publishers, New York, NY, pp. 67–73, 1989.

33. Neal, John H., Apuzzo, M.L.J.: History of Stereotactic Methods and Devices in Neurologic Surgery. In: Apuzzo, M.L.J., Chandrasoma, P. (eds) *Stereotactic Brain Biopsy*. Igaku-Shoin Medical Publishers, New York, NY, Chapter 1, pp. 1–21,1989.

34. Neal, John H., Apuzzo, M.L.J.: Modern Stereotactic Biopsy Methods. In: Apuzzo, M.L.J., Chandrasoma, P. (eds) *Stereotactic Brain Biopsy*. Igaku-Shoin Medical Publishers, New York, NY, pp. 5–6, 1989.

35. Zee, Chi, Apuzzo, M.L.J., Neal, John H.: Imaging Targeting for the Stereotactic Biopsy. In: Apuzzo, M.L.J., Chandrasoma, P. (eds) *Stereotactic Brain Biopsy*. Igaku-Shoin Medical Publishers, New York, NY, pp. 45–63, 1989.

36. Apuzzo, M.L.J.: Clinically Relevant Issues Attendant to Pathology. *In*: (ed.) Apuzzo, M.L.J., *Malignant Cerebral Glioma.* AANS Publishers, Chicago, IL, pp. 19–21, 1990.

37. Apuzzo, M.L.J.: Biological Unravelings. *In*: (ed.) Apuzzo, M.L.J., *Malignant Cerebral Glioma.* AANS Publishers, Chicago, IL, pp. 59, 1990.

38. Apuzzo, M.L.J.: The Initial and Subsequent Surgical Endeavors *In*: (ed.) Apuzzo, M.L.J., *Malignant Cerebral Glioma.* AANS Publishers, Chicago, IL, pp. 155, 1990.

39. Apuzzo, M.L.J.: Applications of Energy Sources: Harvesting the Electromagnetic Spectrum *In*: (ed.) Apuzzo, M.L.J., *Malignant Cerebral Glioma*. AANS Publishers Chicago, IL, pp. 203, 1990.
40. Apuzzo, M.L.J.: Supratentorial Exposures of the Pineal Region. *In*: Setti S. Rengachary (ed) *Atlas of Neurosurgical Techniques*. AANS Publishers, Chicago, IL , 1990.
41. Young, Harold F., Apuzzo, M.L.J.: Immuno competence of Patients with Brain Tumors. *In*: Williams and Wilkins, Publishers, Baltimore, *Neurobiology of Brain Tumors*, Chapter 12, pp. 211–227, 1991.
42. Apuzzo, M.L.J.: Pineal Region Meningiomas *In:* Ossama Al-Mefty (ed) *Meningiomas*. Raven Press, New York, NY, pp. 583–591, 1991.
43. Apuzzo, M.L.J.: Surgical Management of Craniopharyngioma and Third Ventricular Tumors. *In*: N.F. Kassell and D.G. Vollmer (eds.) *Advances in Neurosurgery*. F.A. Davis Publishers, 1991.
44. Apuzzo, M.L.J., Levy, M.L., Tung, H.: Surgical Strategies and Technical Methodologies inOptimal Management of Craniopharyngioma and Masses Affecting the Third Ventricular Chamber. In: Koos, W., Richling, B. (eds) *Processes of the Cranial Midline*. Springer-Verlag Wien-New York, pp. 77–88, l991.
45. Levy, M.L., Tung, H., Couldwell, W.T., Hinton, D.R. and Apuzzo, M.L.J.: Neurosurgery, Molecular Medicine, and the Pandora-Panacea Continuum: Future Implications for Glioma Therapy. *Clinical Neurosurgery*, 39: 421–462, 1992.
46. Apuzzo, M.L.J.: Pineal Masses Supra-and Transtentorial Approaches, Vol. I.: *Brain Surgery, Complication Avoidance and Management.* (ed) Apuzzo, M.L.J., Churchill Livingstone, New York, NY, pp. 486–540,1992.
47. Apuzzo, M.L.J.: Anterior and Mid Third Ventricular Masses, Vol. I.: *Brain Surgery, Complication Avoidance and Management.* (ed) Apuzzo, M.L.J., Churchill Livingstone, New York, NY, pp. 541–579, 1992.
48. Apuzzo, M.L.J., Black, P., Apuzzo, J.A.: What is a Complication?, Vol. I.: *Brain Surgery, Complication Avoidance and Management* (ed) Apuzzo, M.L.J., Churchill Livingstone, New York, NY, pp. 3–9, 1992.
49. Apuzzo, M.L.J., Chin, L.S., Chen, T. and Valencia, P.: Neurosurgery: A Futuristic Prospectus In *Neurosurgery for the Third Millinneum ;* American Association of Neurological Surgeons Neurosurgical Topics (ed) Apuzzo, M.L.J., Chapter 2, pp. 11–23,1992.
50. Apuzzo, M.L.J., Rabb, C., Levy, M., Couldwell, W. T. and Zelman, V.: Cerebral ProtectionIn *Neurosurgery for the Third Millinneum*; American Association of Neurological Surgeons Neurosurgical Topics (ed) Apuzzo, M.L.J., pp. 117–147, 1992.

xliv   BIBLIOGRAPHY

51. Apuzzo, M.L.J.: Turning the Page In *Neurosurgery for the Third Millinneum*; American Association of Neurological Surgeons Neurosurgical Topics (ed) Apuzzo, M.L.J., pp. 199, 1992.
52. Levy, M.L., Tung, H, Couldwell, W.T., Hinton, D.R. and Apuzzo, M.L.J.: Neurosurgery, Molecular Medicine, and the Pandora-Panacea Continuum: Future Implications for Glioma Therapy? Proceedings of the Congress of Neurological Surgeons 1991 *Clinical Neurosurgery*, Vol. 39; Warren Selman, Williams & Wilkins, Baltimore, pp. 421–462, 1992.
53. Apuzzo, M.L.J.: Neurosurgical Morbidity and Complications. In *Philosophy of Neurological Surgery*; American Association of Neurological Surgeons Neurosurgical Topics (ed) Issam A. Awad, 1994.
54. Apuzzo, M.L.J. and Rabb, C.H.: Stereotaxis in the diagnosis and management of brain tumors. *Brain Tumors, An Encyclopedic Approach*; Andrew H. Kaye/Edward R. Laws, Jr., Churchill Livingstone, pp. 305–330, New York, NY, 1995.
55. Apuzzo, M.L.J.: At the Edge of the Millennium—A Kaleidoscope Unfolds In *Benign Cerebral Glioma*; American Association of Neurological Surgeons Neurosurgical Topics (ed) Apuzzo, M.L.J., 1995.
56. Apuzzo, M.L.J.: Evolving Dimensions at the Frontiers of Human Cerebral Surgery. In *Benign Cerebral Glioma*; American Association of Neurological Surgeons Neurosurgical Topics (ed) Apuzzo, M.L.J., pp. 1–12, 1995.
57. Rabb, C.H. and Apuzzo, M.L.J.: Options in the Management of Ventricular Masses. *The Practice of Neurosurgery*, Tindall/Cooper/Barrow, William & Wilkins, Baltimore, Maryland, (1), Chapter. 80, 1995.
58. Gruen, P. and Apuzzo, M.L.J.: Third-Ventricle Exposure by the Interhemispheric Corridor, *Neurosurgical Operative Atlas*; Ed., Robert Wilkins, The American Association ofNeurological Surgeons, 4:, No. 1, pp. 37–42, 1995.
59. Chen, T.C., Hinton, D.R. and Apuzzo, M.L.J.: Diagnostic Biopsy for Neurological Disease. *Neurological Surgery, 4th Edition*, Julian R. Youmans, M.D., Ph.D., Editor-In-Chief, W. B. Saunders Co., Philadelphia, PA,. 1:. 315–347, 1996.
60. Chin, L.S., Levy, M.L. and Apuzzo, M.L.J.: Principles of Stereotactic Neurosurgery. *Neurological Surgery, 4th Edition*, Julian R. Youmans, M.D., Ph.D., Editor-In-Chief, W. B. Saunders Co., Philadelphia, PA, . 1: 767–785, 1996.
61. Schneider, J.H., Chandrasoma P., Nedzi, L. and Apuzzo, M.L.J.: Neoplasms of the Pineal anThird Ventricular Region *Neurological Surgery, 4th Edition*, Julian R. Youmans, M.D., Ph.D., Editor-In-Chief, W. B. Saunders Co., Philadelphia, PA, .(IV): 2715–2747, 1996.

62. Apuzzo, M.L.J. and Levy, M.L.: Immunology of Brain Tumors. *Neurosurgery*, Second *Edition*; Wilkins/Rengachary, McGraw-Hill Book Co., New York, NY, . I: Chapter 73, pp. 707–714, 1996.
63. Apuzzo, M.L.J. and Levy, M.L.: Immunotherapy of Human Gliomas. *Neurosurgery*, Second *Edition*; Wilkins/Rengachary, McGraw-Hill Book Co., New York, NY,.(II): Chapter 188, pp. 1943–1956, 1996.
64. Apuzzo, M.L.J. and Gruen, P.: Pineal Physiology. *Neurosurgery, Second Edition*; Wilkins/Rengachary, McGraw-Hill Book Co., New York, NY, 1: Chapter 98, pp. 977–994, 1996.
65. Apuzzo, M.L.J.: Colloid Cysts: The Case for Craniotomy. *Controversies in Neurosurgery*, Ossama Al-Mefty, T.C. Origitano and H. Louis Harkey, Thieme Med. Pub., Inc., New York, NY, Chapter 4, pp. 30–37, 1996.
66. Chen, T.C. and Apuzzo, M.L.J.: "Principles of Stereotactic Neurosurgery". *Cancer of the Nervous System*, Peter McL. Black, Blackwell Science, Malden, Massachusetts, Chapter 8, pp. 156–177, 1996.
67. Apuzzo, M.L.J. (ed.), Amar, A.P.: THE TRANSCALLOSAL INTERFORNICEAL APPROACH. *Surgery of the Third Ventricle, Second Edition*, Williams and Wilkins, Baltimore, MD, Chapter 18, pp. 1–1254, 1998.
68. Apuzzo, M.L.J.(ed.), Zee, C., Breeze, R.E., Day, J.D.: ANTERIOR AND MID-THIRD VENTRICULAR LESIONS: A SURGICAL OVERVIEW. *Surgery of the Third Ventricle, Second Edition*, Williams and Wilkins, Baltimore, MD, Chapter 28, pp. 635–680, 1998.
69. McComb, J.G., Levy, M.L., Apuzzo, M.L.J. (ed.), THE POSTERIOR INTRAHEMISPHERIC RETROCALLOSAL AND TRANSCALLOSAL APPROACHES TO THE THIRD VENTRICLE REGION. *Surgery of the Third Ventricle, Second Edition*, Williams and Wilkins, Baltimore, MD, Chapter 32, pp. 743–777, 1998.
70. McComb, J.G., Apuzzo, M.L.J. (ed.): OPERATIVE MANAGEMENT OF MALFORMATIONS OF THE VEIN OF GALEN. *Surgery of the Third Ventricle, Second Edition*, Williams and Wilkins, Baltimore, MD, Chapter 33, pp. 779–785, 1998.
71. Albuquerque, F.C., Apuzzo, M.L.J. (ed.), Mendel, E.: PINEAL-REGION MASSES: A UNIFIED APPROACH. *Surgery of the Third Ventricle, Second Edition*, Williams and Wilkins, Baltimore, MD, Chapter 36, pp. 787–799, 1998.
72. Chen, T.C., Krieger, M., Hinton, D.R., Zee, C., Apuzzo, M.L.J. (ed.): THE COLLOID CYST. *Surgery of the Third Ventricle, Second Edition*, Williams and Wilkins, Baltimore, MD, Chapter 47, pp. 1071–1132, 1998.

73. Apuzzo, M.L.J., Chen, T.C.: Biopsy Techniques and Instruments. *Textbook of Stereotactic and Functional Neurosurgery*; Philip L. Gildenberg/Ronald R. Tasker, McGraw-Hill, Inc., New York, NY, Section 5, Chapter 47, pp. 397–412, 1998.

74. Amar, A.P. and Apuzzo, M.L.J.: "Transcallosal Approach to the Third Ventricle".

75. Schmidek H.H. (Editor-in-Chief): *Operative Neurosurgical Techniques: Indications, Methods and Results, Fourth Edition.* Harcourt Brace & Co. Ltd, London, UK, Philadelphia: WB Saunders, 2000, pp. 852–861.

76. Albuquerque, F.C., Amar, A.P. and Apuzzo, M.L.J.: "Pineal Region Tumors". *Neuro-Oncology: The Essentials.* Mark Bernstein & Mitchel S. Berger (Editors), Thieme Medical and Scientific Publishers, Chapter 34, pp. 338–351, 2000.

77. Amar, A.P., (Zee, C., Go, J.) and Apuzzo, M.L.J.: "Treatment of CNS Infections: A Neurosurgical Perspective". *Neuroimaging Clinics of North America.* W. B. Saunders Co., Philadelphia, PA, 2:445–459, 2000.

78. Apuzzo, M.L.J.: TITLE: *Combined Modality Therapy of Central Nervous System Tumors.* Z. Petrovich, L.W. Brady, M.L.J. Apuzzo and M. Bamberg (Editors), Springer pp. 279–315, 397–412, 2000.

79. Amar, A.P. and Apuzzo, M.L.J.: "Intraventricular Tumors: Third Ventricle". *Textbook of Neurological Surgery.* H.H. Batjer and C.M. Loftus (Editors), Lippincott-Raven Publishers; Philadelphia, PA, 2000.

Contents

Manuscripts not submitted:
Arteries and Veins: Handcuffs or Roadmaps?
Albert L. Rhoton, Jr., M.D.

Surgery of the Supratentorial Ventricles: Vectors and Innovations
Axel Perneczky, M.D.

Bypass Surgery: Indications and Expectations
Neil A. Martin, M.D.

Guidelines: An Introduction
Paul C. McCormick, M.D.

I

General Scientific Session I Reinventing Neurosurgery: Surgery of the Cerebrum

1

Introduction of the CNS President: Issam A. Awad

DOUGLAS KONDZIOLKA, M.D.

It is a great honor for me to present to you the 51st president of the Congress of Neurological Surgeons, Dr. Issam Awad. I would like to tell you about Issam from the standpoint of him as a person, a neurosurgeon, an educator, an investigator, a neurosurgical leader and a friend. Dr. Awad was born in 1956 to a Lebanese family with roots tracing to the 15th century. His childhood was shattered by the death of his father when he was 11 years old, but the strength and devotion of his mother and siblings as well as their strong religious values, led to the development of a fine young man. The landscape outside Beirut allowed him to learn the languages and cultures of different nations.

As a youngster, Issam excelled in school and enjoyed outdoor activities. He completed his high school education at the College De La Sagesse in Beirut, distinguishing himself in mathematics and science and graduated as class valedictorian. He was also a distinguished ham radio operator and caught on to the CB radio craze of the 1970s. He arrived in the United States to begin university studies in biochemistry and received his Doctor of Medicine degree from Loma Linda University in 1980.

He began training in neurological surgery at the Cleveland Clinic but more importantly met Cathy Amport, who has become his life-long partner. Cathy obviously had a lot of thinking to do after Issam proposed but made the right decision, and they now have been married for 16 years. Their 12-year-old son Armand, whom some of you know to be a wonderful young man, has shared in many of their travels and exploits. Issam is an avid sportsman and frequently can be seen riding his bike wherever he may travel.

Issam Awad the neurosurgeon began his career at the Cleveland Clinic as a resident and completed training in 1985. At the Cleveland Clinic he made many friends and was mentored by Dr. Joseph Haan and Dr. John Little. He also was influenced by Dr. Tony Furlan and

Dr. Hans Luders as he developed an interest in cerebrovascular disease. He studied at the Royal Infirmatory of Edinburgh with the late Professor Douglas Miller and in 1983 received the neuroscience resident research prize and Crile traveling fellowship.

Between 1985 and 1986 he pursued fellowship training in neurovascular surgery at the Barrow Neurological Institute. He began neurosurgical practice at Stanford in 1986 but returned to Cleveland in 1987 where he became head of the section of epilepsy surgery and later surgical director of the cerebrovascular center, and Vice-Chairman of the department. No doubt, his rapid rise through the academic ranks garnered the interest of other programs and in 1993 Dr. Awad joined the faculty at Yale University as Director of the neurovascular surgery program. Energetic recruitment efforts were put forth by Dr. Spencer in order to get Issam to come to Yale.

His time at Yale was productive on many fronts. Most importantly he gained many new friends (and at least his son learned how to fish from Dr. Collins). In 1994 he was promoted to Professor of Neurosurgery and received an honorary Master of Arts degree from Yale. In 1997, he received the endowed Nixdorff-German professorship, which allowed him to focus his efforts in cerebrovascular surgery. His administrative and research skills as well as techniques in the operating room continued to gain the interest of others across the country.

In January 2001 Dr. Awad became Professor and Chairman of the Department of Neurosurgery at the University of Colorado School of Medicine and serves as the Ogsbury-Kindt Professor of Neurosurgery, Neurology and Pathology. He truly has come back to the mountains.

Issam Awad the professor, has been a leading contributor to neurosurgical education and innovation. He is the author of over 250 scientific papers and book chapters, has edited 11 books, several of which I do own myself, and has presented over 300 lectures at major meetings and symposia. He has been a Visiting Professor at institutions across the world and importantly has taught at all levels of medical training, from medical students to courses in advanced neurosurgical techniques.

Dr. Awad is the director of the RUNN course (Research Update in Neurobiology for Neurosurgeons) at the Marine Biology laboratory in Woods Hole, Massachusetts. As part of his commitment to international neurosurgery, Issam has participated in the development of training programs in many countries. In this image he attended the opening of the Saudi Arabian Epilepsy Center and recently was the special guest of the Japanese Congress of Neurological Surgeons, a meeting that I also attended. At that meeting, Dr. Awad's name was written in English and Japanese in a banner over 30 feet high, so you can see how one's ego can get a little boosted. It sometimes is difficult for Cathy to have Issam take the garbage out when he gets home after these international meetings. Dr. Awad has always conducted himself honorably on the international stage and has welcomed interactions between North American neurosurgeons and those in other countries. A good glass of sake can always help to forge new relationships between societies. The Congress of Neurological Surgeons and the Japanese Congress of Neurological Surgeons have worked hard to develop a strong working relationship.

Issam Awad the investigator, has been a prominent contributor to the science of vascular malformations and in particular, to the genetics of cerebral cavernous malformations. His work in this regard includes research support from the National Institutes of Health, and publication in noted journals as the New England Journal of Medicine and the Proceedings of the National Academy of Sciences. This work has been of landmark status—a true contribution to science.

Issam Awad the leader, has volunteered his time and efforts on behalf of neurosurgeons for over a decade. His work with the Joint Section on Cerebrovascular Surgery culminated with his position as recent chairman of that section. Here at a typical vascular "think tank" he is seen with friends at a 1997 executive committee meeting and at a meeting of past CV Section presidents in 1999. Within the Congress of Neurological Surgeons, Issam has held many positions including education chairman, scientific program chairman, annual meeting chairman, strategic planning chair, and president. He has volunteered many hundreds of hours of his time on your behalf, and he has brought intelligence, energy, and wisdom to the table. Most importantly, Issam has continued to foster joint initiatives with the American Association of Neurological Surgeons. As a true leader, Issam not only has set trends in science and medicine, but also in fashion! Although not originally from Texas, he embraced last year's San Antonio meeting in full cowboy regalia. The problem comes when he starts to push his fashion statements on others who may not be so willing.

Issam and Cathy also have worked on behalf of neurosurgeons with key individuals in our government agencies, such as with Senator John Glenn and recently in a discussion with President Bush regarding the debate on stem cell research. Cathy and Issam truly have been leaders in neurosurgery and have represented the Congress admirably.

Finally, Issam Awad is a true friend to all of those who know him. He is at home in classical music, in the arts, in a discussion of philosophy and culture, handling intraoperative catastrophes, at the microscope, and at a back yard barbecue. He has been a true friend to me personally. Both he and Cathy have also been good friends to my wife and family.

The name Issam Awad is recognized throughout the neurosurgical world, although it is sometimes miswritten and sometimes mispronounced. Nevertheless, this true renaissance man and international figure is a person of integrity, hard work and good humor. Ladies and gentleman, friends and colleagues, I give to you the 51st President of the Congress of Neurological Surgeons, Dr. Issam Awad.

2

Presidential Address: Ode to Meaning and Relevance

ISSAM A. AWAD, M.D., M.SC., F.A.C.S., M.A. (HON)

OPENING COMMENTS REGARDING RECENT EVENTS OF SEPTEMBER 11, 2001

Thank you, Doug, for such a humbling introduction, and thanks to your whole Annual Meeting team—the most creative and diligent in the history of neurosurgery. Dear colleagues, friends and guests, we have come here under difficult conditions, carrying a burden of sadness and uncertainty. The neurosurgeons of America and the world, like our country and its citizens, have shown an incredible determination to prevail. The tragedy of recent weeks is truly immense, and calls for our prayers and deepest reflections, but also for solidarity and determination. As Israeli author Amos Oz commented in the *New York Times* on September 14, this war was launched against civilization, and not between civilizations (Editorial, *The New York Times*, September 14, 2001). Our enemies are fanaticism and hatred, wherever they hide their ugly heads. Our enemies are those who preach intolerance, and those, in every society, who execute extremist means toward whatever goals they feel justified.

To the pundits who wished the retreat and paralysis of our society in the face of terror, we remind them that the colors in the American flag do not run even when it is soaked in tears. By being here, exploring every facet of *Reinventing Neurosurgery* (the theme of the 51st Annual Meeting of the Congress of Neurological Surgeons) in the service of humanity, neurosurgeons have chosen to lead in the defining battle against these forces of darkness, and in a small way, in the rebuilding of what was destroyed in our society that terrible morning.

PERSONAL ACKNOWLEDGMENTS

On a personal note, I am given reason to feel *so* honored and *so* grateful today, acknowledging all the help I've been given over the years and the incredible opportunities provided by this truly wonderful homeland. Indeed I owe countless gratitude to a million faces along my journey to this podium. I am grateful to the professional families at Loma Linda University, at the Cleveland Clinic, at Yale, and most recently in Colorado, and the scores of other neurosurgeon colleagues throughout the world who have contributed to my training and continuing education. I wish to thank my many friends and partners in organized neurosurgery. Together we have helped shape the neurosurgical agenda, keeping faith in its most noble ideals. I acknowledge my many students and trainees, for their sacred trust and inquisitive minds. And a deep gratitude goes to my patients, whose confidence and courage at times of utmost vulnerability truly reflect the most noble face of the human race.

And I take this opportunity to acknowledge the roots and the nurturing values provided to me by my family, early schooling, and church. Sadly, my father and mother have long departed me, but I am sure that they would be proud and pleased today, as are the relatives and many wonderful friends who have traveled from far to be here with us. And particular thanks to my wife Catherine and son Armand, for their continued inspiration, and for their partnership and companionship through challenges and triumphs. You have all helped give meaning and relevance to my life.

MEANING AND RELEVANCE

Meaning and Relevance. Much has been written and expressed, and much has been pursued in our efforts to achieve them. *"Ode to Meaning and Relevance"* is the title of my Address to you today as the 51st President of the Congress of Neurological Surgeons.

"Ode To Meaning" is the title of a poem, written by Robert Pinsky—twice Poet Laureate of the United States—in his masterly and intimate collection of lyrics *Jersey Rain*. A few verses from this poem read as follows:

> Dire one and desired one,
> Savior, sentencer—
> In an old allegory you would
> carry a chained alphabet of tokens:
> Ankh Badge Cross . . .
> Untrusting I court you. Wavering
> I seek your face.
>   . . . What is imagination
> but your lost child born to give birth to you?
>   . . . You are the wound. You
> be the medicine (12)

Elsewhere in the same collection, Pinsky sings another poem, itself entitled "Jersey Rain." The first verses are appropriate for the middle stretch of road, a stage where neurosurgery inarguably is braced at the dawn of the 21st century. The first verses read as follows:

Now near the end of the middle stretch of road
What have I learned? Some earthly wiles. An art.
That often I cannot tell good fortune from bad,
that once had seemed so easy to tell apart (13)

Meaning remains elusive even as we accumulate experience, a track record, accomplishments and feats along the way. Professional accomplishments do not automatically translate into Meaning, or Relevance. Ancient masons had mastered extraordinary crafts with workmanship truly amazing to this day. But their magnificent monuments remain a witness to their lost Relevance in subsequent generations. Yet a simple act, as illustrated by the parable of a Good Samaritan lending a hand to a stranger, continues to explode with Meaning and Relevance across the ages. And this was vividly demonstrated again by countless Good Samaritans in New York and Washington in the aftermath of September 11, 2001.

Meaning and Relevance embody two cardinal elements: (1) contribution or accomplishment, and (2), impact or enduring value. Both elements are essential, and neither alone guarantees Meaning or Relevance. Contribution is judged contemporaneously; while impact is judged over time, by history, as in the view of the old Louvres Museum collection through the modernist glass pyramid of I.M. Pei.

Throughout history, the medical professional was defined by and identified with the current thoughts dominant in that age (2, 14) (*Table 2.1*). From the earliest articulations of professionalism by Hippocrates, to the emphasis on philosophy as a tenet of medicine by Galen, or the theological and ethical implications evoked by Avicenna and Maimonides, and later the explosion of medicine as a scientific discipline culminating in the work of Claude Bernard and others. And some would argue that we are now entering a new age, where information and technology will be the dominant systems of society, and hence the physician of the future must be a true master of information management and technology applications. But these historical layers of Meaning and Relevance are continuous, overlapping and nonexclusionary. Even as medicine evolved in its scientific dimensions, it never fully shed its past emphases on Hippocratic ideals, philosophy or religion. The broad field of ethics, straddling both philosophy and religion, is now being sought more than ever as we tackle the limits of what we will do with genomics, molecular engineering, and transplantation.

TABLE 2.1
Historical Snapshots of Physician Personae

- Empirical professionalism (Hippocrates)
- The physician-philosopher (Galen)
- The physician-theologian (Avicenna, Maimonides)
- The physician scientist (Bernard, "experimental medicine")
- The physician as information manager (?)

SOCIETAL PERCEPTIONS

Meaning and Relevance embody both a perception and a reality. The importance of the physician persona to the value with which medicine is held cannot be overemphasized. When Nobel laureate novelist Sinclair Lewis published *Arrowsmith* (11) in 1925, a caricature of the American medical establishment at the turn of the twentieth century, it most irritated Harvey Cushing, one of the leading physicians of the day, whose own vision of medicine was more idealistic and elitist, consistent with what Porter would later call "The Greatest Benefit to Mankind" (14). We have recently studied the correspondence between Cushing and Lewis, both Yale graduates (Courtesy of research with Mr David Harris and the collection of Harvey Cushing's Correspondence, History Section, Cushing-Whitney Medical Library, Yale University Medical School, New Haven, Connecticut) and were struck by the profound clash of how these two respective icons of medicine and literature each wished medicine to be viewed. Indeed, the concept of reputation remains a most important asset of a physician, and in a collective sense, of our profession. Harvey Cushing recognized this and was willing to confront the leading novelist of the day to preserve medicine's collective image. Lewis, in turn, autographed Cushing's personal copy of *Arrowsmith* with the inscription, both conciliatory and also cynical— "To Harvey Cushing; if he isn't the best physician in the world, I'd like to know who is" (History Section, Cushing-Whitney Medical Library, Yale University Medical School, New Haven, Connecticut).

A half century later, sociologist Elliot Krause of Northwestern University attributed a failure to sustain Relevance in a changing world to the "Death of the Guilds" in the second half of the twentieth century (9). Krause invokes a triangle of balances among the *professional guilds, market capital,* and *state forces.* This triangle illustrates an ongoing loss of power to the expanding influence of regulatory and corporate sectors, leading to the Professions' weakened present position in Western society.

Alford outlined an equally unfavorable conflict between *corporate rationalizers* and *professional monopolizers* (1). It is clear that medicine and neurosurgery are destined to lose this fight in earnest if we are truly perceived as professional monopolizers. Our only opportunity in this balance of power is through renewed professionalism (7), and a strong bond with society based on our advocacy and the weight of our contributions (14).

In an emerging horizontal society (8) rebelling against regulatory forces, the advocacy and contribution of professionals can represent a formidable force against rationalizers and regulators. The age-old values of professionalism, the ideals which have served medicine well and shaped its persona through the centuries, would appear to be our best weapons in future battles for Meaning and Relevance (7, 14).

THE FUTURE OF NEUROSURGERY

Let us now turn to the specific challenges and opportunities facing neurosurgery in the years ahead. Given the premises that we articulated, how do we best position our discipline for prominence and impact? The science of predicting the future (5) would tell us that we will face inevitable progress through growing knowledge and advancing technology (*Table 2.2*). But there will also be paradigm shifts and new epochs, the unplanned and the unexpected. And there will be progress in response to specific societal pressures.

The expansion of knowledge in neurobiology and genomics will likely continue, and we must be prepared to embrace its applications to neurosurgery. Neurosurgeons should probe the basic mechanisms explaining and predicting the clinical behavior of neurosurgical diseases. They should revisit our classification schemes of tumors, malformations and degenerative diseases, through phenotype and genotype correlations. These in turn will enhance risk prediction models, as we incorporate knowledge on deterministic and predisposition genes, impacting the management of individual patients.

Surgical technique will continue to evolve through more facile localization and navigation, and the seamless integration of functional mapping and real time intraoperative imaging. Imaging will also be used for enhanced diagnosis, revealing in vivo spectroscopic signatures of disease, staging and outcome prediction and assessment. And we will be facing the incredible opportunities of nanotechnology, remote tracking, robotics, and the simulation of surgery in virtual reality. The Visible Human Project (Center for Human Simulation, University of Colorado Health Sciences Center, Denver, Colorado; www.uchsc.edu/sm/chs) and other human simulation programs are incorporating real anatomical datasets as well as the touch and feel of tissues during dissections in a virtual stereotactic domain, replacing phantoms and cadaver

TABLE 2.2
Forces Likely to Shape the Future of Neurosurgery

Progress Through Knowledge (Neurobiology and Genomics)
- Mechanisms explaining and predicting disease behavior, healing, recovery
- Disease classification, genotype-phenotype correlations
- Risk prediction, deterministic and predisposition genes, genetic modifiers of disease behavior, healing, recovery

Progress Through Evolving Technology
- Surgical guidance, localization, navigation, mapping, intraoperative imaging
- Imaging for diagnosis, spectrospcopic signatures of disease, staging, outcome assessment
- Robotics, nanotechnology, surgical simulation

Functional and Restorative Neurosurgery
- Augmentative and restorative biologic intervention
- Pacing and triggered neurostimulation
- Transplantation, stem cells, biologic vector modifiers, organogenesis

Epidemiology and Informatics
- Enhanced efficiency of trials, meta-analyses
- The "new statistics" (Bayesian and other methodologies)
- Confidence intervals and measures of certainty
- Megadatabases, pooled outcomes sets, outlier tracking
- Individualized risk management, risk prediction, risk modifiers, profiling

Paradigm Shifts, the Unplanned and the Unexpected
- New and unexpected discoveries, knowledge, technologies

Progress in Response to Societal Pressures
- Pressure toward high technology integration, minimal invasiveness
- Pressure toward added value, impact on quality of life

specimens—and these projects are awaiting specific neurosurgical applications limited only by the realm of our creativity and diligence.

We are truly at the threshold of a golden era in functional neurosurgery, with real possibilities of augmentative and restorative neurosurgery, pacing and triggered neurostimulation, and sensitized and biotargeted radiotherapy. The field of neurotransplantation holds real promise through stem cells, biologic vector modifiers and organogenesis.

And we will progress our knowledge in epidemiology and informatics, with more efficient clinical trial methodologies, information management systems, and clever applications of "new" statistics involving Bayesian and other models. Mega-databases will provide pooled outcome sets and effective outlier tracking. Risk modifiers through profiling and individualized risk management will allow us to determine relative and absolute risks of disease behavior and treatment interventions, along with accurate measures of uncertainty. The computer technology of IBM's "Big Blue," which triumphed in chess over Gary

Kasparov, can be used to articulate differential diagnoses, management decisions, and outcome predictions.

TRANSLATIONAL RESEARCH: A CRITICAL BOTTLENECK

In the face of these incredible opportunities, there is a dire shortage of clinicians involved in the scientific enterprise, and this is being recognized as a critical bottleneck in biomedical research (6). The percentage of American physicians reporting research as their primary career has dropped from 4.2% t o 1.8% between 1984 and 1999, or less than 15,000 physician-scientists, with only a minority of these conducting patient-oriented research. Physicians are unable to capitalize on the explosion of available research dollars, a whopping 48% increase in NIH budget alone between 1999 and 2001. Physicians are effectively excluding themselves from a biomedical research industry representing more than $21 billion dollars annually in Federal funds alone, and countless other monies through foundations and industry. At the same time, the biomedical research establishment cannot survive without physicians. Will neurosurgery get lost in these dizzying trends? Neurosurgeons have a strong scientific tradition, and often enter our field with superb scientific preparation; and our work presents continued opportunities for making seminal observations and testing relevant hypotheses. There are incredible opportunities in neurosurgical research and the resources to realize them—we must aim to promote neurosurgical research by preserving the resident research experience, protecting and encouraging young faculty's research time, and by staunchly supporting neurosurgical role models who inspire and engage in science. Neurosurgery is well equipped to shatter the bottleneck, and we would all be rewarded by the benefits to our field and to mankind.

It is true that neurosurgeons, as busy professionals, cannot be the sole engineers and scientists who develop these advances. Yet, neurosurgeons cannot afford the trend of becoming illiterate observers in an age of expanding knowledge. The neurosurgical perspective and intraoperative and bedside experiences with specific diseases are essential to effective translation of scientific advances to the benefit of our patients (3, 17). Neurosurgeons of the future must set aside protected time to study other fields of knowledge. They must then use other fields' tools and methodologies to study neurosurgical problems. And neurosurgeons should then translate this new knowledge into practical and novel neurosurgical applications. This is a simple but

TABLE 2.3

A Paradigm of Neurosurgical Translational Inquiry

- Study other fields of science and technology (literacy)
- Use other fields' tools to study neurosurgical problems
- Translate into novel neurosurgical applications

guaranteed formula for success in academic neurosurgery (*Table 2.3*). And what a splendid opportunity for future neurosurgeons, learning the language of other disciplines and translating it to the benefit of neurosurgical patients. There are significant career rewards, along with an incredible sense of self-fulfillment awaiting those who choose this path of professional development.

And we will necessarily face unplanned and unexpected developments. Many of these will be driven by societal demands and entrepreneurialism. We cannot leave innovation to modern snake oil salesmen—claiming to have the inside story. As in the whole body scan, now offered in several cities in the United States (for cash only), for under $1,000; promising to detect occult diseases (from cancer to atherosclerosis) before they become clinically manifest. Our task is to grasp these opportunities and understand their appeal. We should drive responsible innovations, and engage, evaluate—and then embrace or discard them, using objective question-driven technology assessment (4). Neurosurgeons should be leaders in defining a new framework for the cost effectiveness of innovation, in terms of economics as well as quality of life.

In these endeavors, science will continue to serve us well as a professional conscience (15), guarding against the ever-present threats of quackery and fraud; protecting us from bias and myth; and helping us understand mechanisms of disease, translational applications, and the efficiency of evidence.

THE WEIGHTED RELEVANCE OF NEUROSURGERY

In aiming to enhance our weighted Relevance we must be committed to factors that strengthen neurosurgeons' contribution and impact (*Table 2.4*). Surrealist painters have admonished us to look beyond the shallow and the obvious. In his famous painting of a pipe with an underlying note *Ceci n'est pas une pipe* (this is not a pipe) , René Magritte seemed to scream that a picture of a pipe cannot capture the full significance of a pipe—the integrated experience of touch, taste, smell and associated memories, friendships and thoughts. Similarly we must grasp the full dimensions of meaning and relevance in our work.

TABLE 2.4
The "Weighted Relevance" of Neurosurgery

Breadth
- Prevention, access, critical care, diagnosis, therapy, restoration, outcome

Depth
- Relevance, rigor, impact

Diversity
- Human resources
- Diseases, questions, techniques
- Models of care, multidisciplinary interface

Benefit to Society
- "Value", generalization, "reach"

Paradigm of Ideals
- Size as an advantage (small specialty, easier to integrate change)
- Model of innovation, progress, credibility

We must not fear *breadth* in neurosurgery. Neurosurgeons should be engaged in every arena of prevention, access, critical care, diagnosis, therapy, restoration, and outcome. Our manpower needs, and our collective strength will depend on, our leadership in every aspect of the care of trauma, stroke, cancer, epilepsy, pain, and degenerative diseases. We should be available, knowledgeable, innovative and engaged—rather than being perceived as busy, shallow, recalcitrant or aloof—lest neurosurgery gradually lose its relevance in the treatment of those respective facets of disease. We must also aim toward *depth* in our endeavors, looking for rigor and impact of our contributions. We should not be afraid of tackling the big questions of society and finding a role for neurosurgery in solving these problems. We must embrace *diversity* and open a million doors out of our insularity. Our teams should be diverse, and our questions, techniques and models of care should also be diverse. We should enrich multidisciplinary interface through countless bridges, seeking a seat for neurosurgery at every table in our hospitals, communities, and academic institutions. And we should strive for a broad and generalizable benefit to society through both value and reach. Neurosurgical advances cannot be limited to rich urban metropoles, but we should strive to leverage our knowledge, technology, and information in models of neurosurgical development relevant throughout the country and the world. Neurosurgery should incorporate the contributions and values of diverse societies, and should benefit from their diverse perspectives. We are indeed a small discipline, but *our size is an advantage* when raising the mean of our weighted Relevance. We can be a small but effective model for innovation, progress, and credibility. Neurosurgery should be viewed by society and by the rest of medicine as a true paradigm of these ideals.

As we increase the weight of our collective Relevance, we must remain committed to our traditional surgical values. The surgeon has always been viewed as a paragon of credibility, compassion, and advocacy. Whether in Udalpho Oppi's painting of *Three Surgeons* in 1926, Walter Dandy's timeless photograph teaching at the bedside, Harvey Cushing's scholarly office at Yale, or the images of a surgeon repairing the human brain under the microscope, the surgeon is regarded by society as a scholar and an intellectual, and also as a technical virtuoso. These images of our ideals should not be taken for granted or marginalized, as they will serve us well in enhancing the impact of our contributions.

Dependent as ever on the trust of our patients and society, we should remain cognizant of the dangers threatening our professionalism ("Business Thrives on Unproven Care, Leaving Science Behind," *The New York Times*, October 3, 1999). In particular, conflict of interest can weaken our collective credibility and reduce us to a vulnerable and indefensible position as self-serving monopolizers. Business practices can and do enhance our efficiency, leveraging our resources and helping us accomplish our professional and academic missions. *But the business model and the corporate ethic cannot be allowed to dominate our professional purpose.* The professional is above all an intellectual, and the intellectual must recognize the sources of bias and conflict of interest, must articulate these to one's self, and must disclose them to society, even at the risk of compromising one's own gains.

And the intellectual should use every opportunity to speak truth to power (16), as in recent debates on stem cell research and patients' Bill of Rights; to influence political priorities—rather than subjecting professional ideals to *realpolitic.*

ODE TO RELEVANCE

I started this Address with an ode to Meaning. I wish to conclude with another lyric, entitled "The Sea, That Has No Ending . . . ", a true ode to Relevance by Stanley Kunitz, who in the middle of his nineties remains a master of contemporary poetry:

Who are we? Why are we here,
huddled on this desolate shore,
so curiously chopped and joined?—
Broken totems, a scruffy tribe!
How many years have passed

since we owned keys to a door,
had friends, walked down familiar streets
and answered to a name? We try
not to remember the places
where we left pieces of ourselves
along the way . . .
What is to become of us?
. . . If only we had strength enough
or nerve for a grand heroic action.
Habit has made it easier for us
to wait for the blessing of the tide . . .
Why is the Master knocking at our ears,
demanding immediate attention?
In the acid of his voice we sense
the horns swelling at his temples
and little drops of spittle
bubbling at the corners of his mouth.
This is not an exhibition, he storms, *It's a life!* (10)

As a professional guild, may our tribe repair its broken totems. May
we remember the places where we left pieces of ourselves. May we
have the strength and nerve for grand heroic actions. And may Neurosurgery understand that this is not an exhibition; *it is a life*.

REFERENCES

1. Alford R. *Health care politics. Ecological and interest group barriers to reform.* Chicago: University of Chicago Press, 1975.
2. Awad IA. Preface. In: Awad IA, Ed. *Philosophy of neurological surgery.* Park Ridge: American Association of Neurological Surgeons, 1995, pp. ix–xii.
3. Awad IA. Neurological surgery and clinical science. In: Awad IA, Ed. *Philosophy of neurological surgery.* Park Ridge: American Association of Neurological Surgeons, 1995, pp. 117–124.
4. Caplan LR. Question-driven technology assessment. **Neurology** 41:187–191; 1991.
5. Casti JL. *Searching for Certainty. What scientists can know about the future.* New York: William Morrow and Company, 1990.
6. Cech TR, Egan LW, Doyle C, et al. The biomedical research bottleneck (Editorial). **Science** 293:573; 2001.
7. Cruess RL, Cruess SR, Johnston SE. Renewing professionalism: An opportunity for medicine. **Acad Med** 74:878–883; 1999.
8. Friedman LM. *The horizontal society.* New Haven: Yale University Press, 1999.
9. Krause E. *The death of the guilds. Professions, states, and the advance of capitalism, 1930 to the present.* New Haven: Yale University Press, 1996.
10. Kunitz S. "The Sea That Has No Ending." In: *Passing through. The later poems new and selected.* New York: W.W. Norton and Company, pp. 153–155, 1997.
11. Lewis S. *Arrowsmith.* New York: Harcourt Brace Jovanovich, 1925 (Reprinted as an HBJ Modern Classic 1990).

12. Pinsky R. "Ode to Meaning." In: *Jersey rain. Poems.* New York: Farrar, Strauss and Giroux, 2000, pp. 5–7.
13. Pinsky R. "Jersey Rain." In: *Jersey rain. Poems.* New York: Farrar, Strauss and Giroux, 2000: 52.
14. Porter R. *The greatest benefit to mankind. A medical history of humanity.* New York: W.W. Norton and Company, 1998.
15. Sagan C. *The demon-haunted world. Science as a candle in the dark.* New York: Ballantine Books, 1996.
16. Said EW. Speaking truth to power. In: *Representations of the intellectual.* New York: Vintage Books, 1996, pp. 85–102.
17. Spencer DD. Neurological surgery and biological science. In: Awad IA, Ed. *Philosophy of neurological surgery.* Park Ridge: American Association of Neurological Surgeons, 1995, pp. 105–115.

3

Black Holes of the Brain: How to Reach Challenging Areas of the Cerebrum

JEFFREY S. HENN, M.D.

G. MICHAEL LEMOLE, JR., M.D.

MAURO A. T. FERREIRA, M.D.*

MARK SCHORNAK, M.S.

MARK PREUL, M.D.*

ROBERT F. SPETZLER, M.D.

The success of any neurosurgical procedure is the result of extensive training, exquisite knowledge of anatomy, precision instruments, modern imaging techniques, and the cumulative efforts of an entire team of healthcare providers. However, even with this armamentarium, particular approaches remain especially challenging. The most challenging areas are those farthest from the surface of the brain, sheltered by the complex anatomy of the bony skull and intimately associated with eloquent neurologic structures. Perhaps the ultimate example is the basilar region, which fulfills all three criteria.

The basilar region consists of the basilar artery, the anterior brain stem, cranial nerves, and closely associated structures. This location is sheltered by the clivus and facial structures anteriorly, the brain stem and cerebellum posteriorly, and the cranial nerves laterally. Access to the region is extremely difficult. Anterior approaches to the basilar region are often associated with complications such as meningitis and cerebrospinal fluid leakage(1). Furthermore, these exposures tend to be deep and provide limited working area. Posterior approaches to the region are precluded by the brain stem. As a result, the basilar region usually must be accessed through various lateral approaches. These approaches were developed and refined to provide safe, effective access to the lower, middle, and upper basilar regions.

PRINCIPLES FOR ACCESSING THE BLACK HOLES OF THE BRAIN

To access the most challenging areas, neurosurgeons must combine fundamental techniques with the capabilities offered by contemporary technology. The basic tenets, which apply to any neurosurgical procedure, are to maximize exposure while minimizing morbidity. These goals are accomplished through meticulous surgical technique and exquisite knowledge of anatomy.

Optimal exposure is obtained through a combination of bone removal and brain relaxation techniques (for example, dissection of the Sylvian fissure, CSF drainage, basal cistern fenestration, mannitol, barbiturates). Although maximizing exposure is essential, it must be accomplished through bone removal and brain relaxation rather than with aggressive brain retraction. Functional exposure also can be improved by decreasing the surgical working distance, which is partially achieved through bone removal. Simple surgical techniques, such as using fishhook retraction to flatten the edges of the wound rather than applying self-retaining retractors, are helpful. Any exposure should be exploited fully using the keyhole techniques of contemporary neurosurgery, including the capabilities of the operating microscope (coaxial illumination, magnification, and stereoscopic vision through a small corridor).

Another component of exposure is to select the approach that provides the best angle for treating a specific pathology. For example, an aneurysm may easily be clipped from one angle but may be much more difficult to treat otherwise. Another example is the *two-point method*, which we use to determine the best surgical approach to lesions of the brain stem (2). A point is placed in the center of the lesion, and a second point is placed where the lesion reaches closest to the surface. A straight line connecting the two points indicates the best angle of attack, which, in turn, dictates the optimal surgical approach. In addition to providing access to a region, an ideal exposure also provides an optimal angle for treating the pathology.

Neurosurgeons must have an extensive knowledge of the anatomy of not only the cerebrum but also the surrounding bony, neural, and vascular structures. Neurosurgeons can then best exploit natural corridors and thereby maximize exposure and the likelihood of success while minimizing the possibility of morbidity.

Several surgical adjuncts are especially useful when approaching the most challenging areas of the cerebrum. The operating microscope is critical for the reasons discussed above. Frameless stereotaxy, which provides valuable feedback about location and trajectory, is particularly helpful when accessing deep, eloquent structures. Electrophysiological monitoring, including electroencephalography (EEG), brain stem auditory evoked potentials (BAEPs), and cranial nerve monitoring, can likewise provide valuable feedback for neurosurgeons working in and around eloquent structures. Barbiturates relax the brain and protect it from ischemia. When treating large and giant aneurysms of the posterior circulation, hypothermic circulatory arrest is another valuable tool. Besides offering the ultimate form of proximal vascular control, this technique allows the dome of an aneurysm to be decompressed so that perforating arteries can be dissected free and the aneurysm optimally clipped.

APPROACHES USED TO ACCESS THE BASILAR REGION

Three approaches, the far lateral, the transcochlear, and the orbitozygomatic, are used to access the lower, mid-, and upper basilar region *(Fig. 3.1)*.

Far-Lateral Approach

The far-lateral approach is a workhorse procedure that provides access to the lower two-fifths of the basilar artery, the anterior pontomedullary region, and the lower clivus (1). This posterolateral approach provides the necessary angle to work successfully in front of the brain stem, with minimal need for retraction. The far-lateral also offers the advantage of early proximal control of the ipsilateral vertebral artery.

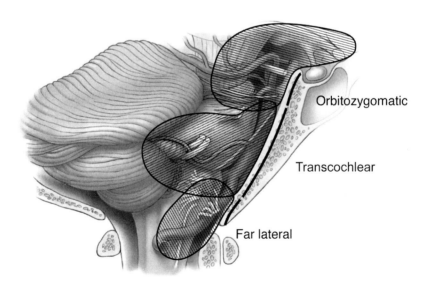

Fig. 3.1 Three approaches provide excellent exposure to the basilar region. The far-lateral approach is used to access the lower two-fifths of the basilar region; the transcochlear approach is used to access the middle fifth of the basilar region; and the orbitozygomatic approach is used to access the upper two-fifths of the basilar region. *With permission from Barrow Neurological Institute.*

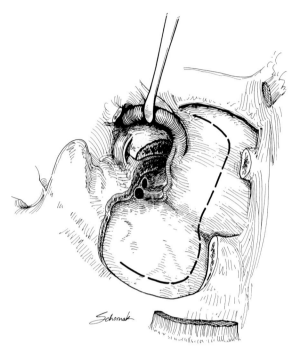

FIG. 3.2 The far-lateral approach includes a lateral extension of a suboccipital craniotomy with removal of the lateral rim of the foramen magnum, the lateral arch of C1,
and the posterior third of the occipital condyle. The dura *(dotted line)* is opened in a C-
shaped fashion to maximize exposure. From Baldwin HZ, Miller CG, van Loveren HR
et al: The far lateral/combined supra- and infratentorial approach. A human cadaveric
prosection model for routes of access to the petroclival region and ventral brain stem.
J Neurosurg 81:60–68, 1994. *With permission from Journal of Neurosurgery.*

First described by Heros (4) and later modified by Spetzler and
Grahm *(Fig. 3.2),* (7) the far-lateral approach is an extension of a lateral suboccipital craniotomy. Three important modifications increase
operative exposure (6). First, the arch of C1 is removed laterally to
the level of the sulcus arteriosus. Next, the lateral rim of the foramen
magnum is removed to the occipital condyle. Finally, the posterior
third of the condyle is removed using a high-speed drill and rongeurs.
Care is taken to protect the extracranial vertebral artery when the
condyle is being drilled. Other potential modifications of the far-
lateral craniotomy include complete mobilization of the extracranial
vertebral artery and drilling of the jugular tubercle. After bone removal is complete, the dura is opened in a "C"-shaped fashion with
the flap based laterally. By working between the nerve roots, the neu-

rosurgeon can gain exposure to both vertebral arteries, the lower basilar artery, the ipsilateral posterior inferior cerebellar artery, and the anterior brain stem.

Transcochlear Approach

The transcochlear approach provides access to the midbasilar artery, the region of the anterior inferior cerebellar artery, and the anterior pons. The transcochlear approach is the most extensive of several transpetrous approaches *(Fig. 3.3)*. It requires extensive drilling of the petrous bone and requires expert knowledge of the temporal bone and related anatomy. At our institution, this drilling is performed by a neuro-otologist. The transcochlear approach causes ipsilateral hearing loss and is typically associated with temporary facial weakness due to exposure and mobilization of the facial nerve (3).

In general, the transcochlear approach can be considered in a series of steps, with each step representing part of the continuum of the transpetrous approaches. The first is the retrolabyrinthine approach, which includes exposure of the sigmoid sinus, presigmoid posterior fossa, and inferior middle fossa. This exposure is extended to a translabyrinthine approach by drilling the semicircular canals and removing the surrounding bone. Finally, the extension to a transcochlear approach includes exposure and transposition of the facial nerve and drilling of the bony external auditory canal, middle ear, and cochlea (9).

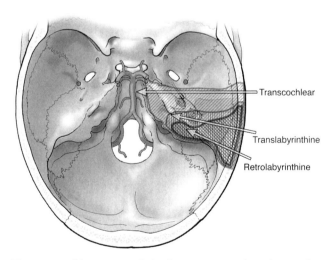

FIG. 3.3 The transcochlear approach is the most extensive of several transpetrous approaches, including the translabyrinthine and retrolabyrinthine approaches. The transcochlear approach provides access to the middle fifth of the basilar region. *With permission from Barrow Neurological Institute.*

After this extensive drilling has been completed, a relatively small and deep corridor is available to the region of the midbasilar artery. Because of its inherent morbidity and limited exposure, the transcochlear approach is reserved for lesions extending into the prepontine area and for aneurysms involving the middle fifth of the basilar artery that cannot be accessed from above or below.

The Orbitozygomatic Approach

The orbitozygomatic approach is an extremely flexible, powerful approach that provides access to the anterior fossa, middle fossa, and upper posterior fossa. This approach can be used to approach the upper two-fifths of the basilar artery.

The orbitozygomatic approach represents an extension of the pterional craniotomy *(Fig. 3.4)*. In fact, some surgeons remove the or-

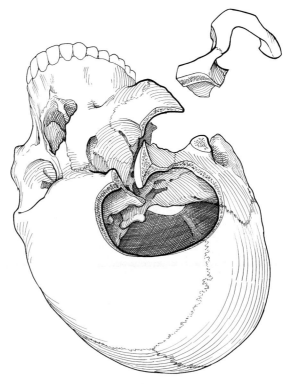

FIG. 3.4 The orbitozygomatic approach is an extension of the pterional craniotomy. This extension increases exposure, decreases working distance, and improves the angle of attack to the upper basilar region. *With permission from Barrow Neurological Institute.*

bitozygomatic bone along with the pterional craniotomy as a single piece. We prefer a two-stage method: the pterional craniotomy is performed first followed by the orbitozygomatic osteotomy in a separate step. After the craniotomy has been performed, the pterion is partially removed to facilitate the orbitozygomatic osteotomy and to gain operative exposure. Much of this bone is removed during the orbitozygomatic osteotomy and later replaced during closure.

The orbitozygomatic osteotomy is performed with a reciprocating saw and includes five cuts (8). Before the cuts are made, the soft tissue and dura are freed from the bone and surrounding structures are protected carefully. The first cut is made through the lateral zygoma, just medial to the root. The second cut crosses the malar eminence from its lateral side to its midpoint. The third cut, made from within the orbit, extends from the inferior orbital fissure up through the malar eminence to the second cut. The fourth cut is made through the orbital roof and inferior frontal fossa and extends around toward the superior orbital fissure. The final cut is made extracranially from the inferior orbital fissure and extends back to either the superior orbital fissure or the previous cut. At this point, the orbitozygomatic osteotomy is removed. Additional bone is removed extradurally as needed to gain maximal exposure.

The dura is opened in a "C"-shaped fashion and held anteriorly with sutures. To fully exploit the bony removal, several sutures are used to flatten the portion of dura over the exposed orbit. The approach can be tailored to the area being accessed: Options include removing the complete orbitozygomatic bar or the orbit or zygoma alone. For access to the upper basilar artery, a full orbitozygomatic approach is used.

After the dura has been opened, the sylvian fissure is widely dissected. Depending on patient's anatomy, the approach to the upper basilar region can be facilitated by drilling the anterior clinoid, the posterior clinoid, and the upper clivus.

The orbitozygomatic approach offers several advantages. Removal of the orbitozygomatic bar increases exposure and limits the need for brain retraction. The working distance is minimized. The lower angle of approach provided by the orbitozygomatic osteotomy also is advantageous for aneurysm clipping (5).

SUMMARY

Numerous techniques and tools can be used to access difficult areas of the cerebrum: skull base techniques, modern operating room equipment, and a unified team approach. Using these principles, challenging areas of the cerebrum can be approached with maximal success and minimal morbidity. These techniques are powerful tools in the armamentarium of neurosurgeons and can improve any neurosurgical approach.

The basilar region remains one of the most difficult areas to approach. Despite its inherent complexity, lesions of the basilar region can be treated successfully. The far-lateral approach is used to access the lower two-fifths of the basilar region; the transcochlear approach is used to access the middle fifth of the basilar region; and the orbitozygomatic approach is used to access the upper two-fifths of the basilar region. Each approach beautifully exemplifies the principles of skull base surgery.

REFERENCES

1. Alleyne CH, Jr, Spetzler RF: The transcondylar approach. **Operative Techniques in Neurosurgery** 2:74–86, 1999.
2. Brown AP, Thompson BG, Spetzler RF: The two-point method: Evaluating brain stem lesions. **BNI Quarterly** 12:20–24, 1996.
3. Friedman RA, Brackmann DE: Transcochlear approach. **Operative Techniques in Neurosurgery** 2:39–45, 1999.
4. Heros RC: Lateral suboccipital approach for vertebral and vertebrobasilar artery lesions. **J Neurosurg** 64:559–562, 1986.
5. Lemole GM, Jr., Henn J, Spetzler RF, et al: Surgical management of giant aneurysms. **Operative Techniques in Neurosurgery** 3:239–254, 2000.
6. Porter RW, Detwiler PW, Spetzler RF: Surgical approaches to the brain stem. **Operative Techniques in Neurosurgery** 3:114–123, 2000.
7. Spetzler RF, Grahm TW: The far-lateral approach to the inferior clivus and the upper cervical region: Technical note. **BNI Quarterly** 6:35–38, 1990.
8. Zabramski JM, Kiris I, Sankhla SK, et al: Orbitozygomatic craniotomy: Technical note. **J Neurosurg** 89:336–341, 1998.
9. Zubay G, Porter RW, Spetzler RF: Transpetrosal approaches. **Operative Techniques in Neurosurgery** 4:24–29, 2001.

CHAPTER

4

Honored Guest Presentation:
Surgery of the Human Cerebrum:
A Collective Modernity

MICHAEL L. J. APUZZO, M.D., CHARLES Y. LIU, M.D., PH.D.,
DANIEL SULLIVAN, M.DIV. AND RODRICK A. FACCIO, B.S.

Safe and beneficial surgery of the human cerebrum is arguably one of mankind's most notable achievements and one of the great testimonials to human creativity, intelligence, and character. It, in many ways, is a testimony to the climates of civilization that have marked human history. In historical terms cranial surgery in the year 2001 is celebrating its twelve thousandth birthday, with cranial manipulation for various religious, mystical, and therapeutic reasons being evident in Africa more than ten millennia before the birth of Christ. It is of interest for all to trace the major developments and attitudes that have laid the foundations of modernity in what is currently surgery and medicine's most exciting and complex technical exercise. It is in fact a twelve thousand year prelude to the modernity that we currently enjoy. Before attempting to define our modernity and emerging futurism with reinvention, examination of the prolonged and tedious invention is appropriate for perspective. Let us examine and recount the accrual of data and attitude changes over the stream of history that has allowed refined surgery of the human cerebrum to become a reality.

THE INVENTION: HISTORICAL FOUNDATIONS— THE EVOLUTION OF CRANIAL SURGERY

For literally thousands of years cranial surgery was principally extradural. Historical evidence suggests that perhaps man's very first attempt at surgical manipulation involved the removal of pieces of the bony coverings of the brain (10, 23, 45, 69, 89, 91, 96, 108). Since these very first attempts by Neolithic man, surgery of the brain and its coverings has evolved slowly over some twelve thousand years, with elements of refinement in instrumentation, but with similar end results.

In fact, the past few decades bear sole witness to the rapid acceleration and expansion in the scope and breadth of neurosurgery.

Prehistoric Cranial Surgery

Trepanation describes the removal of sections of bone from the skull (69). The instrument used to accomplish this procedure is the *trepan*, which derives from the Greek *trypanon*, or borer *(Fig. 4.1)*. *Trephination*, on the other hand, refers to the specific creation of a circular saw, *trephine*, or a more modern instrument (96). Although others may have made earlier reference to trepanation, Paul Broca is generally credited as being the catalyst for the widespread acknowledgement of this practice in ancient cultures (19). He was made aware of a skull discovered by E. G. Squier, a French diplomat to Peru, and after careful examination of the specimen, suggested that the procedure had been performed on a living patient who subsequently survived. Prior to Broca's assertion, it had always been believed that the bony defects found in French skulls since the late 1600s had been the result of post-mortem rituals (10). At present there is almost universal acceptance of ante-mortem skull surgery in pre-history, and archeological evidence supports that the practice was indeed widespread, with skull specimens found in Europe, Asia, Africa, North/Central/South America, and Oceania (10, 45, 69, 77, 89, 91, 96, 104, 110). In fact, the practice sur-

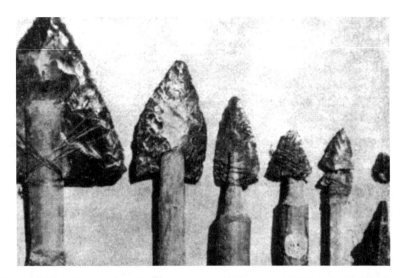

FIG. 4.1 Primitive trephination instruments made of stone blades attached to wooden shafts. (From Laws ER Jr, Udvarhelyi GB: *The genesis of neuroscience by A. Earl Walker, M.D.* Park Ridge, IL: AANS, 1998, p. 5.)

vives to modern times in certain East-African and South American tribes (76).

To date more than 1500 specimens have been found and examined. The oldest examples of trepanation may be specimens found in North Africa, dating back to 10,000 BC. Excavations in the Jericho area in the Near East and Asia have produced specimens from about 8000 to 6000 BC. The earliest European examples are over 10,000 years old, dating perhaps to the late Paleolithic period, but certainly to the Neolithic age (69, 91). Early Danubians were performing skull surgery in 3000 BC, and ancients from the Seine-Oise-Marne area of France were similarly active in 2000 BC. Based on the number of skulls that have been found in France, it is probable that a veritable "surgery center" existed there between 1900 and 1500 BC. Trepanation specimens have also been found in other regions of Neolithic Europe, the Balkans, and Russia. New World specimens of trepanation are much more recent, with the oldest examples found in the South coast of Peru dating to 400 BC. Nevertheless, more trepanned skulls have been found in this region than in the rest of the world combined. It is possible that the practice spread from Peru to what is now Mexico and North America. In the Far East and China, however, no specimens have been found so far.

Despite the plethora of physical evidence of pre-historic trepanation, insight into the motivation to the practice has been much more problematic and controversial (69, 88, 91). In the absence of written records, scholars are left to speculate, invoking a combination of motives as varied as therapeutic, magico-therapeutic, and magico-ritual. For example, given the tendency of Peruvian and Danish skulls to have openings in the left tempero-parietal region, it follows that trepanations had therapeutic intentions for injuries from blows by a right-handed assailant. Ritual was felt to be an important motivation for the development of the trepanation "center" in Neolithic France. In postmortem operations, *roundelles* of cranial bone were presumably obtained for use as charms, amulets, or talismans *(Fig. 4.2)*. These speculations are somewhat supported by observations of the practice of 20th century East African tribes, where the Kisii Tribe perform trepanations primarily to alleviate headache after a blow, while the nearby Lugbara Tribe desires to release evil spirits. A novel speculation proposes that operations on the head were aimed at resurrecting the dead (88). The author argues that Neolitic man appreciated the contrasting outcomes of "fatal" blows by piercing weapons to the chest or abdomen and blunt instruments to the head. For example, "death" by piercing the chest or abdomen was generally permanent, while victims often recovered from ostensibly fatal blows to the head. Thus Neolithic man attempted to revive the dead by surgically manipulating

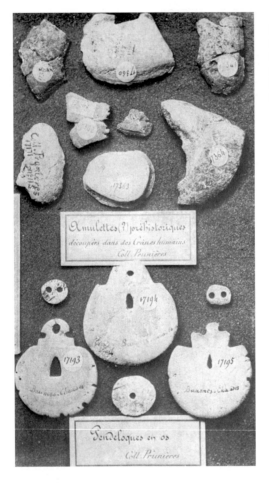

FIG. 4.2 Prehistoric amulets: Bone disks removed by trephination were polished into various shapes and worn around the neck as protection against disease. (From Leonardo RA: *History of surgery*. New York: Froben Press, 1943.)

the head. However, this elegant theory suffers from lack of concrete evidence and has faced the same criticism as prior speculations.

However motivated, pre-historic surgeons invoked essentially four different techniques to remove pieces of cranial bone: (1) scraping, (2) grooving, (3) boring-and-cutting, and (4) rectangular intersecting incisions (69, 91, 110) *(Fig. 4.3)*. The earliest instruments were made of flaked stone, flint, obsidian, and bone. Later on, the ancient Peruvians used curved *tumi* blades to incise soft tissue and to make rectangular cuts in the bony skull *(Fig. 4.4)*. Sharp instruments were used to make grooves and drill holes that could then be connected. Flat scrapers were also used with good effect, while in Mexico, a bow and obsidian drill may have been used. While the primitive surgical instruments have survived to the present day, there is a lack of specific evidence

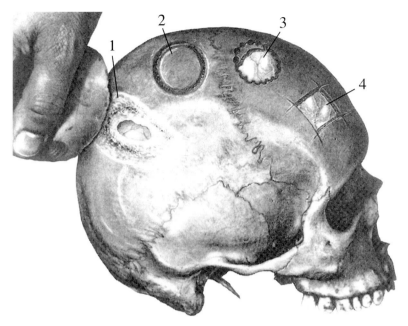

FIG. 4.3 Methods of trephination included (1) scraping, (2) grooving, (3) boring and cutting, and (4) rectangular intersecting incisions. (From Lisowski FP: Prehistoric and early historic trepanation. In Brothwell D, Sandison AT (eds.): *Diseases in antiquity: A survey of the diseases, injuries and surgery of early populations.* Springfield, IL: Charles C Thomas, 1967, pp 651–672.)

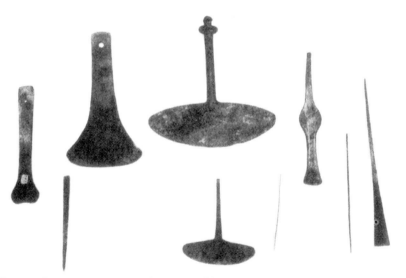

FIG. 4.4 Bronze instruments (*champi*) used by the Incas in craniotomies, including a bone elevator, crescent tumi knives, dissectors and needles. (From Raul Marino, Jr., Marco Gonzales-Portillo: Preconquest Peruvian neurosurgeons: A study of Inca and Pre-Columbian trephination and the art of medicine in ancient Peru. **Neurosurgery** 47: 940–950, 2000.)

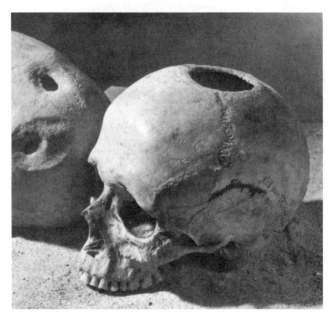

FIG. 4.5 This skull shows evidence of bone healing for trephination. Despite primitive instrumentation and crude methodology, the pre-historic surgeons were surprisingly successful. (From Nationalmuseet, Copenhagen.)

of anesthetic use. Scholars have speculated that alcohol, narcotics, or coco products were administered to alleviate pain. However contemporary East African patients undergo trepanation without anesthesia, and a survivor in Bolivia admitted that while the incision of the soft tissue is painful, analgesia is not an overriding issue once the bony skull is stripped of the pericranium (10).

Despite their primitive instruments and lack of fundamental medical knowledge, pre-historic surgeons were surprisingly successful (10). Evidence of healing in the archeological specimen indicates that patients survived *(Fig. 4.5)*. In some groups of ancient skulls, up to 80% of Neolithic and Melanesian patients survived the operation. In present day Africa, operators claim less than 5% mortality. The ancient Peruvian faced upwards of 50% mortality. However, it is believed that many of their patients were victims of trauma, and the confounding contribution of the traumatic injury could account for their poorer results.

Evolution of Neurosurgery in Ancient and Medieval History

The legacy of cranial surgery by their pre-historic ancestors was embraced as humans began to record their activities. In fact, the importance of operations on the head and bony coverings of the brain is recognized by the prominent movements and personalities that have shaped the evolution of medicine through ancient and medieval history (46, 69). During this period, head trauma appeared to be the principle indication for cranial manipulations.

EGYPT AND CHINA

The ancient Egyptians can claim to have produced both the earliest known practicing physician, *Imhotep (2600 BC) (Fig. 4.6)* and the earliest known medical text, the Ebers papyrus (46). This document, along with the Hearst and Edwin Smith Papyri documented the awareness of the Egyptian of the importance of neurosurgery. For example, the Edwin Smith papyrus *(Fig. 4.7)* dates to 1700 BC and is felt to be the oldest book on surgery; included on its 15 by 1 feet dimensions are descriptions of 48 cases, including those involving the spine and cranium; this document also recognized that injuries resulting in exposed brain

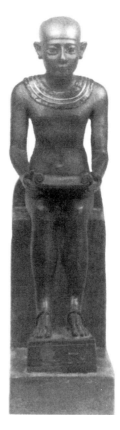

FIG. 4.6 Statute of Imhotep, reputed father of Egyptian medicine. He served as physician to the King Zoser in the Third Dynasty, c. twenty-eighth to late twenty-sixth centuries B.C. In addition to being a medical doctor, Imhotep served as a royal architect, designing the step-pyramid of Sakkara. (From The Egyptian Museum, Cairo.)

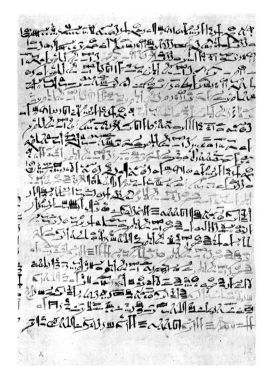

FIG. 4.7 A portion of the Edwin Smith Papyrus, showing the original hieratic script. Named after the pioneer American Egyptologist who purchased the scroll from a dealer in Luxor in 1862, the original text of the treatise dates back to the early part of the Old Kingdom (c. 3000–2500 B.C.). The copy shown here dates to c. 1700 B.C. It is descriptive of clinical methods then in use as well as accurate observations in anatomy, physiology, and pathology. (From Breasted JH (trans.): *The Edwin Smith Surgical Papyrus.* Chicago: University of Chicago Press, 1930.)

often resulted in nuchal rigidity (18, 34). Physical evidence of their practice exits, the earliest dating to the XVIIIth to XIXth Dynasties (1200 BC) found in Sesebi, Sudan. Furthermore, a specimen dating to the XXVth Dynasty (600 BC) was found in Sakkara. Perhaps a contemporary to Imhotep, classical Chinese literature make mention to a legendary physician Yu Fu in the great classic of medicine *Huang Ti Nei Ching Su Wen*; Yu Fu allegedly had the ability to expose the brain (112).

GREEK AND ROMAN TIMES

Despite the earliest murmurings in ancient Egypt and China, medical historians credit the ancient Greeks with the origin of the intellectual evolution of neurological surgery with the founding of the Alexandrian School in 300 BC (46). The ancient Greeks and the Romans/early Byzantines provided the first major movement in the evolution of neurosurgery. Wars provided ample clinical material, and *Hippocrates (460–370 BC) (Fig. 4.8)* provided the earliest writings from this period, demonstrating a surprising understanding of head injury and providing one of the earliest descriptions of subarachnoid hemorrhage. Another contribution of the Hippocratic School was the auger-

A

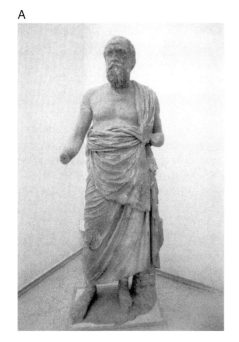

B

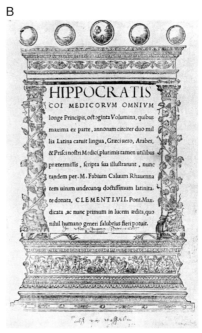

FIG. 4.8 (A) The earliest known statue of Hippocrates (460–370 B.C.). Hippocrates was able to trace directly his ancestry back fifteen generations to Asclepius. (From Cos Museum, Island of Cos, Greece.) (B) Frontispiece of the first edition of the Latin translation of Hippocrates, printed in Rome in 1525. The publication of the Latin translation preceded by one year the publication of the original Greek text, which was printed in Venice in 1526.

shaped instrument resembling the contemporary crown trephine. Hippocrates warned against both using the instrument over a suture to risk injuring the underlying dura as well as incising the brain itself. He advised irrigation during the trephination to avoid warming and organized set principles in his volume *De capitis vulneribus (Head Injury)* that established the foundations for 2000 years of practice (50).

Shortly after Hippocrates, *Herophilus of Chalcedon (335–280 BC)* provided vital anatomic knowledge based on detailed dissections of humans, including that of the nervous system; he is credited with recognizing the brain as the central organ of the nervous system (46). *Rufus of Ephesus (AD 98–117)* expanded upon the knowledge of neuroanatomy gained from Herophilus' dissections. The writings of Rufus provided classic descriptions of the membranes of the brain, distinguished the cerebrum from the cerebellum, described the corpus callosum, and detailed the extent of the ventricular system, the pineal and pituitary glands, the fornix, as well as the quadrigeminal plate. Prominent Greek and Byzantine physicians who followed held true to the theme of improving the management of head-injured patients while concurrently gaining insight to the function of the brain and nervous system. *Aulus Aurelius Cornelius Celsus (25 BC–AD 50) (Fig. 4.9)*, celebrated as the counselor to the emperors Tiberius and Caligula, contributed a book *De re medicina* which became the first medical manuscript to be printed in 1478 after the introduction of the movable type. Along with his famous four cardinal signs of inflammation *rubor, tumor, calore, and dolore*, Celsus contributed observations vital to neurosurgery as well as methods for trephination. *Galen of Pergamon (AD 129–210) (Fig. 4.10)* was the most prolific among the medical writers of antiquity; his preserved works fill over 12,000 pages, the greatest being *De usus partium (the useful parts of the body)*. Galen lived under emperors Antonius Pius and Marcus Aurelius and took maximum advantage of his role as physician to the gladiators of Pergamon. This clinical material along with thoughtful scientific study resulted in voluminous contributions in the areas of neuroanatomy and neurosurgery, including descriptions of the aqueduct of Sylvius, the

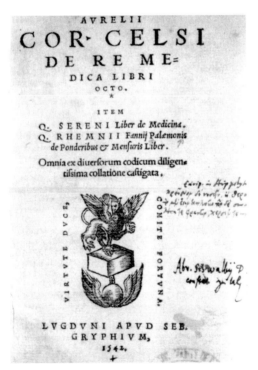

FIG. 4.9 Frontispiece of an early edition of the works of Celsus (Aulus Aurelius Cornelius Celsus), printed in Lyden in 1542. Although his anatomical knowledge was not outstanding, his descriptions of surgery were outstanding, with every step methodically, clearly and exactly presented. His Latin writing was so elegant that he was called "The medical Cicero"; furthermore, his texts provide an excellent source of knowledge on surgical instruments of his day.

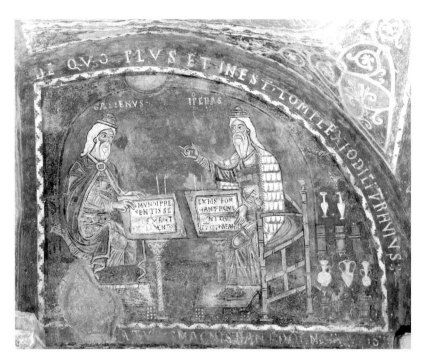

FIG. 4.10 A 13th century fresco of Galen (left) and Hippocrates. Here the two greats are portrayed in a discussion, even though Galen lived almost 500 years after Hippocrates. (From Duomo, Anagni, Italy.)

cranial nerves, hydrocephalus, spinal cord injury, neurotrauma, as well as appreciating the higher functions of the brain. Galen's work formed the basis of knowledge regarding the nervous system until at least the Renaissance, and his influence would extend well into the 18th Century. Following Galen, *Paul of Aegineta (AD 625–690)* was a prolific author and surgeon. His classic text *The Seven Books of Paulus Aegineta* contained an excellent section on head injury and trephination. Paul also classified skull fractures and developed many instruments for cranial surgery, and recognized the importance of birth trauma and hydrocephalus. By using wine in his wound dressings, Paul took advantage of the as yet unknown concept of antisepsis. Paul was the last of the great Byzantine physicians and marked the end of an exceptionally fruitful era of medical and neurosurgical development.

THE ARABIC PERIOD

As Europe descended into turmoil and was overrun by various barbarians, the intellectual centers of medicine shifted to the Arabian and

Byzantine cultures (750–1200) (46). This period was marked by fastidi-
ous and systematic organization and copying of Greek and Roman writings. The physician of this period rarely performed surgery, relegat-
ing the actual tasks to persons of lower rank. Furthermore, the Koran
discouraged dissections, contributing to suppress the development
of the surgical discipline. Prominent Arabic physicians include *Rhazes
(865–930)*, the influential philosopher and physician of Baghdad *Avicenna (979–1037) (Fig. 4.11)*, and *Albucasis* (936–1013) who was credited with designing the non-sinking trephine to reduce the risk of plung-

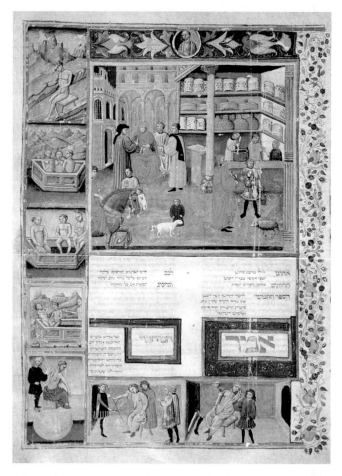

FIG. 4.11 Scene from an open-air pharmacy and other scenes of health care, illustrations from a 15th century Hebrew edition of Avicenna's *Canon of Medicine*. Jewish
physicians were among the best in the Middle Ages, and were instrumental in trans-
mitting Arabic medicine to the rest of Christian Europe. (From Biblioteca Universitaria,
Bologna.)

ing. In contrast to the Greeks and Romans, the Arabic physicians contributed relatively few original ideas. However, their catalogue of existing prior knowledge continued to be influential into the medieval period.

THE MEDIEVAL PERIOD

Despite the barbarian invasions in medieval Europe, a medical school thrived in Salerno (46). *Constantinus Africanus* (1015–1087) learned Arabic medicine in Baghdad and introduced it to the scholars at Salerno and thus to the rest of Europe. He translated Arabic texts on the teachings of Galen and Hippocrates back to Latin, although at times inaccurately. The influence of the Salerno school gave rise to *Roger of Salerno (1170) (Fig. 4.12)* whose work *Practica chirurgiae* (90) was the first writings on surgery in Italy and was tremendously influential in the medieval period. Roger described a novel method of inspecting patients with skull fractures for CSF leak using the Valsava maneuver and encouraged the use of trephination for the treatment of epilepsy. Roger promoted the use of the cruciate incision for depressed fracture management and employed wool and feathers for hemostasis and wormwood soaked in rose water and egg for dressings. He also encouraged the use of soporifics in the preoperative period. In the 13th century, *Theodoric of Cervia (Borgognoni) (1205–1298)* described the conditions for optimal wound healing to include hemostasis, removal of dead space and necrotic tissue, and careful dressing of wounds with material soaked in wine. It was also in this period that surgeons were faced with new wounds resulting from the introduction of gunpowder. *William of Saliceto (1210–1277), Lanfranchi of Milan (d. ca. 1306) (Fig. 4.13),* and *Leonard of Bertapalia (1380–1460)* were other prominent Italian surgeons. In France, the school of Montpellier produced *Henri de Mondeville (1260–1320)* and *Guy de Chauliac (1300–1368) (Fig. 4.14).* Lanfranchi described and refined trephination techniques employing the knife for sharp dissection rather than the cautery for incision. He emphasized anatomical planes and suture repair. Guy de Chauliac stressed the need to shave the head prior to surgery using egg albumin for hemostasis and wine for antisepsis. Furthermore, he offered a refined categorization for head injuries.

Prelude to Modern Times—Early Birthpains

Despite having an increasing body of medical literature and improved surgical instruments, surgeons continued to deal primarily with head trauma and its aftermath, limited by a distinct lack of understanding of neurological function and antisepsis, and the surgeries remained principally epidural. This theme would continue into the Renaissance period. However, a fundamental body of knowledge was being achieved that would lead to the paradigm change that would occur four centuries later.

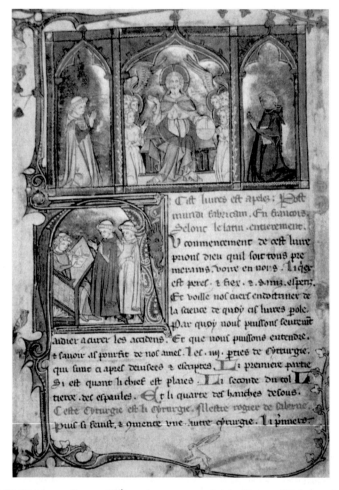

FIG. 4.12 This page from a 13th century manuscript by Roger of Salerno shows surgical scenes regarding head injury. Ruggiero Frugardi (Roger, c. 1210) in general was an original writer; in contrast to the monks of his day, Roger abstained from magic spells and incantations in his medical writings.

Sixteenth century surgeons continued to operate on head wounds on the basis of its physical appearance, without consideration of symptoms, much as Hippocrates described (38). Until the description of the method of interconnecting burr holes to create a bone flap for a craniotomy by *Leonardo Botallo (1530–1588)*, surgeons were limited to working through small apertures created by trephines (17). Furthermore, *Giacomo Berengario da Carpi (1470–1530)* and *Andreas Vesalius (1514–1564)* reintroduced the concept of evidence-based anatomical studies from direct ob-

FIG. 4.13 A woodcut of Lanfranchi of Milan. He was the first to describe cerebral concussion and his writings on skull fractures are considered classics. Among other things, he recommended esophageal intubation, nerve suture, and surgery for empyema. (From Zimmerman LM, Veith I: *Great ideas in the history of surgery.* Baltimore: Williams & Wilkins, 1961, p. 125.)

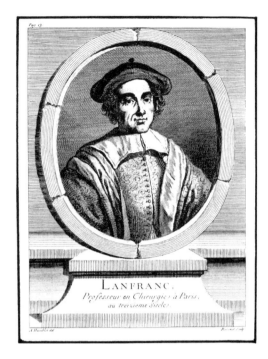

FIG. 4.14 Guy de Chauliac's *Great Surgery* was the foremost surgical text in Europe for nearly 200 years until it was displaced by the work of Ambrose Paré. The first printed edition appeared in 1478, followed by 70 later editions. (From Zimmerman LM, Veith I: *Great ideas in the history of surgery.* Baltimore: Williams & Wilkins, 1961, p. 150.)

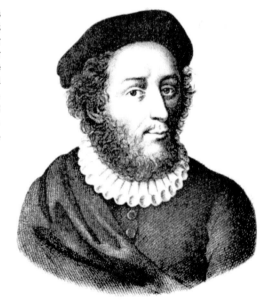

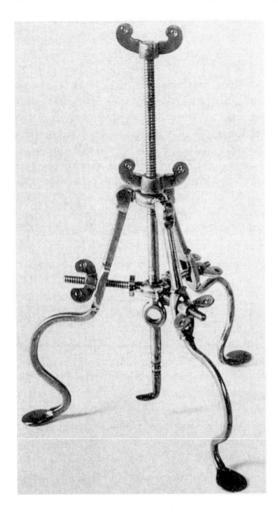

FIG. 4.15 Trephine instrument from the 16th century.

servation (87). Beregarios' *Tractatus de fractura*, published twice in 1518 and then 1535, provided concepts of staged surgeries, gravity drainage of intracranial abscesses, and the first detailed illustrations of surgical instruments (13, 14) *(Fig. 4.15)*. In *Fabrica*, Vesalius gave an account of the corpus callosum superior to that of Galen, suggesting that it connected the two halves of the brain (105). Furthermore, Berengario and Vesalius disputed the existence of the *reté mirabilé* that had been accepted since the time of Galen.

Into the 17th century, refinements of surgical instruments continued, but more importantly to the evolution of neurosurgery, *Rene Descartes (1596–1650) (Fig. 4.16), Thomas Willis (1621–1675) (Fig.*

A

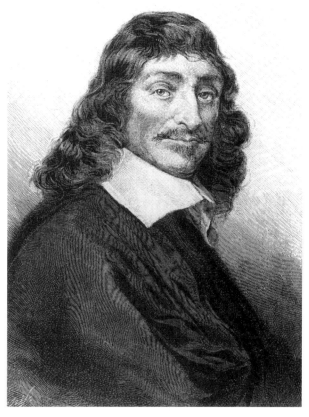

B

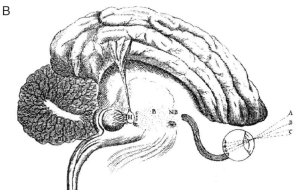

Fig. 4.16 (A) Portrait of René Descartes. (B) Descartes' perception of the soul's control over the body and the soul's location in the pineal region. Descartes, one of the most influential post-Renaissance philosophers, proposed his solution to the mind-body problem in his book *De homine,* published posthumously in 1662.

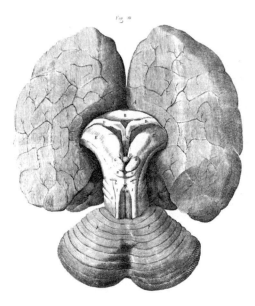

FIG. 4.17 An illustration, by Sir Christopher Wren, of the posterior view of the brain which appeared in Thomas Willis' *The Anatomy of the Brain*. The tectal region appears somewhat elongated, and the pulvinar region is oversimplified. (From Willis T: *Cerebri Anatome*, Londini, Typis Ja. Flesher, impensis Jo. Martyn & Ja. Allestry, 1664.)

4.17), Marcello Malpighi (1628–1694), Humphrey Ridley (1653–1708), Raymond de Vieussens (1641–1716), Steno (Niels Stenson, 1638–1686), and *Johan J. Wepfer (1620–1695)* made numerous important observations in the neurosciences (87). It is important to emphasize that through this period surgeons were hampered by the lack of fundamental knowledge of cerebral physiology and ability to localize processes as well as a complete dearth of the practicalities of anesthesia and comprehension of infection.

THE EMERGENCE OF CEREBRAL CONCERN AND
CONCEPT OF THE FUNCTIONAL BRAIN

The 18th century marked the separation of the surgeon from the barbers in both England and France. However, more importantly, it witnessed the emergence of the consideration for the effect of trauma on the brain itself and not simply on the skull (38). This represents a crucial step to the eventual incorporation of the neurological exam to guide surgical intervention. The French surgeons of the period are credited with the genesis of this important concept. *Jean Louis Petit (1674–1750)*, the first Director of the Royal Academy of Surgery in Paris, was the first to define the *"lucid interval."* He attributed the immediate loss of consciousness after a blow to the head to concussion, and the drowsiness that developed later to compression (85). Petit's contemporary in Paris, *Henri François Le Dran (1685–1770)*, concurred and pointed out that the drowsiness was the result of injury to the brain and not the surrounding skull, and that delayed drowsiness was a sign of compression from an intracranial blood clot (65). *Percivall Pott (1713–1788) (Fig. 4.18)* was an English surgeon who contributed greatly to the early development of neurosurgery as a distinct specialty; his writings on head and spine injuries clearly indicate his acceptance of the novel concepts from France. *Benjamin Bell (1749–1806)* further emphasized the importance of the new neurosurgical principle by recommending against the use of preventative trephination (11).

Acceptance and development of the concept of the brain in trauma as well as general awareness of the cerebrum continued into the first part of the 19th century. *John Abernathy (1764–1831)*, a pupil of Percivall Pott, identified the association between a fixed and dilated pupil with cerebral compression in a patient with an epidural hematoma

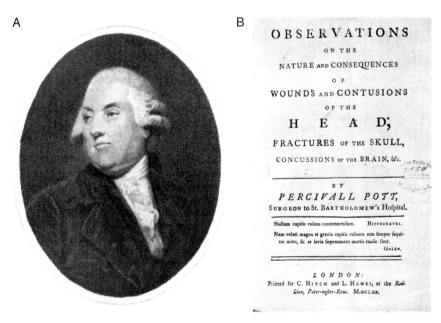

A

B

OBSERVATIONS

ON THE

NATURE AND CONSEQUENCES

O F

WOUNDS AND CONTUSIONS

OF THE

H   E   A   D;

FRACTURES OF THE SKULL,

CONCUSSIONS OF THE BRAIN, &c.

B Y

PERCIVALL POTT,
SURGEON to St. BARTHOLOMEW's Hospital.

Nullum capitis vulnus contemnendum.   HIPPOCRATES.

Nam veluti magna et gravia capitis vulnera non semper sequi-
tur mors, sic et levia sæpenumero mortis causæ sunt.
GALEN.

LONDON:
Printed for C. HITCH and L. HAWES, at the Red-
Lion, Pater-noster-Row. M,DCC.LX.

FIG. 4.18 (A) The English surgeon Percival Pott was the greatest English surgeon during the middle of the 18th century. His collected works contain a vast wealth of significant material. Among the most familiar of his works is his excellent description of the clinical symptoms of tuberculous caries in the vetebra, which has been since known as Pott's disease. (From Zimmerman LM, Veith I: *Great ideas in the history of surgery.* Baltimore: Williams & Wilkins, 1961, p. 325.) (B) The frontispiece of Pott's book *Observations on the Nature and consequences of Wounds and Contusions of the Head.* Pervading themes in Pott's therapy are gentleness, simplicity, unencumbered apparatus, and high ethical standards.

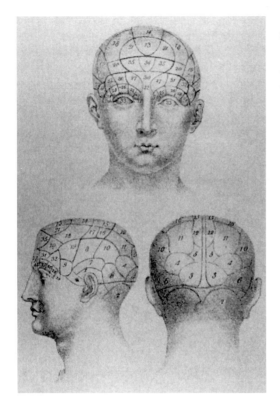

FIG. 4.19 Spurzheim's localization of the faculties on the
scalp and underlying skull. Both
Spurzheim and Gall believed
that for each psychological faculty there existed a corresponding area of the brain and overlying skull. Because the brain
areas are inborn, the individual's characteristics are fixed to
some extent. Potential improvement, however, was possible
through the strengthening of a
deficient faculty by giving it
educated "exercise." (From
Spurzheim JG: *Phrenology, or
the doctrine of the mental phenomena*. Philadelphia: J.P. Lippincott, 1908.)

(1). *Astley Paston Cooper (1768–1841)*, surgeon to King George IV, re-
iterated that dilation of one or both pupils is a sign of cerebral compression (25). In fact, by 1841, *William Sharp (1805–1896)* published
a monograph entitled *Practical Observations on Injuries of the Head*,
where he demonstrated widespread acceptance of the original principles put forth by Le Dran, Petit, and Bell (92). In 1867, *Jonathan
Hutchinson (1828–1913)* defined the third nerve palsy, perhaps one of
the most useful modern signs of head injury and increased intracranial pressure (60). *Franz Josef Gall (1758–1828)* and his colleague *Jo-
hann C. Spurzheim (1776–1832) (Fig. 4.19)* brought widespread attention to the cerebral convolutions and helped firmly establish the
brain as the organ of the mind by the end of the 18th Century (62, 87).
Unfortunately, Gall is perhaps more infamous for the misguided notions of *phrenology* than recognized for his contributions in neuroanatomy and cerebral function.

The conceptual revelation of the functional brain eventually evolved
to definitions of cerebral localization. The 19th Century witnessed the

flourishing of *Paris Medicine*, or the process of correlation of disease state observations with findings at autopsy. Using this concept, *Jean-Baptiste Bouillaud (1796–1881)* localized language function to the frontal lobes in 1825 (47). Bouillaud also understood the dichotomy of aphasia and dysarthria in disorders of speech. Also correlating autopsy findings with pre-mortem observations, *Pierre Paul Broca (1824–1880) (Fig. 4.20)*, a pioneering anthropologist as well as a prominent surgeon, astutely localized the language function to the 3rd left frontal convolution in a series of studies from 1861–1865 (21, 22).

Epilepsy and the physical manifestations of seizure disorders formed a natural model system for the study of brain function. *John Hughlings Jackson (1835–1911) (Fig. 4.21)* studied large numbers of patients with focal motor seizures and other unilateral disorders and described the systematic and consistent *march* of symptomatic involvement of the face and limbs in focal motor seizures. These studies are considered to be of landmark importance in the understanding of cerebral localization (61).

In addition to observations on humans, experimental studies also contributed tremendously to understanding cerebral localization. Frenchman *Marie Jean Pierre Flourens (1794–1867)* conducted ablation and stimulation experiments to elegantly demonstrate the general localization of intelligence, volition, and sensation to the cerebral hemispheres, a concept he termed the *action proper* (40). In Germany, phys-

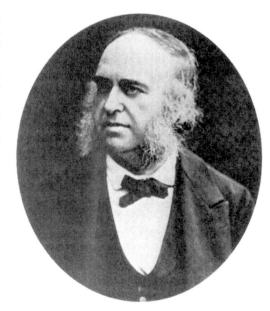

FIG. 4.20   Paul Broca. His famous "Tan" case, and his subsequent pronouncement about the localization of a faculty for articulate speech which differed from that of the phrenologists, made him the leading scientific advocate for the cortical localization of function in the early 1860s. (From Académie de Médecine, Paris.)

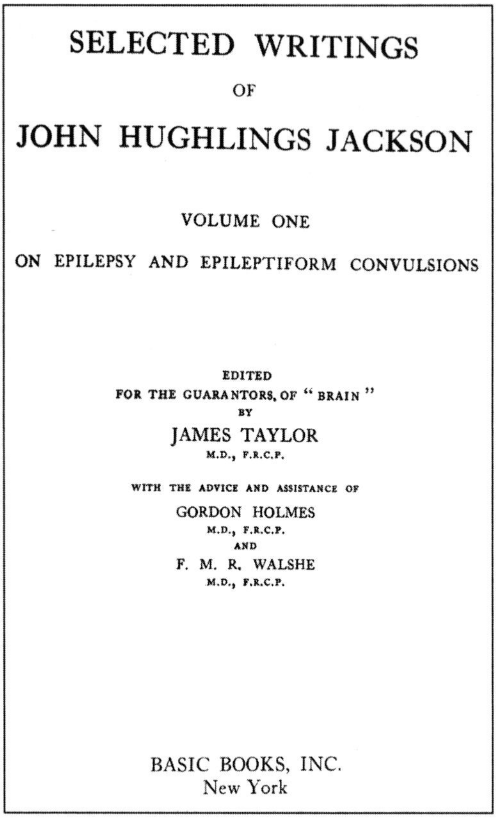

SELECTED WRITINGS

OF

JOHN HUGHLINGS JACKSON

VOLUME ONE

ON EPILEPSY AND EPILEPTIFORM CONVULSIONS

EDITED
FOR THE GUARANTORS, OF " BRAIN "
BY
JAMES TAYLOR
M.D., F.R.C.P.

WITH THE ADVICE AND ASSISTANCE OF
GORDON HOLMES
M.D., F.R.C.P.
AND
F. M. R. WALSHE
M.D., F.R.C.P.

BASIC BOOKS, INC.
New York

FIG. 4.21 Frontispiece of John Hughlings Jackson's *Selected Writings . . . On Epilepsy and Epileptiform Convulsions.* Jackson combined his limitless capacity to elicit very detailed histories and conduct meticulous neurological examinations with a tenacious attention to his patients. He then correlated pathological findings at autopsy with his bedside observations. What separated him from his contemporaries was his ability to distill his observations into a conceptual framework that revolutionized current thinking about the function of the central nervous system.

iologists *Gustav Theodor Fritsch (1838–1891)* and *Eduard Hitzig (1838–1907)* carried out studies in a canine model and provided evidence of cortical control of motor function (41). Building upon the efforts of Jackson and Fritsch and Hitzig, *David Ferrier (1843–1928) (Fig. 4.22)* published detailed studies of cortical localizations starting in 1873, including *The Functions of the Brain* in 1876 (37). He thus established stimulation mapping as an acceptable experimental method.

GENESIS OF MODERN NEUROSCIENCE

During the periods leading up to the 19th Century, neuroscience consisted essentially of gross anatomical studies on adult specimens, with Galenic beliefs providing the dominant influence (62). Several developments in science and neuroscience beginning in the late 18th Century marked a fundamental change in the conceptual view of the causation of disease, providing crucial ingredients to the evolution of neurosurgery. This period was exceptionally fertile for the evolution

A

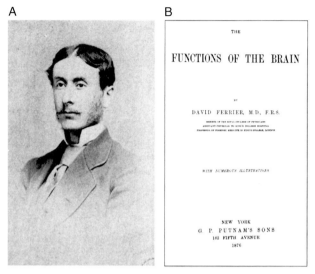

B

THE

FUNCTIONS OF THE BRAIN

BY

DAVID FERRIER, M.D., F.R.S.

NEW YORK
G. P. PUTNAM'S SONS
182 FIFTH AVENUE
1876

C

THE LOCALISATION
OF
CEREBRAL DISEASE

BEING THE

GULSTONIAN LECTURES OF THE ROYAL COLLEGE
OF PHYSICIANS FOR 1878

BY

DAVID FERRIER, M.D., F.R.S.

LONDON
SMITH, ELDER, & CO., 15 WATERLOO PLACE
1878

D

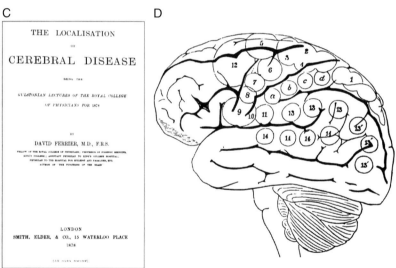

FIG. 4.22 David Ferrier (A), a young Scottish physician, refined the technique of cerebral cortical stimulation by employing faradic (alternating) current and proceeded to perform detailed cortical mapping. The culmination of Ferrier's research publications was the publication in 1876 of *Functions of the Brain* (B). Two years later *The Localisation of Cerebral Disease* (C) was dedicated to Charcot, " . . . in recognition of his pre-eminent services in the localisation of cerebral disease." Figure (D) shows the first human brain map, by Ferrier in 1876. This map, however, was derived from animal brain stimulation studies.

of new ideas, especially with respect to the nervous system, which was seen to serve as an interface between the mind and the body. First, more sophisticated techniques of brain *tissue fixation and sectioning* yielded an even better understanding of the gross three-dimensional anatomy of the brain. *Felix Vicq d'Azyr (1759–1794)* and *Johan Christian Reil (1759–1813)* played crucial roles in this development. Secondly, *comparative anatomy*, originally described by Thomas Willis, was re-popularized. This practice was at least conceptually supported by Darwin's *Theory of Evolution*, which was outlined in 1859. The microscopic architecture of the brain also became visible with the adaptation of the *achromatic microscope* in the 1800s, giving birth to the field of *histology* in the 1840s. In 1839, *Theodor Schwann (1810–1882)* proposed the *cell theory*. German histologist *Robert Remak (1815–1865)* focused his energies on the nervous system. In 1906, the Nobel Prize in Physiology and Medicine was awarded to *Camillo Golgi (1843–1926)* and *Santiago Ramon y Cajal (1852–1934) (Fig. 4.23)*. Finally, interest in the developing nervous system led to the birth of *embryology*, with *Friedrich Tiedemann (1781–1861)* playing a seminal role and adding another perspective to the study of neuroanatomy.

In addition to the improvements in the understanding of the physical architecture of the nervous system, advancements in physiology pro-

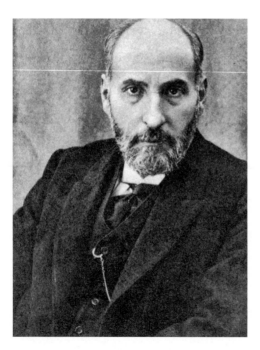

FIG. 4.23 Ramon y Cajal, neuroanatomist and contributor to the neuron doctrine. In contrast to Golgi's beliefs that axons and dendrites underwent anastomosis to form nets, he maintained that neurons remained independent elements and communicated, somehow, across their synapses.

A

B

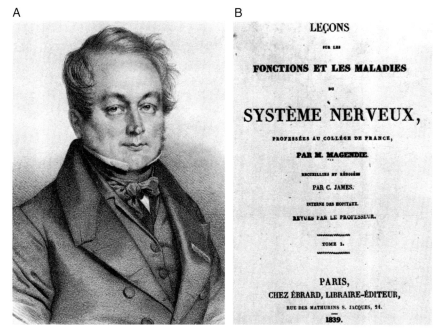

LEÇONS

SUR LES

FONCTIONS ET LES MALADIES

DU

SYSTÈME NERVEUX,

PROFESSÉES AU COLLÈGE DE FRANCE,

PAR M. MAGENDIE.

RECUEILLIES ET RÉDIGÉES

PAR C. JAMES.

INTERNE DES HOPITAUX.

REVUES PAR LE PROFESSEUR.

TOME I.

PARIS,

CHEZ ÉBRARD, LIBRAIRE-ÉDITEUR,

RUE DES MATHURINS S. JACQUES, 24.

1839.

FIG. 4.24 (*A*) François Magendie, one of the most aggressive and versatile of the pioneer experimental physiologists of France. He demonstrated the sensory function of the posterior roots of the spinal cord. Many of his contributions to neurophysiology, including studies of the cerebrospinal fluid, are summarized in his book of 1839 (*B*).

vided insight to function. Despite strenuous public objections, *François Magendie (1783–1855) (Fig. 4.24)* conducted animal vivisection experiments leading to the publication of *Précis Élémentaire de Physiologie* (75). Despite objections on both humanitarian and technical grounds, vivisection was the premier avenue to understanding the function of the nervous system. *Rolando Luigi* introduced the use of electrical currents to conduct stimulation and ablation studies on the brain of animals, making important first steps towards cerebral localization. Subsequent physiologists such as those mentioned previously further refined these techniques. *Charles Scott Sherrington (1857–1952) (Fig. 4.25)* was a central figure in the development of neurophysiology. His work *Integrative Action of the Nervous System* published in 1906 formed the basic paradigm for the rest of the 20th Century (93).

PRACTICAL CONSIDERATIONS–ANESTHESIA

As much as any other singular factor, the development of anesthesia was essential for the evolution of surgery and neurosurgery. An-

A

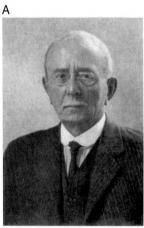

B

THE

INTEGRATIVE ACTION

OF THE

NERVOUS SYSTEM

BY

CHARLES S. SHERRINGTON
D.Sc., M.D., Hon. LL.D. Tor., F.R.S.
Holt Professor of Physiology in the University of Liverpool,
Honorary Member of the American Physiological Society,
&c.

WITH ILLUSTRATIONS

NEW YORK
CHARLES SCRIBNER'S SONS
1906

C

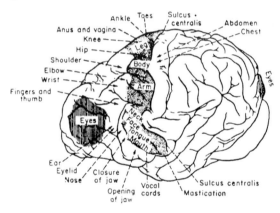

D

Man on his Nature

by

SIR CHARLES SHERRINGTON

THE GIFFORD LECTURES
EDINBURGH
1937-8

CAMBRIDGE
AT THE UNIVERSITY PRESS

E

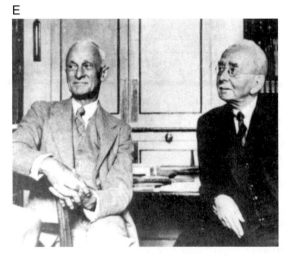

52

cient surgeons likely made use of the anesthetic qualities of alcohol and early narcotics (102). Opium was available in Egypt by 1500 BC. *Hyoscine* was also available in Egypt shortly thereafter and was known to exist in Ancient Greece and Rome. The Sythians used cannabis. In China, *Pien Ch'ia Chow* used anesthesia and the famous surgeon *Hua T'o* (AD 190–265) used *ma-fei-san* dissolved in wine. The first documented neurosurgical application is credited to the Hindus, who in AD 927 used *samohimi* in the trephination of the King of Dahr.

From these developments in antiquity arose *general anesthetic agents*. In 1772, *Joseph Priestly (1733–1804)* discovered *nitrous oxide*, which *Sir Humphry Davy (1778–1829)* suggested might be useful in surgery. In fact, by 1831 all three of the main anesthetic agents of the 19th Century had been discovered: *ether, chloroform*, and nitrous oxide. In 1842, *Crawford W. Long (1815–1878)* of Georgia first applied nitrous oxide to minimize pain in a surgical patient. In 1846, *John Collins Warren (1778–1856)* and fellow dentist *William T. G. Morton (1819–1868)* gave the first public demonstration of painless surgery using sulfuric ether. By 1853, the *hypodermic needle* was invented by *Alexander Wood (1817–1884),* allowing the development of injectable agents to be used. Injectable morphine was used in the American Civil War. Forty years later, *Oliver Wendell Holmes* coined the term *anesthesia*. The early pioneers of neurosurgery were instrumental in applying these new techniques with appropriate modifications to surgery of the brain. In fact, William Macewan was the first to employ an *endotracheal tube* for anesthesia in 1878 (73).

ANTISEPSIS AND THE CONTROL OF INFECTION

Perhaps the singular most important barrier to manipulation inside the dural covering of the brain was the overwhelming infection that resulted. Prior to the 19th Century, the dura was felt to be a prohibitive barrier, to be deliberately violated only as a last resort. In fact,

FIG. 4.25 Charles S. Sherrington (*A*), contributor to the fields of neurophysiology, neurology, and neurosurgery. In one of his early works (*B*), Sherrington discussed the importance of the functional relationship between the terminal axonal boutons and the dendrites of the adjacent neurons (i.e., the synapse, a term coined by Sherrington in 1897). He worked with Gruenbaum on cerebral localization; the map of the chimpanzee brain shown here (*C*), indicates that the motor area is confined strictly in front of the sulcus centralis (Rolandic fissure). This map became the standard for teaching that the Rolandic fissure served as the dividing line, with motor cortex in front of it and sensory cortex behind it. Sherrington's interests ranged far beyond the biological sciences. A lecture series delivered in 1937 and 1938 and later published in 1940 (*D*), ranged on topics of "natural theology," discussing the connection between the mind and brain. (*E*) Sherrington (right) sitting with Harvey Cushing, probably at Harvard. (A, B, D from Horwitz NH: Library: Historical perspective. *Neurosurgery* 41:1442–1445, 1997. C, E from Uematsu S, Lesser R. Gordon B: Localization of sensorimotor cortex: The influence of Sherrington and Cushing on the modern concept. *Neurosurgery* 30:904–912, 1992.)

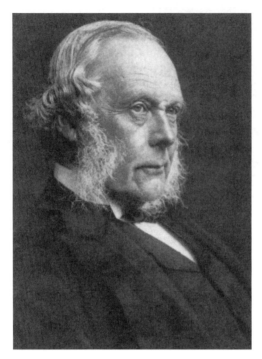

FIG. 4.26   Joseph Lord Lister was indebted to the work of Louis Pasteur. By 1867 Lister had formulated a system of antisepsis based on the use of carbolic acid. For over forty years he worked on creating an antiseptic operative theater, focusing his efforts on the atmosphere (he was convinced that dust particles in the air contained pathogenic germs) and also antiseptic wound dressings. (From Godlee RJ: *Lord Lister*. London: Macmillan and Co., 1917.)

even in cases where the appropriate surgery was performed, patients often succumbed to surgical infections in the form of wound infection, subdural and epidural empyema, and intracerebral abscess (109). The work of *Joseph Lord Lister (1827–1912) (Fig. 4.26)* provided the final key to allow *William Macewan (1848–1924) (Fig. 4.27)*, guided by the new concepts of cerebral localization, to perform successful pioneering craniotomies.

By the time William Macewan entered medical school at the University of Glasgow, Lister was Professor and Head of the Department of Surgery. Lister was keenly aware of the work of Louis Pasteur and the development of the *Germ Theory* and its implications for surgical infections. After trying numerous preparations, Lister used *carbolic acid* in aerosol form in 1865. Carbolic acid saw its initial application soaked into wound dressings in the American Civil War. Lister extended its utility to the antiseptic treatment of surgical instruments, the surgeon's hands, the patient's skin, and finally as a spray over the surgical field (70, 71). Lister's work is recognized as a landmark achievement in the development of surgery.

Motivated by the work of Lister, William Macewan focused tremendous energies to improve and refine the antiseptic technique. Furthermore, guided by the advancement in the field of cerebral local-

A

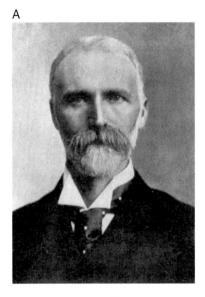

B

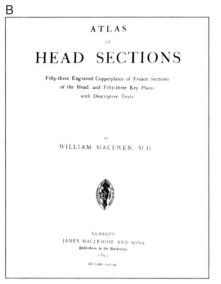

ATLAS
OF
HEAD SECTIONS

Fifty-three Engraved Copperplates of Frozen Sections
of the Head, and Fifty-three Key Plates
with Descriptive Texts

BY

WILLIAM MACEWEN, M.D

GLASGOW
JAMES MACLEHOSE AND SONS
Publishers to the University
1893
All rights reserved

C

PYOGENIC
INFECTIVE DISEASES
OF THE
BRAIN AND SPINAL CORD

MENINGITIS
ABSCESS OF BRAIN
INFECTIVE SINUS THROMBOSIS

BY

WILLIAM MACEWEN, M.D.
GLASGOW

NEW YORK
MACMILLAN AND CO.
1893

FIG. 4.27 (*A*) William Macewen strongly advocated Lister's beliefs on antisepsis. Macewen redesigned instruments so they would not harbor bacteria, and utilized steam sterilization techniques developed by the German surgeon, Ernst von Bergmann. Macewen initiated many firsts in general surgery and neurosurgery in particular, including endotracheal anesthesia, original bone grafting techniques, and the first documented removal of an intracranial neoplasm (a meningioma in 1879). In 1893, he published two monumental works (*B, C*). The Atlas was less well known, but remained the standard atlas for 55 years. *Pyogenic Infective Diseases* . . . records the results of his treatment of 94 patients with intracranial infections. His remarkable surgical success remained unequaled until the era of computed tomography. Even Harvey Cushing admitted that "To Macewen belongs perhaps the distinction of having been the chief pioneer of cranio-cerebral surgery."

ization, in 1879 he performed a successful craniotomy for a subdural hematoma in a boy presenting with a seizure that initiated with left sided symptoms that subsequently generalized to involve the right side. In the same year, he performed another successful surgery to remove an en-plaque meningioma in a young woman. These represent the first modern neurosurgical operations. Building on these initial successes, Macewan continued to surgically treat primarily infectious intradural brain lesions. In 1893 he published the classic entitled *Pyogenic Infective Diseases of the Brain and Spinal Cord: Meningitis, Abscess of Brain, Infective Sinus Thrombosis*, describing his personal surgical series of 94 patients (74).

EARLY PIONEERS

Prior to 1880, neurosurgical cases were aimed primarily at treating traumatic wounds, performed by general surgeons *(Fig. 4.28)*. The critical amalgam formed by the evolution of cerebral localization, functional neuroscience, anesthesia, and antisepsis opened the doors to the refinement of the surgical techniques and instruments aimed at treating intracranial disease processes unrelated to trauma. Several of these pivotal developments and personalities deserve mention.

In 1884, *Rickman Godlee (1849–1925)* was guided by the neurodiagnostic skills of *Alexander Hughes Bennett (1848–1901)* to remove a right hemispheric glioma in a 25-year-old man (12). The patient survived the immediate post-operative period, but succumbed to massive cerebritis one month later. Fourteen months later, *J. O. Hirschfelder (1854–1920)* of San Francisco reported a similar case (52). In the same year, *Francesco Durante (1844–1934)* reported a long-term survival in a patient who underwent resection of an olfactory groove meningioma (33).

In 1886, *Sir Victor Horsley (1857–1916) (Fig. 4.29)* reported the long-term survival of a patient in whom he had removed a brain tumor (53). In that same year, he was appointed First Surgeon at the *National Hospital for Nervous and Mental Diseases, Queen Square*, in London. There his leadership was instrumental to the institution's rise to international prominence. Horsley can also be credited with performing the first craniotomy for epilepsy in 1886. He also made seminal contributions to the early development of stereotactic neurosurgery (54). The original stereotactic frame along with the subsequent contributions by Spiegel, Wycis, and coworkers eventually led to the safe, minimalistic access to deep recesses of the brain (94) *(Fig. 4.30)*. Later, Edwin M. Todd and Trent H. Wells, Jr. would develop a stereotactic system that would be the most widely used in the world *(Figs. 4.31 and 4.32)*.

In Germany, building on a rich legacy of neuroscience developments, *Ernst von Bergmann (1836–1907) (Fig. 4.33)* produced the first mod-

A

B

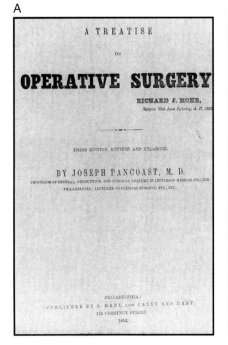
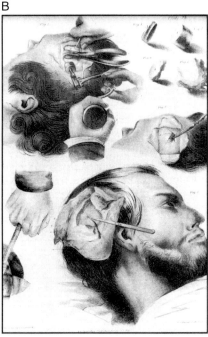

FIG. 4.28 (A) Frontispiece of Joseph Pancoast's *Operative Surgery*; this edition is a rare, hand-colored copy. A professor of surgery and anatomy at Jefferson Medical College, he gained fame as a plastic surgeon, teacher and anatomist. He devised the operative procedure for sectioning of the second and third branches of the fifth pair of nerves as they emerge from the base of the brain. A plate from *Operative Surgery* (B) shows the surgical treatment of depressed cranial fractures. (Courtesy, Special Collections, Norris Library, Keck School of Medicine, University of Southern California, Los Angeles, California.)

ern text on neurosurgery in 1889. A prominent Berlin surgeon especially interested in the nervous system, von Bergmann was celebrated as one of the Kaiser's personal physicians. He was instrumental in the transition from the clumsy antiseptic technique to the more modern *aseptic* technique. In his landmark text, he discussed the factors associated with successful brain surgery. Specifically, he called attention to the high operative mortality rate associated with brain surgery, which at the time was as high as 50% (107).

In 1888, William Keen in Philadelphia made the first recorded access to the ventricular system of a living patient, tapping the lateral ventricle with a hollow needle. Keen was professor of surgery at Jefferson Medical College and is credited with performing the first successful brain tumor removal in America. He also went on to perform some of the first elective craniotomies (72).

A

B

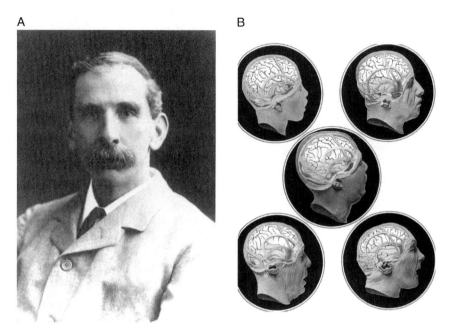

Fig. 4.29 (A) Because of his enthusiasm for brain and spinal cord surgery, his time dedicated to it, and the scope of his work, Victor Horsley is often regarded as the "father of neurological surgery" rather than Macewen or Godlee. Horsley helped endow brain surgery with its modern look, based upon laboratory experiments, cortical localization, and aseptic procedures. In a treatise entitled "Topographical relations of the cranium and surface of the cerebrum," which appeared as a chapter in *Cunningham Memoirs*, Horsley addressed the subject of variations in the relationship of the enveloping skull to the underlying sulci and gyri as a consequence of age, race, sex, and cephalic indices. Taken from heads of various ages and both sexes, Figure (B) shows bars of bone left along the lines of the sutures, and in some cases, also along the fore part or the whole length of the temporal ridge. (From Horwitz N: Library: Historical perspective. **Neurosurgery** 36:428–432, 1995.)

In France, *Antoine M. J. N. Chipault (1866–1920) (Fig. 4.34)* was probably the first surgeon to be completely dedicated to the nervous system. In 1894–1895 he published a 1564 page two-volume text entitled *Chirugie Opératoire du Système Nerveux*, an encyclopedic description of the development and contemporary practice of neurosurgery, including osteoplastic craniotomy, cranioplasty, and surgical aspects of tumor, epilepsy, infection, hydrocephalus, and trigeminal neuralgia (24). He was also responsible for the short-lived *Travaux de Neurologie Chirugicale*, the first journal of neurosurgery that was published from 1896-1901.

In 1898, *Leonardo Gigli* developed a wire saw that would make the actual process of opening the cranium safer (43). These early successes

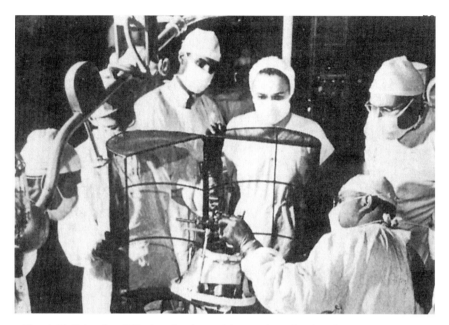

FIG. 4.30 Spiegel and Wycis, who along with coworkers developed a stereotactic frame that eventually led to the safe, minimalistic access to deep recesses of the brain

FIG. 4.31 Trent H. Wells, Jr., pioneer in modern stereotaxy. Along with Edwin M. Todd, he developed a stereotactic system that became the most widely used in the world.

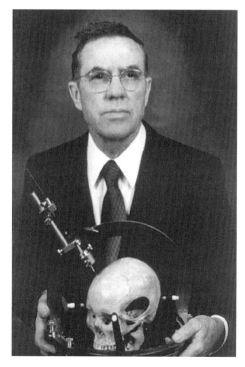

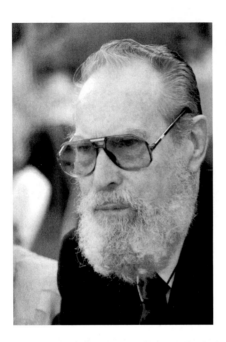

FIG. 4.32 Edwin M. Todd, modern stereotaxy pioneer.

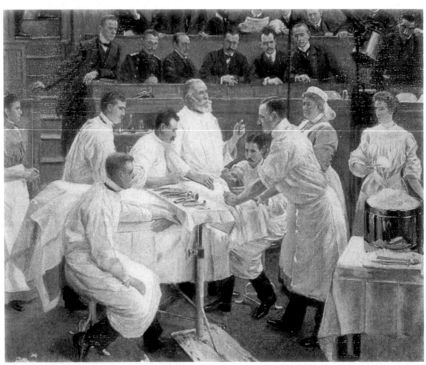

FIG. 4.33 Ernst von Bergman in his operative theater in the University Clinic of Berlin. This painting by Franz Skarbina, painted in 1906, captures the essence of the state-of-the-art operative theater at the turn of the century.

A

B

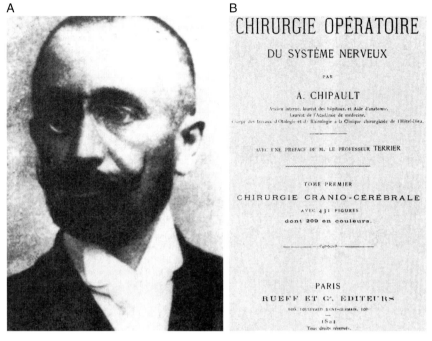

FIG. 4.34 (A) Anthony Chipault and the frontispiece of his *Chirurgie Opératoire du Système Nerveux* (B).

led many would-be neurosurgeons to attempt brain operations. Very few were successful. In fact, during the decade of 1886–1896 following the successful removal of a brain tumor by Victor Horsley, over 500 general surgeons reported attempting brain operations. That number dropped to less than 80 during the following decade, and to a mere handful from 1906 to 1916, demonstrating the challenges ahead and the treacherous nature of surgery on the human cerebrum (109). It is upon this legacy, starting perhaps 12,000 years ago with our Neolithic ancestors, that *Harvey Cushing (1869–1939)* built to initiate the final evolution of modern neurosurgery.

THE AMERICAN INFLUENCE

Until 1900, the developments in Western Europe had a dominant influence in the emerging field of neurosurgery. However, the contributions of the Americans, starting with Harvey Cushing *(Fig. 4.35)*, exerted a definitive force (49). Cushing was born in Cleveland, Ohio in 1869 and educated at Yale College and Harvard Medical School (42). His interest in surgery and neurology was initiated at the Massachusetts General Hospital and the Convalescent Home at Waverly and

A
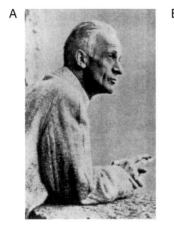

B
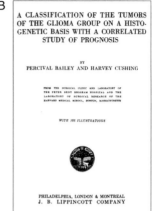

A CLASSIFICATION OF THE TUMORS
OF THE GLIOMA GROUP ON A HISTO-
GENETIC BASIS WITH A CORRELATED
STUDY OF PROGNOSIS

BY

PERCIVAL BAILEY AND HARVEY CUSHING

FROM THE SURGICAL CLINIC AND LABORATORY OF
THE PETER BENT BRIGHAM HOSPITAL AND THE
LABORATORY OF SURGICAL RESEARCH OF THE
HARVARD MEDICAL SCHOOL, BOSTON, MASSACHUSETTS

WITH 108 ILLUSTRATIONS

PHILADELPHIA, LONDON & MONTREAL
J. B. LIPPINCOTT COMPANY

C
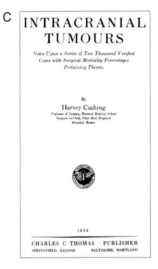

INTRACRANIAL
TUMOURS

*Notes Upon a Series of Two Thousand Verified
Cases with Surgical-Mortality Percentages
Pertaining Thereto*

By

Harvey Cushing
*Professor of Surgery, Harvard Medical School
Surgeon-in-Chief, Peter Bent Brigham
Hospital, Boston*

1932

CHARLES C THOMAS · PUBLISHER
SPRINGFIELD, ILLINOIS   BALTIMORE, MARYLAND

B
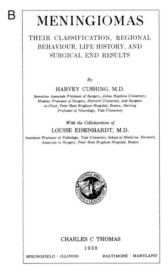

MENINGIOMAS

THEIR CLASSIFICATION, REGIONAL
BEHAVIOUR, LIFE HISTORY, AND
SURGICAL END RESULTS

By

HARVEY CUSHING, M.D.
*Sometime Associate Professor of Surgery, Johns Hopkins University;
Moseley Professor of Surgery, Harvard University, and Surgeon-
in-Chief, Peter Bent Brigham Hospital, Boston; Sterling
Professor of Neurology, Yale University*

With the Collaboration of
LOUISE EISENHARDT, M.D.
*Assistant Professor of Pathology, Yale University School of Medicine. Formerly
Associate in Surgery, Peter Bent Brigham Hospital, Boston*

CHARLES C THOMAS
1938
SPRINGFIELD · ILLINOIS   BALTIMORE · MARYLAND

FIG. 4.35 Harvey Cushing (*A*). Many of his texts became instant classics in the field of neurosurgery, including his work on the classification of gliomas in 1926 (*B*), intracranial tumors in 1932 (*C*), and meningiomas (*D*) in 1938. (A courtesy of Alan Mason Chesney Archive. C, D from Charles C Thomas, Publishers.)

blossomed under the direction of *William Halsted* at Johns Hopkins where completed his residency. He combined the Halstedian principles with his drive and talents to advance the safe surgical treatments of neurological diseases and made singularly important contributions toward the establishment of neurological surgery as a distinct specialty. Toward the end of his residency in 1900, he began to take a special interest in trigeminal neuralgia. Despite engaging initially in a general practice, he began to focus more of his energies on the nervous system after returning from Europe in 1901, performing his first brain tumor operation in the following year. In 1904, he made a presentation in Cleveland titled *"The Special Field of Neurological Surgery"* (26). He had a vision of a field practiced by surgeons specially trained in clinical neurology, neuropathology, and experimental neurophysiology, along with the technical skills of operating on the brain and central nervous system. He was instrumental in the development of methods of hemostasis in all the structures of the head and brain, improved the understanding and control of intracranial pressure, and provided crucial insight to the pathology and natural history of surgically relevant lesions of the nervous system. In 1906, at the request of William W. Keen, Cushing produced a chapter on *"Surgery of the Head"* for the encyclopedic text *Surgery. Its Principles and Practice* (27). This represented the first comprehensive treatise on the subject by an American author. By 1910, he had performed 250 operations on brain tumor patients, with an operative mortality of 13%. In contrast, contemporary surgeons were reporting operative mortalities of around 50%.

This period also witnessed other developments important to American neurosurgery. *Ernest Sachs* was invited to join the faculty of Washington University in St. Louis after completing his training with Victor Horsley at Queen Square in 1910. *Charles A. Elsberg* was appointed surgeon to the New York Neurological Institute in 1909. *Charles H. Frazier*, after spending time with von Bergmann in Berlin, was active in neurosurgery at the University of Pennsylvania. Furthermore, following the publication of the report on *Medical Education in the United States and Canada* by *Abraham Flexner* in 1910 (39), tremendous reforms were initiated in almost every American medical school with Johns Hopkins as the model. Academic neurosurgery programs were evolving.

In 1912, Cushing left Baltimore and assumed the position as Chief of Surgery at the Peter Bent Brigham Hospital in Boston. There, he continued to develop techniques directed toward the surgical treatment of the entire spectrum of neurosurgical diseases, including extrinsic and intrinsic intracranial tumors, trigeminal neuralgia and pituitary tumors. In WWI, Cushing made considerable contributions to the treatment of head trauma. These activities galvanized his position as the leading surgeon in America and lent prominence to the field of neurological surgery. A further legacy of Cushing's impact, many of his residents initiated academic programs of their own. Among these, *John F. Fulton (Fig. 4.36),* was appointed Sterling Professor and Chairman of Physiology at Yale in 1930 (32). Fulton's collaborations with Cushing continued from Boston to New Haven where Cushing spent his final days. Fulton's department was a veritable Mecca for neurophysiology. He published the classic *Physiology of the Nervous System* and helped

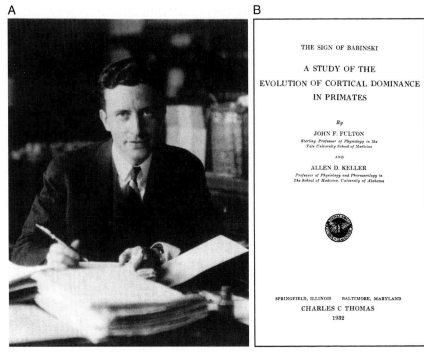

FIG. 4.36 John F. Fulton (A) working on a manuscript at his table in the surgical laboratory of the Peter Bent Brigham Hospital prior to his arrival in New Haven as Sterling Professor and Chairman of the Department of Physiology at Yale University in 1930. The photograph was taken by Harvey Cushing in 1928. (From Horwitz N: Library: Historical Perspective. **Neurosurgery** 43:178–184, 1998.) (B) Frontispiece of Fulton's book published in 1932, dedicated to Harvey Cushing.

found the *Journal of Neurophysiology* in 1938. He was also instrumental in the founding of the *Journal of Neurosurgery* in 1944.

Another giant in the history of neurosurgery in America is *Walter E. Dandy (1886–1946) (Fig. 4.37)*. With Dandy and Cushing, the fun-

FIG. 4.37 Walter E. Dandy (A) (From Fox WL: *Dandy of Johns Hopkins*. Baltimore: Williams & Wilkins, 1984.) (B, C) displays the frontispiece of two of Dandy's seminal works. (D) A lateral view of a normal ventriculogram. (E) Dandy drew countless pathology and intra-operative illustrations, and he was not afraid to employ other talented medical illustrators. This image, by famous artist Max Brödel, shows a tumor of the brain stem causing communicating hydrocephalus owing to the fact that the cisternae are obliterated, thus preventing fluid from reaching the cerebral subarachnoid spaces. (F) Another illustration by Max Brödel, showing the method of attack upon tumors of the pineal and third ventricle. (B from Charles C Thomas, Publishers. E and F from Dandy WE: *The brain*. New York: Hoeber Medical Division, Harper & Row, Publishers, 1969.)

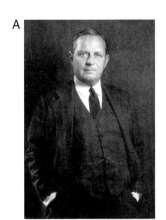

A

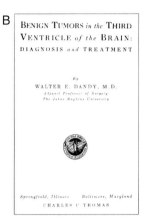

B

BENIGN TUMORS in the THIRD
VENTRICLE of the BRAIN:
DIAGNOSIS and TREATMENT

By

WALTER E. DANDY, M.D.
Adjunct Professor of Surgery
The Johns Hopkins University

Springfield, Illinois   Baltimore, Maryland
CHARLES C THOMAS

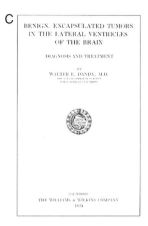

C

BENIGN, ENCAPSULATED TUMORS
IN THE LATERAL VENTRICLES
OF THE BRAIN

DIAGNOSIS AND TREATMENT

BY

WALTER E. DANDY, M.D.

BALTIMORE
THE WILLIAMS & WILKINS COMPANY
1934

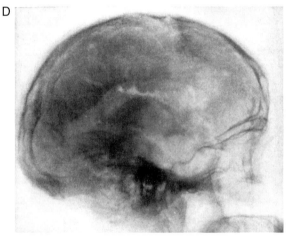

D

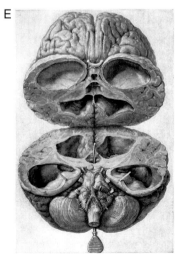

E

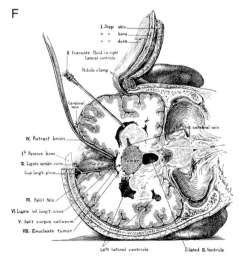

F

damental framework for modern neurosurgery had arrived. Dandy attended medical school at Johns Hopkins and while there he spent a year as a research assistant with Cushing. After Cushing's departure to Boston, Dandy remained at Hopkins were he contributed seminally to the developing field. For example, he developed the technique of *pneumoventrilography* to study ventricular anatomy as it related to hydrocephalus (31). He also developed *pneumoencephalography* to visualize the entire subarachnoid space (30). His studies on cerebral spinal fluid physiology are classic, defining the choroid plexus as the source of CSF production. Dandy also performed the first clip ligation of a cerebral aneurysm while preserving the parent vessel in 1937 (28). His contributions are myriad and elegantly describe in his book *The Brain* (29). His contributions to transcerebral surgeries, particularly intraventricular tumors and rudimentary endoscopic techniques, are particularly noteworthy.

GLOBAL EVOLUTION AND INTERNATIONALISM

With Harvey Cushing and Walter Dandy, the field of neurological surgery gained prominence, especially in America. Outside the United States, however, visionary pioneers were providing leadership for the global evolution of the discipline, adding to the growing critical mass of knowledge and tools that sought to define the field in modern terms. Clearly, to specify each important figure is beyond the scope of this brief synopsis.

In Portugal, *Antonio de Egas Moniz (1874–1955) (Fig. 4.38)* performed rational and methodical studies to define the safe application of *angiography* (79). This technique continues to be indispensable to current neurosurgical diagnostic and interventional practice. Moniz performed the first cerebral angiogram on a living patient in 1926. In addition, Moniz was an instrumental personality in the development of *psychosurgery*, a term that he himself coined (103). He established the *Moniz-Lima prefrontal leukotomy* for which he shared the Nobel Prize in Medicine and Physiology with *Walter Hess (1881–1973)*.

In Berlin, *Fedor Krause (1857–1937) (Fig. 4.39)* built upon the legacy of surgery for epilepsy started by Victor Horsley and Hughlings Jackson, performing operative procedures on 96 seizure patients between 1893 and 1912 (35). Krause recognized two types of epilepsy: general genuine epilepsy (known today as generalized tonic-clonic seizures) and focal Jacksonian motor seizures. He also recognized the deleterious effects of untreated epilepsy on the brain and advocated early surgical treatment for these patients.

In Canada, the *Montreal Neurological Institute (MNI)* founded by *Wilder Penfield (1897–1959) (Fig. 4.40)* in 1934 became an interna-

A

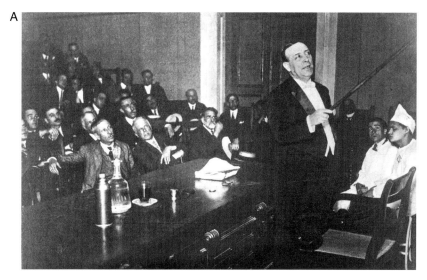

B

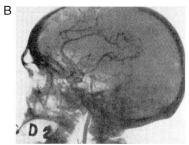

C

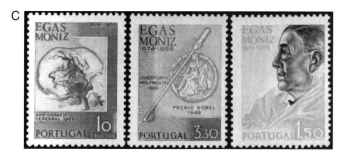

FIG. 4.38 (*A*) Egas Moniz demonstrating the first cerebral arteriograph (June 28, 1927) to the Faculty of Medicine, University of Lisbon. (*B*), Arterial network derived from the internal carotid artery, with injection of 30% NaI. (From Wilkins RH: Neurosurgical Classic: XVI Translation of L'encephalographie arterielle, son importance dans la localisation des tumeurs cerebrales. **Revue Neurologique**. 2:72–89, 1927). (*C*) Portuguese postage stamps issued in honor of Moniz (A and C, courtesy of Elliot Valenstein, Ph.D., Department of Psychology, The University of Michigan, Ann Arbor, Michigan.)

A

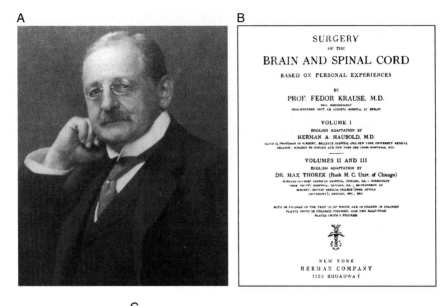

B

SURGERY
OF THE
BRAIN AND SPINAL CORD
BASED ON PERSONAL EXPERIENCES

BY

PROF. FEDOR KRAUSE, M.D.
GEH. MEDIZINALRAT
DIRIGIERENDER ARZT AM AUGUSTA HOSPITAL ZU BERLIN

VOLUME I
ENGLISH ADAPTATION BY
HERMAN A. HAUBOLD, M.D.
CLINICAL PROFESSOR IN SURGERY, BELLEVUE HOSPITAL AND NEW YORK UNIVERSITY MEDICAL
COLLEGE; SURGEON TO HARLEM AND NEW YORK CROSS HOSPITALS, ETC.

VOLUMES II AND III
ENGLISH ADAPTATION BY
DR. MAX THOREK (Rush M. C. Univ. of Chicago)
MEDICO-IN-CHIEF AMERICAN HOSPITAL, CHICAGO, ILL.; CONSULTANT
COOK COUNTY HOSPITAL, CHICAGO, ILL.; EX-PROFESSOR OF
SURGERY, BENNET MEDICAL COLLEGE (PRES. LOYOLA
UNIVERSITY), CHICAGO, ETC., ETC.

WITH 109 FIGURES IN THE TEXT (17 OF WHICH ARE IN COLORED, 44 COLORED
PLATES (WITH 128 COLORED FIGURES), AND TWO HALF-TONE
PLATES (WITH 5 FIGURES)

NEW YORK
REBMAN COMPANY
1123 BROADWAY

C

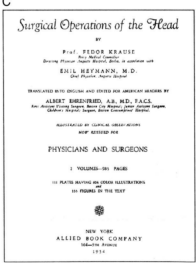

Surgical Operations of the Head

BY

Prof. FEDOR KRAUSE
Privy Medical Councillor
Directing Physician Augusta Hospital, Berlin, in association with

EMIL HEYMANN, M.D.
Chief Physician, Augusta Hospital

TRANSLATED INTO ENGLISH AND EDITED FOR AMERICAN READERS BY

ALBERT EHRENFRIED, A.B., M.D., F.A.C.S.
First Assistant Visiting Surgeon, Boston City Hospital; Junior Assistant Surgeon,
Children's Hospital; Surgeon, Boston Consumptives' Hospital.

ILLUSTRATED BY CLINICAL OBSERVATIONS
NOW REISSUED FOR

PHYSICIANS AND SURGEONS

2 VOLUMES—985 PAGES

111 PLATES HAVING 606 COLOR ILLUSTRATIONS
and
155 FIGURES IN THE TEXT

NEW YORK
ALLIED BOOK COMPANY
104—5TH AVENUE
1934

FIG. 4.39 Fedor Krause (A), his magnum opus, *Surgery of the Brain and Spinal Cord* (B) published in 1912, and a later work (C) *Surgical Operations of the Head*.

tionally celebrated center for epilepsy surgery. Penfield's mentors included Harvey Cushing and the neurophysiologist Charles Scott Sherrington. Along with *Edwin Boldrey (1906–1988)*, Penfield analyzed the results from 163 craniotomies in which electrical stimulation of the exposed cerebral cortex was carried out, generating cortical maps that

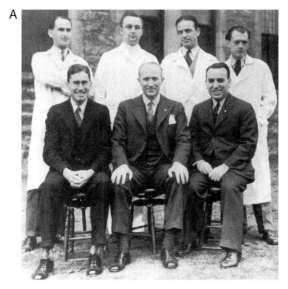

B

Epilepsy and the
Functional Anatomy
of the Human Brain

by

WILDER PENFIELD, O.M., C.M.G.
M.D. (Johns Hopkins)
B.Litt., and D.Sc. (Princeton), B.Sc., Hon. D.Sc., Hon. D.C.L. (Oxon)
F.R.C.S. (Canada), Hon. F.R.C.S. (England), F.R.S. (London)

and

HERBERT JASPER
M.D., C.M. (McGill), B.A. (Reed), M.A. (Oregon)
Ph.D. (Iowa), D. ès Sci. (Paris)

Chapter XIV by Francis McNaughton
B.A. and M.D., C.M. (McGill)

8 color plates and
314 black and white illustrations

Little, Brown and Company . Boston

C

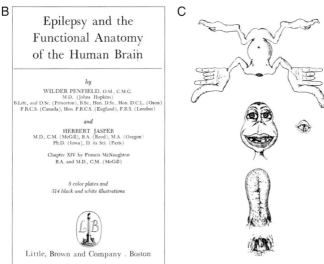

FIG. 4.40 (*A*) Wilder Penfield with members of neurosurgical unit, Royal Victoria Hospital, 1932. Front row, left to right: Arthur Elvidge, Wilder Penfield, William Cone. Back row, left to right: Arne Torkildsen (Norway), Lyle Gaage (U.S.A.), Joseph Evans (U.S.A.), Jerzy Chorobski (Poland). (From the Wilder Penfield Archive, Osler Library, McGill University and the Neuro Archives, Montreal Neurological Institute.) (*B*) Frontispiece to Penfield's classic work. (*C*) Sensory and motor homunculus. This was prepared as a visualization of the order and comparative size of the parts of the body as they appear from above down upon the Rolandic cortex. The larynx represents vocalization, the pharynx swallowing. The comparatively large size of thumb, lips and tongue indicate that these members occupy comparatively long vertical segments of the Rolandic cortex as shown by measurements in individual cases. Sensation of genitalia and rectum lie above and posterior to the lower extremity but are not figured. (After Penfield and Boldry, 1937.) (From Horwitz N: Library: Historical Perspective. **Neurosurgery** 41:314–318, 1997.)

A

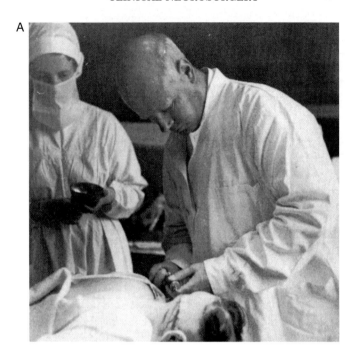

B

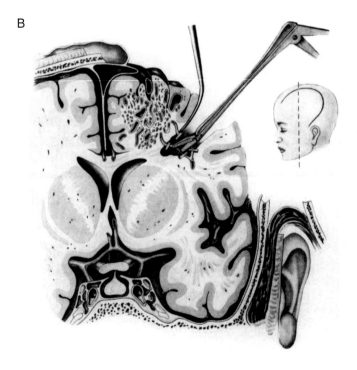

FIG. 4.41 Herbert Olivecrona (From Greenblatt SH (ed.). *A history of neurosurgery in its scientific and professional contexts*. Park Ridge, IL: AANS, 1997. p 527.) (*B*) Illustration showing the removal of an arteriovenous malformation from a 15-year-old boy. The dissection is gradually carried deeper, and the blood vessels are occluded by silver clips as they enter the lesion. (From Olivecrona H, Ladenheim J: *Congenital arteriovenous aneurysms of the carotid and vertebral arterial systems*. Berlin: Springer-Verlag, 1957.)

yielded the familiar sensory and motor *homunculus* (82). It was also at the MNI that *Herbert Jasper* introduced the *electroencephalogram* in 1937. Their book *Epilepsy and the Functional Anatomy of the Human Brain* remains a classic contribution to the topic (83).

In Scandanavia, *Herbert Olivecrona (1891–1980) (Fig. 4.41),* after spending time with Cushing and Dandy in the United States, returned to Stockholm to develop an influential program at the Royal Serafimer Hospital and then at the *Karolinska Institute*. It was at the Karolinska Institute that *Lars Leksell (1907–1986) (Fig. 4.42)* contributed to

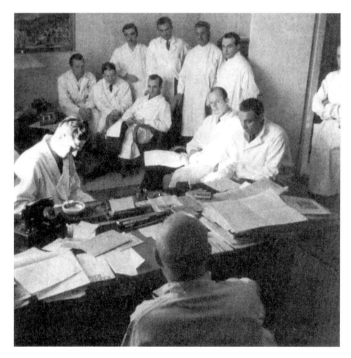

FIG. 4.42 Photograph of Herbert Olivecrona's "Academy." Gösta Norlén (left) and Lars Leksell (right) are in the foreground by the tutor's desk. (From Lindquist C, Kihlström L: Department of Neurosurgery, Karolinska Institute, 60 Years. **Neurosurgery** 39:1016–1021, 1996.)

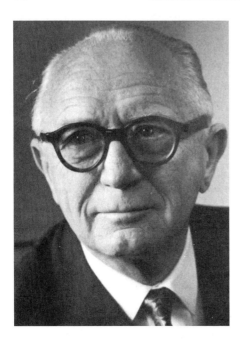

FIG. 4.43 Hugo Krayenbühl (From *The Society of Neurological Surgeons, 75th* Annniversary Volume. p 446.)

define the application of focused beam radiosurgery applied to neuro-surgical processes.

In Switzerland, *Hugo Krayenbühl (1902–1985) (Fig. 4.43)* was the catalyst for a program in Zurich that fostered the development of *M. Gazi Yaşargil*, whose contributions to microneurosurgery are very familiar.

By the mid-20th Century, the specialty of neurological surgery and the concept and practice of surgery of the human cerebrum were firmly established but clearly in a state where a paradigm shift was neces-sary to create dimensions of safety and precision that would expand its effectiveness and capabilities. Technical factors and support would present themselves to allow reinvention of the newly invented surgi-cal specialty.

1965–2001 THE PERIOD OF CYCLICAL REINVENTION

As we enter the new millennium, modernity exerts forces, one of which is a desire to be "modern," particularly as a professional (3). We are pressed to evolve and required to define modernity in terms per-sonal and otherwise. However, all of medicine does not exist in a vac-uum but is developed and practiced on large national and global stages that are fueled and directed by forces that drive medical progress.

These can be seen to include national economic vitalities, popular attitudes and demands, emerging intellectual, effectual and economic buoyancies, parallel progress in transferable, technical and biological areas and crisis situations real and perceived (5).

Neurosurgery is part of the larger global microcosm of medicine. It can be defined as an intellectual and physical exercise in the functionally complex three-dimensional space. The major objectives within the evolution of the field include the expansion of its capability, the minimizing of morbidity and the decreasing of cost involved in the treatment of the individual case or disorders.

With very little doubt, neurosurgery more than any of the other surgical specialties is dependent upon technology for its evolution and the level of its presence. Recently the *Los Angeles Times* polled notable scientists and sociologists worldwide to develop a concept and ranking of the major inventions and discoveries that have changed the way that we have lived in modern times *(Table 4.1)* (86). The disclosures of this poll are as follows: (1) *electricity*, 1873; (2) *the microprocessor*, 1971; (3) *the computer*, 1946; (4) *DNA*, 1953; (5) *the telephone*, 1876; (6) *the automobile*, 1886; (7) *the internet*, 1991; (8) *television*, 1926; (9) *refrigeration*, 1913; (10) *the airplane*, in 1903. All of these have had influence on the evolution and practice of neurosurgery as it exists at this time, but perhaps none has more of an influence on the future than the *microprocessor (Table 4.2)*. This device has been responsible for a number of paradigm shifts in a variety of fields. Its importance relates to the capabilities that it offers and the applications that may

TABLE 4.1
Top Discoveries: The Top Ten
Inventions and Discoveries That
Have Changed the Way We Live

Rank	Year
1. Electricity	1873
2. Microprocessor	1971
3. Computer	1946
4. DNA	1953
5. Telephone	1876
6. Automobile	1886
7. Internet	1991*
8. Television	1926
9. Refrigeration	1913
10. Airplane	1903

*Became available publicly.

Source: Los Angeles Times, Tuesday, June 10, 1997.

TABLE 4.2
The Future Is Now: Ten of the New Technologies Made Possible by the Microprocessor

• Lasers	• Amplifying light through emission of radiation
• Virtual reality	• Simulating human experiences
• Genomics	• Studying genes and their place in DNA structure
• Integration technology	• Linking cable, satellites, radio, TV
• Biotechnology	• Applying knowledge of natural biology
• Smart products	• Using microwaves to control machines and sensors
• Nano-technology	• Manipulating matter at an atomic level
• Bionics	• Merging biological, mechanical systems
• Global positioning	• Using satellites to pinpoint positions
• Micro-machines	• Manufacturing tiny gears, motors, etc.

influence the field of neurosurgery. These areas include (1) *lasers* (the application of light through emission irradiation); (2) *virtual reality* (simulation of human experiences); (3) *genomics* (the study of genes and their place in DNA structure); (4) *integration technology* (linking of cable, satellites, radio and television, as well as the seamless melding of computing and communication); (5) *biotechnology* (technically applying knowledge of natural biology); (6) *smart products* (important developments whereby artificial intelligence is incorporated into products to enable them to perform such cognitive functions as learning [i.e., improving performance with practice] and reasoning [i.e., using sensory information to deduce appropriate responses]); (7) *nanotechnology* (manipulating matter at an atomic level); (8) *bionics* (merging biological and mechanical systems); (9) *global positioning* (using satellites to pinpoint positions); and (10) *micromachines* (the manufacturing of tiny gears, motors, etc.).

A Generation of Progress

It can be argued that the advent of modern neurosurgery occurred approximately a generation ago with the introduction of the operating microscope. In defining "modernity" as it currently exists, it is of value to examine the development of trends of technical neurosurgery during the period of 1965 through 1990. This was a critical quarter century during which there was remarkable escalation in our diagnostic and therapeutic capabilities. These topics were examined in depth during the course of a symposium held at the annual meeting of the American Association of Neurological Surgeons in 1991 and subsequently published in the monograph *Neurosurgery for the Third Millennium* (4). During the course of the symposium and as documented in the monograph, during the period there was a refinement of the preoperative definition of the structural substrate, a minimization of operative corridors, a reduction of operative trauma, increased effectiveness at the target site and incorporation of improved technical adjuvants as physical tools. During this period major points of technical impact included *magnification, computers*, and through the introduction of computers sophisticated structurally related *medical imaging*. The concatenation of all of these effects was the production of an evolution in neurosurgery, which offered a precision of orientation and manipulation that presented and achieved progressive *minimalism*.

The Last Decade

During the decade of the 1990s there was unusual escalation in capabilities for neuroscience. These were highlighted and represented in remarkable achievements in the scientific sectors manifested by the landing of the Pathfinder on Mars with its subsequent exploration of the Martian surface (78) and the remarkable biological event of sheep cloning experiments (84). During this period of evolution in neurosurgery there was a progression of influence and focus related to the use in the more sophisticated sense of the microscope through a more precise definition of the anatomical substrate, the introduction of more refined elements of imaging modes including magnetic resonance, PET, etc., acceptance of the computer as a neurosurgical tool, and more sophisticated monitoring modes both for intraoperative assessment of neurological function as well as the general soma.

The introduction of the *penetrating imaging modalities*, which allowed surgeons to see beyond the visible and to define both structural and functional elements of the operative substrate, was essential for progress. This was carried forward to the use of magnetic resonance imaging devices within the operating theatre with methodology defined initially by Black (15) and other later investigators. This remarkable and sophisticated use of refined imaging modes presented problems in relation to cost and the adaptability of the surgeon within the environment of the unit. Further developments in technology in relation to both size and capabilities of the magnetic resonance concept are currently underway which will allow smaller, more adaptable units *(Fig. 4.44)* to be used for "real time" intraoperative imaging with the definition of both the structural and functional substrate (80).

The incorporation of the computer as a neurosurgical tool during the course of this evolution has been striking. During this past decade, full advantage was taken for the capabilities for imaging and the amalgam with various mechanical and non-mechanical linkages for both point and volume *stereotaxy* for intracranial navigation and localization. Advanced concepts of stereotaxy are now beginning to emerge with the use of *voice control*, real time holography, *robotics* for both

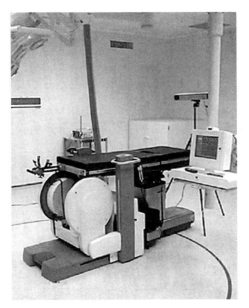

FIG. 4.44 Intraoperative magnetic resonance imaging-guided system useful in a conventional neurosurgical operating room, the PoleStar N-10 (Odin Technologies, Yokneam, Israel). The compact magnet fits under the operating room table, and standard instruments can be used. This scanning and navigational system eliminates the drawback of brain shift, which limits conventional neuronavigational systems. (Reprinted from, Moshe H, Spiegelmann R, Feldman Z, Berkenstadt H, Ram Z: Novel, compact, intraoperative magnetic resonance image-guided system for conventional neurosurgical operating rooms. **Neurosurgery** 48:799–809, 2001.)

positioning and micromanipulation (16, 22, 66, 97–101), and the concept of *telerobotics* for the performance of remote surgeries with the surgeon operating with the adjuvant surgeon working in a *virtual reality* environment and the secondary robotic transfer taking place within the actual patient care area *(Figs. 4.45, 4.46, and 4.47)*. Naturally this also includes the use of the virtual reality concept that is becoming more valuable from a standpoint of simulation of operative events, training and, as noted, the actual surgical event (63).

Neurostimulation particularly for deep brain targets has become popular and is currently undergoing intensive study because of its considerably attractive elements, which include reversibility, variable targeting, and variable modulation. Its adverse elements appear to be its inherent complexity and the cost in time in relation to reimbursement, particularly for the neurologist. However, its application for movement disorders for essential tremor, intention tremor, dystonia, Parkinson's disease, Huntington's disease, and Gilles de la Tourette's disease is generally embraced, while studies for the methods application in epilepsy, obsessive-compulsive disorder, eating difficulties, brain injury and facilitation of restoration are underway.

During the decade of the 1990s there has been no doubt that the application of the amalgam between imaging and the use of high energy forms through both *rotational* and *fixed beam radiosurgical systems* has become an integral part of the standard armamentarium of neurologi-

A

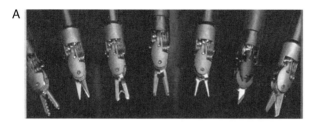

B

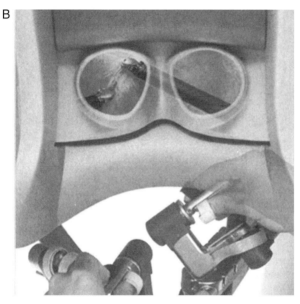

FIG. 4.45 Robotic system for open-heart surgery. Hand motion at a remote computer console is robotically transferred to effect surgical maneuvers. Shown are the robotically manipulated surgical instruments (A). Also shown is the view from the surgeon's perspective, revealing two instruments inserted through the thoracic wall guided by a camera system similarly applied (B). Although the practical application is still limited by a steep learning curve, this represents an important first commercial system aimed at robotic assisted minimalization. (Reprinted from Borst C: Operating on a beating heart. **Sci Am** 283:58–263, 2000.)

cal surgery. Robotic devices have been incorporated into the more "traditional" fixed beam systems, arguably reducing surgeon fatigue and increasing the overall accuracy and safety of such systems (*Fig. 4.47*). Functional neurosurgery is being explored with this noninvasive radiosurgical method; protocols for movement disorders, pain, epilepsy, and psychiatric disorders are widely underway. In fact, because of the failure of drug protocols and growing patient awareness, it appears that a surgical role in psychiatric disorders may reemerge in importance (36).

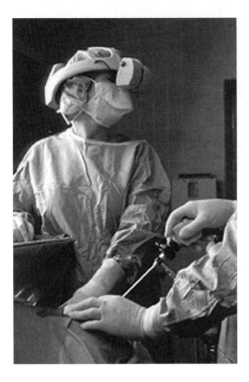

FIG. 4.46 Virtual reality apparatus. Heads-up display and headset,
connnected to operative instruments,
provides the surgeon with precision
control without ever physically touch-
ing the patient.

The future in this area would appear to be a *frameless imaging-guided robotic rotational radiosurgical system* that has been developed by John Adler and the group at the Stanford University Medical Center *(Fig. 4.48)* (2). One of the principal benefits of this machine is the prospect for being able to treat not only intracranial lesions but also virtually all body regions through its methodology. Being fundamentally based on standard principles of linear accelerator techniques, no requirement for reloading of sources or dependency and alteration of treatment times related to half-life of isotopes are other factors of benefit with this device.

In keeping with a theme of minimalism, the reintroduction of the *endoscope* as a very positive and useful surgical adjuvant has become commonplace, and utilization of simulation units for virtual endoscopy is a new avenue of capability which offers further promise to this element of minimalism within the field (9).

Continuing in this same theme, the discipline of *endovascular surgery* has maintained a rapid and now escalating pace of inroads into the management of intracranial aneurysms, arteriovenous malformations and vascular occlusive disorders. Not only the development of the *GDC coil*

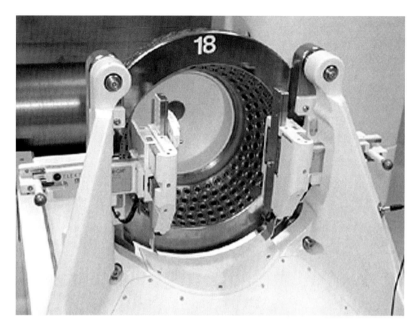

FIG. 4.47 Automatic positioning system of the Model C Leksell gamma knife. A robotic device carries out complex stereotatic radiosurgery treatment plans involving multiple isocenters, greatly improving overall accuracy and reducing human error as a result of fatigue. The computer and robotic system stimulates every step of the movement of a patient's head within the helmet before treatment is initiated. (From Apuzzo MLJ, Liu CY: 2001: Things to come. **Neurosurgery**, 49(4):765–778, 2001.)

FIG. 4.48 CyberKnife, a frameless imaging-guided robotic rotational radiosurgical system. This device is based on standard principles of linear accelerator techniques and has the potential to treat not only intracranial lesions but also virtually all body regions. (Reprinted from Adler JR Jr, Murphy MJ, Chang SD, Hancock SL: Image-guided robotic radiosurgery. **Neurosurgery** 44: 1299–1307, 1999.)

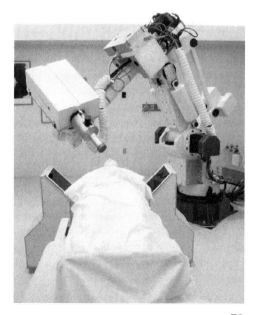

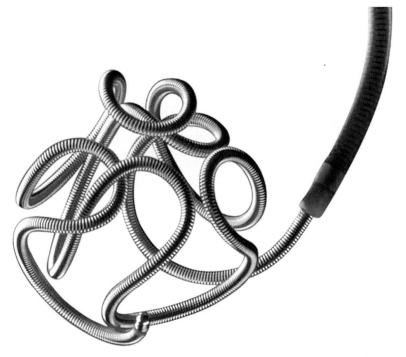

FIG. 4.49 Three-dimensional Guglielmi detachable coil. (Courtesy, Boston Scientific/Target.)

(Fig. 4.49) but also now intravascular *stenting* has shown elements of capability which will make significant inroads in the management of extracranial vascular disease as well as intracranial vascular problems. New occlusive materials for arteriovenous malformations and incorporation of biological components into mechanical devices hold great promise for resolving current technical difficulties (52, 106).

During the latter portion of the decade of the 1980s the idea of *molecular* or *cellular neurosurgery* was conceived. This represented the surgical introduction of genetic information or genetically modified cells for functional augmentation, restoration or ablation. Later, significant expansion of this concept and some element of practical reality were realized. It is apparent that there are now clearly a number of possibilities for cellular or *gene therapies* of central nervous system disorders (114, 115) *(Fig. 4.50)*. These include the use of gene or cellular therapies for *global neurodegenerative deficiencies* (recessive mutation in a single gene). The possible modes of therapy for this type of disorder include viral bacteria mediated gene enzyme replacement

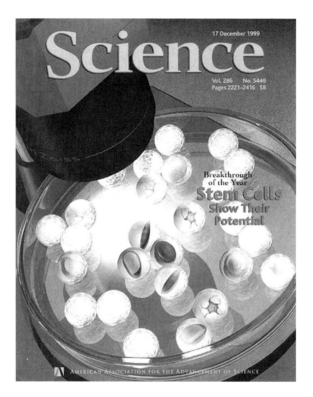

Fig. 4.50 Cover of the December 17, 1999 issue of **Science**, highlighting the break-through of stem cell research and other genetic therapies.

with a single normal allele or the use of genetically transformed neu-roprogeneter cells. Another category of central nervous system disease that may be treated includes *localized neurodegenerative disorders* which may be affected by the use of viral vector mediated transfer of a therapeutic gene or the use of embryonic implants or the trans-plantation of stem cells, genetically modified cells or direct transfer of a plasmid DNA-lipofectin complex. *Brain tumors* will also potentially be the focus of treatment of gene or cellular therapy through the trans-fer of drug susceptibility suicide genes or the transduction with toxic genes or transduction with antisense cell cycle genes or adoptive im-munotherapy. Interestingly, *stroke* is another area for cellular or gene therapy with the introduction of therapeutic stem cells, genes or ge-netic manipulations within the fibrolitic system. There has now been annotation of the human genome assembly, the significance of which can with time only be enormous (58, 59). This is a particularly excit-ing area, which will no doubt change the practice of neurosurgery in a practical way as the years unfold. The dawn of true *functional restoration* within the central nervous system is at hand!

Within the *operative environments* new directions would appear to be the introduction of more specialized developments within the operating room setting, robotics, sensors, and more sophisticated methodology for data accrual, visualization, monitoring and simulation (8).

On a more global scale, we are living in a revolutionary period of information transfer in which the fundamental body of knowledge doubles every six years. Enterprises are turning over at a rate of 10% per year, and it is felt that only 20–30% of professionals will have the ability to remain current. Of particular importance with regard to the entire framework of scientific capability and their applications to neurosurgery are the field of *informatics* and the operational tool of the *internet* (6). This remarkable capability for facilitation of information access, which offers multimedia access and allows exchange of information that promotes ease of biological searches, access to databases, educational opportunities, professional interface, and protocol collaboration, truly offers a positive force for neurosurgery. However, there are concerns associated with the internet process in which anyone has access. The ease of entering information within the system promotes misinformation, misrepresentation and abuse. In consideration of the use of this tool, it is important that scientific statements are provided with the assurance of *complete quality peer review*. This is the only fundamental reassurance to the reader that data is verified and a true statement. The scientific community must in general have an absolute way to discern meaningful data, and it is important for us to manage this element of media to decrease the volume of data and increase the significance of new information presented, thereby providing the public with some sort of measure of the validity and credibility of internet information on topics such as those concerning surgery.

The Collective Modernity

In 2001, mankind is afflicted with numerous categories of diseases related to the cerebrum. These maybe categorized within the frameworks of *traumatic, congenital, infectious, neoplastic, vascular, functional, and degenerative disorders*, all of which may be devastating to life and function in the given individual.

It may be considered that for the neurosurgeon the principle *tools of modernity* include the *operating microscope*, the comprehension of *neuroanatomy* and *function*, modes of *imaging*, the *computer, ionizing radiation*, elements of *biomedical technology*, and *biomolecular science*. These represent the epitome of the neurosurgical armamentarium and are in essence devised to be applied to the phalanx of cerebral disorders.

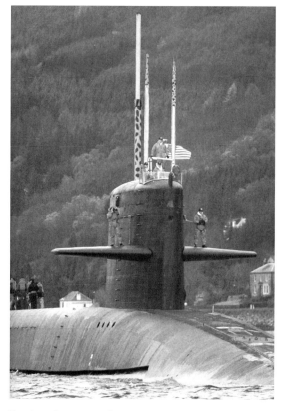

FIG. 4.51 Application of concepts of navigation such as satellite global positioning systems useful in submarines represents one form of technology transfer to neurosurgical application.

The application is effected with *concepts of modernity* which may be considered to be the following: (1) *Individual comprehension*, that is the precise appreciation of the individual anatomic and physiological substrate altered in fact by the given pathological process. (2) *Minimalism*, the application of therapeutic modes and tools with minimal physical and functional disruption of cerebral architecture and function. (3) *Guidance* as a navigational concept *(Fig. 4.51)* allows for minimalism and represents enhanced precision of establishing corridors and access to target areas. Although usually restricted to imaging-directed computer-aided orientation in the larger sense, it may represent the oriented control afforded by receptor biology or robotic enhancement of precision of achieved endpoints through (4) *biomechanical integration* in the operative process. (5) *Rehearsal* of operative events with image-based individualized computer-aided graphics of structure and function likewise enhances the economy of actions involved in the concept of minimalism. The concept allows for freedom of trial and error that true operative events do not permit. (6) *Restoration* presents a developing concept within the frame of cellular and molecular neurosurgery for action to realize structural and functional reconstruction on either focal or more general cerebral scales.

These tools and concepts represent the collective modernity of surgery of the human cerebrum as it has been reinvented during the past decade. It represents a new and totally integrated clinical science that may be viewed as *"Cerebral Surgery,"* as the integration of tools and unity allows for cross-fertilization regardless of the underlying disorder that initiated the need for therapy.

REFERENCES

1. Abernethy J: *Surgical observations on injuries of the head and on miscellaneous subjects.* London: Longman, Hurst, Rees, Orme, & Brown, 1810.
2. Adler JR, Murphy, Martin J, Chang S, Hancock SL: Image-guided robotic radiosurgery. **Neurosurgery** 44(6):1299–1306, 1999.
3. Apuzzo MLJ: Modernity and the emerging futurism in neurosurgery: tempora mutantur nos et mutamur in illis. **J Clin Neurosci** 7(2):85–87, 2000.
4. Apuzzo MLJ (ed.): *Neurosurgery for the third millennium: American Association of Neurological Surgeons neurosurgical topics.* Park Ridge I:, AANS, 1992.
5. Apuzzo MLJ: SCHNEIDER LECTURE – New dimensions of neurosurgery in the realm of high technology: Possibilities, practicalities, realities. **Neurosurgery** 38(4):625–639, 1996.
6. Apuzzo MLJ, Hodge CJ Jr: The metamorphosis of communication, the knowledge revolution, and the maintenance of a contemporary perspective during the 21st century. **Neurosurgery** 46(1):7–15, 2000.
7. Apuzzo MLJ, Liu CY: 2001: Things to come. **Neurosurgery**, 49(4):765–778, 2001.
8. Apuzzo MLJ, Weinberg RA: The architecture and functional design of advanced neurosurgical operating environments. **Neurosurgery** 33(4):663–673, 1993.
9. Auer LM, Auer DP: Virtual endoscopy for planning and simulation of minimally invasive neurosurgery. **Neurosurgery** 43(3): 529–548, 1998.
10. Aufderheide AC: The enigma of ancient cranial trepanation. **Minn Med** 68:119–122, 1985.
11. Bell B: *A system of surgery, Vols 1–6.* Edinburgh, C Elliot, 1783–1788.
12. Bennett AH, Godlee RJ: Case of cerebral tumour. The surgical treatment. **Trans R Med Chir Soc Lond** 68:243–275, 1885 (Reprinted in Wilkins RH (ed.): *Neurosurgical classics.* Park Ridge IL, AANS, 1992, pp 361–371.)
13. Berengario da Carpi J: *Tractatus de fractura calue siue cranei.* Bologna: H de Benedictis, 1518.
14. Berengario da Carpi J: *Tractatus perutilis et completus de fractura cranei.* Venice: Nicolinis de Sabio, 1535.
15. Black PML, Moriarty T, Alexander E III, Steig P, Woodard EJ, Gleason PL, Martin CH, Kikinis R, Schwartz RB, Jolesz FA: Development and implementation of intraoperative magnetic resonance imaging and its neurosurgical applications. **Neurosurgery** 41(4):831–845, 1997.

16. Borst C: Operating on a beating heart. **Sci Am** 283(4):58–63, 2000.
17. Botallo L: *De curandis vulneribus sclopetorum.* Lyon: G Roville, 1560.
18. Breasted JH: *The Edwin Smith surgical papyrus: Published in facsimile and heirogliphic transliteration with translation and commentary in two volumes.* Chicago IL, University of Chicago Press, 1930.
19. Broca P: La trépanation chez les Incas. **Bull Acad Natl Med (Paris)** 32:866–871, 1867.
20. Broca P: Nouvelle observation d'aphémie produite par une lésion de la moitié postérieure de dexième et troisième circonvolutions frontales. **Bulletin et Mémoires de la Société Anatomique de Paris, s.2**, 6:398–407, 1861a.
21. Broca P: Perte de la parole, ramollissement chronique et destruction partielle du lobe antérieur gauche du cerveau. **Bulletins de la Société d'Anthropologie** 2:235–238, 1861b.
22. Cadeddu JA, Stoianovici D, Kavoussi LR: Robotic surgery in urology. **Urol Clin North Am** 23(1):75–85, 1998.
23. Campanillo D: Neurosurgical pathology in prehistory. **Acta Neurochirugica** 70:275–290, 1984.
24. Chipault A: *Chirurgie opératoire du système nerveux, 2 vols.* Paris: Reuff & Cie, 1894–1895.
25. Cooper A: *The lectures of Sir Astley Cooper: On the principles and practice of surgery.* London: Thomas & George Underwood, 1824–1825, pp 252–352.
26. Cushing H: The special field of neurological surgery. **Bull Johns Hopkins Hosp** 16:77–87, 1905.
27. Cushing H: Surgery of the head, in Keen WW (ed.): *Surgery. Its principles and practice.* Philadelphia PA, WB Saunders, 1908, Vol 3, pp 17–276.
28. Dandy WE: Intracranial aneurysm of the internal carotid artery. **Annals of Surgery** 107:654–659, 1938 (Reprinted in Wilkins RH (ed.): *Neurosurgical classics.* Park Ridge IL: AANS, 1992, pp 437–441.)
29. Dandy WE: *The brain.* New York, Evanston, London: Harper & Row, Hoeber Medical Division, reprinted in 1969.
30. Dandy WE: Röntgenography of the brain after the injection of air into the spinal canal. **Ann Surg** 70:397–403, 1919 (Reprinted in Wilkins RH (ed.): *Neurosurgical classics.* Park Ridge IL: AANS, 1992, pp 251–256.)
31. Dandy WE: Ventriculography following the injection of air into the cerebral ventricles. **Ann Surg** 68:5–11, 1918 (Reprinted in Wilkins RH (ed.): *Neurosurgical classics.* Park Ridge IL: AANS, 1992, pp 244–250.)
32. Davey LM: John Farquhar Fulton. **Neurosurgery** 43:185–187, 1998.
33. Durante F: Contribution to endocranial surgery. **Lancet** 2:654–655, 1887 (Reprinted in Wilkins RH (ed.): *Neurosurgical classics.* Park Ridge IL: AANS, 1992, pp 375–376.)
34. Elsberg CA: Edwin Smith Surgical Papyrus and the diagnosis and treatment of injuries to skull and spine 5000 years ago. **Ann Med Hist** 3:271–279, 1931.
35. Feindel W, Leblanc R, Villemure JG: History of the surgical treatment of epilepsy, in Greenblatt SH (ed.): *A history of neurosurgery in its scientific and professional contexts.* Park Ridge, IL: AANS Publications, 1997, pp 465–488.
36. Feldman RP, Goodrich JT: Psychosurgery: a historical overview. **Neurosurgery** 48(3):647–659, 2001.
37. Ferrier D: *The functions of the brain.* London: Smith, Elder & Co., 1876.
38. Flamm ES: From signs to symptoms: the neurosurgical management of head trauma from 1517–1867. In Greenblatt SH (ed.): *A history of neurosurgery in its scientific and professional contexts.* Park Ridge, IL: AANS Publications, 1997, pp 65–81.

86   CLINICAL NEUROSURGERY

39. Flexner A: *Medical education in the United States and Canada: A report to the Carnegie Foundation for the Advancement of Teaching.* New York, NY: Carnegie Foundation for the Advancement of Teaching, 1910.
40. Flourens P: *Recherches expérimentales sur les propiétés et les fonctions du systeme nerveux dans les animaux vertébrés.* Paris: Crevot, 1824.
41. Fritsch GT, Hitzig E: Ueber die elektrische erregbarkeit des grosshirns. **Arch Anat Physiol Wissenchaft Med** 37:300–332, 1870. (Translated as "On the electrical excitability of the cerebrum," in Von Bonin G (ed.): *Some papers on the cerebral cortex.* Springfield IL: Charles C Thomas, 1960, pp 73–96.) (Reprinted in Wilkins RH (ed.): *Neurosurgical classics.* Park Ridge IL: AANS, 1992, pp 16–27).
42. Fulton JF: *Harvey Cushing. A biography.* Springfield IL: Charles C Thomas, 1946.
43. Gigli L: Zur technik der temporären schädelresection mit meiner drahtsäge. **Centralbl Chir** 25:425–428, 1898. (Reprinted in Wilkins EH (ed.): *Neurosurgical classics.* Park Ridge IL: AANS, 1992, pp 380–382.)
44. Godlee RJ: *Lord Lister.* London: Macmillan and Co., 1917.
45. Gomez JG: Paleoneurosurgery in Columbia. **J Neurosurg** 39:585–588, 1973.
46. Goodrich JT: Neurosurgery in the ancient and medieval worlds. In Greenblatt SH (ed.): *A History of neurosurgery in its scientific and professional contexts.* Park Ridge, IL: AANS Publications, 1997, pp 37–64.
47. Greenblatt SH: Cerebral localization: From theory to practice (Paul Broca and Hughlings Jackson to David Ferrier and William Macewen). In Greenblatt SH (ed.): *A history of neurosurgery in its scientific and professional contexts.* Park Ridge, IL: AANS Publications, 1997, pp 137–152.
48. Greenblatt SH (ed.): *A history of neurosurgery in its scientific and professional contexts.* Park Ridge, IL: AANS Publications, 1997.
49. Greenblatt SH, Smith DC: The emergence of Cushing's leadership: 1901–1920. In Greenblatt SH (ed.): *A history of neurosurgery in its scientific and professional contexts.* Park Ridge, IL: AANS Publications, 1997, pp 167–190.
50. Hippocrates: On injuries of the head. **Med Classics** 3:145–160, 1938.
51. Hirschfelder JO: Removal of a tumor of the brain. **Pacific Med Surg J** 29:210–216, 1886.
52. Hopkins LN, Lanzino G, Guterman LR: Treating complex nervous system vascular disorders through a "needle stick": Origin, evolution, future of neuroendovascular therapy. **Neurosurgery** 48(3):463–475, 2001.
53. Horsley V: Brain surgery. **Br Med J** 2:670–675, 1886.
54. Horsley V, Clarke RH: The structure and functions of the cerebellum examined by a new method. **Brain** 31:45–124, 1908. (Reprinted in Wilkins RH (ed.): *Neurosurgical classics.* Park Ridge IL: AANS, 1992, pp 162–185.)
55. Horwitz N: Library: Historical Perspective. **Neurosurgery** 36:428–432, 1995.
56. Horwitz N: Library: Historical Perspective. **Neurosurgery** 41:314–318, 1997.
57. Horwitz N: Library: Historical Perspective. **Neurosurgery** 43:178–184, 1998.
58. Human Genome issue. **Nature** 409:813–960, 2001.
59. Human Genome issue. **Science** 291:1145–1434, 2001.
60. Hutchinson J: Four lectures on compression of the brain. **Clin Lectures Reports Lond Hosp** 4:10–55, 1867–1868.
61. Jackson JH: A study of convolutions. **Transactions St. Andrews Med Grad Assoc** 3:162–204, 1870.
62. Jacyna LS: The neurosciences: 1800–1875. In Greenblatt SH (ed.): *A history of neurosurgery in its scientific and professional contexts.* Park Ridge, IL: AANS Publications, 1997, pp 131–136.
63. Kockro RA, Serra S, Tseng-Tsai Y, Chan C, Yih-Yian S, Gim-Guan C, Lee E, Hoe

LY, Hern N, Nowinski WL: Planning and simulation of neurosurgery in a virtual reality environment. **Neurosurgery** 46(1):118–137, 2000.

64. Laws ER Jr, Udvarhelyi GB: *The genesis of neuroscience by A. Earl Walker, M.D.* Park Ridge IL: AANS, 1998.

65. Le Dran HF: *Observations de chirurgie ,Vols 1–2.* Paris: C Osmont, 1731.

66. Le Roux PD, Das H, Esquenazi S, Kelly PJ: Robot-assisted microsurgery: A feasibility study in the rat. **Neurosurgery** 48(3):584–589, 2001.

67. Leonardo RA: *History of surgery.* New York: Froben Press, 1943.

68. Lindquist C, Kihlström L: Department of Neurosurgery, Karolinska Institute, 60 Years. **Neurosurgery** 39:1016–1021, 1996.

69. Lisowski FP: Prehistoric and early historic trepanation In Brothwell D, Sandison AT (eds): *Diseases in antiquity*, Springfield, IL: Charles C Thomas, 1967, pp 651–672.

70. Lister J: Illustrations of the antiseptic system of treatment in surgery. **Lancet** 2:668–669, 1867.

71. Lister J: On the antiseptic principle in the practice of surgery. **Lancet** 2:353–356, 1867.

72. Lyon AE: The crucible years 1880 to 1900: Macewen to Cushing. In Greenblatt SH (ed.): *A history of neurosurgery in its scientific and professional contexts.* Park Ridge, IL: AANS Publications, 1997, pp 153–166.

73. Macewen W: Clinical observations on the introduction of tracheal tubes by mouth instead of performing tracheostomy or laryngotomy. **Br Med J** 2:122–124, 1880.

74. Macewan W: *Pyogenic infective diseases of the brain and spinal cord: Meningitis, abscess of brain, infective sinus thrombosis.* Glasgow: James Maclehose & Sons, 1893.

75. Magendie F: *Précis elémentaire de physiologie.* Paris: Méquignon-Marvis, 1836.

76. Magetts EL: Trepanation of the skull by the medicine-men of primitive cultures, with particular reference to present-day native East African practice. In Brothwell D, Sandison AT (eds): *Diseases in antiquity*, Springfield, IL: Charles C Thomas, 1967, pp 673–701.

77. Marino R Jr., Gonzales-Portillo M: Preconquest Peruvian neurosurgeons: A study of Inca and pre-Columbian trephination and the art of medicine in ancient Peru. **Neurosurgery** 47:940–950, 2000.

78. Mars Pathfinder issue. **Science** 278:1734–1774, 1997.

79. Monaz E: L'encéphalographie artérielle, son importance dans la localization des tumeurs cérébrales. **Rev Neurol** 2:72–89, 1927. (Reprinted in Wilkins RH (ed.): *Neurosurgical classics.* Park Ridge, IL: AANS, 1992, pp 265–276.)

80. Moshe H, Spiegelman R, Feldman Z, Berkenstadt H, Ram Z: Novel, compact, intraoperative magnetic resonance image-guided system for conventional neurosurgical operating rooms. **Neurosurgery** 48(4):799–809, 2001.

81. Olivecrona H, Ladenheim J: *Congenital arteriovenous aneurysms of the carotid and vertebral arterial systems.* Berlin: Springer-Verlag, 1957.

82. Penfield W, Boldrey E: Somatic motor and sensory representation in the cerebral cortex of man as studied by electrical stimulation. **Brain** 60:389–443, 1937.

83. Penfield W, Jasper H: *Epilepsy and the functional anatomy of the human brain.* Boston: Little Brown & Co., 1954.

84. Pennisi E: Breakthrough of the year: The lamb that roared. **Science** 278:2038–2039, 1997.

85. Petit JL: *Principe de chirurgie.* Paris, 1730.

86. Pine A: "Economists see rosy long-term U.S. future", *Los Angeles Times,* June 10, 1997, Home Edition, Part A, Page A-1.

87. Preul MC: A history of neuroscience from Galen to Gall. In Greenblatt SH (ed.): *A history of neurosurgery in its scientific and professional contexts*. Park Ridge, IL: AANS Publications, 1997, pp 99–130.
88. Prioreschi P: Possible reasons for Neolithic skull trephining. **Perspect Biol Med** 34:296–303, 1991.
89. Rifkinson-Mann S: Cranial surgery in ancient Peru. **Neurosurgery** 23:411–416, 1988.
90. Roger of Salerno: Practica chirugiae, in Guy de Chauliac (de Vitalibus BV, trans): *Cyrurgia et cyrugia bruni. Teodorici. Rolandi. Lanfranci. Rogerii. Bertapalie. Noviter impressus*. 1591.
91. Saul FP, Saul JM: Trepanation: Old world and new world. In Greenblatt SH (ed.): *A history of neurosurgery in its scientific and professional contexts*. Park Ridge, IL: AANS Publications, 1997, pp 29–35.
92. Sharp W: *Practical observations on injuries of the head*. London: Churchill, 1841.
93. Sherrington CS: *The integrative action of the nervous system*. New Haven: Yale University Press, 1906.
94. Spiegel EA, Wycis HT, Marks M, Lee AJ: Stereotaxic apparatus for operation on the human brain. **Science** 106:349–350, 1947.
95. Spurzheim JG: *Phrenology, or the doctrine of the mental phenomena*. Philadelphia: J.P. Lippincott, 1908.
96. Stone JL, Miles ML: Skull trepanation among the early Indians of Canada and the United States. **Neurosurgery** 26:1015–1020, 1990.
97. Taylor RH: Robotics in orthopaedic surgery. In Nolte LP, Ganz R (eds.): *Computer assisted orthopedic surgery (CAOS)*. Seattle: Hogrefe and Huber, 1999, pp 35–41.
98. Taylor RH, Funda J, Eldridge K, Gruben D, LaRose D, Gomory S, Talamini M: A telerobotic assistant for laparoscopic surgery. In Taylor RH, Lavallee S, Burdea G, Mosges R (eds.): *Computer-integrated surgery*, Cambridge, MA: MIT Press, 1996, pp 581–592.
99. Taylor R, Jensen P, Whitcomb L, Barnes A, Kumar R, Stoinovici D, Gupta P, Wang Z, de Juan E, Kavoussi L: A steady-hand robotic system for microsurgical augmentation. In *Medical image computing and computer-assisted interventions (MICCAI)*. Cambridge, England: Springer Lecture Notes in Computer Science, 1999.
100. Taylor RH, Lavallee S, Burdea G, Mosges R (eds.): *Computer-integrated surgery*. Cambridge, MA: MIT Press, 1996.
101. Taylor RH, Paul HA, Kazandzides P, Mittelstadt BD, Hanson W, Zuhars JF, Williamson B, Musits BL, Glassman E, Bargar WL: An image-directed robotic system for precise orthopedic surgery. **IEEE Trans Robotics Automation** 10(3):261–275, 1994.
102. Tracy PT, Hanigan WC: History of neuroanesthesia, in Greenblatt SH (ed.): *A history of neurosurgery in its scientific and professional contexts*. Park Ridge, IL: AANS Publications, 1997, pp 213–221.
103. Valenstein ES: History of psychosurgery. In Greenblatt SH (ed.): *A history of neurosurgery in its scientific and professional contexts*. Park Ridge, IL: AANS Publications, 1997, pp 499–516.
104. Velasca-Suarez M, Martinez JB, Oliveros RG, Weinstein PR: Archeological origins of cranial surgery: Trephinations in Mexico. **Neurosurgery** 31:313–319, 1992.
105. Vesalius A: *De humani corporis fabrica libri septem*. Basel: Johannes Oporinus, 1543.
106. Vinuela F, Murayama Y, Duckwiler GM, Gobin YP, Jahan R: "Unreachable" peaks of the neurointerventional mountaineers. **Neurosurgery** 48(3): 698–699, 2001.

107. von Bergmann E: *Die Chirurgische Behandlung von Hirnkrankheiten. Zweitte, Vermehrte und Umgearbeitete Auflage.* Berlin: A Hirshwald, 1851.
108. Walker AE: Primitive trepanations: the beginning of medical history. **Trans Stud Cell Phys Phila** 26:99–102, 1958.
109. Wilkins RH: Treatment of craniocerebral infection and other common neurosurgical operations at the time of Lister and Macewan. In Greenblatt SH (ed.): *A history of neurosurgery in its scientific and professional contexts.* Park Ridge, IL: AANS Publications, 1997, pp 83–96.
110. Wilkinson RG: Trephination by drilling in ancient Mexico. **Bull NY Acad Med** 51:838–850, 1975.
111. Willis T: *Cerebri Anatome,* Londini, Typis Ja. Flesher, impensis Jo. Martyn & Ja. Allestry, 1664.
112. Wong K, Chi-Min, Wu LT: *History of Chinese medicine: Being a chronicle of medical happenings in China from ancient to present period,* 2nd edition. Shanghai: National Quarantine Service, 1936.
113. Zimmerman LM, Veith I: *Great ideas in the history of surgery.* Baltimore: Williams & Wilkins, 1961.
114. Zlokovic BV, Apuzzo MLJ: Cellular and molecular neurosurgery: Pathways from concept to reality—Part I: Target disorders and concept approaches to gene therapy of the central nervous system. **Neurosurgery** 40(4):789–804, 1997.
115. Zlokovic BV, Apuzzo MLJ: Cellular and molecular neurosurgery: Pathways from concept to reality—Part II: Vector systems and delivery methodologies for gene therapy of the central nervous system. **Neurosurgery** 40(4):805–813, 1997.

ACKNOWLEDGMENTS

All pictures are reprinted with the permission of the publishers. Figures 4.8B, 4.9, 4.12, 4.15, 4.16A, B, 4.17, 4.18B, 4.19, 4.21, 4.22 A–D, 4.24B, 4.26, 4.27A–C, 4.28A, B, 4.34A, B, and 4.39 A–C are used courtesy of the Rare Book Room, Norris Medical Library, Keck School of Medicine, University of Southern California, Los Angeles, California.

CHAPTER

5

Minimalist Approach: Functional Mapping

PETER BLACK, M.D., PH.D., JUHA JAASKELAINEN, M.D.,
ALEXANDRA CHABRERIE, M.S., ALEXANDRA GOLBY, M.D.,
AND LAVERNE GUGINO, M.D.

INTRODUCTION

It is increasingly important that neurosurgeons know precisely the functions of brain tissue surrounding a lesion. For low grade gliomas, for example, the goal is to achieve maximal resection while preserving normal brain tissue and function (1, 2). The surgeon should be able to exactly localize the lesion, know which brain areas must be avoided, and have an ongoing concept of possible post-surgical deficits (3). The capacity to achieve this goal can be greatly enhanced by mapping brain function in and around a lesion. Preoperative and intraoperative mapping, which delineates normal and abnormal functions, allows the resection of lesions in and adjacent to eloquent areas which were formerly regarded as inoperable.

In the human cortex, the function is clustered so that in certain areas, cortical excision will cause a permanent neurological deficit (primary motor, sensory, and visual cortices, and language areas of Broca and Wernicke), transient deficit (e.g., supplementary motor area) or no detectable deficit. Anatomical MRI of the brain fails to reliably identify eloquent cortical areas according to landmarks for several reasons:

1. There is individual variability in gyral and sulcal architecture so that no two cortices are exactly similar, except in monozygous twins (4). Even the detection of the central sulcus is uncertain in MR images, especially when there is adjacent pathology which distorts the brain architecture. Moreover, MRI does not allow homuncular separation of leg, hand, and head, except in the omega-shaped 'hand knob'.
2. Laterilization of functions such as language or memory may cause surprises. In right-handed persons, language is in most cases represented in the left hemisphere, but in left-handed and both-handed persons, language areas may locate in either hemisphere.
3. Slowly growing lesions such as meningiomas, low grade gliomas,

and arteriovenous malformations (AVMs) may shift eloquent cortical areas in unexpected directions. In some AVM cases, function is
shifted to the contralateral hemisphere (5). As a result, low grade
gliomas or AVMs in eloquent cortical areas should not be declared
inoperable before cortical mapping.

Anatomical MRI of the brain also fails to present the delicate white
matter architecture. Neurosurgeons tend to consider white matter as
a bundle of mini-cables connecting the cortex to the periphery, rather
than a three-dimensional network. However, the functional density of
this area varies greatly allowing for very little manipulation and great
risk. This is particularly the case for the system of tracts and nuclei
from the medulla to the thalamus, as well as tracts up to the cortex
including the corticospinal tract and the optic tract.

There are presently at least six minimally invasive methods of mapping brain function:

1. Functional MRI (fMRI)
2. Magnetoencephalography (MEG)
3. Transcranial magnetic or electrical stimulation (TMS)
4. Direct cortical stimulation
5. Evoked responses
6. Positron emission tomography (PET) (not discussed here).

1. FUNCTIONAL MAGNETIC
RESONANCE IMAGING (FMRI)

fMRI is a powerful method for mapping the brain and it is increasingly used in neurosurgical planning (6). fMRI is based on blood oxygen level dependent (BOLD) endogenous contrast (7, 8), detecting small
changes in the concentration of deoxyhemoglobin, a paramagnetic substance, to infer information about focal neuronal activation. After increased neural activity, a surplus of oxygenated hemoglobin is delivered, resulting in a net increase in the oxy- to deoxyhemoglobin ratio,
which is detected as an increase in regional signal intensity in MR. An
activation task or paradigm typically compares the signal intensities
during a control task with a specific stimulation task to determine the
location(s) of functional activation related to that paradigm.

fMRI offers several advantages in the preoperative mapping of eloquent cortical areas. It is noninvasive, temporal resolution is 2 to 3
seconds, and spatial resolution is a few millimeters. 1.5 Tesla systems
with BOLD techniques are widely distributed, and there is extensive
experience from basic neuroscience. Activation tasks can be repeated
multiple times with several variations, as each activation paradigm

can be executed in a few minutes. Most neurosurgical cases require MRI evaluation, and functional imaging can be performed in the same session. Furthermore, diffusion tensor imaging (DTI) data can be acquired after fMRI session to visualize functionally important white matter tracts adjacent to the lesion.

However, fMRI does rely on expertise in radiology, neurology, neurophysiology, and neuropsychology, and requires additional effort and dedication to make it run smoothly for neurosurgical purposes. While neuroscientists achieve clean fMRI data by repetition and averaging over subjects, these data usually have to be acquired in one session in the neurosurgical setting. Furthermore, the data may be obscured by neurological deficits of the patient, previous surgeries, effects of the lesion, uncertainty of threshold levels, or unexplained activation. As a result, increasing efforts have been underway to make fMRI a more reliable peri-operative method of functional mapping.

Several groups have reported on the usefulness of fMRI for mapping of primary motor cortex, with good correlation to direct cortical stimulation mapping during awake craniotomy (9, 10, 11). These studies are usually conducted by visually comparing a cortical reconstruction showing fMRI activity to stimulations in the surgical field. Recent studies have focused on factors which may influence the degree of activation obtained with fMRI, such as handedness and motor dominance and rate of motor movement (12, 13). Mapping of language-related areas is more complicated. One group correlated language fMRI to direct cortical language mapping in 23 patients and found that language fMRI can provide accurate mapping of eloquent cortex (14). Golby et al. compared fMRI with WADA testing in predicting memory dominance in patients with mesial temporal sclerosis. They found good correlation in eight out of nine patients (15). The reason for the lack of correlation in the remaining patient was not clear, and points to the need for further study of fMRI and its relation to direct cortical stimulation.

Few studies correlate findings from cortical stimulation to fMRI activation in other areas than the primary motor and sensory cortices. Further data on areas related to language and memory, and on associative areas such as the supplementary motor area are needed. In the Surgical Planning Laboratory at Brigham and Women's Hospital, automated registration of the fMRI data to a high resolution anatomical scans, including the lesion and vessels, and frameless registration to the patient allows for a routine way to compare preoperative functional imaging and intraoperative stimulation data. In the interventional MRI scanner (0.5 T) at Brigham and Women's Hospital, direct correlation can be made with the brain anatomy. Patients are operated on with intravenous sedation, while the neuronavigational system allows direct correlation of the stimulation sites and the preoperative functional map of the brain. The performance of the patient is monitored by computerized tasks simultaneously.

2. MAGNETOENCEPHALOGRAPHY (MEG)

MEG directly monitors the cortical electric activity in milliseconds, unlike fMRI, which measures the BOLD response, a secondary phenomenon. MEG is a noninvasive high-resolution EEG with the remarkable advantage that MEG monitors the cortical electric activity through magnetic fields which are not affected by the skull. However, MEG does require a shielded room and strict measures to eliminate any sources of current induction affecting the weak cortical magnetic fields (10^{-12} to 10^{-14} T). In neurosurgery, MEG can be used to study eloquent cortical areas (16, 17) or lateralization similarly to fMRI, though the spatial resolution is somewhat weaker, several millimeters at best. MEG data is registered to high-resolution MR images of the patient's brain to be presented in 2D slices or 3D reconstruction of the cortex. It may also be included in the pre-surgical evaluation of epilepsy patients. However, it does only allow a brief period of monitoring as compared to days of invasive cortical grip and depth electrode monitoring.

3. TRANSCRANIAL MAGNETIC AND/OR ELECTRICAL STIMULATION (TMS)

Gugino et al. summarized the history and principles of transcranial magnetic or electrical stimulation (18). In 1980 Merton and Morton described a noninvasive single pulse electrical transcranial stimulation technique for activation of the human corticospinal tract (19, 20). Levy et al. demonstrated that transcranial electrical stimulation can be used to elicit spinal cord and neurogenic motor potentials in anesthetized patients (21).

The magnetic stimulator consists of two components: a current source which produces, stores, and releases a large current; and a stimulating coil to which the current is passed *(Fig. 5.1)*. The coils are insulated to protect the operator and the patient from direct contact with the conductive material. A pulsed magnetic field induces an electric field around the coil, which is proportional to the rate of change of the pulsed magnetic field (22). The induced current loop is proportional to the induced electric field intensity and conductivity, and the distance from the coil. Several coil sizes are available. Small coils produce a more intense magnetic field close to the windings than larger coils,

A

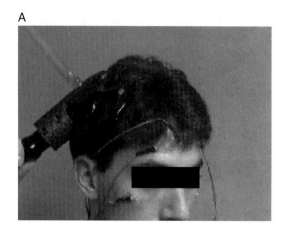

B

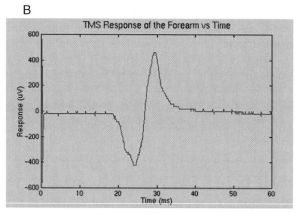

C

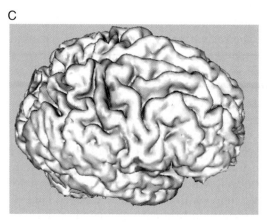

FIG. 5.1 (*A*) Illustration of the double coil positioned on the patients' scalp. The Light Emitting Diodes (LEDs) attached to the coil and the patient's face track the position of the head and establish correspondence with the three-dimensional reconstruction (3D) of the patient's MRI. (*B*) Compound muscle action potential (CMAP) obtained from muscle sensors during a single TMS pulse. The response is defined as peak to peak amplitude of greater than 50 microvolts, take-off latency, area under the response, baseline to peak amplitude and peak to trough amplitude. (PC Assisted Neurophysiology Data Analysis, Boston, MA). (*C*) 3D reconstruction of the patient's brain with normalized amplitude color coding corresponding to TMS excited cortical surface loci. The lateral foci (blue, purple) correspond to response to orbicularis oris stimulation, while medial foci (green, yellow, red) denote upper limb muscle responses.

←————————————————————————————————————

but have a more rapid falloff (22). Large coils are used in general for stimulation of large areas of motor cortex.

TMS can be used to stimulate the brain in awake patients and to identify motor cortex. It may have some pain associated with it. Recent studies suggest that TMS can induce direct excitation of corticospinal tract neurons within the motor cortex (23–28). Monophasic TMS pulses seem optimal for discrete excitation of the cortex, whereas biphasic, or attenuated sine wave pulses, are better for excitation of the CST-anterior horn cell pathway that is depressed during general anesthesia. The goal of a recently developed localization system at Brigham and Women's Hospital is to correlate external scalp TMS loci with direct intraoperative cortical stimulation. 3D reconstruction and co-registration of stimulated scalp loci to cortical surface loci are integrated into a single reference frame, thus providing a means for the quantification of coil placement error while allowing near-real time identification of cortical surface simulated by the TMS (4) *(Fig. 5.2).*

FIG. 5.2 Three-dimensional aggregate motor map derived using minimum response latencies for biceps, flexor carpi radialis (FCR), first dorsal interossei (FDI), left and right orbicularis oris (L & R oris).

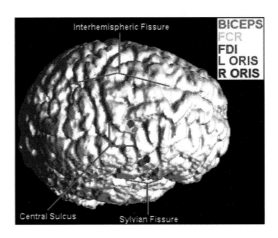

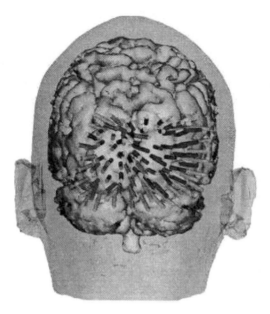

FIG. 5.3 Visual suppression cortical map: Occipital cortex showing areas where TMS train stimuli caused visual suppression. Green pegs denote failure of TMS to elicit suppressions. Red and blue pegs correspond to right and left visual field suppression, respectively.

TMS is useful primarily for localization of the motor and visual cortices *(Fig. 5.3)*.

4. DIRECT CORTICAL STIMULATION

Direct electrical stimulation of the cortical surface may produce either excitation or inhibition. It can be performed through cortical grids implanted in epilepsy patients at the bedside, or during craniotomy under local anesthesia. Stimulation of the primary motor cortex is also possible under general anesthesia when muscle relaxants are not used (29). Stimulation of the primary motor cortex usually leads to contractions of contralateral agonists, or at times agonist and antagonist muscles, which do not resemble normal voluntary movements. In the human homuncular pattern, described by Cushing and Penfield (30, 31), oral facial contractions are noted laterally. Large cortical surface medial to the face area gives rise to hand contractions, and stimulation more medially activates proximal upper limb musculature which blends into trunk and lower limb responses. It is important to note that when localizing the primary motor cortex through excitatory responses, an overlapping cortical representation of body parts is usually found such that the face is overlapping the distal upper limb. There is considerable variability in motor maps across individuals (32,

33), and individual maps may also change with time, as seen after training musical instruments or amputation.

In awake patients, inhibitory effects of cortical stimulation can be used for mapping motor and speech areas. Discrete electrical stimuli applied to the cortex while the patient is making voluntary movements or speaking, lead to depression of ongoing motor activity (33, 34). Mechanisms include excitation of inhibitory neurons and/or depolarization block of the motor clusters beneath the stimulating electrode. However, little experimental work is available to determine their role in this phenomenon.

Direct cortical stimulation can be done at the bedside in epilepsy patients with subdural grids and strips for preoperative evaluation. The grids and strips, sites of eloquent cortical areas located by stimulation, and possible lesion(s) can be superimposed on 3D MRI reconstructions of the cortex and the brain, thus creating a full "road map" for surgery (35, 36). Functional cortical mapping is often carried out on patients whose craniotomies are done under local anesthesia. Sedation as opposed to general anesthesia allows the patient to report the location of paresthesiae elicited when stimulating primary sensory areas. Mapping of cortical language areas requires patient participation, for example, naming objects or reading written material aloud. Most general anesthetic techniques profoundly depress motor-neuron synaptic excitability, precluding visual assessment of muscle contractions when primary motor areas are stimulated (37). Aglio et al. recently reviewed sedation techniques for use during cortical mapping procedures (38).

Similar stimulation parameters are used for all cortical areas. Biphasic pulses of 200 to 500 microsecond duration are presented as trains lasting 2 to 5 seconds with pulse frequencies of 50 to 70 Hz *(Fig. 5.4)*. Constant current stimulator intensities of 2 to 12 milliamps are usually required for mapping (39, 40). The stimulation intensity is increased gradually to find a stimulating current sufficient for mapping but which do not cause after-polarizations or seizures. Cortical grids or strips can be used to monitor the after-polarizations, and sterile ice water can be used for irrigation to prevent seizures. It is important to identify post-seizure paresis which makes motor mapping temporarily unreliable.

Monopolar technique uses a single stimulating electrode for probing the cortical surface, and a second electrode placed on exposed muscle or scalp to allow a return path for the current. In bipolar technique, the stimulating current path is restricted between two closely spaced electrodes connected to a handheld probe. Bipolar stimulation is pre-

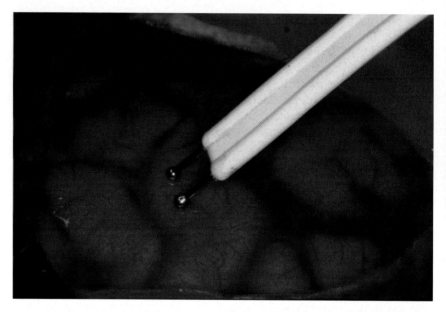

FIG. 5.4 Bipolar electrical stimulator: Localization of the eloquent cortex is conducted by moving the probe directly across the exposed brain surface. Biphasic pulses of 200 to 500 microseconds are presented as trains of 2 to 5 seconds with pulse frequencies of 50 to 70 Hz.

ferred at our institution. Nathan et al., using a finite element modeling for stimulus spread within the cortex, showed theoretically that the most focal excitation of cortical tissue would be obtained with the bipolar technique (41). Cortical stimulation can also be carried out using cortical grids with an array of platinum contacts, usually at 1cm intervals. A constant biphasic stimulation current can be routed between any two contacts in the grid, either through a switch box or by hand. The switch box also allows EEG monitoring of seizures when a handheld stimulator is used.

Localization is carried out by moving the stimulating probe across the exposed cortex, in a systematic manner. At each stimulation point, the presence of muscle contractions (distinguished from focal epilepsy), inhibition of on-going motor function or speech, or development of paresthesiae are noted. Cortical regions giving positive or negative functional responses can be labeled by small placecards. After mapping, the surgeon should know the areas of eloquent cortex to plan the resection accordingly. If a seizure occurs during the stimulation, ice water irrigation of cortex will stop it. We have carried out brain mapping with bipolar stimulation in 600 patients and have found it reliable and simple (39).

5. EVOKED POTENTIALS

Evoked potentials can be used to assess the functional integrity of the primary sensory, auditory and visual pathways, but they are not particularly useful for functional mapping as described above (43, 44). However, when surgery in children or adults is possible only under general anesthesia, somatosensory potentials become important for the localization of the central sulcus. Cortical surface recording grids, consisting of either platinum or stainless steel electrodes embedded in a flexible plastic material, are used. Platinum contacts are used when both localization of the central sulcus as well as cortical stimulation are planned, since platinum does not polarize or deposit toxic metallic ions onto the cortical surface. It is important that the surgeon maximize the electrical contact of the grid electrodes and the cortical surface *(Fig. 5.5)*.

We have limited experience this technique in adults. In children however, we have found it to be extremely useful.

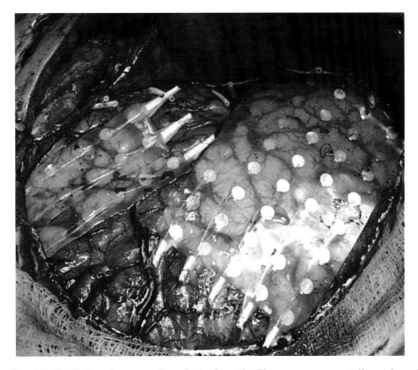

FIG. 5.5 Cortical surface recording electrode grids: These are commercially made and consist of either platinum or stainless steel electrodes embedded in a flexible plastic material. Stimulation may be carried out by connecting a biphasic constant current electrical stimulation output to a switch box, which routs the stimulus trains to a combination of any two electrodes within the grid.

SUMMARY AND CONCLUSION

The ability to accurately map functional cortex both preoperatively and intraoperatively is an important neurosurgical challenge for the next decade. The central concept of preoperative mapping is to superimpose blood flow and electrical activation data on a three-dimensional matrix created by MR imaging and image processing. The gold standard, at present, is direct cortical stimulation, which can identify primary motor, sensory, speech, and visual cortices. Cortical mapping can be performed intraoperatively or through implanted subdural electrodes at the bedside. The tasks for the next decade include the validation of these preoperative techniques (fMRI, MEG, TMS, EP):

1. Correlation of direct cortical stimulation with advanced perioperative stimulation/ monitoring systems, in a wide variety of cases. In addition, extension of these applications into intraoperative imaging systems like the GE Signa unit should also be envisaged.
2. Evaluation of how various pathologies such as AVMs, well-circumscribed tumors, and infiltrative tumors affect the data obtained by these techniques.
3. Expansion of mapping to areas outside the primary motor and sensory cortices, including those referred to as "associative" and to higher functions collectively termed as "cognition."

REFERENCES

1. Black PM, DaNikas D: Neurosurgical considerations in low grade gliomas. 11th International Congress of Neurosurgery, 1997.
2. Berger MS, Rostomily RC: Low grade gliomas: functional mapping resection strategies, extent of resection, and outcome. **J Neurooncol** 34(1):85–101, 1997.
3. Black, PM: Surgery for cerebral gliomas: Past, present and future, MA Howard, JP Elliott, MM Haglund, FM McKhann (eds): **Clin Neurosurg** 47:21–45, 2000.
4. Thompson PM, Cannon TD, Narr KL, van Erp T, Poutanen VP, Huttunen M, Lonnqvist J, Standertskjold-Nordenstam CG, Kaprio J, Khaledy M, Dail R, Zoumalan CI, Toga AW: Genetic influences on brain structure. **Nature Neuroscience** 4:1253–8, 2001.
5. Lazar RM, Marshall RS, Pile-Spellman J, Duong HC, Mohr JP, Young WL, Solomon RL, Perera GM, DeLaPaz RL: Interhemispheric transfer of language in patients with left frontal cerebral arteriovenous malformation. **Neuropsychologia** 38(10):1325–32, 2000.
6. Hirsch J, Ruge MI, Kim KH, Correa DD, Victor JD, Relkin NR, Labar DR, Krol G, Bilsky MH, Souweidane MM, DeAngelis LM, Gutin PH: An integrated functional magnetic resonance imaging procedure for preoperative mapping of cortical areas associated with tactile, motor, language, and visual functions. **Neurosurgery** 47:11–21, 2000.
7. Ogawa, S. & Lee, T. M. Magnetic resonance imaging of blood vessels at high fields: in vivo and in vitro measurements and image simulation. **Magn Reson Med** 16:9–18, 1990.

8. Kwong KK: Dynamic magnetic resonance imaging of human brain activity during primary sensory stimulation. **Proc Natl Acad Sci** (USA) 89:5675–5679, 1992.

9. Puce A: Comparative assessment of sensorimotor function using functional magnetic resonance imaging and electrophysiological methods. **J Clin Neurophysiol** 12(5):450–459, 1995.

10. Mueller WM, Yetkin FZ, Hammeke TA, Morris III GL, Swanson SS, Reichert K, Cox R, Haughton V: Functional magnetic resonance imaging mapping of the motor cortex in patients with cerebral tumors. **Neurosurgery** 39(3):515–521, 1996.

11. Pujol J, Conesa G, Deus J, Vendrell P, Isamat F, Zannoli G, Marti-Vilalta JL, Capdevila A: Presurgical identification of the primary sensorimotor cortex by functional magnetic resonance imaging. **J Neurosurg** 84:7–13, 1996.

12. Springer JA, Binder JR, Hammeke TA, Swanson SJ, Frost JA, Bellgowan PS, Brewer CC, Perry HM, Morris GL, Mueller WM: Language dominance in neurologically normal and epilepsy subjects: A functional MRI study. **Brain** 122:2033–2046, 1999.

13. Pujol J, Deus J, Losilla JM, Capdevila A: Cerebral lateralization of language in normal left-handed people studied by functional MRI. **Neurology** 52(5):1038–1043, 1999.

14. Benson RR, FitzGerald DB, LeSueur LL, Kennedy DN, Kwong KK, Buchbinder BR, Davis TL, Weisskoff RM, Talavage TM, Logan WJ, Cosgrove GR, Belliveau JW, Rosen BR: Language dominance determined by whole brain functional MRI in patients with brain lesions. **Neurology** 52(4):798–809, 1999.

15. Golby AJ, Poldrack RA, Brewer JB, Spencer D, Desmond JE, Aron AP, Gabrieli JD: Material-specific lateralization in the medial temporal lobe and prefrontal cortex during memory encoding. **Brain** 124(9):1841–1854, 2001.

16. Fahlbusch R, Ganslandt O, Nimsky C: Intraoperative imaging with open magnetic resonance imaging and neuronavigation. **Childs Nerv Syst** 10-11:829–831, 2000.

17. Mäkelä J, Seppä M, Hämäläinen M, Forss N, Kirveskari E, Avikainen S, Salonen O, Salenius S, Kovala T, Randell T, Jääskeläinen J, Hari R: Three-dimensional imaging of functional brain anatomy to facilitate intraoperative navigation around the somatomotor strip. **Human Brain Mapping** 12:182–190, 2000.

18. Gugino LD, Potts G, Aglio LS, et al: Localization of eloquent cortex using transcranial magnetic stimulation. In Alexander E, Maciunas RJ (eds): *Advanced Neurosurgical Navigation.* New York, Thieme Publishers, 1998, pp163–199.

19. Merton PA, Morton HB: Stimulation of the cerebral cortex in the intact human subject. **Nature** 285(5762):227, 1980.

20. Merton QA, Hill DK, Morton HB, et al: Scope of a technique for electrical stimulation of the human brain, spinal cord, and muscle. **Lancet** 2(8298):597–600, 1982.

21. Levy WJ, Oro J, Tucker D, et al: Safety studies of electric and magnetic stimulation for the production of motor evoked potentials. In Chokroverty S (ed): *Magnetic Stimulation in Clinical Neurophysiology.* Boston, Butterworth, 1990, pp 165–172.

22. Jalinous R: Technical and practical aspects of magnetic nerve stimulation. **J Clin Neurophysiol** 8(1):10–25, 1991.

23. Amassian VE, Quirk GJ, Stewart M: Magnetic coil versus electrical stimulation of monkey motor cortex. **J Physiol** (Lond) 394:119, 1987.

24. Amassian VE, Cracco RO, Macabee PJ, et al: Matching focal and non-focal magnetic coil stimulation to properties of human nervous system. Mapping motor unit fields in motor cortex contrasted with alternating sequential digit movements by premotor SMA stimulation. **Electroencephalogr Clin Neurophysiol** Suppl 43:3–28, 1991.

25. Rothwell JC: Physiological studies of electric and magnetic stimulation of the human brain. **Electroencephalogr Clin Neurophysiol** Suppl 43:29–35, 1991.

26. Rothwell JC, Thompson PD, Day BL, et al: Stimulation of the human motor cortex through the scalp. **Exp Physiol** 76(2):159–200, 1991.
27. Day BL, Dick JPR, Mardsen CD: Differences between electrical and magnetic stimulation of the human brain. **J Physiol** 37:836–842, 1986.
28. Berardelli A, Inghiller M, Cruccu G, et al: Corticospinal potentials after electrical and magnetic stimulation in man. **Electroencephalogr Clin Neurophys** Suppl 43:147–154, 1991.
29. Kombos T, Suess O, Ciklatekerlio O, Brock M: Monitoring of intraoperative motor evoked potentials to increase the safety of surgery in and around the motor cortex. **J Neurosurg** 95:608–14, 2001.
30. Cushing H: A note on the faradic stimulation of the human brain. **Brain** 32:44–53, 1939.
31. Penfield W, Bolder P: Somatic motor and sensory representation in the cerebral cortex of man as studied by electrical stimulation. **Brain** 60:389–443, 1937.
32. Penfield W, Welsh K: Instability of response to stimulation of the sensorimotor cortex of man. **J Physiol** (Lond) 109:358–365, 1949.
33. Dogali M: Sensorimotor cortical mapping and physiological response localization. In Devinski O, Beric A, Dogali M (eds): *Electrical and Magnetic Stimulation of the Brain and Spinal Cord.* New York, Raven Press, pp 141–148, 1993.
34. Ojemann GA: Functional mapping of cortical language areas in adults: Intraoperative approaches. In Devinski O, Beric A, Dogali M (eds): Electrical and Magnetic Stimulation of the Brain and Spinal Cord. New York, Raven Press, pp155–163, 1993.
35. Chabrerie A, Ozlen F, Nakajima S, Leventon ME, Atsumi H, Grimson E, Keeve E, Helmers S, Riviello J Jr, Holmes G, Duffy F, Jolesz F, Kikinis R, Black PM: Three-dimensional reconstruction and surgical navigation in pediatric epilepsy surgery. **Pediatr Neurosurg** 27(6):304–310, 1997
36. Ozlen F, Nakajima S, Chabrerie A, Leventon ME, Grimson E, Kikinis R, Jolesz F, Black PM: Excision of cortical dysplasia in the language area with use of a surgical navigator: a case report. **Epilepsia** 39(12):1361–1366, 1998.
37. Tung HL, Drummond JC, Bickford RG: The effects of anaesthetic sedative agents on magnetic motor responses (Abstract). **Anaesthesiology** 69:313, 1988.
38. Aglio LS, Gugino LD: Consicous sedation for intraoperative neurosurgical procedures. In Loftus CM, Batjer HH (eds): *Techniques in Neurosurgery,* New York, Lippincott-Raven, 2001.
39. Danks RA, Aglio LS, Gugino LD, Black PM: Craniotomy under local anesthesia and monitored conscious sedation for the resection of tumors involving eloquent cortex. **J Neurooncol** 49(2):131–139, 2000.
40. Mehta V, Danks A, Black PM: Cortical mapping under local anaesthesia for tumor resection. **Semin Neurosurg** 11(3):387–299, 2000.
41. Nathan L, Lesser R, Gordon B, Thanker NV: Electrical stimulation of the human cerebral cortex: Theoretical approach. In Devinski O, Beric A, Dogali M (eds): Electrical and magnetic stimulation of the brain and spinal cord. New York, Raven Press, 1993, pp 61–86.
42. Haglund M, Ojemann G, Hoichmann D: Optical imaging of epileptiform and functional activity in human cerebral cortex. **Nature** 358:668–671, 1992.
43. Hahn J, Lüders H: Placement of subdural grid electrodes at the Cleveland Clinic. In Engel J Jr (ed): *Surgical Treatment of the Epilepsies.*
44. New York, Raven, 1987, pp 621–627.
45. Wood CC, Spencer DD, Allison T, McCarthy G, Williamson PD, Goff WR: Localization of human sensorimotor cortex during surgery by cortical surface recording of somatosensory evoked potentials. **J Neurosurg** 68(1):99–111, 1988

II

General Scientific
Session II
Reinventing Neurosurgery:
Technical and Scientific
Advances for the
21st Century

CHAPTER

6

Surgical Guidance Now and in the Future: The Next Generation of Instrumentation

JOHN R. ADLER, JR., M.D.

INTRODUCTION

Arguably more than any other surgical specialty, neurosurgery has developed hand-in-hand with medical imaging. This phenomenon began with simple x-rays, grew with the arrival of ventriculography and angiography, and has now become a dominant reality with the development of modern computerized imaging, i.e., computerized tomographic (CT) and magnetic resonance (MR) imaging. During the initial utilization of each new imaging modality, a neurosurgeon's inherently imperfect spatial reasoning remained interposed between "diagnostic" images and the actual performance of a surgical procedure. However, with time, neurosurgeons have developed ingenious ways of merging 3-D operative space with historical medical images. This field of endeavor is broadly termed *surgical navigation*. The rapidly evolving collection of techniques within surgical navigation has the potential to dramatically change the way all neurosurgeons operate.

Stereotactic frames were the first surgical instruments designed to transpose the spatial information acquired from diagnostic images onto a patient's anatomy. While such frames provide a straightforward yet accurate method for targeting, these instruments are only readily applicable to a restricted set of procedures, primarily "intracranial" operations for which a neurosurgeon need only target a small number of predetermined points in space. A critical limitation of stereotactic frames is that they are not practical outside the cranium, e.g., within or adjacent to the spine. In contrast, more recently developed image-guided surgical navigation is interactive and provides a surgeon with continuous feedback regarding spatial localization (1, 2, 3). Furthermore, these principles can also be applied to the spine (4). For these reasons, and the growing power of machine computation, intraoperative image guidance is becoming ever more commonplace.

INTRAOPERATIVE IMAGING

A principle drawback of surgical navigation is its reliance on "historic" image sets whose information may not reflect the anatomic changes produced by the operative intervention itself. Largely because of this limitation, real-time intraoperative imaging remains an attractive concept. For example, real-time intraoperative fluoroscopy continues to be an invaluable guide for many transsphenoidal and complex spinal operations. Meanwhile, the growing movement towards intraoperative magnetic resonance imaging (MR) seeks to achieve an analogous objective for intracranial surgery (5, 6, 7). However, with both of these forms of intraoperative guidance, their implementation can be technically awkward, and in the case of MR, quite expensive. Fluoroscopy and MR also require shielding of either the operating room staff or the room itself. Meanwhile, because the information provided by these imaging modalities is either 2-D (fluoroscopy) or not truly real time (MR), there are benefits to tightly referencing the information with "historic" 3-D image data; one can argue persuasively that practical constraints preclude the use of true "real time" MR imaging, and as a result, this technology is primarily used to facilitate the rapid intraoperative acquisition of MR scans as opposed to delivering true dynamic feedback. It is for these reasons that even when imaging is used during surgery, neurosurgeons continue to be confronted with the challenge of merging the 3-D operative space with historical medical images, a task best embodied by the principles of image-guided surgical navigation.

IMAGE-GUIDED SURGICAL NAVIGATION

The past 15 years have witnessed the flourishing of computerized tools that allow surgeons to accurately merge patient-specific computerized image sets with the surgical anatomy at hand (1, 2, 8, 9). To date, the primary benefits of image-guided surgical navigation are that it both permits neurosurgeons to use smaller and more strategically placed incisions and provides intermittent reorientation should brain or skull-base anatomy be markedly abnormal or otherwise disorienting. As a consequence, computerized image-guidance, when combined with ever-improved imaging, has made surgical "exploration" an antiquated notion. Despite these substantial benefits, such technology has only refined our surgical approaches. Moreover, one might argue that many skilled neurosurgeons had innate 3-D localization skills that were comparable substitutes for much of current image-guidance technology. Now, however, the next generation of image-guidance technology, which is already starting to arrive, promises to do much more (8). These new tools for navigation have the potential to be used in ways that lead to a complete redesign of how surgeons operate, and some of these concepts may call into question the very definition of surgery itself (1).

3-D Volume Rendering

By presenting neurosurgeons with visual depictions of the patient's CT or MR scan, and providing tools for the accurate 3-D registration of this data with the operative site, image-guided surgical navigation has made it possible to perform smaller and more precise operations. Probably the most important practical function provided by these systems is that a surgeon can understand the anatomy that lurks beneath a visible operative surface, i.e., image-guidance gives a surgeon a form of "Superman-like x-ray vision." However, almost exclusively, the visual information relayed to surgeons on the computer monitor is represented in 2 dimensions. In other words, a surgeon is called upon to mentally transpose a 2-dimensional image space onto a 3-D operative site. To in part compensate for this situation, image-guidance systems typically provide a "surface-rendered" 3-D depiction of the anatomy at hand. While such visual information has some uses, it often does not give the surgeon a critical mental picture of what lies beneath a visible surface, which as stated above, should be the ultimate benefit of surgical navigation.

The major reason why current surgical navigation systems only provide surface rendered images to display 3-D information stems from the combined inability of software algorithms and computer processors to perform fast enough calculations for more sophisticated and helpful depictions. However, recent improvements in these technologies have made real-time volume rendering possible, and with it, an opportunity to immerse surgeons in a complex, visually rich, 3-dimensional world. As a result, a world of possibilities for rethinking many operative procedures is opening (8).

By combining surgical navigation software that includes volume rendering with new, and most likely highly specialized endoscopic hardware, it will become possible in the near future to create radically new minimally invasive surgical approaches to many neurosurgical conditions (9, 10). For example, volume rendering of MR or CT angiographic data can be merged with real-time endoscopic imagery to guide the occlusion of aneurysms using specialized hardware for retraction, dissection and vascular occlusion/clipping *(Fig. 6.1)*. Not only can such "endoscopic assisted" procedures be less invasive than current operations, but they also promise to give neurosurgeons a more complete

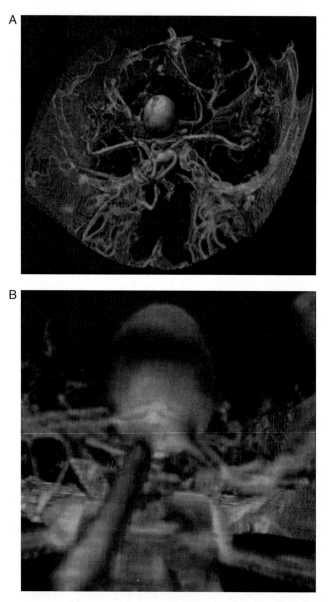

FIG. 6.1 A single perspective image obtained from a volume rendered CT angiogram and depicting both basilar and anterior communicating artery aneurysms (A). This rendered image set can be manipulated in real time to reflect a surgeon's ever-changing perspective (B), and when merged with advanced endoscopic tools, has the potential to guide minimally invasive therapy for aneurysms.

intraoperative understanding for the spatial location of otherwise difficult to discern perforating arteries, e.g., those present on the often invisible back side of some aneurysms. There are analogous and perhaps even greater gains to be had in merging volume-rendered image guidance with numerous endoscopic spinal procedures, especially in the thoracic spine (10). Here too, there is considerable potential to develop less-invasive operations for decompression and even fusion. Although these new tools for image-guidance tools are only now starting to appear commercially, it will require neurosurgical inventiveness to develop the next generation of practical surgical applications.

IMAGE-GUIDED STEREOTACTIC RADIOSURGERY

Radiosurgery utilizes stereotactic principles of localization and multiple cross-fired beams to deliver a large radiation dose to a well-defined target with limited fractionation. Over the past $1^1/_2$ decades frame-based radiosurgery, beginning with the Gamma Knife®, has transformed the treatment of nearly all types of brain tumor and even many non-neoplastic neurological diseases. Nevertheless, the need for a stereotactic frame has precluded the use of true radiosurgical methods either when treatment fractionation was warranted or for non-intracranial lesions. Now, with the emergence of technology that combines image-guidance with mechanical systems that precisely target therapeutic radiation, it is finally possible to extend radiosurgical ablation to virtually any anatomic location (1). This frameless radiosurgical technology, which is still available only at a small number of institutions worldwide, makes it possible to precisely target radiation at lesions of the head and neck and more recently the spinal axis. Eventually, this technology promises to make radiosurgery a generic surgical tool that is used for ablation virtually anywhere in the body (2).

Image-Guided Robotic Radiosurgery System (IGRR) Description

Image-guided robotic radiosurgery (The CyberKnife Radiosurgical System® manufactured by Accuray Incorporated, Sunnyvale, CA.) utilizes an orthogonal pair of digital cameras to capture near real-time stereo x-rays of the skeleton or implanted fiducials (1) *(Fig. 6.2)*. During radiosurgery, these images are automatically referenced against computer-synthesized digitally reconstructed radiographs (DRRs) "generated on the fly" from previously obtained CT scans; meanwhile, the treatment plan is designed from the same CT. This computational process makes it possible for the IGRR system to precisely establish patient position and orientation with near millimeter accuracy (11, 12). A miniature and lightweight 6 MV X-band linear accelerator

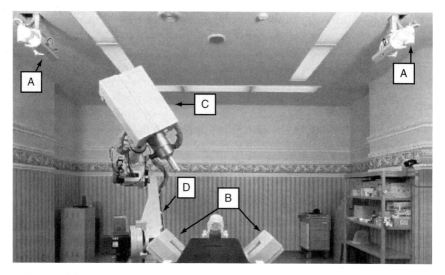

FIG. 6.2 The CyberKnife Radiosurgical System that includes: (A) Dual diagnostic energy x-ray sources. (B) Paired amorphous silicon cameras. (C) 6 mV X-band LINAC. (D) Robotic manipulator with 6 degrees of freedom.

(LINAC) provides a source of high-energy radiation. Because of its size and weight, it is possible to aim and dynamically reposition the LINAC by means of a robotic manipulator with 6 degrees of freedom (3 translational degrees of freedom as well as roll, pitch, and yaw). The current generation of IGRR includes an inverse treatment planning algorithm which takes advantage of the flexibility afforded by robotic targeting, and in doing so, provides for a high degree of dose conformality when treating non-spherically shaped lesions (13).

Clinical Outcome with IGRR

Three hundred and thirty-eight patients with brain tumors have been treated with a prototype system for IGRR at Stanford University. Patients were treated most commonly with single fraction radiosurgery, but in those cases where a large lesion was immediately adjacent to or involving critical brain structures, such as the optic apparatus, hypofractionated radiosurgery in 2–5 fractions was administered. To date, overall results after image-guided radiosurgical ablation of brain tumors are comparable to other more invasive radiosurgical approaches. More importantly for many of the treated patients, alternative therapies, whether involving radiosurgery, open surgery, or radiation therapy, have been limited (14) *(Fig. 6.3)*.

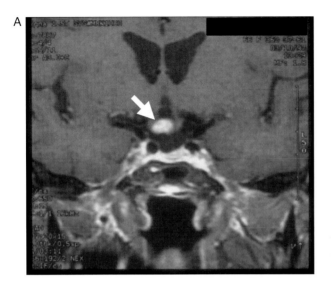

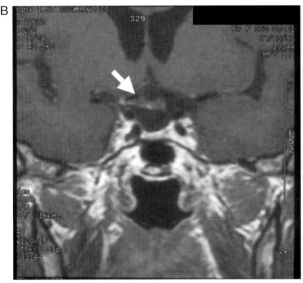

FIG. 6.3 (*A*) A 66-year-old female with a 25-year history of cranial radiotherapy and multiple surgically resected parasellar meningiomas presents with a constriction of her visual field and, on enhanced MRI, a recurrent lesion within her optic chiasm. (*B*) Patient was treated with fractionated stereotactic radiosurgery using IGRR to a total dose of 30 Gy in 5 fractions prescribed at the 80th percentile. Subsequent MRI at 6 months revealed complete disappearance of the previously noted lesion. Five years after the fractionated radiosurgery the patient's vision is unchanged.

Clinical Experience with Spinal Radiosurgery at Stanford

Given the grave potential consequences of either ineffective or overly aggressive treatment for lesions of the spinal axis, management of such lesions is a continuing challenge. However, besides targeting the position of a brain tumor from skull x-rays, IGRR can be used to track the vertebral bodies of the neck or embedded stainless steel markers. This capability has been used to treat 31 patients at Stanford University with tumors in various regions of the cervical, thoracic, and lumbar spine as well as the spinal cord itself (15). The types of spinal pathology treated to date with the CyberKnife include hemangioblastoma, arteriovenous malformation, metastatic carcinoma, schwannoma, a meningioma, and chordoma. Although the accuracy of such treatment is dependent on certain key technical details and, in particular, CT slice thickness, the average measured root-mean-square targeting error in phantoms ranges between 1.0 and 1.1 mm, which

B

A

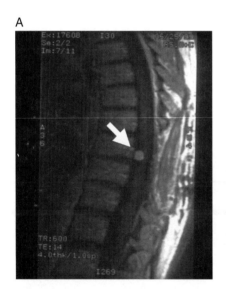
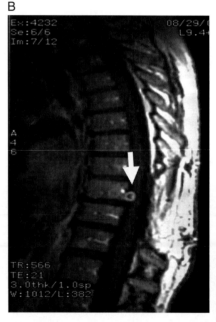

FIG. 6.4 (A) Six years after resection of a T9-T10 schwannoma, this 62-year-old female developed a new onset myelopathy. Contrast-enhanced thoracic MRI revealed recurrent tumor at T9 with spinal cord compression. (B) Patient was treated with IGRR to total dose of 21 Gy in 3 fractions as prescribed to the 85th percentile. Over 1 year of follow-up, there was resolution of the patient's myelopathy and follow-up MRI revealed loss of central contrast enhancement within the tumor as well as a significant decrease in size.

compares favorably with frame-based intracranial stereotactic localization (15, 16).

Clinical and radiological follow-up for the spinal lesions treated at Stanford ranges from 4 to 74 months. Only 1 patient with a multiply recurrent chordoma treated with a total dose of 25 Gy (prescribed to the 80th percentile) in 5 fractions demonstrated MRI evidence of tumor progression. Since most patients had either benign tumors or vascular malformations, clinical and radiologic follow-up is still rather preliminary. Despite the relatively short follow-up, clear-cut evidence of radiosurgical efficacy could be documented in many patients *(Fig. 6.4)*. There have been no treatment-related complications to date.

Extraneural Radiosurgery

Although still in its infancy, IGRR is starting to be used to ablate tumors of the lung, pancreas, and, most recently, prostate (12). In treating all of these soft tissue lesions, the IGRR imaging system utilizes gold fiducials embedded percutaneously in or around the target through an 18-gauge needle. These x-ray visible landmarks provide a system for spatial reference. Because IGRR uses a robotic manipulator, it is even possible for this technology to accurately treat tumors that are near the diaphragm and move throughout respiration. In such cases, the beam is dynamically retargeted to compensate for respiratory movements of as much as 2 cm. With increasingly faster response times for such robots, targeting accuracies promise to compare favorably with present-day stereotactic radiosurgical standards.

Radiosurgical Revolution

IGRR has the potential to evolve into a generic surgical tool that is used by increasing numbers of surgeons for an ever-wider array of indications. For example, new molecule marker or spiral CT and PET imaging technologies are resulting in significantly earlier diagnosis of early stage systemic cancers. These generally very small lesions represent ideal targets for minimally invasive radiosurgical ablation. Meanwhile, some patients with slow-growing metastatic cancer that involves a few organs are now routinely treated with expensive and morbid chemotherapy regimens that have limited efficacy. By having a tool that can noninvasively and cost-effectively ablate small tumors throughout the body, it will be possible to re-explore the limits of "surgical" management for such cancers. These possibilities should in part change neurosurgical notions of what is beneficial for many of our patients. Meanwhile, the realization that neurosurgeons have pioneered techniques that will eventually find widespread application among our other surgical colleagues and help countless patients should instill a special sense of pride within our specialty.

REFERENCES

1. Adler JR, Murphy MJ, Chang SD, Hancock SL: Image-guided robotic radiosurgery. **Neurosurgery** 44(6):1299–1307, 1999.
2. Guthrie B, Adler JR: Frameless stereotaxy: Computer interactive neurosurgery. **Perspect Neuro Surg** 2(1):1–22, 1991.
3. Smith KR, Frank KJ, Bucholz RD: The NeuroStation—A highly accurate,minimally invasive solution to frameless stereotactic neurosurgery. **Comput Med Imaging Graph** 18(4):247–256, 1994.
4. Kalfas IH: Image-guided spinal navigation (Review). **Clin Neurosurg** 46:70–88, 2000.
5. Black PM, Alexander E 3rd, Martin C, et al: Craniotomy for tumor treatment in an intraoperative magnetic resonance imaging unit. **Neurosurgery** 46(5):1270, 2000.
6. Nabavi A, Black PM, Gering DT, et al: Serial intraoperative magnetic resonance imaging of brain shift. **Neurosurgery** 48(4):787–798, 2001.
7. Woodard EJ, Leon SP, Moriarty TM, Quinones A, Zamani AA, Jolesz FA: Initial experience with intraoperative magnetic resonance imaging in spine surgery. **Spine** 26(4):410–417, 2001.
8. Shahidi R, Tombropoulos R, Grzeszczuk RP: Clinical applications of three-dimensional rendering of medical data sets. **Proc IEEE** 86(3):555–568, 1998.
9. Shahidi R, Wang B, Epitaux M, Grzeszczuk R, Adler J: Volumetric image guidance via a stereotactic endoscope. In: Wells WM, Colchester ACF, Delp S, Eds. *Medical Image Computing & Computer-Assisted Intervention—MICCAI '98.* New York: Springer-Verlag, 1998, Vol. 1496, pp 241–252.
10. Abbasi H, Chin S, Kim D, Shahidi R, Steinberg G: Computerized lateral endoscopic approach to spinal pathologies. In *International Congress Series 2001;* Vol. 1230 pp 240–247.
11. Murphy MJ: The importance of computed tomography slice thickness in radiographic patient positioning for radiosurgery. **Med Physics** 26(2):171–175, 1999.
12. Murphy M, Adler JR, Bodduluri M, Dooley J, Forster K, Hai J, Le Q, Luxton G, Martin D, Poen J: Image-guided radiosurgery for the spine and pancreas. *Computer-Aided Surgery* 5(4), 278–288, 2000.
13. Schweikard A, Bodduluri M, Adler JR: Planning for camera-guided robotic radiosurgery. **IEEE Trans Robotics Automation**14(6):951–962, 1998
14. Mehta VK, Le QL, Chang SD, et al: Fractionated image-guided stereotactic radiosurgery for lesions in proximity to the anterior visual pathways. Submitted for publication to **J Rad Onc Phys Med,** 2001.
15. Ryu SI, Kim DH, Murphy MJ, Le Q, Martin DP, Chang SD: Image-guided frameless robotic stereotactic radiosurgery to spinal lesions. **Neurosurgery,** in press, 2001.
16. Maciunas RJ, Galloway RL Jr, Latimer JW: The application accuracy of stereotactic frames. **Neurosurgery** 35:682–695, 1994.

7

Endovascular Tools for the Neurosurgeon

ROBERT H. ROSENWASSER, M.D.

INTRODUCTION

Vascular neurosurgery is in evolution, as are many other subspecialties, as new and minimally invasive techniques evolve. This parallels other subspecialties of neurosurgery, such as image guidance for tumor surgery, instrumentation and understanding of biomechanics and spinal surgery, and the application of radiosurgical techniques to the armamentarium of the neurosurgeon. There is no question that the nature of the vascular neurosurgical practice is changing. Our philosophy has been disease-oriented rather than procedure-oriented, with the purpose being to grasp and master all of the tools necessary to treat the particular disorder.

The question to be asked is what tools and skills are necessary to completely treat cerebrovascular disease. It is known that the tools and skills of the cerebrovascular physician and surgeon include basic neurosurgical skills, critical care medicine, a complete knowledge of medical therapy of ischemic and hemorrhagic disease and hence, to become a "stroke doctor." The tools and skills of the cerebrovascular physician and surgeon include the aneurysm clip and the bipolar for extraluminal approaches to intracranial cerebrovascular disease and spinal vascular disease. Other tools such as coils, balloons, liquid embolic materials, and stents have become cornerstones in the endovascular management of these same diseases. Overlaps exist to other subspecialties of neurosurgery to master techniques of cortical mapping for AVM resection and to enhance the safety and reduce morbidity. Stereotactic radiosurgery has clearly found its place in the armamentarium of certain vascular diseases of the central nervous system.

The environment of the neurovascular surgeon has become well-known in terms of the operating room, the operating microscope, and microsurgical tools, but intraoperative angiography has also become very important in the neurosurgical operating theatre *(Fig. 7.1)*. Tools which are very common include the array of aneurysm clips and appliers, which have become essential and invaluable in treating very

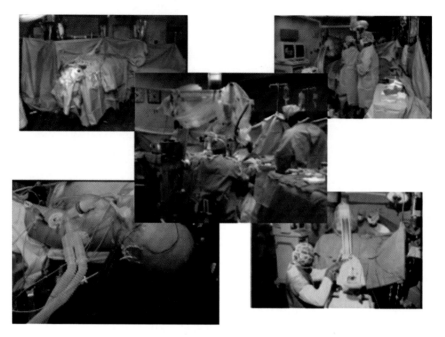

FIG. 7.1 The environment that neurovascular surgeons are at home in: The operating microscope and the operating room set up for intraoperative angiography.

complex aneurysms and arteriovenous malformations of the central nervous system *(Fig. 7.2)*.

However, a new operating room environment has become essential to treat cerebrovascular disease. Biplane digital angiography has made endovascular navigation safe. In addition, it is necessary for the cerebrovascular surgeon who decides to embark on this new specialty to learn a completely new set of tools and skills. Knowledge of radiation physics and radiation biology are essential in understanding and dealing with this very useful but potentially very dangerous equipment *(Fig. 7.3)*. Just as the classically trained vascular neurosurgeon is familiar with all of the microsurgical instrumentation, liquid embolic materials such as N-butyl cyanoacrylate and other embolic materials are the new set of tools. In place of clip appliers and clips, there is an array of syringes used to mix the embolic material to various concentrations prior to an injection into an arteriovenous malformation. Most of the time endovascular surgeons are using dilute concentrations of NbCA in order to permeate the nidus and close the pedicle of an arteriovenous malformation. The setup is very similar at most institutions and is illustrated in *Fig. 7.4*. Microcatheter technology has al-

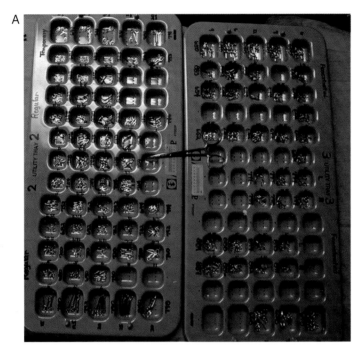

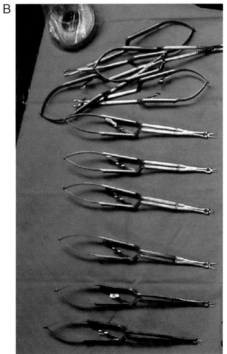

FIG. 7.2 Tools of the trade: Aneurysm clip assortment and clip appliers.

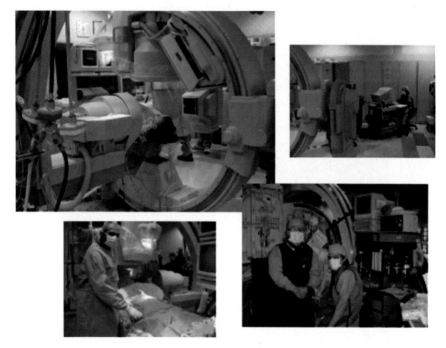

FIG. 7.3 The new operating room environment: A new view into the central nervous
system with a new set of tools to combat the enemy. Biplane digital angiography unit
with rotational capabilities.

lowed navigation into the distal cerebral circulation. Systems can be
either wire-driven systems or flow-directed catheters and range in size
from 0.01 mm to 0.18 mm in their external diameter *(Fig. 7.5)*.

The treatment of arteriovenous malformations has progressed to the
point that small numbers of these malformations may now even be
cured with embolic intervention. *Fig. 7.6* illustrates a parasagittal arteriovenous malformation embolized with N-butyl cyanoacrylate and
cured, based on a 6-week follow-up angiogram. This is a rare event,
however, and occurs only approximately 10% of the time. The goal in
this patient was to embolize prior to surgery; however, with aggressive embolization the lesion was able to be cured *(Figs. 7.6 and 7.7)*.
One must be cautious in assuming complete cure and it is advised that
all patients come back for additional follow-up to be certain that recanalization has not taken place. This becomes even more of a concern when dilute glue mixtures are utilized.

Balloon and stent technology has become useful in the treatment of
cervical carotid disease, both for traumatic stenosis and atheroscle-

LIQUID EMBOLIC MATERIALS

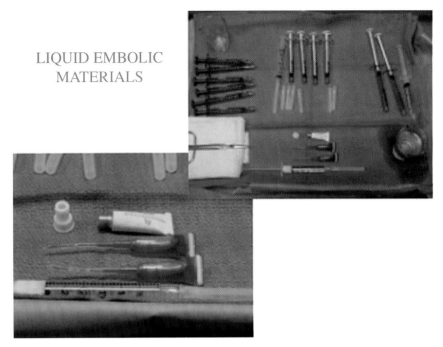

FIG. 7.4 Liquid embolic materials, NbCA, and the array of syringes used to mix the material to various concentrations prior to injection into an AVM. Most endovascular surgeons use 10% to 30% concentrations in order to permeate the nidus and close the pedicle. For fistulae, a much higher concentration is often used for a faster polymerization rate.

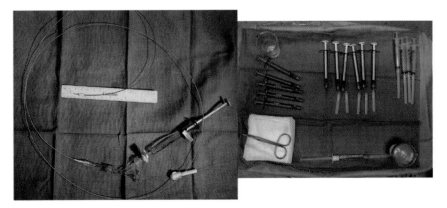

FIG. 7.5 Microcatheter technology allows navigation into the distal cerebral circulation. Systems are wire-driven and flow-directed. The sizes vary from 0.10 to 0.18 external diameter.

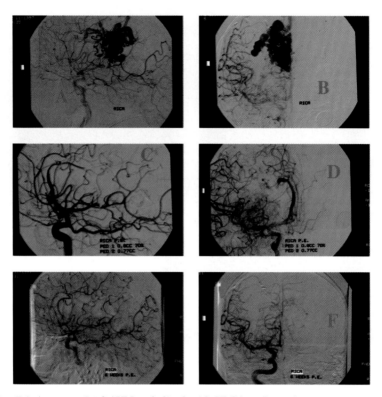

Fig. 7.6 A parasagittal AVM embolized with NbCA and cured – a rare event occurring approximately 10% of the time. This was initially a presurgical embolization, but even a 6-week follow-up demonstrated no shunting. (*A and B*) Midarterial phase demonstrating arteriovenous malformation, AP, lateral. (*C and D*) Immediate postembolization demonstrating complete obliteration of the AVM. Posterior circulation injection also demonstrated no filling of the lesion. (*E and F*) 6-week follow-up confirming complete obliteration of the lesion.

rotic disease in patients who may not be candidates for open surgical correction of their high grade symptomatic or asymptomatic lesion. *Fig. 7.8* illustrates examples of self-expanding stents used in the cervical carotid circulation and proximal intracranial circulation. *Fig. 7.9* illustrates examples of noncompliant balloon systems utilized in angioplasty procedures both of the extracranial circulation and the intracranial circulation.

Angioplasty for cerebral vasospasm has become a useful modality in treating one of the most common causes of in-hospital neurologic morbidity following aneurysmal subarachnoid hemorrhage and successful correction of the offending lesion either by transcranial sur-

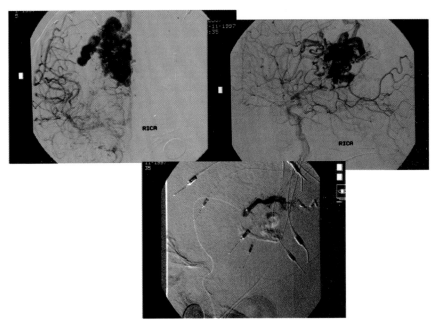

FIG. 7.7 The lower image demonstrates the glue cast in the AVM.

gery or endovascular means. *Fig. 7.10* illustrates examples of wire-driven and flow-directed balloon systems utilized in intracranial angioplasty for cerebral vasospasm or lesions of atherosclerotic origin.

Clearly one of the major revolutions in the treatment of aneurysmal

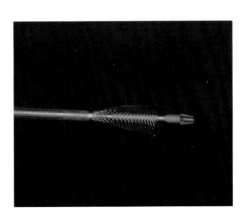
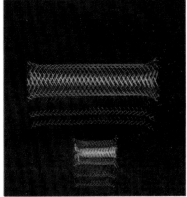

FIG. 7.8 Examples of self-expanding stents used in the cervical carotid circulation and proximal intracranial vessels.

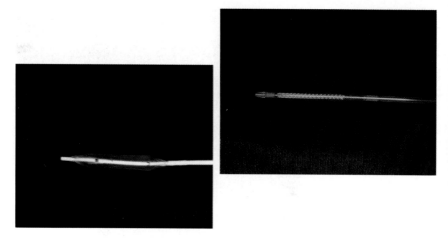

FIG. 7.9 Examples of noncompliant balloon systems utilized in angioplasty procedures.

subarachnoid hemorrhage has been the development of the Guglielmi detachable coil. This is the first device that can be safely delivered into an aneurysm through a microcatheter based delivery system and detached *(Figs. 7.11 and 7.12).* If the placement is not suitable, the coil material can be withdrawn prior to detachment and replaced with a different size or shape coil. Coils come in various 3-D configurations,

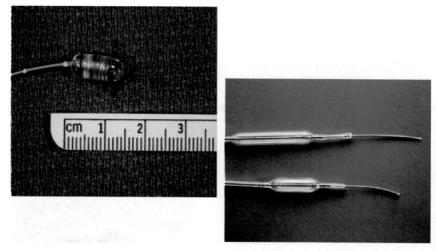

FIG. 7.10 Examples of wire-driven and flow-directed balloon systems utilized in intracranial angioplasty for cerebral vasospasm and atherosclerotic occlusive disease.

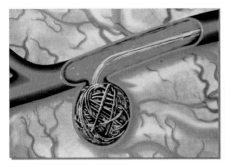
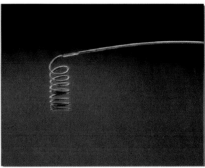

FIG. 7.11 A revolution in the treatment of intracranial aneurysms: An illustration of Guglielmi detachable coils in an artist's representation of a treated aneurysm. The coil shown in its unsheathed state.

2-D configurations and stiffness from what is termed a standard coil to an ultrasoft variety. *Fig. 7.13* illustrates a patient with a wide neck basilar aneurysm treated with what is termed balloon remodeling technique in order to create a neck and help to contain the coil complex. Although the use of endovascular coils is controversial in the treat-

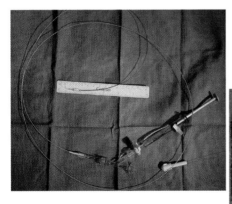
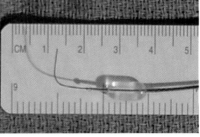

FIG. 7.12 The new tool/technique for cerebral vasospasm, which is now the leading cause of death and disability in patients surviving to treatment.

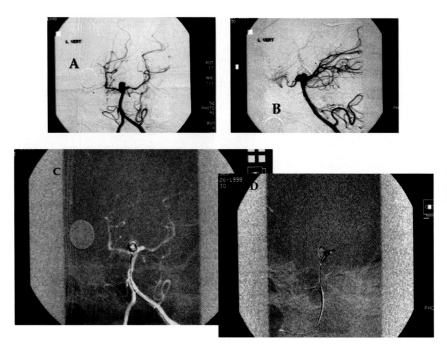

FIG. 7.13 (*A and* B) A patient with a wide-necked basilar apex aneurysm treated with "balloon remodeling technique" to create a neck to help contain the coil complex. (*C*) Prolapse of the coil complex into the parent vessel. (*D*) The balloon is inflated in the left P1 segment during coil deployment.

ment of aneurysmal subarachnoid hemorrhage, certain subpopulations of patients are being defined as benefiting from this modality of treatment. Elderly patients or patients in poor neurological grade are currently the patients most commonly treated with this modality. As the technology improves, younger patients and patients of good neurological grade are also currently being treated with this modality. Problematic is the occurrence of recanalization of these aneurysms and extensive follow-up must be carried out, generally with angiography at 6 and 18 months or MRI angiography with or without gadolinium. Aggressive re-treatment of recurrence is essential to prevent re-hemorrhage. *Fig. 7.14* illustrates the preoperative and postoperative images of a patient treated with the endovascular technique and balloon remodeling.

Stent assisted coiling of aneurysms is something that has been popularized recently. There are no dedicated intracranial stents, therefore coronary stents have been used, not only for occlusive disease but for aneurysm therapy, to bridge broad-necked aneurysms and certain fusiform lesions. *Fig. 7.15* illustrates a patient who presented with a

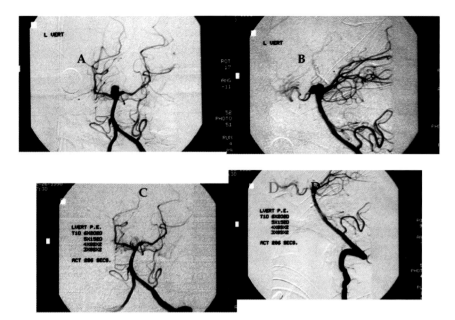

FIG. 7.14 (*A and B*) Pretreatment AP and lateral angiograms. (*C and D*) Postoperative AP and lateral images with the activated clotting time indicating full anticoagulation and no filling of the aneurysm.

STENT ASSISTED
COILING

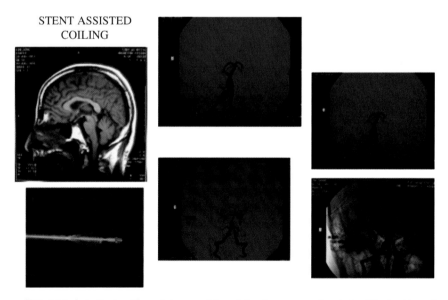

FIG. 7.15 A patient with an intracranial vertebral aneurysm treated with stenting of the vessel followed by coiling through the stent. Use of coronary stents intracranially for occlusive disease and aneurysm Rx. Stents are currently in trial for intracranial use. (*A*) MRI demonstrating the lesion with thrombus. (*B and C*) Preoperative AP and lateral angiograms. (*D and E*) The post-treatment angiogram and the nonsubtracted image. (*F*) A partially deployed self-expanding stent.

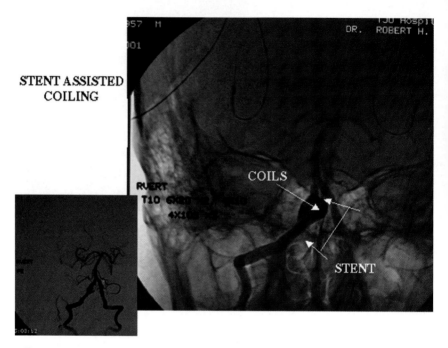

STENT ASSISTED
COILING

FIG. 7.16 Enlarged view of the stent crossing the neck of the aneurysm with coils in the aneurysm.

subarachnoid hemorrhage from an intracranial vertebral aneurysm treated with stenting across the lesion, followed by coiling through the interstices of the stent. *Fig. 7.16* is the enlarged view of the stent crossing the neck of the aneurysm with the coils within the aneurysm thereby avoiding sacrifice of this vessel.

Another example is in *Fig. 7.17,* which shows a patient with a basilar trunk aneurysm, clearly a lesion that would have significant surgical morbidity with an open surgical procedure. This is treated with a coronary stent across the neck of the aneurysm which encompasses 180 degrees of the basilar artery below the superior cerebellar system. Panels C and D in Fig. 7.17 illustrate the placement of the stent, which is a balloon expandable stent, placed across the neck of the aneurysm. *Fig. 7.18* illustrates the final result after the stent has been deployed and the lesion coiled through the interstices of the stent, resulting in occlusion of the aneurysm and preservation of the parent vessel. Follow-up of these patients is clearly essential to determine if recanalization will occur.

Intracranial thrombolysis is an advance in the treatment of occlusive disease due not only to atherosclerotic lesions but also embolic

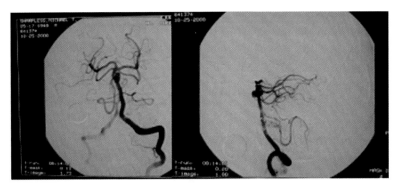

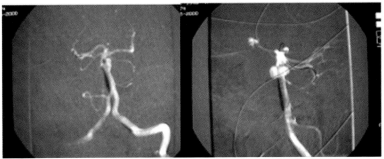

FIG. 7.17 Patient with a basilar trunk aneurysm treated with placement of a stent across the neck of the aneurysm and coiled through the cells of the stent. (*A and B*) AP and lateral angiograms demonstrating the aneurysm of the basilar trunk below the superior cerebellar arteries. (*C and D*) AP and lateral views showing the stent being deployed by balloon inflation.

events. *Fig. 7.19* illustrates a patient who presented with a right hemiplegia with a known left internal carotid artery occlusion. The patient's left hemisphere was being supplied through the anterior communicating artery and, due to a cervical carotid lesion, an embolic event occurred with blockage of the anterior communicating artery as illustrated in Fig. 7.19 AP and lateral views. *Fig. 7.20* illustrates the right common carotid angiogram demonstrating a high grade stenosis with an ulcer. The patient was treated with angioplasty and then stent placement to recanalize and reopen the cervical carotid circulation. *Fig. 7.21* illustrates progressive reopening of the cerebral circulation using intraarterial TPA and Reopro, which is a 2 beta 3 platelet antagonist.

Certain advances have been made in problematic cases of subarachnoid hemorrhage. *Fig. 7.22* illustrates a 50-year-old patient who presented on day 7 after a subarachnoid hemorrhage from an anterior

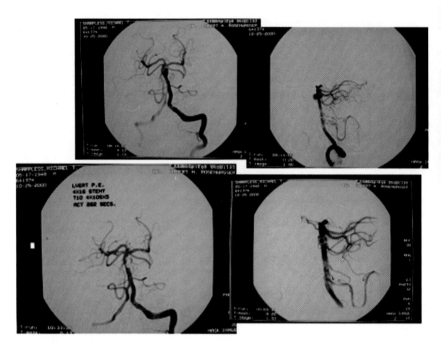

FIG. 7.18 (*A and B*) Preoperative AP and lateral angiograms. (*C and D*) Postoperative AP and lateral angiograms.

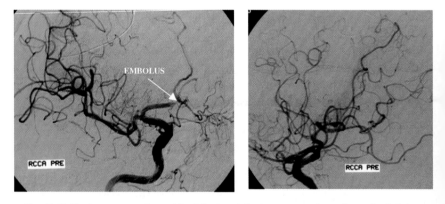

FIG. 7.19 Patient presenting with right hemiplegia, source of supply to the left hemisphere, occluded at ACOM by embolus from a right internal carotid stenosis. (*A*) AP oblique view. (*B*) Lateral view.

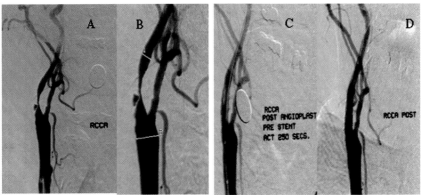

FIG. 7.20 (*A and B*) Pretreatment lateral images. (*C*) Post angioplasty, pre stent deployment. (*D*) Post stent placement.

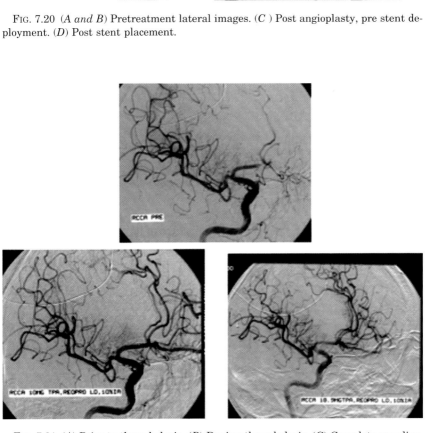

FIG. 7.21 (*A*) Prior to thrombolysis. (*B*) During thrombolysis. (*C*) Complete canalization of ACOM and contralateral circulation utilizing TPA and Reopro.

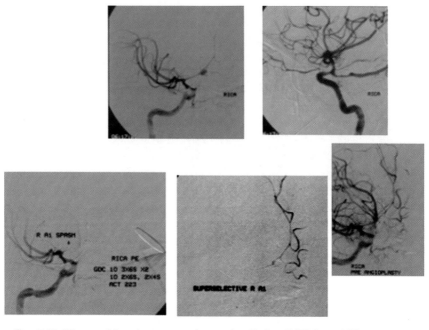

FIG. 7.22 50-year-old patient presenting on day 7 after SAH from ACOM aneurysm. Treated with endovascular occlusion of the aneurysm and angioplasty to treat the spasm at the same sitting. (*A and B*) Right oblique view and right lateral view. (*C*) The microcatheter occluding the A1 segment during the coiling procedure. (*D and E*) Superselective angiogram after coiling, prior to angioplasty.

communicating artery aneurysm. From an anatomical standpoint, this would be a fairly straightforward surgical case but, due to the fact that she had significant cerebral vasospasm, the decision was made to treat the aneurysm and the vasospasm at the same sitting. A case could be made for surgery followed by immediate angioplasty and that is certainly a reasonable approach. Panels A and B in Fig. 7.22 illustrate the preoperative angiogram. Panel C illustrates that with catheterization of the A1 segment, there is complete occlusion of the anterior cerebral circulation due to the vasospasm. Panel B illustrates a superselective angiogram performed in the distal A1 segment demonstrating occlusion of the aneurysm and preservation of the distal cerebral circulation. This was followed by progressive angioplasty as illustrated in *Fig. 7.23*. Panel B is the fluoroscopic image of the coil complex within the aneurysm and the balloon in the A1 segment over the wire system. Panel C and D illustrate the postoperative angiogram demonstrating complete occlusion of the aneurysm and improvement in the cerebral circulation after angioplasty.

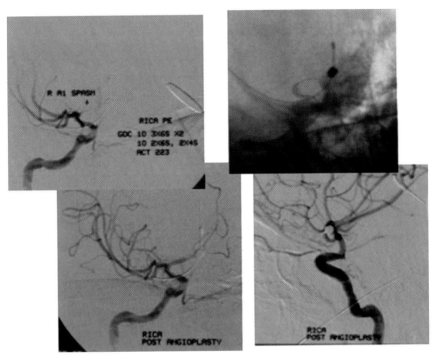

FIG. 7.23 *(A)* Right oblique view post coiling and pre angioplasty. *(B)* Fluoroscopic image showing the coiled aneurysm and the angioplasty balloon in the A1 segment. *(C and D)* Oblique and lateral images post coiling and post angioplasty.

ENDOVASCULAR TRAINING

The ACGME has established Fellowship training requirements, which have been agreed upon by the RRC in Neurosurgery and the RRC in Radiology *(Fig. 7.24)*. Residents who complete a neurosurgical program must have completed 12 consecutive months of neuroradiology, catheter skills, radiobiology and physics. This may be acquired during the elective time during residency training. Residents who decide to pursue this specialty from a radiology program must have completed an ACGME approved residency in radiology followed by 12 months of neuroradiology. The Fellowship in endovascular surgery for the neuroradiologist also requires three months of clinical neurosurgery and intensive care management.

The question has arisen whether individuals can pursue both open microsurgical training and endovascular training. The Fellowship at Thomas Jefferson University is a 2-year Fellowship which encompasses both microsurgical training and endovascular training. *Fig.*

ENDOVASCULAR TRAINING

RESIDENTS—NEUROSURGERY

- 1 COMPLETED ACGME ACCREDITED RESIDENCY IN NEUROLOGICAL SURGERY
- 2. COMPLETED 12 MONTHS, PREFERABLY CONSECUTIVE, OF NEURORADIOLOGY, CATHETER SKILLS, RADIOBIOLOGY, PHYSICS. MAY BE ACQUIRED DURING ELECTIVE TIME DURING RESIDENCY TRAINING

RESIDENTS—RADIOLOGY

- 1. ACGME RESIDENCY IN RADIOLOGY
- 2. 12 MONTHS NEUROBIOLOGY
- 3. MONTHS OF CLINICAL NEUROSURGERY

FIG. 7.24 ACGME requirements for fellowship training.

Case Record for Thomas R. Forget, Jr., MD
Cerebrovascular/Interventional Neuroradiology Fellow
Thomas Jefferson/Wills Eye Hospital July 15, 1999-Sept 8, 2000

Craniotomies with Intra-operative Angiograms

ANEURYSMS (83)
    ACOM-21
    MCA-26
    ICA Bifurcation-7
    PCOM-16
    OPHTHALMIC-6
    BASILAR-1
    PICA-4
    SCA-1
    PERICALLOSAL-1
AVM-3

MENINGIOMAS-3

TRAUMA-6

Cranioplasty-5

Carotid Endarterectomy-11

Chiari Decompression-1

Spinal AVF-1

TSH-3

Glycerol Rhizotomy-3

VPS-23

LP Shunt-1

Evacuation Cerebellar Hematoma-6

Exposure superior division Ophthalmic Vein-2

Endovascular Case Record for Thomas R. Forget, Jr., MD
Cerebrovascular/Interventional Neuroradiology Fellow
Thomas Jefferson/Wills Eye Hospital July 15, 1999-Sept 8, 200

Diagnostic Angiograms

Cerebral-105
Spinal-3

GDC Coiling Aneurysm (64)

PCOM-13
ACOM-16
BASILAR-14
PICA-3
MCA-3
AICA-1
ICA BIFURCATION-4
OPHTHALMIC-5
SCA-1
PCA-2
VERT-2
C-C Fistula-4

Balloon Assist-2

Angioplasty For Vasospasm-8

Agram for GAMMA Knife of AVM-8

Angioplasty & Stenting (7)
    Carotid-4
    Vertebral-3

Temporary Balloon Occlusion-7

Detachable Balloon for Spinal AVF-1

Embolization
    AVM-21
    Tumor-3
    Spinal AVF-1
    Epistaxsis-2
    Vein of Galen-2

FIG. 7.25 Data of fellow indicating numbers of surgical and endovascular cases.

Subject: stats
   Date: Fri, 8 Sep 2000 02:39:03 +0000
From: ron_benitez@hotmail.com
    To: robert.h.rosenwasser@mail.tju.edu

```
Dr. R
   Here are my stats for the period 1/1/2000-9/7/2000.

Crani
   aneurysm- 46
   AVM- 4
CEA- 8

GDC- 27
Embo
   AVM- 19
   Tumor- 2
diagnostic agrams- 58
IVC filter- 6
epistaxis- 2
TBO- 6
PBO- 3
Thrombolysis- 3
angioplasty for spasm- 4
carotid stent- 7
gamma knife foe AVM- 11
```

FIG. 7.26 Data of fellow indicating numbers of surgical and endovascular cases.

7.25 indicates the data of previous fellows and the types of cases they have performed both from a microsurgical standpoint and endovascular intervention. With proper training, individuals can pursue both areas if they desire but, obviously, competency must be maintained by performing adequate numbers of both types of procedures once they finish their training and enter practice *(Fig. 7.26)*. This is no different from any other type of procedure, where competency is maintained based on volume.

SUMMARY

In summary, the treatment of cerebrovascular disease is markedly changing and neurosurgeons interested in this area of neurosurgery must adapt and evolve. This requires mastering a new set of tools and skills; however, the future is very bright for vascular neurosurgery, interventional neuroradiology and most importantly, our patients.

BIBLIOGRAPHY

Armonda RA, Thomas JE, Rosenwasser RH: Therapeutic options for endovascular therapy for intracranial aneurysms. **Neurosurg Focus** 5: 4, 1998.

Adams HP Jr, Brott TG, Furlan AJ, et al: Guidelines for thrombolytic therapy for acute stroke: a supplement to the guidelines for the management of patients with acute ischemic stroke. A statement for healthcare professionals from a Special Writing Group of the Stroke Council, American Heart Association. **Circulation** 94: 1167–1174, 1996.

Albuquerque FC, Teitelbaum GP, Giannotta SL: Carotid angioplasty and stenting in high-risk patients [abstract]. **Neurosurgery** 43: 685, 1998.

Barnwell SL, Higashida RT, Halbach VV, et al: Transluminal angioplasty of intracerebral vessels for cerebral arterial spasm: Reversal of neurological deficits after delayed treatment. **Neurosurgery** 25: 424–429, 1989.

Brown RD, Wiebers DO, Forbes G, et al: The natural history of unruptured intracranial arteriovenous malformations. **J Neurosurg** 68: 352–357, 1988.

Brown RD, Wiebers DO, Forbes G: Unruptured intracranial aneurysms and arteriovenous malformations: Frequency of intracranial hemorrhage and relationship of lesions. **J Neurosurg** 73: 859–863, 1990.

Crawford PM, West CR, Chadwick DW, et al: Arteriovenous malformations of the brain: Natural history in unoperated patients. **J Neurol Neurosurg Psychiatry** 49: 1–10, 1986.

Debrun G, Vinuela F, Fox A, et al: Embolization of cerebral arteriovenous malformations with bucrylate. **J Neurosurg** 56: 615–627, 1982.

del Zoppo GJ: Thrombolytic therapy in the treatment of stroke. **Drugs** 54(suppl 3): 90–98, discussion 98–99, 1997.

del Zoppo GJ, Ferbert A, Otis S, et al: Local intra-arterial fibrinolytic therapy in acute carotid territory stroke: A pilot study. **Stroke** 19: 307–313, 1988.

del Zoppo GJ, Higashida RT, Furlan AJ, et al: PROACT: A phase II randomized trial of recombinant pro-urokinase by direct arterial delivery in acute middle cerebral artery stroke. PROACT Investigators. Prolyse in Acute Cerebral Thromboembolism [see comments]. **Stroke** 29: 4–11, 1998.

Eskridge JM, McAuliffe W, Song JK, et al: Balloon angioplasty for the treatment of vasospasm: Results of first 50 cases. **Neurosurgery** 42: 510-516, discussion 516–517, 1998.

Eskridge JM, Song JK and Participants: Endovascular embolization of 150 basilar tip aneurysms with Gugliemli detachable coils: Results of the Food and Drug Administration multicenter clinical trial. **J Neurosurg** 89: 81–86, 1998.

Eskridge JM, Newell DW, Pendleton GA: Transluminal angioplasty for treatment of vasospasm. **Neurosurg Clin North Am** 1: 387–399, 1990.

Gobin YP, Laurent A, Merienne L, et al: Treatment of brain arteriovenous malformations by embolization and radiosurgery. **J Neurosurg** 85: 19–28, 1996.

Guglielmi G, Vinuela F, Dion J, et al: Electrothrombosis of saccular aneurysms via endovascular approach: Part 2. Preliminary clinical experience. **J Neurosurg** 75: 8–14, 1991.

Guterman LR, Budny JL, Gibbons KJ, et al: Thrombolysis of the cervical internal carotid artery before balloon angioplasty and stent placement: Report of two cases. **Neurosurgery** 38: 620–624, 1996.

Higashida RT, Halbach VV, Dowd CF, et al: Intravascular balloon dilatation therapy for intracranial arterial vasospasm: patient selection, technique, and clinical results. **Neurosurg Rev** 15: 89–95, 1992.

Higashida RT, Hieshima GB, Tsai FY, et al: Transluminal angioplasty of the vertebral and basilar artery. **AJNR** 8: 745–749, 1987.

Higashida RT, Smith W, Gress D, et al: Intravascular stent and endovascular coil place-ment for a ruptured fusiform aneurysm of the basilar artery : Case report and review of the literature. **J Neurosurg** 187: 944–949, 1997.

Joint Officers of the Congress of Neurological Surgeons and the American Association of Neurological Surgeons: Carotid angioplasty and stent: An alternative to carotid en-darterectomy. **Neurosurgery** 40: 344–345, 1997.

Kondziolka D, McLaughlin MR, Kestle JR: Simple risk predictions for arteriovenous malformation hemorrhage. **Neurosurgery** 37: 851–855, 1995.

Lanzino G, Wakhloo AK, Fessler RD, et al: Intravascular stents for intracranial inter-nal carotid and vertebral artery aneurysms: preliminary clinical experience. **Neuro-surg Focus** 5: 1998.

Lüessenhop AJ, Kachmann R, Shevolin W, et al: Clinical evaluation of artificial em-bolization in the management of large cerebral arteriovenous malformations. **J Neu-rosurg** 23: 400–417, 1965.

North American Symptomatic Endarterectomy Trial (NASCET) Collaborators: Benefi-cial effect of carotid endarterectomy in symptomatic patients with high-grade steno-sis. **N Engl J Med** 325: 445–453, 1991.

Ondra S, Troupp H, George ED, et al: The natural history of symptomatic arteriove-nous malformations of the brain: A 24 year follow-up assessment. **J Neurosurg** 73: 387–391, 1990.

Richling B: Homologous controlled viscosity fibrin for endovascular embolization: Part I. Experimental development of the medium. **Acta Neurochir** 62: 159–170, 1982.

Richling B: Homologous controlled viscosity fibrin for endovascular embolization: Part II. Catheterization technique, animal experiments. **Acta Neurochir** 64: 109–124, 1982.

Richling B: The current state in endovascular treatment of cerebral arteriovenous mal-formations. In Aichinger F, Gerstenbrand F, Grcevic N, et al (eds): *Neuroimaging II.* New York: Gustav Fisher, 1988, pp 309–315.

Rosenwasser RH, Thomas JE, Gannon P, et al: Management of cerebral vasospasm: timing of endovascular options [abstract]. **J Neurosurg** 88: 386, 1998.

Spetzler RF, Martin NA, Carter LP, et al: Surgical management of large AVMs by staged embolization and operative excision. **J Neurosurg** 67: 17–28, 1987.

Sundt TM Jr, Sandock BA, Whisnant JP: Carotid endarterectomy: Complications and preoperative assessment of risk. **Mayo Clin Proc** 50: 301–306, 1975.

Thomas JE, Armonda RA, Rosenwasser RH: Endosaccular thrombosis of cerebral aneurysms: Strategy, indications and technique. **Neurosurg Clin North Am** 11(1): 101–121, 2000.

Vinuela F, Duckwiler G, Guglielmi G, et al: Intravascular embolization of brain arteri-ovenous malformations. In Maciunas RJ (ed): *Endovascular Neurological Interven-tion.* Park Ridge, IL: The American Association of Neurological Surgeons, 1995, pp 189–199.

Vinuela F, Duckwiler G, Mawad M: Guglielmi detachable coil embolization of acute in-tracranial aneurysm: Perioperative anatomical and clinical outcome in 403 patients. **J Neurosurg** 86: 475–482, 1997.

Willinsky RH, Lasjaunias P, TerBrugge K, et al: Brain arteriovenous malformations: Analysis of the angioarchitecture in relationship to hemorrhage. **J Neuroradiol** 15: 225–237, 1988.

Yadav JS, Roubin GS, Iyer S, et al: Elective Stenting of the extracranial arteries. **Cir-culation** 95: 376–381, 1997.

8

Neurosurgical Robotics

PATRICK J. KELLY, M.D., F.A.C.S.

INTRODUCTION

At the 1939 World's Fair, Westinghouse unveiled Electro. Electro was what was then called a "Mechanical Man"—a robot controlled by relays and actuators. Electro couldn't do much. He could keep up a verbal repartee as long as the answers were prerecorded. He could turn his head and respond to gross visual stimuli by means of "electric eyes"—photovoltaic cells. Electro could also walk along a short track. And he could smoke a cigarette.

In 1940, Westinghouse provided Electro with a companion: a robotic dog named "Sparko." Sparko did little more than raise up on hind legs, turn its head, and bark. Neither of these robots had any practical use whatsoever. They were for entertainment value only. And they were a "hit" in this regard. Nonetheless, that they existed at all was tribute to the ingenuity of the electronic engineers at the time. All of this was possible without a host computer—something inherent in today's robotic devices. The Electronic Numerical Integrator and Calculator or ENIAC was not developed until 1946.

The public's fascination with robots continued. Robots became heroes or villains in science fiction stories, books, and movies. These had either human form or at least human attributes. Technology, however, was not, and is still not, up to the creation of complex machines that would simulate biological systems.

ROBOTS IN INDUSTRY

As computers became more powerful and less expensive in the 1970s, simple robotic applications became practical for straightforward industrial applications. A series of four basic robot designs developed as illustrated in *Fig. 8.1*.

PERSONNEL ROBOTS

In a joint venture between the companies Unimation and Kawasaki, the Japanese were the first to develop and exploit practical industrial

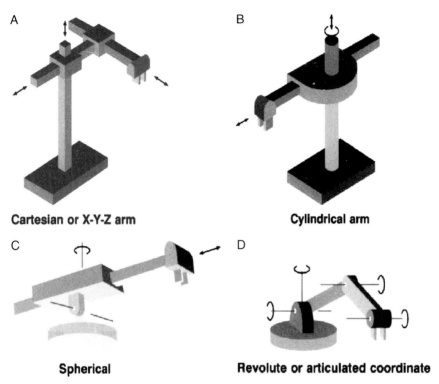

A

Cartesian or X-Y-Z arm

B

Cylindrical arm

C

Spherical

D

Revolute or articulated coordinate

FIG. 8.1 Four robotic types. Each employs Cartesian or polar coordinate systems to define the work envelope.

robots. In their factories, robots performed menial repetitive tasks on assembly lines, freed humans from these tasks but put them out of jobs. By reducing manufacturing labor costs, particularly in the automobiles and electronics industries, Japanese companies were able to compete successfully in the international marketplace by supplying superior products at lower costs. To remain competitive, other nations had to scramble to catch up in the automation of their factories.

Personnel costs are a significant expense in the operating budget of most companies, particularly in the service industry. This includes hospitals. The average hospital allocates 75% of its annual budget for employee salaries and benefits. Some of this expense could be reduced by robotics in food service, cleaning, and nursing to deliver patient meals and collect trays, clean floors and pass medications, respectively. Robots could also pass surgical instruments, as illustrated in *Fig. 8.2.*

In laporoscopic applications such as cholecystectomy, robots are already being used to replace the surgical assistant who must keep the

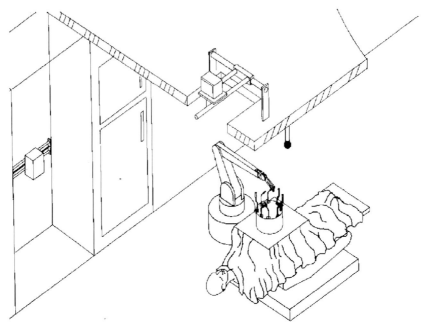

FIG. 8.2 Voice activated robotic scrub "nurse" which would pass specific instruments to a surgeon based on voice commands. This is similar to a tool server used on industrial assembly lines.

endoscope aligned with the area of interest within the surgical field as shown in *Fig. 8.3*. Studies have shown that robots can do this task occasionally better and certainly cheaper than a human assistant.

ACCURACY AND PRECISION

Stereotactic surgery experienced a renaissance in the early 1980s with the incorporation of computer-based medical imaging; particularly computed tomography and magnetic resonance imaging. These modalities provided precise three-dimensional datasets which could be used to guide biopsies and even open stereotactic procedures for tumors and other intracranial pathologies. Stereotactic frames employed a coordinate system as o robots and these provided an accurate method for translating between imaging defined three-dimensional space and the real-world space of the patient on the operating table.

However, stereotactic frames were cumbersome when imaging-based stereotactic surgical procedures extended beyond simple point-in-space target applications such as tumor biopsy to procedures which considered a target volume and hundreds or even thousands of points (voxels) in space. Computer interactive frameless stereotactic devices were less cumbersome but less accurate (application accuracies on the order of 3 to 5 mm). Industrial robots, on the other hand, easily dealt with volumetric tasks within a defined work envelope. Registration issues aside, robots had accuracy and repeatability specifications measured in microns (typically plus/minus 25 microns). One logical step, therefore, was to adapt industrial robots to human stereotactic surgery.

"Off the shelf" robots have been used as stereotactic frames for the biopsy and the resection of intracranial tumors (10, 29). These efforts did not persist for practical reasons, including significant safety issues. It was an industry standard that no human being should be within the work envelope of an operational robot as the possibility of malfunction and personal injury. Industrial robots are powerful devices built for the rapid movement of heavy payloads. A computer glitch could send the robotic arm to one of the outer rings of Saturn as it passed through the patient's or the surgeon's skull! It soon became clear that industrial robots had to be modified significantly or totally redesigned before they would be suitable for human surgery.

The COMPASS system *(Fig. 8.4)* was one of the first purpose-built human stereotactic robots (16). It comprised a simple Cartesian (X,Y

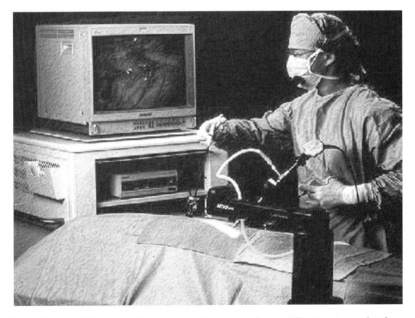

FIG. 8.3 Aesop (Automated Endoscopic System for Optimal Positioning) robot has replaced endoscope holding assistant in this laparoscopic abdominal procedure.(Courtesy Computer Motion, Goleta, Ca).

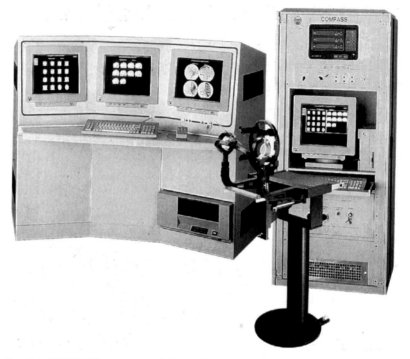

FIG. 8.4 COMPASS system consisting of 3 screen workstation, control rack and three dimension Cartesian robotic slide with fixed arc quadrant. (Courtesy COMPASS International, Inc., Rochester, Minnesota).

and Z) mechanical slide which moved the patient's head within a fixed arc quadrant. The stereotactic coordinates were set on the slide by computer-activated stepper motors. These moved the headholder by means of worm gears. Optical encoders provided feedback of stereotactic coordinates to the host computer which also functioned as an imaging-based surgical planning workstation. A mechanical backup was also a feature: the worm gears could be turned by hand cranks; the stereotactic coordinates could be read off mechanical scales on the three axes.

There were other stereotactic robotic systems. These included the IMMI robot system developed in Grenoble, France (2, 3). This featured an articulated coordinate robotic system with a significant speed scale down for safety reasons. The system provided a convenient interaction with a preoperative imaging database.

Robots could also hold an operating microscope in a known position in stereotactic space (*Fig. 8.5*) (16, 22). An indexing registration system was used to translate the coordinate systems of the robot's work envelope, the patient's head and the imaging database. "Heads-up"

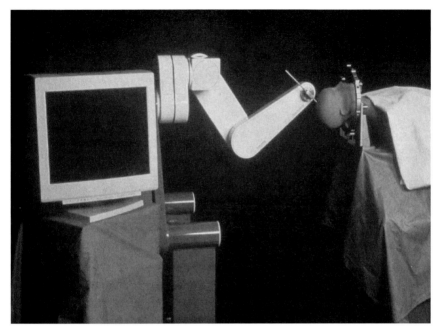

FIG. 8.5 NeuroMate stereotactic robotic system developed by Benebid and colleagues at the University of Grenoble. This features an articulated arm and frame-based or frameless registration by means of skull mounted fiducials. (Courtesy Integrated Surgical Systems, Inc.; Davis, Ca)

display units on the robot mounted microscope superimposed a computer generated image of the patient's tumor (interpolated from the imaging database) over the actual surgical field viewed through the microscope. Prototype systems were developed by our group (16), the Grenoble group, and others. The Grenoble group, working with a French robotics company, developed a new robot type: the so-called spider robot , which provided increased accuracy and safety *(Fig. 8.6)*.

Commercial versions of this concept have been employed at several institutions with reported success. As with any frameless stereotactic system, however, registration is the key issue in determining accuracy.

TEDIOUS TASKS

The most common use of robotics in industry is the performance of tedious repetitive tasks such as moving a part from a storage bin to a conveyor belt, painting, or welding. These tasks, which are usually too boring for human workers, are perfect for robots, which will do

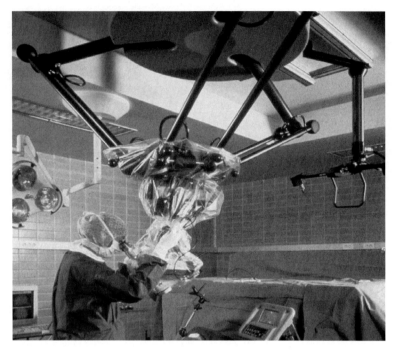

FIG. 8.6 The spider robot, originally introduced by DeeMed, now marketed as the Surgiscope by another vendor. The microscope is indexed to the patient's head by means of a LED sensor system. (Courtesy of Elekta, Inc; Atlanta, Ga.)

them well over and over again. Although neurosurgical procedures nay have some aspects which are tedious, few of these are repetitive.

A BLIND ALLEY

In 1982 our group reported a computer-assisted stereotactic technique in which a subcortical tumor was vaporized using a CO2 LASER beam directed from a 400 mm radius stereotactic arc quadrant. The position of the laser was also computer monitored on a display of computer slice images reformatted from stereotactic CT scan slices. The original technique called for slice by slice vaporization with a defocused LASER beam progressing from the most superficial tumor slice to the deepest. Inspired by a cloth-cutting robot used in the garment industry (Hart, Scaffner, and Marks), we fashioned a computer-controlled system in which the LASER would scan the tumor based on the computer slice images *(Fig. 8.7)*.

The so-called Kelly-Goerss system worked flawlessly in tests. However, in surgery, the LASER started up bleeding and had to be stopped in order coagulate the vessel manually. This wasted time. Because of

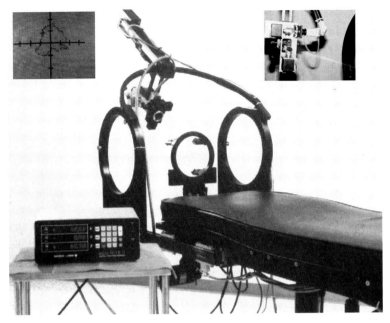

FIG. 8.7 The Kelly-Goerss robotic LASER system in which a CO2 LASER beam was directed by X, Y mirrors controlled by galvanometers whose pitch was set by the digital-to-analog output of the host computer system (Right insert). A computer program would sweep the LASER beam horizontally in X and at the edge of the CT defined tumor boundary, drop down 1 mm (the spot size) in Y and sweep back again in X. The position of the LASER beam with respect to the tumor boundary as indicated as a cursor on the computer display (insert left). A stepper motor would advance the LASER manipulator one millimeter when the LASER had covered the entire slice, the next tumor target slice was displayed by the computer and the process would begin again.

the fact that surgery took longer with the robotic system than without, and that the result was no better than surgery done manually with simple image guidance, it was determined that the system would never be practical and this effort was abandoned.

In fact, few tasks in surgery involve tedious repetitive movements—except for skull base bone removal involved in gaining the necessary surgical exposure. A specialized robotic technology may offer assistance with this task.

ROBODOC

Robots are good for performing repetitive, tedious tasks that are boring to humans. In surgery we have some tedious tasks, which lend themselves to robotic applications. In some surgical specialties, one such task is the removal of large quantities of bone.

Veterinary orthopedic surgeon Hap Paul was dismayed by the available procedures for hip replacements in dogs. He noted that the prostheses did not fit well in the cavity reamed out in the femur and that sometimes the prostheses actually fractured through the shaft of the femur. He conceived of a robotic system, which would excavate a precise cavity in the femur in which a commercial implant would fit precisely. Working in collaboration with the robotics division of IBM, he developed a system, which utilized CT data from the animal's hip joint and proximal femur. Cross-sectional images of the implant would then be positioned within reformatted CT slice data of the hip joint and this was then incorporated into a robotics routine in which a robot would guide a drill and automatically ream out the inside of the femur to fit the implant. The registration between the imaging data was achieved by surgically implanted bone fiducials. These would be digitized in the imaging dataset and registered by the robotic device before the actual drilling began.

This worked so well in dogs that he and his team proposed adapting the system for total hip surgery in humans. IBM wanted to separate itself from the substantial liability. A new company was formed to develop, test in the laboratory and clinical trials, and secure FDA clearance for the device. The new company, Integrated Surgical Systems (ISS), launched the new product called RoboDoc. This consisted of a scaled down industrial robot and a computer workstation called OrthoDoc.

The device performed well in human trials. Although slower than conventional methods for creating a cavity in the femur for a total hip prosthesis, RoboDoc achieved a perfect fit for the hip prosthesis almost every time, acrylic filler was not necessary and the incidence of femoral fractures was far lower than with conventional procedures. Nonetheless, acceptance of this device in the orthopedic surgical community has been slow in coming. This is probably due to the cost of the unit as well as the fact that the surgical procedures take longer with this instrumentation—the "kiss of death" for many promising technologies.

Nonetheless, additional applications have been proposed for RoboDoc. These include preparation of the recipient site for total knee and shoulder implant procedures. The company has tried to transfer RoboDoc applications to other surgical specialties within general hospitals. These applications are basically those which allow the robotic device to perform precise but repetitive and tedious tasks.

Neurosurgical uses have been contemplated. Much of neurosurgery is tedious and many of the tasks require precision. However, few neurosurgical tasks are repetitive and for this reason the applications of RoboDoc to neurosurgery are limited. There is, however, one possible exception—performing bone removal for skull base exposures: translabyrinthine, transcochlear, transpetrous and general temporal bone approaches. Here a surgeon would simply outline, on a stereotactic imaging study, the bone which should be removed. The robot would be registered to bone implanted fiducials. Then the robot would drill out the desired volume of bone at the skull base—automatically and precisely.

Even though the robot could also turn bone flaps, there would be little advantage in this: the robot could not do it significantly faster than a surgeon. A robot could drill out a vertebral body in spinal procedures, but it is unlikely that it could do this better or more rapidly than an experienced surgeon. It is also unlikely that a robot could be used to automatically remove a tumor until there is an automatic method for identifying and controlling bleeding.

DEXTERITY ENHANCEMENT

Important characteristics of most robots are accuracy, precision, and repeatability. In a practical sense this translates to something that robots don't have but humans do: physiological tremor. Physiologic tremor is worse in some surgeons than in others. Nonetheless, this limits our dexterity in performing fine motor tasks. In fact the best microsurgeons working with high power microscopes, forearm stabilization, and short instruments have surgical accuracies no better than 100 microns. If the length of the instruments is increased, physiologic tremor is amplified. However, the average industrial robot can provide an accuracy of 25 microns and purpose-built systems may have an accuracy of 4 microns. It is therefore probable that surgeons working through a robotic interface may be able to reduce physiologic tremor by a factor of 25 (18, 20, 27).

This may not be so important in surface microsurgical procedures where the instrument working length is short. However, the advantage of robotic dexterity enhancement will increase in direct relationship to the working distance; the deeper the surgical target and longer the surgical instruments, the greater the application potential of this technology. This may really be of advantage in endoscopic procedures where the working distance is very long. In these cases instruments are no longer manipulated by fine finger movements but by grosser control of the wrist, forearm, and elbow joints. Here physiologic tremor can be extreme and severely limits the potential of endoscopic surgery.

Dr. Steve Charles, a vitreo-retinal surgeon pointed out the possibilities of dexterity enhancement and was the first to suggest that ro-

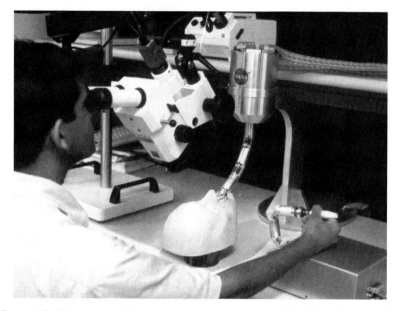

FIG. 8.8 Dr Hari Das of JPL demonstrating use of the RAMS (Robot-Assisted Micro-Surgery) system. The surgeon works at a master control unit that manipulates a slave unit holding the surgical instrument in the surgical field. (Courtesy Dr Das and Jet Propulsion Laboratory, Pasadena, Ca.)

botic interfaces may provide the solution to physiologic tremor (18). He designed a robotic system for his own work and had a prototype built by the Jet Propulsion Laboratory (JPL) in Pasadena, CA. The prototype system is shown in *Fig. 8.8*.

There were several problems with this particular unit: First, cables were used to adjust the position of the effector tip. In time the cables fatigued and the accuracy of tip positioning degraded. Secondly, there was no haptic feedback from the effector tip on the slave unit to the master controller. Thus, positioning of the surgical instrument depended solely on stereoscopic visual placement of the instrument tip in the surgical field viewed through the operating microscope. Lack of proprioceptive and touch (haptic) feedback confounded an intuitive feel to the system. Of course, surgeons could learn to use the system which relied on hand-eye coordination only.

A third short-coming of the RAMS system as regards neurosurgery was that the controller device did not have the look and feel of our usual surgical instruments. Initially the controls on the master unit seemed awkward and cumbersome. Here, again training and practice resulted in surgeons becoming more comfortable with the system (20, 27).

Finally, with no position encoders and the use of cables, it was not possible for the host computer to register the real-time position of the instrument tip within the three-dimensional work envelope of the surgical field. Similarly, the instrument tip position could not be co-registered onto a retrospective or real-time imaging database. This would not pose a problem for the original purpose of the device—canceling out hand tremor in precise microsurgical work requiring high dexterity. However, this system does ignore one of the prime possible utilities of robotics in human neurosurgery: knowing where the instrument tip is in imaging-defined stereotactic space.

REMOTE TELEMANIPULATION

Precise robotic movement of a surgical instrument by means of a slave manipulator controlled by the surgeon working at a master control can be taken one step beyond the RAMS system. In the RAMS system the surgeon views the surgical instrument directly, usually through an operating microscope, while the master control is used to move that instrument in the surgical field. By necessity, therefore, the master control unit and the slave manipulator must be within a few centimeters of each other; certainly within arm's length. The spatial limitation here is imposed by the necessity to view the surgical field directly, say, through an operating microscope. However, if the surgical field could be viewed at a distance by, for example, a direct video system or an endoscope equipped with video camera and monitor, the distance between master control unit and slave manipulator can increase from several centimeters to many miles—as far as the practical limits of the communication time between master and slave.

The concept of telerobotic surgery developed during the early stages of the space program when NASA scientist contemplating manned space stations considered the problems which could be encountered by an astronaut who developed a surgical problem such as appendicitis. The idea of a surgeon on earth manipulating a robotic "surgeon" on a space station seemed, at the time, an attractive, albeit whimsical, solution. Nonetheless, the seeds for telepresence surgery were sewn here. A simple calculation, however, revealed that the time for a signal to pass from the surface of the earth to the space station could be as long as 7 seconds. Any surgeon knows that a great deal can happen in 7 seconds and a 7 second response time would be far too slow for efficient or safe surgery (28).

Nonetheless, the remote surgery concept had down-to-earth potential in at least two specialized applications: on the battlefield and in remote geographical areas where specific surgical expertise was lacking.

ECONOMIC REALITIES AND CIVILIAN APPLICATIONS

The development of a telesurgical system for human surgery is expensive; prototype manufacture and refinement, engineering costs, software development and debugging, trial and error re-engineering, etc, can consume large amounts of money very quickly. And then there's the FDA, the cost of clinical trials, the legal fees, the re-engineering, the training of personnel, marketing, and many other daunting expenses. Projects of this type are so expensive, in fact, that few commercial ventures could undertake such a task. In addition, the civilian market for products of this nature is limited. Recovery of the development costs reflected in the purchase price would render the equipment so expensive that no civilian medical center could justify or even consider it. However, telepresence surgery was pioneered using the vast economic resources of the military and/or the federal government.

MILITARY APPLICATIONS

A casualty's chance of surviving a war wound is much better if he or she can reach the expertise available at a base hospital. In the Vietnam War over 90% of the wounded arriving at a base hospital alive survived their wounds (4, 25). Traditional cold war indoctrinated military thinking embraced the idea of having expensive highly trained surgeons at behind-the-lines base hospitals performing surgery near the front lines with the assistance of less expensive corpsmen or general medical officers.

In concept, the surgeon would manipulate controls at a workstation (a safe distance away from the fighting) and the surgery would be performed in a mobile operating room on the front lines (4, 5, 6, 25). A stereoscopic view of the surgical field would be transmitted back to the surgeon from two mobile video cameras, controlled by the surgeon, to video monitors in the control room behind the lines. The monitors were then replaced by LED (light emitting diode) goggles worn by the surgeon. The master control unit and slave surgical unit is shown in *Fig. 8.9.*

MINIMALLY INVASIVE SURGERY (MIS)

Endoscopic procedures in general surgery, gynecology, orthopedics, and urology have proven that the less invasive the procedure the better the patient does; less postoperative pain, shorter hospital stays, and faster return to work (12, 14, 23, 24). However, for the most part,

B

A

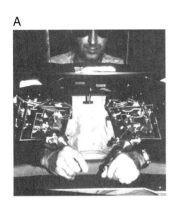
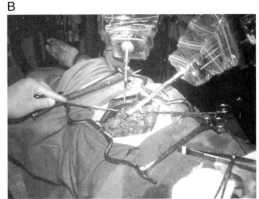

FIG. 8.9 Military-type telesurgical system with the master control unit on the left (note: LED goggles on surgeon with controls) and slave surgical init on the Right. Right and left hands of the surgeon control respective effectors of the "slave" system. (Courtesy: J. Bowersox and SRI International, Menlo Park, California.)

these procedures are usually for pathologies quite close to the surface or within large cavities such as the abdomen or chest. Surgical instruments are short and may not exaggerate a surgeon's physiological tremor. The longer the instrument, the more cumbersome and more time consuming the procedure; witness the dexterity drop in an excellent general surgeon performing a laparoscopic cholecystectomy.

With cardiac and neurosurgical procedures, reduction of dexterity at a distance would be unacceptable, and, perhaps, even dangerous. In addition, a surgeon must be able to see the surgical field, preferably with stereoscopic vision. The development of high quality endoscopes and high resolution video systems has expanded the potential of telesurgery in cardiac and, also, neurosurgery. There are two contemporary commercial systems now on the market which are pursuing cardiac and neurosurgical applications.

THE ZEUS SYSTEM

The Zeus system (Computer Motion Inc, Santa Barbara, CA), illustrated in *Fig. 8.10,* evolved from the popular and successful Aesop system, which was developed to hold the laparoscope in endoscopic procedures. The Zeus system, however, has two effector arms and a workstation with a two-dimensional screen. Its primary application is endoscopic suturing. This makes it useful in cardiac procedures such as valve replacement and coronary bypass procedures. Other disciplines also benefit from this capability: general surgery for laparo-

A   B

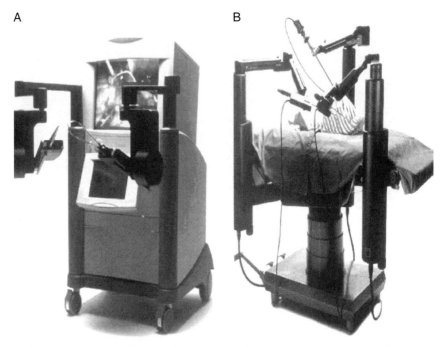

FIG. 8.10 The Zeus telesurgical system which comprises a remote surgical manipulator system with a video monitor and two 6 degrees of freedom control units on the left and the slave surgcal unit, shown on the right, with two surgical manipulator arms and a third arm which holds the endoscope.

scopic cholecystectomies and bowel resections, as well as urology for endoscopic radical prostatectomy and other operations.

In practice, the surgeon sits at a workstation and views the surgical field on a video monitor which transmits the image from an endoscope and camera held by a third robotic arm (see Fig. 8.10, right). Surgical instruments are remotely controlled by the surgeon using the two manipulators on the console of the workstation (Fig. 8.10, left). At the present time the master and slave units are usually in the same area of the operating room (but with the "surgeon here and the patient there") but the surgeon could be many feet away from the patient or in another room or in another country.

In fact, there are recent cases of a laparoscopic cholecystectomies done on a patient in France by a surgeon at a hospital in New York City and on a patient in Singapore done by a surgeon in Baltimore (8, 19). These publicity stunts not only show that such feats are possible but also demonstrate another application: telementoring—the training of surgeons at a remote location (13, 26).

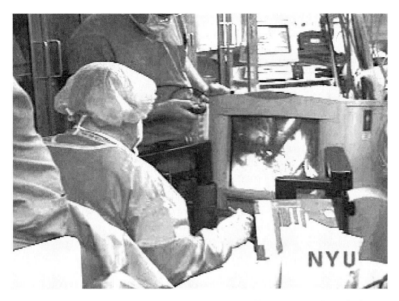

FIG. 8.11 Dr. Gene Grossi, Professor of Surgery (Cardiac) at NYU School of Medicine, performing a heart valve replacement using the Zeus system (Computer Motion, Goleta, Ca). Dr. Grossi is working in a control room with full view of the patient on the operating table. A "scrubbed" surgical team is standing-by next to the patient in the operating room.

At NYU cardiac surgeons have been using the Zeus system for cardiac valve replacements and cardiac revascularization procedures in the laboratory and on human patients *(see Fig. 8.11)*. They have also used telepresence surgery to train surgeons in mainland China. However, their experience has shown two shortcoming of the system: First, surgery is a three-dimensional exercise and the vision of the surgeon should also be stereoscopic. Certainly surgeons can train themselves to use two-dimensional visualization of the surgical field as they did with laparoscopic cholecystectomy and other procedures. However, the "learning curve" for technical competence in these procedures would be shorter and the acceptance of these new procedures quicker if new technology can duplicate the environment to which surgeons are accustomed: stereoscopic vision, haptic (force) feedback, and instruments that have the look and feel of those presently used in surgery.

THE DAVINCI SYSTEM

The DaVinci system (Intuitive Surgical Inc.; Mountain View, CA) evolved out of work done by SRI Inc. on military telesurgical systems

(4–6). It features a remote workstation and a three armed manipulator unit, similar to those of the Zeus device. However, there are three important differences: First, the surgical field is viewed through a stereoscopic endoscope. Stereoscopic vision provides depth cues which enhance the facility with which surgeons work in a surgical field (21). In addition, as with most endoscopes, the light illuminating the surgical field emanates from the end of the endoscope which also improves visualization. The stereoscopic endoscope used by the DaVinci system is pictured in *Fig. 8.12* (left). This is positioned in the surgical field by a manipulator arm which tracks the position of the surgical instruments in the field and the magnification (zoom) and focus of the image from the endoscope is controlled by foot pedals on the workstation.

Secondly, the DaVinci direct fiberoptic feed to the surgical workstation allows an optical image quality at a level equal to the standard operating microscope. The workstation operating controls for the endoscope make it more convenient to use than the usual operating microscope.

Third, each of the manipulator arms of the DaVinci system provide 7 degrees of freedom (DOF) which significantly increases dexterity and the facility with which various microsurgical tasks can be accomplished.

Finally, the DaVinci system has a large variety of instruments which, although originally designed for cardiac surgery, would be easily adaptable to neurosurgical applications. These are shown in *Fig. 8.12* (right).

The surgeon is seated at the ergonomically designed workstation, rests his forehead above the ocular viewing ports, and places all five

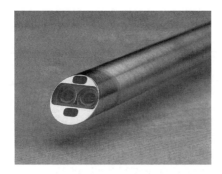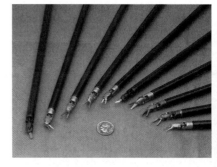

FIG. 8.12 Left: Stereoscopic endoscope used in the DaVinci system. This is manipulated in the surgical field by a third arm of the robot and tracks the position of the surgical instruments within the surgical field. Zoom, focus and pan adjustments are controlled by workstation foot pedals. Right: Variety of instruments manufactured for use with the DaVinci system include knives, scissors, needle holders, graspers (forceps) and bipolar coagulation. (Courtesy Intuitive Surgical Inc., Mountain View, Ca.)

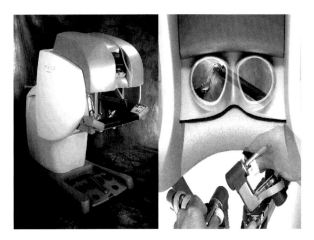

FIG. 8.13 The DaVinci workstation (Left) is ergonomically designed and provides a comfortable and intuitive working situation for the surgeon. Right: The surgeon views the surgical field by means of a direct fiberoptic feed from the stereoscopic endoscope in the surgical field. Surgical instruments are manipulated by finger motions, wrist and hand movements joystick. (Courtesy Intuitive Surgical Inc., Mountain View, Ca.)

fingers of each hand into rings on the master manipulator unit as shown in *Fig. 8.13*. Movements of the endoscope are controlled by a combination of hand movements and foot pedals, which are very intuitive and easy to learn. There is excellent force (haptic) feedback. The combination of haptic feedback and stereoscopic vision greatly shortens the time necessary to learn to use the device.

The author spent a morning working with the DaVinci system and test objects as well as a cadaver head at Intuitive Surgical's development laboratory in Mountain View. The "learning curve" was virtually miniscule and the ergonomics and optical quality at the workstation were, in my opinion, superior to those using a conventional operating microscope in the usual operating room situation.

The system is designed to improve dexterity in minimally invasive procedures. The interfaces are well designed and comfortable to use. Movements of the fingers are transmitted to movements of the instruments in the surgical field *(Fig. 8.14)*.

Long distance telesurgical procedures are also possible with the existing instrumentation, as shown in *Fig. 8.15*, which illustrates the surgical set-up. The workstation and surgeon are on one side of the operating room and the patient is on the other, as with the Zeus system. The workstation could also be outside the operating room or at a distance limited only by the bandwidth of the optical and electronic communications.

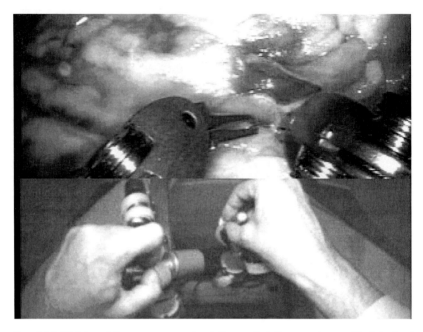

FIG. 8.14 Wrist and finger movements at the workstation are transmitted to the instruments in the surgical field in an intuitive manner. (Courtesy Intuitive Surgical Inc., Mountain View, Ca.)

DISCUSSION

Although endoscopic procedures have been used in neurosurgery since 1923, their applications have been limited to work within the ventricular system: third ventriculostomies, cyst and septum perforations, and the biopsy of tumors. Recently endoscopes have been used in conjunction with the operating microscope in minimally invasive procedures, usually at the skull base. Neurosurgical applications have been limited because, unlike urology, general, or cardiac surgery, neurosurgeons do not have a large fluid or gas filled cavity in which to work. In addition, intra-axial pathologies greatly outnumber extra-axial or intraventricular conditions that may be amenable to endoscopic approaches.

In intra-axial neurosurgery, navigation becomes a problem: finding the lesion and discerning its margins from healthy brain tissue. Indeed, this is sometimes difficult with the large exposures with which neurosurgeons are accustomed. However, we have used image-guided techniques for almost 20 years and as a result, less invasive neurosurgical approaches have become possible. Image-guided stereotactic approaches could, therefore, be adapted to endoscopic surgery for

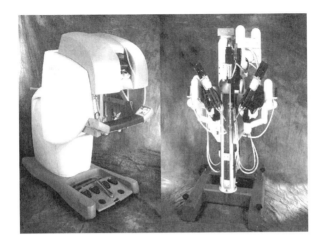

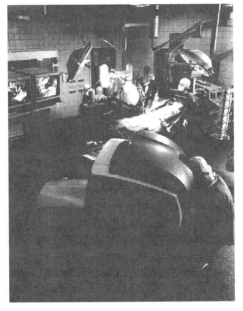

FIG. 8.15 Top. DaVinci system with workstation on left, manipulator system on right. Bottom: Operating room set-up showing surgeon at workstation console in foreground and patient in background. Assistant watches surgery on external monitors. (Courtesy Intuitive Surgical Inc., Mountain View, Ca.)

intra-axial work and provide localization accuracy beyond the dead-reckoning and identification of anatomical landmarks navigational methods used in intraventricular endoscopy.

Working distances in endoscopic procedures are longer than in conventional procedures. This is where dexterity enhancement robotics can be of practical use. Not only can these cancel out a surgeon's physiologic tremor, but it is also possible to have the action part of the instrument close to the pathology but manipulated at some distance through a narrow surgical corridor.

Neurosurgeons require, therefore, two things to advance minimally invasive techniques: image-guided navigation and dexterity enhancement. Both are now available. Most of the robotic devices proposed for neurosurgery have complemented telesurgery/dexterity enhancement robotics with an imaging-based stereotactic coordinate system (2, 3, 10, 11, 17, 29). Addition of real-time MRI targeting and monitoring will be complementary to telepresence robotics as the robotics device will all surgeons to do complex surgical procedures outside of the confining restriction imposed by the MRI aperture (1, 9, 15).

A coordinate system is inherent in all robotic devices. In an industrial robot, the host computer must track the three-dimensional position of the tool tip in its own coordinate space and register this to the coordinate system of the work envelope. The job is based on a three-dimensionally precise mechanical drawing or computer-aided design (CAD) developed beforehand. The commercially available surgical robots developed to date are still line-of-sight telemanipulators that do not yet interface with our CAD of the brain: CT and MRI. However, there is another problem which must be considered.

Uncontrollable bleeding presents a potential problem during all endoscopic procedures. For the moment, a surgical team stands ready to perform a more conventional procedure to control hemorrhage, should it occur. This is little more than an inconvenience when, say, a ruptured cystic artery retracts in a crevice with difficult access; the surgeon simply does a laparotomy and deals with it. A cardiac surgeon can also open a chest in a matter of minutes to deal with bleeding, if necessary.

The situation may not be so straightforward for a neurosurgeon attempting to resect an intra-axial tumor or working in the subarachnoid space. Unlike the abdomen and chest which are large cavities in which blood can accumulate for a time without problems (assuming that an anesthesiologist keeps up with the blood loss), the skull is a closed box and intracranial spaces are relatively small. A developing hematoma causes intracranial pressure to rise and cerebral blood flow to fall with possible ischemic neurological sequelae. In addition, it takes longer to open a head or spinal canal than a chest or abdomen.

No technology will be acquired, much less survive in a civilian hospital without a specific application that results in better patient care, increased income from new billing codes or facility charges, the saving of time or reduction of ancillary personnel. It is not clear that telesurgical dexterity enhancement actually saves operating room time; on the contrary, it probably prolongs it (7, 20). In fact the major expenses in a hospital's annual budget are salaries and benefits for its employees; typically about 75% of the total budget. Any technology intensive equipment which requires the hiring of additional people for its operation will not be looked upon favorably by the leadership of medical centers. As opposed to the military applications for telesurgery, the protection of highly trained surgeons from hostile fire (other than from administrators) is not a priority in civilian health care delivery systems; nor is the rapid institution of a surgical procedure at a remote site.

We must have new reasons to justify the acquisition of expensive novel technology such as telepresence robotics to our hospital administrators. These are: (1) The enhancement of minimally invasive procedures resulting in less operating room time, shorter lengths of stay, less patient morbidity and discomfort, i.e., better patient care. (2) Prestige; hospital image. The general public has the belief that high technology medicine is better medicine. Hospitals can use the acquisition of an expensive piece of high technology equipment in the marketing program to attract patients away from the competitor across town. As such there is a future, in civilian medical centers, for robotics, in general and telepresence surgery, in particular.

REFERENCES

1. Alexander E 3rd, Moriarty TM, Kikinis R, Black P, Jolesz FM: The present and future role of intraoperative MRI in neurosurgical procedures. **Stereotact Funct Neurosurg** 68:10–17, 1997.
2. Benabid AL, Cinquin P, Lavalle S, Le Bas JF, Demongeot J, de Rougemont J: Computer-driven robot for stereotactic surgery connected to CT scan and magnetic resonance imaging. Technological design and preliminary results. **Appl Neurophysiol** 50; 153–154, 1987.
3. Benabid AL, Lavallee S, Hoffmann D, Cinquin P, Demongeot J, Danel F: Potential use of robots in endoscopic neurosurgery. **Acta Neurochir Suppl** (Wien) 54:93–97, 1992.
4. Bowersox JC: Telepresence surgery. **Br J Surg** 83(4):433–434, 1996.
5. Bowersox JC, Shah A, Jensen J, Hill J, Cordts PR, Green PS: Vascular applications of telepresence surgery: initial feasibility studies in swine. **J Vasc Surg** 23(2):281–287, 1996.
6. Bowersox JC, Cordts PR, LaPorta AJ: Use of an intuitive telemanipulator system for remote trauma surgery: an experimental study. **J Am Coll Surg** 186: 615–621, 1998.
7. Cadiere GB, Himpens J, Vertruyen M, Bruyns J, Germay O, Leman G, Izizaw R: Evaluation of telesurgical (robotic) NISSEN fundoplication. **Surg Endosc** 15:918–923, 2001.

8. Cheah WK, Lee B, Lenzi JE, Goh PM: Telesurgical laparoscopic cholecystectomy between two countries. **Surg Endosc** 14:1085, 2000.
9. Chinzei K, Miller K: Towards MRI guided surgical manipulator. **Med Sci Monit** 7: 153–163, 2001.
10. Drake JM, Joy M, Goldenberg A, Kreindler D: Computer- and robot-assisted resection of thalamic astrocytomas in children. **Neurosurgery** 29:27–33, 1991.
11. Glauser D, Fankhauser H, Epitaux M, Hefti JL, Jaccottet A: Neurosurgical robot Minerva: First results and current developments. **J Image Guid Surg** 1:266–272, 1995.
12. Guillonneau B, Jayet C, Tewari A, Vallancien G: Robot assisted laparoscopic nephrectomy. **J Urol** 166:200–201, 2001.
13. Hiatt JR, Shabot MM, Phillips EH, Haines RF, Grant TL: Telesurgery. Acceptability of compressed video for remote surgical proctoring. **Arch Surg** 131:396–401, 1996.
14. Jensen JF, Hill JW: Advanced telepresence surgery system development. **Stud Health Technol Inform** 29:107–117, 1996.
15. Jolesz FA, Nabavi A, Kikinis R: Integration of interventional MRI with computer-assisted surgery. **J Magn Reson Imaging** 13:69–77, 2001.
16. Kelly PJ: *Tumor Stereotaxis.* Philadelphia: Saunders, 1991, p *xxii.*
17. Kelly PJ: Stereotactic surgery: what is past is prologue. **Neurosurgery** 46:16–27, 2000.
18. Kozlowski DM, Morimoto AK, Charles ST: Micro-telerobotic surgical system for microsurgery. **Stud Health Technol Inform** 39:216–223, 1997.
19. Larkin M: Transatlantic, robot-assisted telesurgery deemed a success. **Lancet** 29; 358(9287):1074, 2001.
20. Le Roux PD, Das H, Esquenazi S, Kelly PJ: Robot-assisted microsurgery: a feasibility study in the rat. **Neurosurgery** 48:584–589, 2001.
21. Mitchell TN, Robertson J, Nagy AG, Lomax A: Three-dimensional endoscopic imaging for minimal access surgery. **J R Coll Surg Edinb** 38:285–292, 1993.
22. Nakamura M, Tamaki N, Tamura S, Yamashita H, Hara Y, Ehara K: Image-guided microsurgery with the Mehrkoordinaten Manipulator system for cerebral arteriovenous malformations. **J Clin Neurosci** 7(Suppl 1):10–13, 2000.
23. Rassweiler J, Frede T, Seemann O, Stock C, Sentker L: Telesurgical laparoscopic radical prostatectomy. Initial experience. **Eur Urol** 40:75–83, 2001.
24. Satava RM, Simon IB: Teleoperation, telerobotics, and telepresence in surgery. **Endosc Surg Allied Technol** 1:151–153, 1993.
25. Satava RM: Virtual reality and telepresence for military medicine. **Comput Biol Med** 25:229–236, 1995.
26. Satava RM: Virtual reality, telesurgery, and the new world order of medicine. **J Image Guid Surg** 1:12–16, 1995.
27. Siemionow M, Ozer K, Siemionow W, Lister G: Robotic assistance in microsurgery. **J Reconstr Microsurg** 16:643–649, 2000.
28. Thompson JM, Ottensmeyer MP, Sheridan TB: Human factors in telesurgery: effects of time delay and asynchrony in video and control feedback with local manipulative assistance. **Telemed J** 5:129–137, 1999.
29. Young RF: Application of robotics to stereotactic neurosurgery. **Neurol Res** 9:123–128, 1987.

CHAPTER

9

Honored Guest Presentation: Quid Novi? In the Realm of Ideas– The Neurosurgical Dialectic

MICHAEL L. J. APUZZO, M.D., AND CHARLES Y. LIU, M.D., PH.D.

During the past generation neurosurgery has been reinvented with modern practice bearing little resemblance to that practiced 30 years ago. The metamorphosis has been striking from every dimensional viewpoint. Magnification, computers, and various aspects of medical imaging have created a capacity of sophistication in achieving minimalistic surgical approaches to disease processes (6, 7, 8, 13, 16, 30, 85, 94, 113). This has been further realized with refinements in radiosurgery (see Figs. 9.4 and 9.5) and endovascular techniques (1, 70, 150). We are discussing cellular and molecular neurosurgery in more realistic terms with gene therapy and the concept of neurorestoration apparently nearly within our grasp as we are developing interventions at the cellular and molecular levels (162, 163).

We are currently embroiled in an information revolution with our body of data doubling every 5 to 10 years, with capabilities for information transmission and access virtually exploding in scale daily (10).

With all of this development we are further encumbered with cultural, racial, economical, ethical, and moral concerns (9).

How will we emerge as neurosurgeons during the next evolving century or centuries? Reality is not as yet upon us, but it is clear that to a certain extent history is predictive, and concept eventually proceeds with time to reality.

FUTURE PROSPECTUS

The *impetus for progress* will come from the utilization of combinations of technologies, combinations of disciplines and combinations of industries. The primary areas of influence for the evolution of the field in the future will be (1) *computational science*, (2) *imaging*, (3) *biomedical engineering*, (4) *information processing*, and (5) *molecular science.*

There is no question in consideration of the foregoing presented information that we are indeed reinventing neurosurgery, and in fact

159

over the course of the past 25 years we have seen a reinvention of our concepts and perspectives in relation to the field in an ever-changing kaleidoscopic mode in which the pace and cycle of reinvention is escalating rapidly (8, 11, 12). It is important for us to maintain a contemporary perspective and to maintain an open mind in which we clearly embrace what is substantive from the past but willingly accept and move forward with the revolution of the future.

The words of Le Corbusier from "Toward a New Architecture" (1927) are particularly pertinent (92):

> Man's stock of tools mark out the stages of civilization, the Stone Age, the Bronze Age, the Iron Age. Tools are the result of successive improvement; the effort of all generations is embodied in them. The tool is the direct and immediate expression of progress; it gives man essential assistance and essential freedom, also. We throw the out-of-date tool on the scrap-heap; the carbine, the culverin, the growler, and the old locomotive. This action is a manifestation of health, of moral health, of morale also; it is not right that we should produce bad things because of a bad tool; nor is it right that we should waste our energy, our health, and our courage because of a bad tool; it must be thrown away and replaced.

We can ask ourselves, "Where will this rapidly cyclical reinvention of neurosurgery take us?" We have seen a progressive refinement of action characterized by a progressive minimalization instigated by technology, the microscope, the computer, imaging, and molecular science. What transformations are ahead?

Historically, medicine has seen major transformations. The nineteenth century was characterized by the emergence of refinements of rational and scientific method, and the twentieth century by the development of molecular science with revolution in genomics, proteomics, and bioinformatics. Some have postulated a movement toward a shift to the "molecular" technologic during the twenty-first century, with molecular structure employed to design microscopic machines—a paradigm shift from medical science to medical engineering.

In 1959, Nobel laureate Richard P. Feynman described "the problem of manipulating and controlling things on a small scale" in a lecture titled "There's Plenty of Room at the Bottom" (58). This has been credited as the birth of the concept contemporarily termed "*nanotechnology*" (46, 49, 50).

A nanometer is a billionth of a meter (10^{-9} m) and spans approximately 10 atomic diameters. Nanotechnology is the technology for designing, fabricating, and applying "nanosystems" (52). *Molecular nanotechnology* employs three-dimensional control of atomic and molecular structures to create materials and devices with molecular precision (51). Molecular nanotechnology and molecular manufacturing are conceptually key enabling technologies for the potential emergence of *nanomedicine* as a reality (60). Mature nanomedicine will require the ability to build devices to atomic precision that will be employed to establish and maintain health.

A formal definition for nanotechnology is provided in the 1999 report of the Interagency Working Group on Nanoscience, Engineering, and Technology, presented to the OSTP Committee on Technology (74):

> Nanotechnology is concerned with materials and systems whose structures and components exhibit novel and significantly improved physical, chemical and biological properties, phenomena and processes because of their small nanoscale size. Structural features in the range of about 10^{-9} to 10^{-7} m (1 to 100 nanometers) determine important changes as compared to the behavior of isolated molecules (1 nanometer) or of bulk materials. For comparison, 10 nanometers are 1000 times smaller than the diameter of a human hair.

The influence of nanotechnology will likely be paramount in each of the five areas previously noted for the development in neurosurgery and medicine in the distant future, potentially allowing the emergence of *nanoneurosurgery*.

COMPUTATIONAL SCIENCE

As have been stated, the development of the silicon microchip and modern computers has arguably been the primary driving force in technological advancement and has had a fundamental effect not only on medicine and neurosurgery, but also on every aspect of life (11, 12). This will likely continue but with new nanotechnology derivatives replacing silicon as the basis. According to the Semiconductor Industry Association, silicon based computer chips have and will continue to miniaturize at a rate of four-fold every three years, resulting in significant advantages in processing speed and power requirement (110, 111). This predicts that our very ability to manufacture ever smaller chips will first witness significant escalations in cost, and then subsequently plateau, with processing capability and power usage being similarly limited. For example, consider the replacement technology required as integrated circuit components approach and exceed the 200 nm resolution of ultraviolet light used in current integrated circuit manufacturing. Furthermore, as the nanoscale is approached, quantum mechanical effects begin to hinder the optimal function of silicon-based computers. Finally, the computer scientists and mathematicians have long recognized the fundamental limitations posed by the binary logic that forms the basis of current computer technology.

Quantum computing is one exciting area of future development (20, 48, 57, 61, 97, 101). Computer scientists and engineers are actively elucidating methodologies to read, write, and process information by analyzing alterations in quantum mechanical phenomena. Quantum computers will use *superposition* to utilize a quantum bit ("qubit") of information in multiple concurrent calculations. For example, if the spin state of a particle holds the qubit of information, then multiple states are used concurrently rather than sequentially in calculations, allowing a single processing unit to perform multiple operations at the same time. This yields an exponential advantage in computational power. Error correction is facilitated by the quantum mechanical phenomenon of *entanglement*. For example, a qubit's value is dependent on that of its neighbor's, allowing errors to be identified and rectified using neighboring qubits as a guide.

Another significant conceptual area in computer development is *molecular computation*, where data is stored, accessed, and processed in the primary, secondary, tertiary, and quaternary structure of molecules such as DNA and proteins (17, 18, 67, 104, 120, 126, 127). Molecular switching devices, transistors, memory elements and other components of molecular electronics have been described. For example, *Fig. 9.1* shows a comparative schematic representation of a conventional transistor and its molecular counterpart. A transistor consists of two terminals between which current flows, all controlled by a third terminal. A molecular transistor composed of three benzene ring structures can be used to switch current flow in response to an electric field. The middle benzene ring has asymmetric fragments, enabling electrical fields to alter the alignment of the conjugated pi-bonds of the rings to alter current conduction (126, 127). Clearly, to manufacture such devices will require new fabrication concepts such as *self-assembly*, where atoms, molecules, or groups of molecules spontaneously rearrange into regular or complex patterns. Such technology will make massively parallel processing possible. A fundamental limitation to integrating these new "molecular components" into current technology is the orders of magnitude difference in scale, not only in physical terms but also in power requirement and heat generation/dissipation considerations. In fact, molecular electronic scientists have difficulty imagining large-scale circuits. However, once practical considerations match theory, it would not be difficult to imagine the integration of computers with living tissue in a synergistic fashion, creating hybrid "*biocomputers*," which

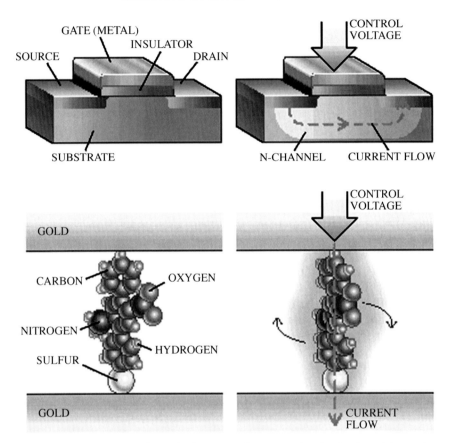

FIG. 9.1 Comparative schematic diagrams of a conventional microtransistor and a molecular counterpart. The conventional transistor (A) has three terminals: the source, gate, and drain. When a voltage is applied to the gate (B), electrons are drawn into the insulator, allowing current to flow from the source to the drain. A molecular transistor (C) consists of three benzene rings with asymmetric fragments. The asymmetry allows the structure to be twisted in the presence of an electrical field (D), altering the alignment of the conjugated pi-bonds and thus altering current flow. (*From* Reed MA, Tour JM: Computing with molecules. **Sci Am** 282:86–93, 2000)

are predicted by some computer scientists to be the dominant mold in next generation computer architecture.

Nanotechnology, quantum computing, and molecular computing could result in computers with orders of magnitude improvements in computing power, of unparalleled efficiency, all seamlessly integrated with living tissue. The effects of these advances in computational science on neurosurgery, medicine, and daily life, will likely dwarf that of silicon-based computers.

IMAGING

It would appear that into the twenty-first century, developments in imaging and microscopy have and will continue to revolutionize medicine and neurosurgery. The invention of the *optical microscope* in the 1600s allowed visualization of micro-scale detail in cells and tissue and continues to be widely applicable with modern refinements. The application of the optical microscope to operative neurosurgery resulted in a veritable "microneurosurgical revolution," improving surgical safety and allowing the development of surgical corridors and access to deep recesses of the intracranial space. This body of accomplishments represents the efforts of an entire generation of neurosurgeons. X-ray technology represented the first form of *medical imaging*. With the development of computers and image processing, high resolution CT scanning is the standard of care in most parts of the world. Novel applications of NMR technology yielded MRI scanning which essentially generates 2-D gray-scale anatomic sections of tissue with minimal patient discomfort. The past two decades have witnessed the continued maturation and clinical application of functional imaging technology such as PET and SPECT. Novel applications of imaging and computer visual processing have been instrumental to advances in the field of neuronavigation and stereotactic neurosurgery. As medicine moves to the sub-micron or nanoscale, imaging and microscopy will likely play a seminal role. Developments in these and related areas are discussed briefly below.

Clearly, our ability to manufacture, manipulate, diagnose, and intervene at the nanoscale will hinge upon concurrent developments in imaging technology. The advent of the *scanning electron microscope* (SEM) in the 1940s circumvented the inherent constraints of optical resolution, but the properties of electromagnetic lenses set the limit of resolution at 50 angstroms, or 5 nm. Furthermore, SEM requires complex sample preparation that prohibits application to living tissue.

The envelope of resolution was pushed to the sub-atomic level in 1981, with the development of *scanning probe microscopy* (SPM) (25–29). The first manifestation of this technology was the *scanning tunneling microscope*, which measured the surface topography of samples to unit angstrom or 0.1 nm resolutions *(Fig. 9.2)*. The basis of this

Fɪɢ. 9.2 Scanning tunneling microscope image of a NiO single crystal demonstrating atomic resolution. Image *a* shows the nickel atoms, and image *b* shows the oxygen atom. The scale represents 4.17 angstroms. Clearly, imaging to atomic detail is possible with this technology.

A

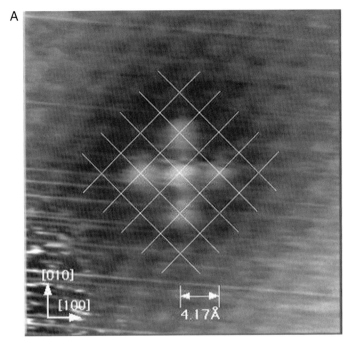

B

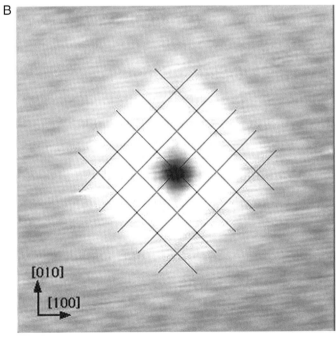

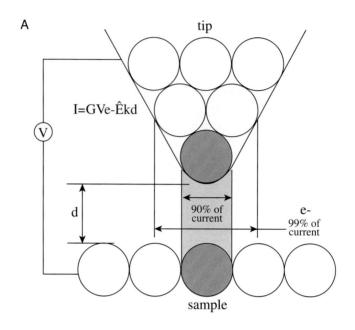

$I = GVe\text{-}\hat{E}kd$

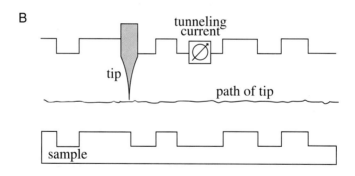

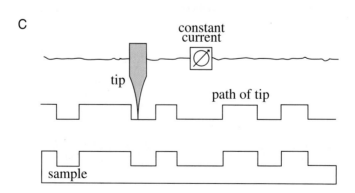

technology is the movement of an extremely sharp conducting probe over a sample between which a current flows. *Figure 9.3* shows a schematic of the probe-sample interaction. This tunneling current varies with the distance between probe and sample in an exponential fashion. Measuring either the variations in tunneling current or the minute deflections of the tip required to maintain a constant tunneling current yields a topographic map as the tip moves over the sample. This particular model has the limitation that the probe and the sample must both be conductive and cannot be used in biological structures (31, 93). Further developments of this technology has yielded the *atomic force microscope*, of similar resolution *(Fig. 9.4),* but based on the mechanical deflection of a cantilever arm attached to the probe (24). Other permutations of scanning probe microscopy include *magnetic force microscopes* and *scanning capacitance microscopy*, which take advantage of the variations of the magnetic forces and surface electrical charges respectively (59, 86, 115, 122, 134). These techniques of nanoscale imaging have the advantage that living biological tissue can be imaged in-vivo (34, 68, 71).

Optical resolution is similarly being improved (22, 23, 114). According to the Nyquist relation, optical resolution is limited by the wavelength of the light source to approximately 0.2 micron, or 200 nm. The basic principle behind this limitation stems from the dual nature of light, specifically its wave nature. In conventional optical imaging, or *far-field optics*, a light source is focused on an object at a distance much greater than the wavelength of light. Know as the far-field diffraction limit, or the *Abbé barrier*, the limit in resolution in these systems is one half the wavelength of the light. Monochromatic lasers and ultraviolet light sources of increasingly higher energy and shorter wavelengths have been applied. However, the development of a new field of optical imaging surpasses the far-field diffraction limit. In *near-field optics*, the distance between the light source and the object to be imaged is much shorter than the wavelength of the light (81). Instru-

---

FIG. 9.3 *(A)* Schematic of a scanning tunneling microscope (STM) tip. In this mode of imaging, an extremely sharp tip is passed over a sample. When the tip is brought to within 10 angstroms of the sample and a bias voltage is applied between the tip and sample, "tunneling current" is observed. This tunneling current varies exponential with the distance between the tip and sample. By measuring the variation of the tunneling current as the tip scans the surface of the sample *(B)*, a topographic image can be generated (constant-height mode). Alternatively, the minute deflections necessary to maintain a constant tunneling current can also be used (constant-current mode)*(C)*. Clearly, this mode of imaging requires that both the tip and sample must be conductive. (*From* www.thermomicro.com)

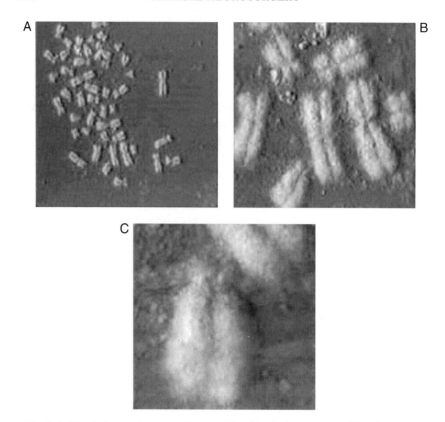

F<small>IG</small>. 9.4 Atomic force microscope image of irradiated chromosomes. The three images show increasing magnification. Images *A, B,* and *C* represent 52 μm by 52 μm, 12 μm by 12 μm, and 5 μm by 5 μm images, respectively. The detail is remarkable, especially in image *C*.

ments based on this principle such as the scanning near-field optical microscope have theoretical limits of resolution twenty times higher than the best conventional microscope. Already, images on sub-0.1 micron resolution have been achieved. As the availability of nanoscale lasers (78) and image/data processing technology improves, the resolution will surely improve upon these achievements.

Other developments in nanoscale imaging including those based on infrared nano-scale spectroscopy have already been described, along with numerous others such as femtosecond near-field pump-probe spectroscopy and stimulated emission depletion systems which yield fluorescent images of living cells with previously unseen resolution (114). Driven by advancements in nanotechnology and computation, molecular details of cell membrane surfaces and intracellular contents and function will likely be possible in vivo, with subsequent novel applications to medical imaging.

BIOMEDICAL ENGINEERING

Engineers have and will continue to make important contributions in the field of medicine and neurosurgery. In their arsenal, the engineer has mathematical modeling and experimental techniques, brought to bear in a synergistic fashion. Already, the field of bioengineering and biomedical engineering are attracting some of the brightest engineering students, and academic institutions are dedicating substantial sums of money in "biological initiatives." Immediate results of their efforts can be seen in novel drug delivery devices, bioprosthetics designed with mechanical engineering principles, novel biomaterials, blood and tissue substitutes, and biomedical instrumentation (63, 107, 140).

Already, tissue and biomaterials engineering have developed tremendous levels of sophistication. Early efforts to synthesize biocompatible materials primarily attempted to generate materials that were immunologically silent and biologically inert. The strategy was to produce materials that were invisible to the human body when implanted. In fact, structural integrity was the primary function served by these materials. The next step was to produce implantable "tissues" that consisted of a synthetic three-dimensional scaffold for structural integrity on which living cells are cultured, resulting in "artificial organs" (109, 116, 146). Currently, biomaterials are being developed that actively interact with the cells with which they contact (53, 153). These materials are amino-acid based polymeric constructs with integrated cell-adhesion specific peptide domains. The added functional activity of these materials represents a distinct elevation in sophistication. Clearly, cells interact with not only neighboring cells but also with their surrounding extracellular matrix. Thus, cellular function is modulated by communication with neighboring cells and environment changes through signaling mechanisms mediated by diffusible factors, both endocrine and paracrine. Furthermore, cellular differentiation, tissue growth, both normal and neoplastic, is controlled by contact-mediated signaling mechanisms, with one cell presenting a membrane-based ligand to a cell-surface receptor on a neighboring cell (117). With the next step-increase in complexity and sophistication, engineered biomaterials will actively interact with both cultured and endogenous host cells, activating appropriate signaling mechanisms in an integrated manner (106, 124). In essence future biomaterials will be appropriately functional rather than biologically inert.

Proteins form a natural bridge between synthetic and living tissue. In the past, scientists and engineers depended on naturally occurring proteins and their amino acid components for building blocks to design structures of complex architecture and function. Traditionally, protein engineers have been limited to using naturally occurring proteins composed of the 20 amino acid building blocks. Over the past few years, a novel strategy has been developed to construct polymeric biomaterials from both naturally occurring amino acids as well as those that are not usually incorporated into proteins (83, 87, 119, 133, 148, 159). Synthetic polymers have function limited to that defined by its physical properties, whereas naturally occurring polymers have the added sophistication of catalytic, informational, and signal transduction properties, due perhaps to the exact definition of lengths, sequences, and stereochemistries in the natural polymers. Constructing artificial genes that encode for both structural and signaling sequences and expressing the artificial proteins in a microbial host, synthetic materials are now being made with the subtle, sophisticated characteristics traditionally limited to natural polymers. To achieve this, the expression machinery of the microbial hosts as well as the genetic templates that define the materials must be specifically and strategically engineered. The potential clinical applications of this technology are likely to be exceptionally broad in scope.

In addition to constructing biomaterials of sophisticated functional capabilities, protein engineers are strategically altering naturally occurring proteins such as enzymes in a coherent fashion to optimize function. The natural force that drives the diversity of subtle variations in enzyme function is evolution. For example, spontaneous mutations are emphasized and propagated by forces of natural selection to create change. However, the time-scale on which these natural forces create change can be prohibitively long to manipulate practically. Unable to accelerate these forces of change, scientists have been traditionally relegated to identifying those proteins with desirable characteristics that have naturally evolved over millions of years. However, agriculturists and animal farmers have increased the relative presence of desirable phenotypes far beyond that possible through natural occurrence by breeding. Using a similar process termed *directed evolution*, protein engineers are accelerating the evolutionary process and essentially breeding molecules and enzymes for desirable characteristics (14, 32). Directed evolution is characterized by first generating molecular diversity and then identifying the improved variants. Random point mutageneses are generated by an error-prone version the polymerase chain reaction at a rate of approximately one amino acid substitution per sequence per generation (35). Beneficial mutations can be further amplified synergistically by *in vitro* recombination (139, 161). The myriad variations are then screened for the desirable characteristic. For example, the optimal temperature of maximum catalytic activity can be lowered by generating mutations in the gene encoding an enzyme variant that functions well at high temperatures and then screening for those that function optimally in low temperatures. This ability represents a powerful new tool in protein engineering.

Despite an improved understanding of cellular structure and function, direct physical and surgical manipulation of intracellular structures is damaging, and extensive maneuvers such as those with micropipettes are not tolerated. New optical techniques have been developed to circumvent those limitations. The basic principle behind this technology is that as light passes an object, momentum is transferred from the light to the object. By Newton's second law, this exerts a force on the object. By appropriate application of micro laser beams, optical traps, or optical tweezers and stretchers can be created (21, 64, 65, 141). These devices allow for the micromanipulation of intracellular organelles as well as molecules, both membrane based or free floating. Another application is the measurement of the mechanical properties of microscopic structures, even down to the nanoscale. Already, intermolecular bonds have been characterized, as well as noncovalent interactions between molecules such as DNA and its binding proteins. This technology will clearly find broader application as the need for noninvasive micromanipulation and nanoscale mechanical properties measurements increase.

Engineers have conceived, constructed, and maintained almost every process that affects daily life. This will likely continue with processes of ever decreasing scale, eventually down to the nanoscale. It is likely that every function of living tissue and cells will be understood, anticipated, manipulated, repaired, and optimized in a fashion currently seen in process engineering. These functions will include the genetic content, gene expression, protein product, cell structure/function, organ structure/function, and eventually the entire organism. Guiding these developments will be the principle of *biomimetics*, or in simple terms, the process of learning tricks and tools from nature and biological systems (2, 131, 135). The resultant products will be "smart" and will "evolve" and "adapt" to environmental conditions and functional necessity using available resources.

Future products of bioengineering will likely have the ability to seamlessly integrate with biological tissue in vivo. Examples of the integration of silicon-based electronics and biological tissues, or biochips, are already available. Biocomputers have also been described in theory, as discussed earlier. Commercial applications of biosensor technology are already available, which will likely make continuous in vivo monitoring of body chemistries and enzymes possible, obviating conventional analysis from phlebotomy (19, 137, 145, 147). The field of *bionics* will likely continue to expand exponentially. Bionics refers to instruments that are part living tissue, part machine (47, 121). Current examples of bionic devices include cochlear implants and bioimplantable, sub-retinal chips that simulate the function of photoreceptors (36, 37, 41, 142, 155). Another novel example of a bionic device is the BION, a hypodermically injected muscle stimulator (38, 98, 99) (Advanced Bionics Corp., Sylmar, CA). These devices are designed to be placed in paralyzed muscles and restore muscle activity to prevent disuse atrophy and even possibly to restore functional activity. These devices form an interface between the muscle and an external controller, in essence, bionic-neurons.

Nanotechnology will surely make important contributions in bioengineering. Manufacturing at the molecular levels is well illustrated by the synthesis of the soccer ball shaped buckminster fullerene molecule (88, 89, 136). Subsequently, nanotubes, nanomanipulators, nanowires, and molecular motors *(Figs. 9.5, 9.6, 9.7, 9.8, 9.9)* have all been described (3, 43, 56, 69, 75, 84, 96, 132, 138, 157). Nanoscientists are able to precisely manipulate single atoms *(Fig. 9.10)*. Even soft materials are becoming suitable substrates for manufacturing to nanometer precision *(Fig. 9.11)* (123). Molecules with molecular imprinting, or "memory" of interactions with other molecules have been synthesized (105, 112). In fact, prototypes of intracellular *nanoprobes* of 20 to 200 nm diameters with both diagnostic and therapeutic potential have already been developed (39, 40). These could serve as components of molecular *nanomachines*. One fundamental limitation in the function of nanomachines is the requirement that they function in the aqueous environment found *in vivo* (76). At these scales, the molecular forces found at the interfaces between machine and water will be relatively more important. Clearly, the field of interfacial phenomenon study will have to develop to include the nanoscale. Development in space technology will allow studies of the effects of low gravity environments on nanoscale events. Molecular manufacturing will likely be facilitated by the development of computer simulation, or *molecular simulation*, of nanoscale events, made possible by advances in computation (62, 66). These simulations will be analogous to the mathematical simulation of a manufacturing process or *computer-aided-design* (CAD) commonly used today (90, 91). Although true micromachines are yet to be produced, nano- and microelectromechanical systems and micron-scale actuators represent a bridging technology *(Figs. 9.12, 9.13)* (42, 77, 129).

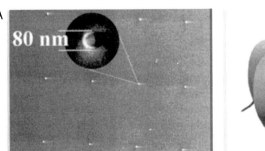
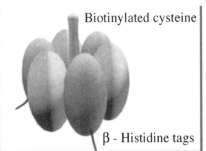
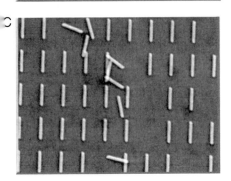
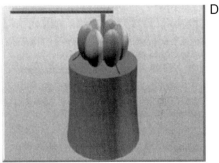

FIG. 9.5 An example of a biomolecular motor-powered nanomechanical device. The schematic shows (A) a Ni post (height 200nm, diameter 80nm), (B) F$_1$-ATPase biomolecular motor, (C) nanopropeller (length 750 to 1400nm, diameter 150nm), and (D) the final assembled device. The motor spins the post, which in turn drives the propeller. (*From* Soong RK, Bachand GD, Neves HP, Olkhovets AG, Craighead HG, Montemagno CD: Powering an inorganic nanodevice with a biomolecular motor. **Science** 290:1555–1558, 2000.)

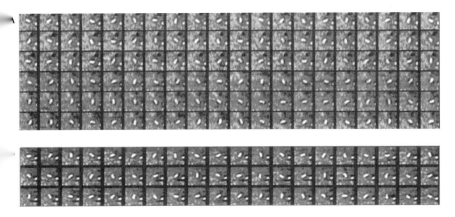

FIG. 9.6 Image sequence of the biomolecular motor-powered nanomechanical device in movement. In images A and B, the F$_1$-ATPase motor counterclockwise is rotating the nanopropeller at 8.3 and 7.7 revolutions per second, respectively. The device operated for 2.5 hours while ATP was maintained in the flow cell. (*From* Soong RK, Bachand GD, Neves HP, Olkhovets AG, Craighead HG, Montemagno CD: Powering an inorganic nanodevice with a biomolecular motor. **Science** 290:1555–1558, 2000.)

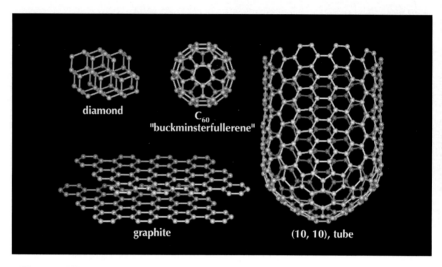

Fig. 9.7 Allotropic forms of carbon include the familiar graphite and diamond forms, as well as a third form, the fullerenes. These single-walled carbon structures form by self-assembly from vapors generated by carbon arcs and lasers. Fullerenes can be modified by altering the interior, the exterior, and the surface of the cage, and they have fascinating structural, mechanical, and conductive properties. The discovery in 1985 of the original fullerene, the C_{60} *buckminsterfullerene*, was of landmark importance in identifying these building blocks of carbon-based nanotechnology. (*From* Smalley RE: Discovering the fullerenes (Nobel lecture). **Rev Mod Phys** 69:723–730, 1997.)

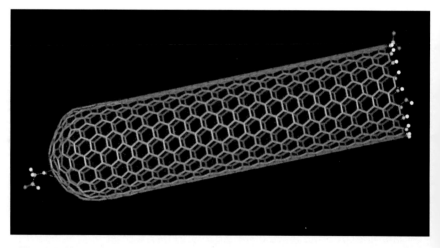

Fig. 9.8 Nanotubes are giant linear fullerenes and represent building blocks of carbon-based nanotechnology. The nanotubes can be open or closed-ended; these ends can be chemically derivitized to achieve specialized properties. The nanotube acts as a quantum waveguide for electrons, allowing communication between the derivatives. (*From* Smalley RE: Discovering the fullerenes (Nobel lecture). **Rev Mod Phys** 69:723–730, 1997.)

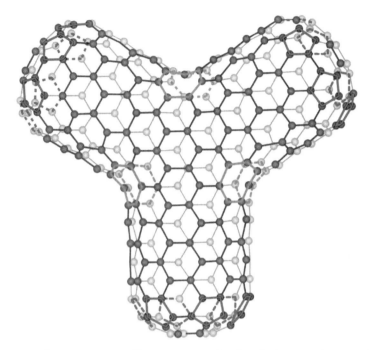

F<small>IG</small>. 9.9 Fullerenes are cage-like structures of carbon in hexagonal arrays. These structures can theoretically attain fantastic morphology by strategic inclusion of pentagonal arrays, for positive curvature, and heptagonal arrays for negative curvature. (*from*, Yakobson BI, Smalley RE: Fullerene nanotubes: $C_{1,000,000}$ and beyond. **Am Scientist** 85:324–337, 1997.)

INFORMATION PROCESSING AND ANALYSIS

The early part of 2001 witnessed the much-anticipated completion of the human genome project. Major scientific journals rushed to publish the result of one of the most ambitious projects in the history of science (72, 73). Critics of the project pointed out at its inception that much effort and expense was to be spent on gathering information without a definitive use. Since then, entire fields of study have emerged that will extract useful information from the vast databases that have been generated. Computational biology initiatives are underway at almost every major academic institution. The study of *genomics* has four major approaches including *bioinformatics*, genetic analysis of extended populations, large-scale expression studies, and functional approaches (79). Bioinformatics is defined as the application of computers, databases, and computational methods to the management of biologic information (80, 125). Workers are scouring the vast DNA sequences for recurrent themes that translate into successful natural strategies for solving biological problems. Understanding these strate-

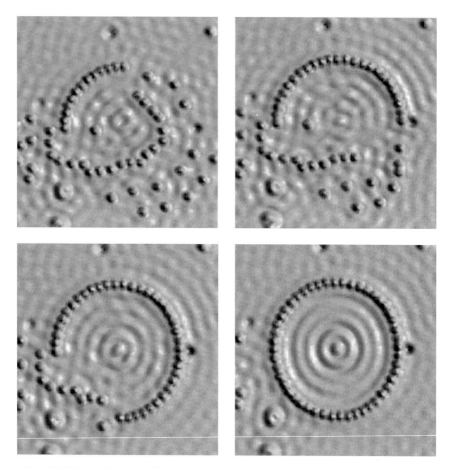

FIG. 9.10 Scanning tunneling microscope image of the construction of a circular corral of Fe on Cu. The images show various stages in the assembly process. This is an excellent example of how scanning probe microscopy technology is relevant not only for imaging, but also for molecular manufacturing. (*From* Crommie MF, Lutz, CP, Eigler DM: Confinement of electrons to quantum corrals on a metal surface. **Science** 262:218–220, 1993; *also*, Issues in nanotechnology. **Science** 290:1523–1545, 2000.)

gies may guide therapeutic interventions for disease processes. Simply organizing and managing these vast databases is a daunting task. The information will form the basis for improved understanding of structural biology (33). Furthermore, the field of *proteomics* will seek to determine the function and structure of proteins defined by the DNA sequences (130).

Epidemiologists are incorporating *statistical genetics* and bioinformatics with traditional tools to localize genes influencing complex phe-

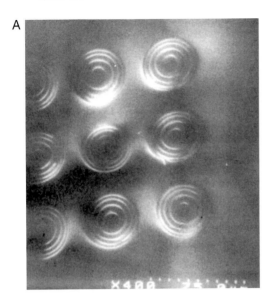

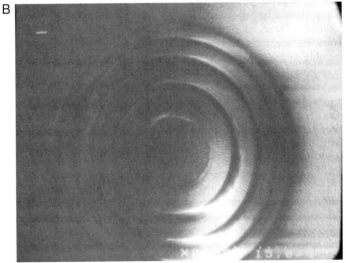

Fig. 9.11 An array of diffractive optical lenses fabricated by replica molding of a soft elastomer (A) and a higher magnification image of an individual lens (B). The smallest line widths are 80nm. The feature sizes are 200nm. These arrays have applications to efficiently couple light into and out of microfluidic chips for biochemical assays. The ability to manufacture these devices demonstrates the evolution of micro- and nanomanufacturing capabilities to include soft materials. (*From* Quake SR, Scherer A: From micro- to nanofabrication with soft materials. **Science** 290:1536–1540, 2000.)

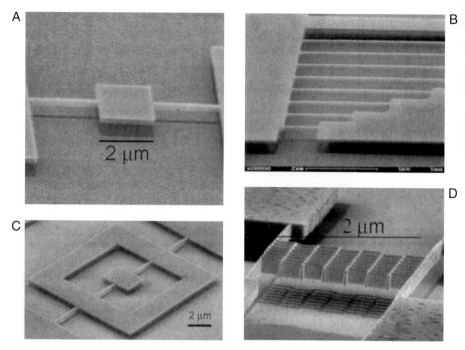

FIG. 9.12 Electron micrograph of a nanoelectromechanical system objects fabricated in single-crystal silicon using electron beam lithography and surface micro machining. Image (*A*) shows a tensional oscillator, (*B*) a compound tensional oscillator, (*C*) a series of silicon nanowires, (***D***) an oscillating silicon mesh mirror. These micron-scale nanoelectromechanical systems represent a bridging technology from current state of the art to true nanoscale devices. (*From* Craighead HG: Nanoelectromechanical systems. **Science** 290:1532–1535, 2000.)

notypic expressions and study the genetic effects on disease susceptibility (55). Informed decisions regarding lifestyle and preventative measures will be possible. Screening procedures that are now felt to be cost inefficient can be targeted to those individuals with genetic predisposition and high risk. Similar applications are being made in the field of *pharmacogenetics*, where the influence of individual genetic variations on the effect, therapeutic or adverse, is being elucidated (103). Genetic polymorphism in drug-metabolizing enzymes, ion channels, drug transporters, and target receptors probably account for these wide variations (108). *Pharmacogenomics* is a branch of pharmacogenetics that carries the analysis at the level of the genome (45, 149). These studies will further guide rational drug design by precisely identifying targets and increasing the efficiency of clinical trials (82).

Potentially useful drugs that have failed prior testing may be revisited. Furthermore, individualization of dosing can be achieved with greater precision. No longer will such crude and imprecise criteria, as age, sex, or weight be the sole guide to drug dosing and selection.

Supported by the concurrent advancement of computational power, it is not too difficult to imagine when individual genetic and genomic data will be available to physicians to guide treatment. For example, a patient's "chart" may include individual predisposition to disease and likely response to therapy as predicted by genetic and genomic

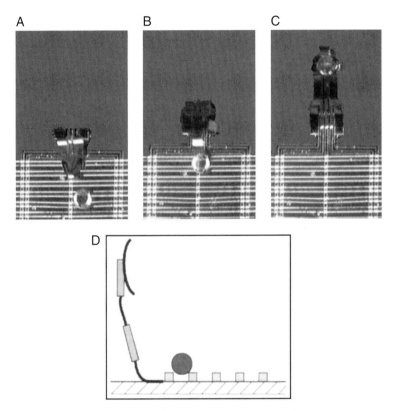

FIG. 9.13 A micro robot arm made of conjugate polymer micro actuators. The arm consists of an "elbow", a "wrist", and a "hand", with "fingers." The whole device measures 670 μm long from base to fingertip. Images (A) through (C) demonstrate the device in the action of grabbing and lifting a 100 μm glass bead. Image (D) shows a schematic of the entire action. The total displacement of the glass bead that could be achieved by the microrobot arm was 270 μm. This device, although not truly nanoscale, represents another example of important bridging technology. (*From* Jager EWH, Smela E, Inganas O: Microfabricating conjugated polymer actuators. **Science** 290:1540–1545, 2000.)

analysis, along with other traditional elements of the history and physical. Free access to this sensitive data raises some serious ethical questions, especially in the area of medical insurance where prediction of risk is paramount. Concerns about the use of such information as selective criteria in other arenas have also been voiced. Clearly, one of the important challenges of managing the vast amount of information that is being generated is to set acceptable guidelines for its ethical use.

MOLECULAR SCIENCE

The influence of molecular biology and science has been identified in the popular as well as scientific press, including the neurosurgical literature (118, 162, 163). It is difficult to discuss this topic in isolation from the others above, as they are almost inextricably mated. However, several general areas are worth discussing specifically. *Gene therapy*, for example, has generated enormous interest (4, 154). The promise of gene therapy has not been met, and several barriers have been identified. There is a lack of safe and efficient gene-delivery systems. It is in this area that bioengineers will likely make significant contributions. The patients that will benefit from gene therapy will span the spectrum of ages, from prenatal to adulthood (160). However, although animal experiments yield promising results, human clinical trials of in-utero gene therapy have yet to be conduced. Currently, gene therapy is actively sought for cardiovascular diseases, cancer, HIV, hemophilia, and neurodegenerative disease. Other potential areas of interest will include mental illness, preventative medicine, and in-utero gene therapy.

The manipulation of human genetic material has also led to the development of genetic vaccines. These include both DNA and RNA vaccines aimed at such varied disease processes as AIDS, ebola infection, measles, tuberculosis, and cancer (15, 54, 95, 100, 144, 152, 158). Furthermore, DNA vaccines have shown potential for enhancing the immune response (151).

The manipulation of human and mammalian genetic material presents many ethical questions, especially in the eyes of the public (143). Molecular biological developments in plants have enjoyed a more muted response. Almost every major player in the chemical industry has made considerable investments in the area of molecular biology and agriculture (128). Plants have the complex post-translational machinery to produce complex protein products that are of use to human disease processes, either therapeutically or preventatively. Furthermore, they are easy to produce in large quantities at lower cost (102).

However, ecological and environmental considerations must be made and anti-biotechnology groups pacified before there is widespread acceptance of this technology (156).

The concepts presented would seem to have a Jules Verne quality, but history has demonstrated that concept is the seed for future practical reality. Mankind exists in a continuum of time and space with forces of discovery creating evolution and advancement, which are repetitively evident as cyclical reinvention recurs in the quest for utopia (5).

REFERENCES

1. Adler JR, Murphy, Martin J, Chang S, Hancock SL: Image-guided Robotic Radio-surgery. **Neurosurgery** 44(6):1299–1306, 1999.
2. Alivisatos AP: Naturally aligned nanocrystals. **Science** 289:736–737, 2000.
3. Amato I: Fomenting a revolution, in miniature. **Science** 282:402–405, 1998.
4. Anderson WF: Human gene therapy. **Nature** 392(6679 suppl):25–30, 1998.
5. Apuzzo MLJ: Brave new world: reaching for utopia. **Neurosurgery** 46(5):1033, 2000.
6. Apuzzo MLJ: Modernity and the emerging futurism in neurosurgery: tempora mutantur nos et mutamur in illis. **Journal of Clinical Neurosciences** 7(2):85–87, 2000.
7. Apuzzo MLJ (ed): *Neurosurgery for the Third Millennium: American Association of Neurological Surgeons Neurosurgical Topics.* USA, AANS, 1992.
8. Apuzzo MLJ: Reinventing neurosurgery: Entering the third millennium. **Neurosurgery** 46(1):1–2, 2000.
9. Apuzzo MLJ: SCHNEIDER LECTURE–New dimensions of neurosurgery in the realm of high technology: Possibilities, practicalities, realities. **Neurosurgery** 38(4):625–639, 1996.
10. Apuzzo MLJ, Hodge CJ Jr: The metamorphosis of communication, the knowledge revolution, and the maintenance of a contemporary perspective during the 21st century. **Neurosurgery** 46(1):7–15, 2000.
11. Apuzzo MLJ, Liu CY: 2001: Things to come. **Neurosurgery** 49: (in press), 2001.
12. Apuzzo MLJ, Liu CY, Sullivan SD, Faccio RA: Reinventing neurosurgery-Surgery of the human cerebrum: a collective modernity. **Clin Neurosurg** (in press), 2001.
13. Apuzzo MLJ, Weinberg RA: The architecture and functional design of advanced neurosurgical operating environments. **Neurosurgery** 33(4):663–673, 1993.
14. Arnold FH, Wintrode PL, Miyazaki K, Gershenson A: How enzymes adapt: lessons from directed evolution. **Trend Biochem Sci** 26:100–106, 2001.
15. Arvin AM: Measles vaccine – a positive step toward eradicating a negative strand. **Nature Med** 6(7):744–745, 2000.
16. Auer LM, Auer DP: Virtual endoscopy for planning and simulation of minimally invasive neurosurgery. **Neurosurgery** 43(3): 529–548, 1998.
17. Aviram A: A view of the future of molecular electronics. **Molecular Crystals and Liquid Crystals** 234(1):13–28, 1993.
18. Aviram A, Ratner M (eds): Molecular electronics: Science and technology. **Ann NY Acad Sci** 852, 1998.
19. Barker SL, Kopelman R, Meyer TE, Cusanovich MA: Fiber-optic nitric oxide-sensitive biosensors and nanosensors. **Anal Chem** 70(5):971–976, 1998.

20. Bennett CH: Quantum information and computation. **Physics Today** 48(10): 24–30, 1995.
21. Bennink ML, Leuba SH, Leno GH, Zlatanova J, de Grooth BG, Greeve J: Unfolding individual nucleosomes by stretching individual chromatin fibers with optical tweezers. **Nat Struct Biol** 8:606–610, 2001.
22. Betzig E, Chichester RJ: Single molecules observed by near-field scanning optical microscopy. **Science** 262:1425–1427, 1993.
23. Betzig E, Trautman JK, Harris TD, Weiner JS, Kostelak RL: Breaking the diffraction barrier: optical microscopy on a nanometric scale. **Science** 251:1468–1470, 1991.
24. Binnig G, Quate CF, Gerber Ch: Atomic force microscopy. **Physics Review Letters** 56:990–993, 1986)
25. Binnig G, Rohrer H: Scanning tunneling microscopy. **Helv Phys Acta** 55:726–735, 1982.
26. Binnig G, Rohrer H, Gerber C, Weibel E: Surface studies by scanning tunneling microscopy. **Physics Review Letters** 49:57–61, 1982.
27. Binnig T, Rohrer H: The scanning tunneling microscope. **Sci Am** 253:50–56, 1985.
28. Binnig T, Rohrer H: Scanning tunneling microscopy. **IBM Journal of Research Development** 30:355–369, 1986.
29. Binnig T, Rohrer H: Scanning tunneling microscopy from birth to adolescence. **Review of Modern Physics** 59:615–625, 1987.
30. Black PML, Moriarty T, Alexander E III, Stieg P, Woodard EJ, Gleason PL, Martin CH, Kikinis R, Schwartz RB, Jolesz FA: Development and implementation of intraoperative magnetic resonance imaging and its neurosurgical applications. **Neurosurgery** 41(4): 831–845, 1997.
31. Boland T, Ratner BD: Direct measurement of hydrogen bonding in DNA nucleotide bases by atomic force microscopy. **Proc Natl Acad Sci USA** 92:5297–5301, 1995.
32. Brown K: Biotech speeds its evolution. **Technology Review**, November/December 2000.
33. Burley SK, Almo SC, Bonanno JB, Capel M, Chance MR, Gaasterland T, Lin D, Sali A, Studier FW, Swaminathan S: Structural genomics: beyond the human genome project. **Nature Genetics** 23(2):151–157, 1999.
34. Butt HJ, Wolff EK, Gould SA, Northern BD, Peterson CM, Hansma PK: Imaging cells with the atomic force microscope. **J Struc Biol** 105:54–61, 1990.
35. Caldwell RC, Joyce GF: Mutagenic PCR. **PCR Methods and Applications** 2:28–33, 1994.
36. Chen JM, Farb R, Hanusaik L, Shipp D, Nedzelski JM: Depth and quality of electrode insertion: a radiologic and pitch scaling assessment of two cochlear implant systems. **Am J Otology** 20(2):192–197, 1999.
37. Chen J, Hanusaik L, Ramses P, Schipp D, Anderson J, McLean A, Nedzelski J: Comparative psychophysical evaluation in cochlear implantation: electrical and magnetic stimulation. **Am J Otology** 18(1):39–43, 1997.
38. Cheng E, Brown IE, Loeb GE: Virtual muscle: A computational approach to understanding the effects of muscle properties on motor control. **J Neurosci Methods** 101:117–130, 2000.
39. Clark HA, Hoyer M, Philbert MA, Kopelman R: Optical nanosensors for chemical analysis inside single living cells. 1. Fabrication, characterization, and methods for intracellular delivery of PEBBLE sensors. **Anal Chem** 71(21): 4831–4836, 1999.
40. Clark HA, Kopelman R, Tjalkens R, Philbert MA: Optical nanosensors for chemical analysis inside single living cells. 2. Sensors for pH and calcium and the intracellular application of PEBBLE sensors. **Anal Chem** 71(2):4837–4843, 1999.
41. Cleland B: Helping the blind see. **Aust N Z J Opthalmology** 26(3):193–194, 1998.

42. Craighead HG: Nanoelectromechanical systems. **Science** 290:1532–1535, 2000.
43. Cummings J, Zettl A: Low-friction nanoscale linear bearing realized from multi-wall carbon nanotubes. **Science** 289:602–604, 2000.
44. Crommie MF, Lutz, CP, Eigler DM: Confinement of electrons to quantum corrals on a metal surface. **Science** 262:218–220, 1993.
45. Destenaves B, Thomas F: New advances in pharmacogenomics. **Curr Opin Chem Biol** 4(4):440–444, 2000.
46. Dewdney AK: Nanotechnology—wherein molecular computers control tiny circulatory submarines. **Sci Am** 258:100–103, 1988.
47. Dickinson MH: Bionics: biological insight into mechanical design. **Proc Natl Acad Sci USA** 96(25):14208–14209, 1999.
48. DiVincenzo DP: Quantum computation. **Science** 270(5234):255–261, 1995.
49. Drexler KE: Molecular engineering, an approach to the development of general capabilities for molecular manipulation. **Proc Natl Acad Sci USA** 78:5275–5278, 1981.
50. Drexler KE: *Engines of Creation: The Coming Era of Nanotechnology*. New York, Anchor Press/Doubleday, 1986.
51. Drexler KE, Peterson C, Pergamit G: *Unbounding the Future: The Nanotechnology Revolution*. New York, William Morrow/Quill Books, 1991.
52. Drexler KE: Nanosystems: *Molecular Machinery, Manufacturing, and Computation*. New York, John Wiley & Sons, 1992.
53. Drumheller PD, Hubbell JA: Polymer networks with grafted cell-adhesion peptides for highly biospecific cell adhesive substrates. **Anal Biochem** 222:380–388, 1994.
54. During MJ, Symes CW, Lawlor PA, Dunning LJ, Fitzsimons HL, Poulsen D, Leone P, Xu R, Dicker BL, Lipski J, Young D: An oral vaccine against NMDAR1 with efficacy in experimental stoke and epilepsy. **Science** 287(5457):1453–1460, 2000.
55. Ellsworth DL, Nanolio TA: The emerging importance of genetics in epidemiologic research III: Bioinformatics and statistical genetic methods. **Ann Epidemiol** 9(4):207–224, 1999.
56. Feringa BL: In control of molecular motion. **Nature** 408:151–154, 2000.
57. Feynman RP: Quantum mechanical computers. **Foundations of Physics** 16(6): 507–531, 1986.
58. Feynman RP: There's plenty of room at the bottom, in Crandall BC, Lewis J (eds): *Nanotechnology: Research and Perspectives*. Boston, MIT Press, 1992, pp347–363.
59. Foss S, Dahlberg ED, Proksch R: Measurement of the effects of the localized field of a magnetic force microscope tip on a 180-degree domain wall. **Journal of Applied Physics** 81(8):5032–5034, 1997.
60. Frietas RA Jr.: *Nanomedicine, Volume I: Basic Capabilities*. Austin, TX, Landes Bioscience, 1999.
61. Gershenfeld NA, Chuang IL: Bulk spin-resonance quantum computation. **Science** 275(5298):350–356, 1997.
62. Globus A, Baushlicher CW Jr, Han J, Jaffe FL, Levit C, Srivastava D: Machine phase fullerene nanotechnology. **Nanotechnology** 9:192–199, 1998.
63. Greco RS: Body parts: in vivo veritas. **J Biomed Material Res** 34(4):409–410, 1997.
64. Greulich KO, Pilarczyk G, Hoffmann A, Meyer Zu Horste G, Shafer B, Uhl V, Monajembashi S: Micromanipulation by laser microbeam and optical tweezers: from plant cells to single molecules. **J Microscopy** 198:182–187, 2000.
65. Guck J, Ananthakrishnan R, Mahmood H, Moon TJ, Cunningham CC, Kas J: The optical stretcher: A novel laser tool to micromanipulate cells. **Biophys J** 81:767–784, 2001.
66. Han J, Globus A, Jaffe R, Deardorff G: Molecular dynamics simulations of carbon nanotube-based gears. **Nanotechnology** 8:95–102, 1997.

184   CLINICAL NEUROSURGERY

67. Heath JR, Keukes PJ, Snider GS, Williams RS. A defect-tolerant computer architecture: opportunities for nanotechnology. **Science** 280:1716–1721, 1998.
68. Henderson E, Haydon PG, Sakaguchi DS: Actin filament dynamics in living glial cells imaged by atomic force microscopy. **Science** 257:1944–1946, 1992.
69. Honjie D, Hafner JH, Rinzler AG, Colbert DT, Smalley RE: Nanotubes as nanoprobes in scanning probe microscopy. **Nature** 384:147–151, 1996.
70. Hopkins LN, Lanzino G, Guterman LR: Treating complex nervous system vascular disorders through a "needle stick": origin, evolution, future of neuroendovascular therapy. **Neurosurgery** 48(3): 463–475, 2001.
71. Horber JKH, Haberle W, Ohnesorge F, Binnig G, Liebich HG, Czerny CP, Mahnel H, Mayr A: Investigation of living cells in the nanometer regime with the scanning force microscope. **Scanning Microscopy** 6:919–930, 1992.
72. Human Genome issue. **Science** 291:1145–1434, 2001.
73. Human Genome issue. **Nature** 409:813–960, 2001.
74. Interagency Working Group on Nanoscience, Engineering, and Technology: Nanotechnology—a revolution in the making – vision for R&D in the next decade. Presented to the OSTP Committee on Technology, March 10, 1999.
75. Issues in nanotechnology. **Science** 290:1523–1545, 2000.
76. Jager EWH, Inganas O, Lundstrom I: Microrobots for micrometer-size objects in aqueous media: potential tools for single cell manipulation. **Science** 288:2335–2338, 2000.
77. Jager EWH, Smela E, Inganas O: Microfabricating conjugated polymer actuators. **Science** 290:1540–1545, 2000.
78. Jewel JL, Harbison JP, Scherer A: Microlasers. **Sci Am** 265:86–94, 1991.
79. Jordan BR: 'Genomics': buzzword or reality. **J Biomed Sci** 6(3):145–150, 1999.
80. Kaminski N: Bioinformatics: a user's perspective. **Am J Respir Cell Mol Biol** 23(6):705–711, 2000.
81. Keller O: Near-field optics: the nightmare of the photon. **Journal of Chemical Physics** 112(18):7856–7863, 2000.
82. Kennedy GC: The impact of genomics on therapeutic drug development. **EXS** 89: 1–10, 2000.
83. Kiick KL, van Hest JCM, Tirrell DA: Expanding the scope of protein biosynthesis by altering the methionly-tRNA synthetase activity of a bacterial expression host. **Angew Chem Int Ed** 39:2148–2152, 2000.
84. Kim P, Lieber CM: Nanotube nanotweezers. **Science** 286:2148–2150, 1999.
85. Kockro RA, Serra S, Tseng-Tsai Y, Chan C, Yih-Yian S, Gim-Guan C, Lee E, Hoe LY, Hern N, Nowinski WL: Planning and simulation of neurosurgery in a virtual reality environment. **Neurosurgery** 46(1):118–137, 2000.
86. Kopanski JJ, Marchiando JF, Lowney JR: Scanning capacitance microscopy measurements and modeling: progress towards dopant profiling of silicon. **Journal of Vacuum Science and Technology B** 14(1):242–247.
87. Krejchi MT, Atkins EDT, Waddon AJ, Fournier MJ, Mason TL, Tirrell DA: Chemical sequence control of β-sheet assembly in macromolecular crystals of periodic polypeptides. **Science** 265:1427–1432, 1994.
88. Kroto HW: The stability of the fullerenes C_n with n = 24, 28, 32, 36, 50, 60, and 70. **Nature** 329:529–531, 1987.
89. Kroto HW, Heath JR, O'Brien SC, Curl RF, Smalley RE: C-60 buckminster fullerene. **Nature** 318:162–163, 1985.
90. Leach G: Advances in molecular CAD. **Nanotechnology** 7:197–203, 1996.
91. Leach GI, Merkle RC: Crystal clear: a molecular CAD tool. **Nanotechnology** 5: 168–171, 1994.
92. LeCorbusier. *Towards a New Architecture*. Architectural Press, London, 1927.

93. Lee GU, Chrisey LA, Colton RJ: Direct measurement of the forces between complementary strands of DNA. **Science** 266:771–773, 1994.

94. Le Roux PD, Das H, Esquenazi S, Kelly PJ: Robot-assisted microsurgery: a feasibility study in the rat. **Neurosurgery** 48(3): 584–589.

95. Letvin NL: Progress in the development of an HIV-1 vaccine. **Science** 280(5371): 1875–1880, 1998.

96. Liu J, Rinzler A, Dai H, Hafner J, Bradley R, Lu A, Shelimov K, Huffman C, Rodriguez-Macias F, Boul P, Iverson T, Colbert DT, Smalley RE: Fullerene pipes. **Science** 280:1253, 1998.

97. Lloyd S: Universal quantum simulators. **Science** 273(5278):1073–1078, 1996.

98. Loeb GE: Neural prosthetics, in Arbib MA (ed): *The Handbook of Brain Theory and Neural Networks.* Cambridge, MIT Press, 2000, ed 2.

99. Loeb GE, Peck RA, Moore WH, Hood K: BION system for distributed neural prosthetic interfaces. **Med Eng Phys** 23(1):9–18, 2001.

100. Lowrie DB, Tascon RE, Bonato VL, Lima VM, Faccioli LH, Stavropoulos E, Colston MJ, Hewinson RG, Moelling K, Silva CL: Therapy of tuberculosis in mice by DNA vaccination. **Nature** 400(6741):269–271, 1999.

101. Maddox J: Toward the quantum computer? **Nature** 316:573, 1985.

102. Mahoney RJ: Opportunity for agricultural biotechnology. Science 289(5478):392–393, 2000.

103. Maitland-van der Zee AH, de Boer A, Leufkens HG: The interface between pharmacoepidemiology and pharmacogenetics. **Eur J Pharmacol** 410(2–3):121–130, 2000.

104. Mao C, LaBean TH, Relf JH, Seeman NC: Logical computation using algorithmic self-assembly of DNA triple-crossover molecules. **Nature** 407:493–496, 2000.

105. Markowitz MA, Kust PK, Deng G, Schoen PE, Dordick JS, Clark DS, Gaber BP: Catalytic silica particles via template-directed molecular imprinting. **Langmuir** 16:1759–1765, 2000.

106. Martins-Green M: The dynamics of cell-ECM interactions with implications for tissue engineering, in Lanza RP, Langer R, Chick WL (eds.): *Principles of Tissue Engineering.* R. G. Landes Co., Austin, 1997.

107. McGrath P: Building a better human. **Newsweek** 136(26A):46–49, 2000.

108. Meyer UA: Pharmacogenetics and adverse drug reactions. **Lancet** 356(9242):1667–1671, 2000.

109. Mooney DJ, Mikos AG: Growing new organs. **Sci Am** 280(4):60–65, 1999.

110. Moore GE: Cramming more components onto integrated circuits. **Electronics** 38(8), April 19, 1965.

111. Moravec H: *Mind Children: The Future of Robot and Human Intelligence.* Cambridge, MA, Harvard University Press, 1988.

112. Mosbach K: Molecular imprinting. **Trend Biochem Sci** 19:9–14, 1994.

113. Moshe H, Spiegelman R, Feldman Z, Berkenstadt H, and Ram Z: Novel, compact, intraoperative magnetic resonance image-guided system for conventional neurosurgical operating rooms. **Neurosurgery** 48(4):799–809, 2001.

114. Near-field optics issue. **J Microscopy** 202:1–450, 2001.

115. Neubauer G, Erikson AN, Williams CC, Rodgers M, Adderton D: Two-dimensional scanning capacitance measurements of cross-sectioned very large scale integration test structures. **Journal of Vacuum Science and Technology B** 14(1): 426–432, 1996.

116. Patrick CW Jr, Mikos AG, McIntire LV (eds): *Frontiers in Tissue Engineering.* New York, Elsevier Science, 1998.

117. Pawson T, Scott JD: Signaling through scaffold, anchoring, and adaptor proteins. **Science** 278:2075–2080, 1997)

118. Pennisi E: Breakthrough of the year: The lamb that roared. **Science** 278:2038–2039, 1997.
119. Petka WA, Harden JL, McGrath KP, Wirtz D, Tirrell DA: Reversible hydrogels from self-assembling artificial proteins. **Science** 281:389–392, 1998.
120. Petty MC, Bryce MR, Bloor D: *Introduction to Molecular Electronics*. London, Edward Arnold, 1995.
121. Popescu AI: Bionics, biological systems and the principle of optimal design. **Acta Biotheoretica** 46(4):299:310, 1998–1999.
122. Proksch R, Skidmore GD, Dahlberg ED, Foss S, Schmidt JJ, Merton C, Welsh B, Dugas M: Quantitative magnetic field measurements with the magnetic force microscope. **Applied Physics Letters** 69(17):2599–2601, 1996.
123. Quake SR, Scherer A: From micro- to nanofabrication with soft materials. **Science** 290:1536–1540, 2000.
124. Ratner B: Perspectives and possibilities in biomaterial science, in Ratner BD, Hoffman AS, Schoen FJ, Lemons JE (eds.): *Biomaterials Science: An Introductions to Materials in Medicine*. Academic Press, San Diego, 1996.
125. Rawlings CJ, Searls DB: Computational gene discovery and human disease. **Curr Opin Gen Dev** 7(3):416–423, 1997.
126. Reed MA, Tour JM: Computing with molecules. **Sci Am** 282:86–93, 2000.
127. Reed MA, Zhou C, Muller CJ, Burgin TP, Tour JM: Conductance of a molecular junction. **Science** 278:252–254, 1997.
128. Rotman D: The next biotech harvest. **Technology Review** September/October, 1998.
129. Roy S, Ferrara L, Fleischman A, Benzel EC: MEMS and neurosurgery: A new era in a new millennium. **Neurosurgery**, 44: (in press), 2001.
130. Rutka JT, Taylor M, Mainprize T, Langlois A, Ivanchuk S, Mondal S, Dirks P: Molecular biology and neurosurgery in the third millennium. **Neurosurgery** 46(5):1034–1051, 2000.
131. Sarikaya M: Biomimetics: materials fabrication through biology. **Proc Natl Acad Sci USA** 96(25):14183–14185, 1999.
132. Service RF: Borrowing from biology to power the petite. **Science** 1999; 283:27–28.
133. Sharma N, Furter R, Tirrell DA: Efficient introduction of aryl bromide functionality into proteins *in vivo*. **FEBS Letters** 467:37–40, 2000.
134. Skidmore GD, Dahlberg ED: Improved spatial resolution in MFM. **Applied Physics Letters** 71(22)/3293–3295, 1997.
135. Sleytr UB, Pum D, Sara M: Advances in S-layer nanotechnology and biomimetics. **Advances in Biophysics** 34:71–79, 1997.
136. Smalley RE: Discovering the fullerenes: Nobel lecture. **Review of Modern Physics** 69:723–730, 1997.
137. Song A, Parus S, Kopelman R: High-performance fiber-optic pH microsensors for practical physiological measurements using a dual-emission sensitive dye. **Anal Chem** 69(5): 863–867, 1997.
138. Soong RK, Bachand GD, Neves HP, Olkhovets AG, Craighead HG, Montemagno CD: Powering an inorganic nanodevice with a biomolecular motor. **Science** 290:1555–1558, 2000.
139. Stemmer WPC: Rapid evolution of a protein by *in vitro* DNA shuffling. **Nature** 370:389–391, 1994.
140. Sterkman LG, Riesle J. The frontier of substitution medicine: integrating biomaterials and tissue engineering. **IEEE Eng Med Biol Mag** 19(3):115–117, 2000.
141. Stout AL: Detection and characterization of individual intermolecular bonds using optical tweezers. **Biophys J** 80:2976–2986, 2001.

142. Suaning GJ, Lovell NH, Schindhelm K, Coroneo MT: The bionic eye (electronic visual prosthesis): a review. **Aust N Z J Opthalmol** 26(3):195–202, 1998.

143. Sugarman J: Policy forum: human genetics. Ethical considerations in leaping from bench to bedside. **Science** 285(5436):2071–2072, 1999.

144. Sullivan NJ, Sanchez A, Rollin PE, Yang ZY, Nabel GJ: Development of a preventive vaccine for Ebola virus infection in primates. **Nature** 408(6812):605–609, 2000.

145. Tan W, Kopelman R, Barker SL, Miller MT: Ultrasmall optical sensors for cellular measurements. **Anal Chem** 71(17):606A–612A, 1999.

146. Thomson RC, Mikos AG, Beahm E, Lemon JC, Satterfield WC, Aufdemorte TB, Miller MJ: Guided tissue fabrication from periosteum using preformed biodegradable polymer scaffolds. **Biomaterials** 20:2007–2018, 1999.

147. Turner APF: Biosensors—sense and sensitivity. **Science** 290:1315–1317, 2000.

148. van Hest JCM, Kiick KL, Tirrell DA: Efficient incorporation of unsaturated methionine analogues into proteins *in vivo*. **J Am Chem Soc** 122:1282–1288, 2000.

149. Vesell ES: Advances in pharmacogenetics and pharmacogenomics. **J Clin Pharmacol** 40(9):930–938, 2000.

150. Vinuela F, Murayama Y, Duckwiler GM, Gobin YP, Jahan R: "Unreachable" peaks of the neurointerventional mountaineers. **Neurosurgery** 48(3): 698–699, 2001.

151. Wang R, Doolan DL, Le TP, Hedstrom RC, Coonan KM, Charoenvit Y, Jones TR, Hobart P, Margalith M, Ng J, Weiss WR, Sedegah M, de Taisne C, Norman JA, Hoffman SL: Induction of antigen-specific cytotoxic T lymphocytes in humans by a malaria DNA vaccine. **Science** 282(5388):476–480, 1998.

152. Weiner DB, Kennedy RC: Genetic vaccines. **Sci Am** 281(1):50–57, 1999.

153. Welsh ER, Tirrell DA: Engineering the extracellular matrix: A novel approach to polymeric biomaterials. I. Control of physical properties of artificial protein matrices designed to support adhesion of vascular endothelial cells. **Biomacromolecules** 1: 23–30, 2000.

154. Willard HF: Genomics and gene therapy. Artificial chromosomes coming to life. **Science** 290(5495):1308–1309, 2000.

155. Wilson BS: The future of cochlear implants. **Br J Audiol** 31(4):205–225, 1997.

156. Wolfenbarger LL, Phifer PR: The ecological risks and benefits of genetically engineered plants. **Science** 290(5499):2088–2093, 2000.

157. Yakobson BI, Smalley RE: Fullerene nanotubes: $C_{1,000,000}$ and beyond. **Am Scientist** 85:324–337, 1997.

158. Ying H, Zaks TZ, Wang RF, Irvine KR, Kammula US, Marincola FM, Leitner WW, Restifo NP: Cancer therapy using a self-replicating RNA vaccine. **Nat Med** 5(7): 823–827, 1999.

159. Yu SM, Conticello V, Zhang GH, Kayser C, Fournier MJ, Mason TL, Tirrell DA: Smectic ordering in solutions ad films of a rod-like polymer owing to monodispersity of chain length. **Nature** 389;167–170, 1997.

160. Zanjani ED, Anderson WF: Prospects for in utero human gene therapy. **Science** 285(5436):2071–2072, 1999.

161. Zhao H, Giver L, Shao Z, Affholter JA, Arnold FH: Molecular evolution by staggered extension process (StEP) *in vitro* recombination. **Nat Biotechnol** 16:258–261, 1998.

162. Zlokovic BV, Apuzzo MLJ: Cellular and molecular neurosurgery: Pathways from concept to reality—Part II: Vector systems and delivery methodologies for gene therapy of the central nervous system. **Neurosurgery** 40(4): 805–813, 1997.

163. Zlokovic BV, Apuzzo MLJ: Cellular and molecular neurosurgery: Pathways from concept to reality—Part I: Target disorders and concept approaches to gene therapy of the central nervous system. **Neurosurgery** 40(4): 789–804, 1997.

CHAPTER

10

Revelations in Deformity Correction and Scoliosis Surgery

GEOFFREY P. ZUBAY, M.D., AND VOLKER K.H. SONNTAG, M.D.

The clinical significance of spinal deformity has been recognized for centuries. Hippocrates was the first to discuss the condition extensively and to introduce the use of longitudinal traction to treat scoliotic deformities. As discussed by Alberstone and Benzel (2), Ambrose Paré was later credited as the first physician to use an external orthosis to prevent the progression of a scoliotic curve. However, the inadequacies of such therapies were recognized early. French surgeons, Guerin in 1839 and Malgaigne in 1844, performed paraspinal myotomies to treat scoliosis believing the disease to be a consequence of muscle imbalance (2). With advances in surgical technique, the concept of internal surgical correction of a deformity and stabilization developed. Independently, Albee (1) and Hibbs (35) first reported the use of fusion to stabilize the spine. Hibbs used autologous bone applied over the dorsal elements of the spine to achieve fusion to prevent progressive deformity in patients with Pott's disease.

In the latter half of the 20th century, two paradigm shifts spawned the modern age of spinal surgery: the birth of spinal biomechanics and the birth of modern spinal surgical stabilization. Holdsworth, a British orthopedic surgeon, presented his clinical work with traumatic spinal fractures in the 1950s (36). He introduced a classification scheme for traumatic injuries to the spine based on a two-column model of stability. His systematic classification of traumatic spinal injuries is considered one of the earliest attempts to develop a biomechanical theory of injury and a rational diagnostic algorithm for identifying patients with spinal instability.

In the 1930s the introduction of vitallium, a metal resistant to electrolysis used previously as a material for dental fillings, allowed rapid advances in techniques for internal hardware fixation. In the following decades, Paul Harrington made many of the seminal advances in hardware fixation techniques. An orthopedic surgeon, Harrington worked extensively with scoliotic patients from the 1940s to the 1960s (31, 32). Although his early work with compression and distraction hooks and rods made of stainless steel was highly successful in the early treatment of deformity and posttraumatic instability, the corrections often failed over time. Failure was attributed to hardware-related complications that preceded osseous fusion. By achieving early fusion of the spine, Harrington learned that deformity correction and spinal stabilization could be maintained despite later failure of the instrumentation hardware. For these observations, Harrington is credited with the appreciation of the "race between instrumentation failure and the acquisition of spinal fusion."

Contemporary spinal biomechanics and surgical techniques have enabled a sophisticated understanding of spinal instability and correction of spinal deformities. Most of what we have learned is the result of trial-and-error applications of different treatments for different disease processes affecting the spine. Repeatedly, the failure of different instrumentation techniques has forced re-examination of our understanding of the spinal biomechanics involved in different pathologic processes. Such re-examinations have enhanced our knowledge, improving technical applications for achieving spinal balance and stability.

SPINAL BALANCE

The normal spine, which consists of 33 vertebrae interconnected by ligaments, muscles, and articulating joints, serves to transmit load, to allow motion, and to protect the spinal cord. Derangements in any component can impair the ability of the spine to perform any of these functions.

The normal spine has two primary and two secondary curves. The thoracic kyphosis and the lumbosacral kyphosis are present at birth and persist as relatively fixed structural curves partially formed by the structural wedging of the vertebral bodies. Because these sagittal curves are present at birth and are relatively fixed, they are known as primary curves.

As a child develops and assumes an upright head posture, a secondary cervical lordotic curvature is produced. With the assumption of an erect posture, the lumbar lordosis is developed. Because these curves develop in response to postural changes, they are called secondary curves. Furthermore, because these curves are compensatory, they are formed primarily by angulation of the adjacent vertebral bodies and not by wedging of the vertebral bodies like the thoracic kyphotic curvature.

Normal spinal balance is measured in a Cartesian coordinate system with an x, y, and z axis. Typically, the spine is measured in segmental, local, or global coordinate systems. Within these coordinate systems, translation or angulation can be measured. Translation is a calculation of the magnitude of anterior or posterior segmental subluxation. Angulation is a calculation of the magnitude of bending using the Cobb angle technique either segmentally or regionally. The Cobb angle is a reliable method of measuring segmental or regional angulation. The standard error of this technique is within 2 to 3° (6, 7). With these techniques, normal standards for the cervical, thoracic, and lumbar spine have been established to afford surgeons a reference against which to measure deformity.

The cervical spine is the most complex region because it is capable of a wide range of motion. The craniocervical junction includes the occiput, C1, and C2. The atlantooccipital junction affords 13 to 16° of flexion and extension and 5° of lateral bending. The atlantoaxial joint affords 10 to 13° of flexion and extension and 40° of unilateral axial rotation, representing 40% of total rotation in the cervical spine. The entire cervical spine permits 60 to 75° of flexion and extension. The normal limit of translation in the cervical spine is 2 to 3 mm (13).

The thoracic spine is a relatively fixed curve that affords little motion. The thoracic regional curvature from T1 to T12 measures from 20 to 40°. There is one degree of kyphosis per segment, increasing segmentally to 5° at the apex of the thoracic curve at T6-7 (7, 34). The thoracolumbar junction is straight and extends from T12 to L1. It is an area of transition between the rigid thoracic kyphosis and the mobile lumbar lordosis.

The lumbar lordosis starts at L1 and increases gradually down to the sacrum. Normal lordosis ranges from 20 to 60°. The mean lordosis from L1-S1 is 60° with two-thirds of the curvature contributed from L4-S1. The apex of the curve is at L3-4 (7, 34).

Global spinal balance is measured by using a plumb line and a standing radiograph of the entire spine. When dropped from the dens, the plumb line falls near the S1 spinous process in the coronal plane and through the body of C7, anterior to the thoracic spine, posterior to the lumbar spine, and through the posterior corner of S1 in the sagittal plane (7, 34).

Derangements in normal spinal balance lead to derangements in load transmission. With normal spinal balance gravitational load is transmitted through the spine to the sacroiliac joint. The sacroiliac joint is a fibrocartilaginous amphi-arthrodial joint that couples the pelvis to the spine. The numerous ligaments and muscles that interconnect the lumbosacral spine to the pelvis facilitate the transfer of load from the spine to the pelvis and to the hip joints. Derangements in the normal curvature of the spine lead to abnormal load transmission. Instead of load being transferred vertically through the spine, it is absorbed locally. Abnormal levels of stress and strain result and lead to progressive deformity, instability, or both over time. To accommodate abnormal load transmission, compensatory curvature abnormalities can develop in the cervical and lumbar spine to restore spinal balance.

Although compensatory curves may restore spinal balance, they do not correct the primary pathological process. The spine sometimes accommodates small deformities that remain fixed over time. Many deformities, however, are dynamic and tend to progress as a result of the primary pathological process or cyclic gravitational loading. Surgical treatment is needed when a deformity (1) continues to progress leading to progressive spinal imbalance, (2) impairs or threatens the integrity of the spinal cord, (3) causes significant pain, or (4) impairs the function of basic vital organs such as the cardiopulmonary system.

DEFORMITY

There are numerous causes of deformity, many of which are beyond the scope of this article. Deformity can originate from congenital, idiopathic, and acquired causes. Acquired causes of deformity can be subdivided into causes related to degenerative, infectious, traumatic, and iatrogenic causes. Each will be discussed separately.

I. Congenital and Idiopathic Causes of Deformity

Congenital causes of deformity are grouped into failures of formation (type I) and failures of segmentation (type II) (44). Type I abnormalities tend to arise from the formation of hemivertebrae. Hemivertebra can lead to primary derangements in spinal curvature that may progress over time. Type II abnormalities may occur unilaterally or bilaterally. Unilateral abnormalities can cause curvature abnormalities as a child grows.

Idiopathic scoliosis or deformity is the most common form of scoliosis. The Scoliosis Research Society divides idiopathic scoliosis into three groups based on age of presentation: infantile scoliosis (from birth to 3), juvenile scoliosis (between 4 and 10 years), and adolescent scoliosis (between 10 and 20 years) (22).

Infantile scoliosis is unique. Males dominate, and it is often associated with abnormalities like plagiocephaly, bat-ear deformity, congenital muscular torticollis, and developmental hip dysplasia. This deformity is thought to result from a compressive fetopathy caused by abnormal intrauterine positioning (11).

In contrast, juvenile and adolescent scoliosis is seldom associated with such neonatal deformities. The cause is unknown and there are

TABLE 10.1
Mechanisms of Spinal Deformity

Type of Deformity	Mechanism
Congenital	Segmentation failure
Idiopathic	Unknown
Acquired	
Tumor	Tethering
	Bone erosion
Infection	Bone erosion
	Gradual onset of instability
Trauma	Acute displacement or instability
	Acute loss of load bearing features
Degenerative	Gradual loss of load bearing features
Iatrogenic	Surgical compromise of stability
	Increased stress on adjacent segments

numerous theories. An abnormal curvature can originate from a variety of factors that may include a discrepancy between the anterior and posterior growth of the spine, neuromuscular abnormalities, or a neurohormonal abnormality related to the pineal gland (45).

These causes of deformity are beyond the scope this discussion. Their importance, however, in understanding how to correct a deformity is underscored by the advances in spinal correction and stabilization. Harrington's seminal work was the product of his experience in the treatment of patients with idiopathic scoliosis (31,32).

II. Acquired Deformity

The most frequently treated type of deformity is the acquired deformity. Deformity can be acquired as the result of the normal degenerative process, tumors, infections, and trauma. Each compromises the normal integrity of the spine either segmentally or globally and can lead to a progressive deformity that impairs the load-bearing characteristics of the spine and the spine's ability to protect the spinal cord. In each case the treatment is removal or repair of the abnormality, restoration of spinal balance, and spinal fusion for long-term maintenance of spinal balance.

DEGENERATIVE DEFORMITY

All people undergo degenerative changes in the spine over time. Repetitive cyclic loading of the spine can result in ultrastructural changes to the vertebral bodies. Normal aging and use also leads to loss of the normal water content of the disc materials leading to loss of disc mobility and height. In the healthy spine the primary curves of the thoracic and sacral spine are formed by normal structural wedging of the vertebral bodies. To maintain sagittal balance during the erect posture, the cervical and lumbar lordosis are formed primarily by the wedging of the disc spaces. Wedging of the cervical and lumbar vertebral bodies does not normally occur except in pathologic conditions. With aging, degeneration of the disc spaces in the cervical and lumbar spine leads to loss of the lordosis. Loss of the lumbar lordosis displaces the thoracic curve anteriorly resulting in positive sagittal balance. Without the lumbar lordosis to balance the thoracic kyphosis in the sagittal plane, repetitive gravitational loading will cause the thoracic curve to progress in a debilitating fashion resulting in a pathologic kyphosis. Degenerative changes as such occur in people to varying degrees. Such changes may be responsible for the genesis of degenerative scoliosis which is sporadically identified in the adult population.

Degenerative scoliosis typically occurs primarily in the lumbar spine. Secondary compensatory curves may develop in the thoracic spine. It rarely occurs in patients younger than 40 years. Usually, its course is insidious and is characterized by a combination of leg and back pain. Theoretically, the disc spaces degenerate at a rate that exceeds the rate at which compensatory facet hypertrophy and anterior osteophyte formation can form to stabilize the spine. Subsequently, an abnormal curvature of the spine develops. In contrast to typical patients with a symptomatic degenerative back and stenosis related to facet hypertrophy, these patients manifest symptoms or a progression of symptoms related to a progressive scoliotic deformity.

Most patients with degenerative back disease have some abnormal curvature. Deciding when the degree of deformity is a relevant consideration in the surgical and nonsurgical management of a patient is difficult (24, 41, 47).

Numerous authors have reported their experience in the treatment of such disease. Different classification schemes have been reported in an attempt to standardize the care of such patients. The details of these classification schemes are beyond the scope of this paper, but the principles are considered universal. Globally considered factors are (1) the degree of coronal and sagittal imbalance, (2) the amount of translation (subluxation), (3) the extent of stenosis, and (4) the degree to which the deformity is reducible on bending radiographs (24, 41, 47).

Patients with mild stenosis, mild sagittal and coronal imbalance, and a paucity of symptoms related to the stenosis usually can be managed with conservative means alone. Conservative treatments include physical therapy and low-impact exercise. The senior author recommends walking and swimming for these purposes.

Patients who have significant symptoms related to significant radiographic stenosis, mild coronal and sagittal imbalance, and the absence of radiographic instability usually can be treated with surgical decompression alone. The senior author places patients who also have a significant component of back pain in an orthotic device such as a thoracolumbosacral orthosis for several weeks before surgery. If patients' back pain is reduced significantly in response to external orthotic immobilization, fusion over the segments decompressed is offered with no emphasis on deformity correction.

Patients with significant symptoms related to radiographic stenosis, and significant coronal and sagittal deformities may be candidates for surgical decompression and surgical correction of the deformity. These patients usually have greater degrees of vertebral body subluxation and demonstrate a reasonable amount of correction of their coronal deformities on lateral bending radiographs. The use of posterior pedicle screw fixation systems usually achieves a significant degree of coronal and sagittal deformity correction with in situ rod bending, rod rotation, and three-point bending techniques.

Occasionally, patients exhibit significant symptoms related to radiographic stenosis and significant sagittal and coronal deformities that do not correct on bending radiographs. An anterior and posterior combined surgical approach can be used to treat these patients. Surgery is performed anteriorly to release the disc segments and to enable the placement of spacers to help correct the coronal and sagittal imbalance. The rate of morbidity associated with such procedures is high, and patients need to be selected carefully for such procedures.

In correcting all such deformities, particular care is needed to begin and end the fusion at neutral and stable vertebrae and to avoid ending the fusion at the apex of a major sagittal curve. The apex of the thoracic kyphosis is from T5-9, and the apex of the lumbar curve is at L3-4. Extending the fusion beyond these curvature apices may be prudent to avoid complications such as the development of disabling sagittal imbalance.

TUMOR-RELATED CAUSES OF DEFORMITY

Primary intraspinal tumors, primary intraosseous tumors, and metastatic tumors to the spinal column can cause a spinal deformity. The tumors often become symptomatic with pain or myelopathy related to spinal cord compression. Deformity is usually a late feature of tumor-related pathology. Some tumors, such as lipomas, can tether the spinal cord resulting in a scoliotic deformity. Primary left thoracic and cervicothoracic curves can be associated with primary spinal cord pathology, and when identified a primary neurologic disorder should be screened with spinal magnetic resonance (MR) imaging. A primary intraspinal pathology will be identified in as many as 20% of such patients (5). In these patients treatment of the primary intraspinal pathology can lead to spontaneous correction of the deformity over time.

Resection of tumors often destabilizes the spine dramatically. If left untreated, immediate or late deformity can result. A classic example of the development of a late deformity is postcervical laminectomy kyphosis. Besides the extensive laminectomy needed to remove the tumor, postoperative chemotherapy or radiation therapy may further destabilize the spine. Consequently, when a spinal axis tumor is to be resected, spinal reconstruction should be considered.

Anteriorly in the cervical spine, corpectomies can be performed. Bone should be resected until healthy margins are encountered. The segment can be filled with an autologous or donated bone strut to reconstruct the anterior column of the spine. Similar techniques are used in the thoracolumbar spine, but bone-filled metallic cages are more popular. Posteriorly, lateral mass plates can be used in the cervical spine and pedicle screws can be used in the thoracolumbar spine. Such posterior fixation systems are preferable because the spinous processes and lamina are usually removed to obtain adequate tumor resection.

INFECTION-RELATED CAUSES OF DEFORMITY

The origins of infections to the spinal column are numerous. Most spread to the spine through a hematogenous route. Infection can spread into the subchondral endplates, leading to endplate infarction and osteomyelitis, and can spread to the disc space especially in the young with their prominent vascular supply to the disc.

Typically, infection causes segmental pain. The natural load-bearing viscoelastic properties of the vertebral body are compromised by the infection. In the absence of deformity early in infections, treatment with antibiotics alone can restore the lost load-bearing characteristics of the vertebral body. In these patients, procuring a diagnosis with needle biopsy following intravenous antibiotics and external orthotic immobilization is the treatment of choice.

Surgery is often required. The compromised biomechanical properties of the infected body can lead to progressive deformity that jeopardizes the spinal cord. The infection load in the affected vertebral bodies may require generous debridement to facilitate adequate antibiotic treatment. When surgery is needed, aggressive debridement of the affected tissues is necessary. The surgeon should ensure that normal bleeding bone is encountered at the margins of the debridement to provide an optimal substrate for bone grafts and instrumentation. Instrumentation and fusion are needed when the spine is intrinsically unstable from infection or when instability is acquired from extensive bone debridement.

There has long been a reluctance to apply hardware in the presence of infection although the idea is now discredited (43). However, poor blood supply to the scar tissue at the interface of the hardware and soft tissue acts as a refuge for bacteria escaping the bacteriocidal effects of antibiotics. Consequently, it is mandatory to proceed with dissection of the soft tissue until good, healthy bone is encountered.

TRAUMA-RELATED CAUSES OF DEFORMITY

Perhaps the most extensive experience has been accumulated from correcting trauma-related deformity and instability. In trauma-related cases, fusion and stabilization are the mainstays for affording adequate and immediate protection of the spinal cord, which can be jeopardized by destabilizing injuries to the spinal column. The application of appropriate deformity correction principles and adequate restoration of spinal balance are important for the long-term maintenance of that balance and prevention of delayed deformity progression. Because the treatment of various traumatic injuries to the spine is so complex, the different regions of the spine are considered separately.

THE OCCIPITAL CERVICAL JUNCTION
AND THE SUBAXIAL CERVICAL SPINE

The occipitocervical junction, which includes the base of the occiput, C1 and C2, has unique biomechanical properties. Trauma to this region often requires operative fixation and fusion because of excessive instability. The determination of instability is based solely on radiographic studies that provide information about the morphology of fractures and the integrity of surrounding supporting ligamentous structures.

The base of the occiput articulates with the cervical spine through the occipital condyles. Condylar fractures are classified into three types based on their morphology. Type I fractures have no displacement into the foramen magnum and are usually stable. Type II fractures are extensions of basilar skull fractures and usually stable (3, 55). Type III fractures involve medially displaced fragments and are typically traction injuries related to the alar ligaments. These fractures are potentially unstable. Because of the complex relationships at the occipitocervical junction, fusion, if needed, must extend from the occiput to at least C3. However, most Type III injuries can be treated successfully with a halo apparatus.

In an atlanto-occipital dislocation, the normal ligaments that secure the top of the cervical spine to the occiput are disrupted. Because large forces are required to cause such an injury, patients rarely survive the initial injury. Consequently, diagnosis is often made postmortem (16). Clinically, the diagnosis is based on radiographic criteria measuring the relationship of C1 and C2 to the base of the occiput. To prevent further neurologic injury, this highly unstable injury needs to be repaired surgically as soon as possible.

The C1 fracture was originally described in a study by Sir Geoffrey Jefferson and subsequently became known as Jefferson fractures (38). They result from axial-loading injuries to the spine that burst the vertebral body. When the injury is significant, the transverse ligament, which maintains the relationship of C2 to the C1 body, is compromised making the fracture unstable. The ligamentous injury can be indirectly diagnosed based on radiographs, which can identify more than 6.9 mm of lateral spread of the lateral masses. Or it can be diagnosed directly by MR imaging of the spine, which identifies primary injury to the transverse ligament (53). Unstable injuries require fusion of C1 to C2. If the morphology of the C1 fracture does not allow segmental C1-2 fusion, the fusion needs to be extended to the occiput (4, 27).

The C2 body can be injured in a variety of manners (26, 28). Fractures of the odontoid process are characterized based on the location of the fracture line in the odontoid process. External orthoses are usually sufficient to treat fractures alone. Electively, patients may undergo reduction of the C2 fracture with an anteriorly placed odontoid screw (40). When the transverse ligament is disrupted as seen on MR imaging, a C1-2 fusion is needed if the degree of fracture is displaced more than 5 mm anteriorly or posteriorly (14, 15, 23). C1-2 fusion can be achieved with transarticular screws, posterior interspinous wiring, or both (17, 39, 49). Transarticular screws provide superior stability with respect to rotational stress and strain.

When the C2 body is fractured through the pars interarticularis, the fracture is known as a hangman's fracture. Again, the need for fusion is determined by the degree of deformity (28). Angulation or displacement of the C2 body indicates ligamentous injury as well as possibly a C2-3 disc herniation. Fusion with an anterior cervical discotomy at C2-3 and subsequent fusion and plating should be considered. If reduction cannot be performed preoperatively, the deformity can be reduced intraoperatively under radiographic visualization.

Subaxial cervical spinal injuries resulting in deformity include unilateral and bilateral locked facets, fracture dislocations, and wedge-compression fractures of the vertebral bodies. Appropriate treatment begins with identifying the deformity, restoring spinal balance, and fixating the unstable segment.

The use of anterior or posterior fixation depends on several questions. Is the primary injury to the anterior or posterior elements? Can the deformity be corrected effectively from an anterior or posterior approach? Is an anterior and/or a posterior decompression indicated? Which approach is safer for the patient? Should the patient undergo both approaches for both anterior and posterior fixation?

It is difficult to make generalizations about many of these questions. The mechanism of injury and the forces that need to be applied to reduce the deformity are the most important considerations. Fractures that lead to significant structural compromise of the vertebral body causing kyphotic angulation of the normal cervical lordosis are treated optimally by anterior approaches. Anterior cervical discectomies and/or corpectomy can restore normal cervical lordosis using distracting and load-sharing anterior struts fixated with anterior plating systems (9, 20).

In contrast, posterior injuries often are treated optimally with lateral mass plating or screw-rod systems. As rigid constructs, lateral mass plating or screw-rod systems are superior to older wiring techniques. Lateral mass plating or hook-rod systems also can be applied in the presence of fractured lamina, fractured spinous processes, and extensive decompressive laminectomies (10, 21). Injuries that compromise the dorsal tension band can be treated effectively with such hardware systems. Older wiring techniques depend on the integrity of these components of the posterior spine.

Intuitively, as injuries that affect the facet joint, unilateral and bilateral facet dislocations should be treated effectively with posterior techniques. Reduction and fixation of facet dislocations can be readily achieved by posterior techniques, and short segment fixation with interspinous wiring, lateral mass plates, or hook-rod systems can stabilize the reduced segmental deformity. However, the use of posterior techniques alone may increase a patient's risk of a reduction-related injury. Using posterior reduction techniques in the setting of a large anterior disc herniation associated with a facet dislocation may injure the spinal cord (29).

In one study, MR imaging identified a herniated disc in 46% of patients with facet subluxations and unilateral facet dislocations and in 62% of patients with bilateral facet dislocations (29). If a significant disc herniation is present, the safest option may be an anterior approach for primary decompression of the disc space before open reduction of the deformity is considered. Correction of the deformity related to unilateral or bilateral facet dislocation from an anterior approach is also well described. The senior author prefers using distracting posts in the adjacent vertebral bodies to reduce the subluxation under fluoroscopic guidance. After reduction, fusion and arthrodesis are achieved with an anterior strut graft and a ventral fixation plate. Routine posterior fixation is unnecessary.

THE THORACIC AND LUMBAR SPINE

The early internal reduction and fixation of traumatic fractures of the thoracolumbar spine have been advocated since the time of Holdsworth (36). Early treatment offers patients the opportunity for early rehabilitation. The evolution of fixation techniques involving anterior and posterior approaches has paralleled an increased understanding of the biomechanical issues relevant to the restoration of spinal balance and deformity correction.

The thoracolumbar spine assumes most of the gravitational load-bearing requirements of the spine. Because the center of gravity is anterior to the spine, the predominant stress to the spine is a gravitational bending moment. Traumatically injured segments of the spine can cause deformity as a result of impaired load-bearing capabilities. Deformity results from loss of height, abnormal kyphotic angulation, and subluxation.

The surgical treatment of thoracolumbar fractures is needed for frank instability and deformities causing spinal imbalance and when the risk for delayed progression of a deformity is significant.

Our understanding of spinal stability in the thoracolumbar spine is best summarized by the classical work of Denis. Denis (12) reviewed 412 thoracolumbar fractures and modified Holdsworth's (36) two-column theory by dividing the anterior column into anterior and middle columns. The stability of fractures is often defined based on Denis's classification system. When two or more columns of the spine are impaired, a fracture is classified as unstable.

Deformity is usually defined by angulation in the sagittal and coronal planes. A common parameter is the sagittal index, (7, 37) a segmental Cobb measurement of kyphosis corrected for the normal regional kyphosis of the spine. In the thoracic spine 5° are subtracted, in the thoracolumbar region no adjustment is made, and in the lumbar spine 10° are added to account for the normal lordosis. A sagittal index greater than 15 is associated with an increased risk for segmental instability and progression of kyphosis (24).

Using Denis's classification system and segmental Cobb angle measurements can help surgeons to decide when surgery is needed to stabilize a fracture to prevent delayed deformity (12). In fact, most treatment algorithms for complex thoracolumbar fractures evaluate the morphology of the fracture based on these criteria and the subjective determination of a fracture's ability to participate in anterior load sharing. However, most of these treatment algorithms are based on retrospective clinical data. An equal number of contradictory papers support conservative treatment alone (8, 25). For example, Cantor et al. reported no complications from the nonoperative treatment of thoracolumbar fractures associated with kyphotic deformities as large as 26% and with as much as 60% loss of vertebral height (8). At best, therefore, these measurement techniques serve as guidelines in the management of thoracolumbar fractures.

When the decision to treat a wedge-compression fracture surgically is made, a deformity can be corrected and fixed anteriorly or posteriorly. Correction of the segmental sagittal deformity is essential to restore global sagittal balance. Fixation and fusion in the absence of sagittal plane correction can lead to long-term complications related to sagittal imbalance.

Using posterior approaches, a short segment pedicle screw fixation system can restore segmental stability and allow correction of the segmental sagittal plane. When there is significant injury to the vertebral body anteriorly with significant loss of vertebral height and kyphosis, correction and stabilization posteriorly may be insufficient because the vertebral body is unable to participate in anterior load sharing. If the vertebral body is unable to participate in anterior load sharing after reduction, axial loading transmits the entire load to the hardware posteriorly and its failure is accelerated. To prevent this complication, an anterior load-bearing strut can be placed posteriorly by performing a transpedicular corpectomy, a costotransversectomy approach, or a lateral extracavitary approach. Alternatively, an anterior approach can be performed to place the load-bearing strut, or the fracture can be treated entirely by an anterior approach with the use of an anterior strut and screw-plate system.

Burst fractures often require an anterior approach because the spinal canal is compromised by retropulsed fragments. Retropulsed fragments are poorly treated through midline posterior approaches. Sometimes, more complex lateral and far-lateral posterior approaches afford adequate access to the retropulsed fragment. However, the anterior approach is preferred because it easily affords the ability to decompress the spinal canal, to correct a deformity with a distracting anterior strut to restore the normal curvature of the spine, to confer adequate anterior load-sharing features to the construct, and to allow adequate fixation with an anteriorly placed screw-plate or rod construct.

Fracture dislocations of the spine are unstable injuries that often require the application of significant forces to restore normal alignment. Typically, such forces are applied using posterior techniques. Most of the techniques used in such reductions are adaptations of techniques used to correct scoliosis.

Successful deformity correction depends on achieving the desired curve correction while assembling a construct with evenly distributed forces of low magnitude. If any construct is assembled under significant stress, any or all of its components are likely to fail.

Numerous techniques are used to allow the application of large bending moments to correct a deformity while reducing the likelihood of hardware failure. Because the magnitude of the moment that can be applied is proportional to the length of the system, a longer construct affords more of a mechanical advantage during reduction than a shorter one. The length of a construct depends on the magnitude of the bending moment that must be applied to achieve reduction and on the strength of the fixation of individual points. Hooks and wires have weaker points of fixation than other constructs. Therefore, longer constructs need to be assembled to prevent segmental hardware failure. When pedicle screws are used, individual points of fixation tend to be strong and greater forces can be applied with a shorter segment system without jeopardizing the integrity of the construct. The advantage of lengthening the construct and increasing the number of points of fixation is exemplified by biomechanical studies that show that each additional level of pedicle screws reduces the bending moment applied to the hardware at each level by 20% (19).

To reduce a deformity, one end of the rod is assembled either rostral or caudal to the deformity and a bending moment is applied as the other end of the rod is brought down to the spine and secured. This technique is referred to as rod reduction and can be facilitated by numerous techniques. Segmental sequential sublaminar wire tightening can help reduce the bending moment experienced at any given point of fixation, facilitating successful rod reduction. The use of the crossed rod technique exemplifies the application of this principle. Rods on either side of the spine secured at opposing ends of the construct are reduced to the spine using sublaminar wires. Alternatively, a contoured rod can be fixated at one end of a construct and then rotated during fixation to achieve the required reduction. Finally, a rod can be fixated to the spine above and below a given deformity. In situ rod-contouring techniques are then used to achieve the required reduction. Next, in situ rod bending and segmental compression and distraction are applied to optimize the correction of the deformity in the coronal and sagittal planes.

Each of these techniques is associated with its own set of advantages and disadvantages. Combining techniques can optimize outcomes by minimizing the shortcomings of any one technique. For example, the application of sublaminar wires or hooks in a pedicle screw construct helps reduce segmental screw failure by reducing the instantaneous load applied to a given screw during the reduction. Using a combination of rod rotation and in situ rod bending techniques reduces the magnitude of the bending moment that needs to be applied instantaneously during rod reduction, thereby reducing the likelihood of segmental hardware failure.

IATROGENIC CAUSES OF DEFORMITY

Surgical advances have allowed spine surgeons to treat diseases of the spinal axis aggressively. Today ventral, lateral, and posterolateral approaches are common. Complex approaches also have led to the development of sophisticated techniques for fixating hardware to the spine. Improved hardware has led to the development of more rigid fixation systems that better resist stress and strain over time. Unfortunately, such improvements have been associated with an increase in surgical complications. Some of these complications involve the destabilized segments operated on, and some of these complications involve the segments of the spine adjacent to the operated segments of the spine.

The surgical treatment of spinal cord tumors in children can lead to a postlaminectomy kyphosis. The incidence of postlaminectomy kyphosis in the cervical spine is primarily related to the width of the laminectomy performed. With normal axial loading of the spine, the anterior and middle columns of the spine transmit only 36% of the load while the facets individually transmit 32% of the load (33, 48). Not surprisingly, partial facetectomies performed with decompressive laminectomies predispose patients for the subsequent development of instability. In children the risk for developing postlaminectomy kyphosis in the cervical spine is related to the degree of facet violation, the number of lamina removed, the patient's age, and the baseline curvature of the spine. In some clinical series (33), the reported incidence of postlaminectomy kyphosis in children is as high as 95% but is significantly less in adults (33).

In addition to producing cosmetic deformity, postlaminectomy kyphosis causes complications related to spinal cord compression along the apex of the kyphosis. Surgery is indicated to correct the kyphotic deformity, to decompress the neural elements, and to stabilize the spine. Ideally, an anterior approach is used (34, 56). Closed reduction of postlaminectomy kyphotic deformities rarely achieves significant correction because two of the three columns of support remain. After a corpectomy, the remaining stabilizing columns of the spine are eliminated, and reduction can be achieved with manual traction (35, 46).

Earlier attempts to treat postlaminectomy kyphosis with an anterior strut fusion were complicated by a high incidence of graft subluxation and pseudarthrosis (34). These complications required the postoperative application of a halo brace or a second-stage posterior procedure. In most cases, the use of an anterior plating system provides immediate fixation and obviates the need for postoperative halo fixation. In the authors' experience, the application of the cervical plating system dramatically improves outcomes and is the procedure of choice. In the senior author's series, 20 patients treated for postlaminectomy kyphosis all developed a solid fusion and their curvature improved a mean of 16° of residual kyphosis (34).

In contrast, postlaminectomy kyphosis is best prevented by a posterior fusion. For unclear reasons postlaminectomy kyphosis rarely develops in adults (i.e., in the mature spine). The development of postlaminectomy kyphosis in adults probably increases significantly when partial facetectomies are performed to decompress adjacent nerve roots. Many authors advocate unroofing 8 to 10 mm of the nerve root during a posterior approach for nerve root decompression. To decompress 8 to 10 mm of the nerve root, 60 to 70% of the facet needs to be resected (51). When more than 50% of the facet joint is resected bilaterally, the shear strength of the cervical motion segment is compromised significantly (51). Hence, in adults undergoing multilevel cervical laminectomies accompanied by significant resection of the facet joint, prophylactic fusion should be considered to prevent postlaminectomy kyphosis.

Posterior fusion of the spine after laminectomy can be achieved by placing lateral mass plates or rods and screws or by replacing bone with an osteoplastic laminoplasty. Both strategies work well, and their advantages depend upon clinical conditions and the indications for posterior decompression.

In the lumbar spine, frank kyphosis seldom develops when the facets are disrupted. Rather, complications related to glacial instability arise and lead to the translation of vertebral bodies over each other. This olithesis can cause back pain related to instability and radical symptoms related to compromise of the adjacent neural foramen. A posterior fusion is required to restore the normal alignment and stability of the spine. During decompressive surgery, the facets may be disrupted. However, when prophylactic fusion is indicated is controversial.

Sometimes the indications for fusion are more subtle. Postoperatively, patients who have undergone a microdiscectomy to treat a herniated disc can develop complications related to a recurrent disc herniation. In the authors' experience (unpublished data) when a disc herniation recurs more than two times, segmental instability is likely and best treated with local fusion to prevent subsequent complications.

Although decompressive operations can result in local segmental instability and deformity, fixation techniques can lead to adjacent segment instability or deformity. Fixation and fusion of the spine produce a rigid segment of the spine that translates axial load with an increased moment arm to the adjacent segments. The increased moment arm experienced at adjacent segments can accelerate degeneration and the development of instability. The importance of this principal is underscored by the experience of scoliosis surgeons: Long-segment fusions at or near the apex of spinal curvatures are associated with adjacent level disease and instability.

In a retrospective review of patients who underwent lumbar fusion, Rahm and Hall reported a 35% incidence of adjacent segment degeneration (50). The incidence of this complication and how it relates to long-term clinical outcomes is unclear. Although this complication occurs in patients after cervical and lumbar fusion, its overall incidence is probably low. Patients who develop the complication probably share some predisposing features or clinical conditions. Halliday and colleagues have suggested that the magnitude of the stress on adjacent segments may be attenuated by the application of less rigid fixation techniques at the transitional segments (30). The use of sublaminar hooks at the ends of pedicle fixation constructs may attenuate the load transmitted to the adjacent segments. When adjacent level instability does develop, the surgeon is frequently forced to reoperate to extend the existing fusion and to include the adjacent segment.

Less frequently, fusion leads to local segmental complications such as the crankshaft phenomenon and flat-back syndrome. When a posterior fusion is performed in skeletally immature children, there is a risk of complications related to the crankshaft phenomenon. Spinal growth originates from three areas: the posterior articular processes, the vertebral end plates, and the neurocentral synchondrosis. Posterior fusion arrests growth in the articular processes of the spine. Continued growth in the vertebral end plates and the neurocentral synchondrosis causes progressive curvature and rotation as originally described by Dubousset et al. (18). In a study 40 patients undergoing posterior spinal fusion with posterior instrumentation for idiopathic or neurogenic scoliosis under the age of 12 years, curves progressed an average of 15° and rotated an average of 15.5° in 39 (54).

Judging which skeletally immature patients are at greatest risk for this complication is difficult and cannot be determined accurately using traditional techniques to estimate skeletal maturity such as the Risser sign. The best predictors of outcome appear to be age and radiographic assessment of the triradiate cartilage. Current recommendations are to perform an anterior fusion with posterior fusion to arrest anterior growth concurrently in patients younger than 10 years or in those older than 10 years with an open triradiate cartilage (52).

The development of a swan neck deformity after cervical laminectomy may be the result of similar mechanisms involved in the pathogenesis of the crankshaft phenomenon. The posterior arrest of growth with unopposed growth of the anterior vertebral body end plates can lead to the development of this deformity in children after cervical laminectomy. The causes, incidence, and risk factors for the development of this deformity are less well understood.

Flat-back syndrome was common with the use of long-segment distraction systems such as the Harrington rod system. Overdistraction led to the loss of the normal lumbar lordosis, (42) causing sagittal imbalance. Patients become symptomatic from back pain, forward inclination of the trunk, and the inability to stand erect. The incidence of flat back increases significantly when fusion constructs are extended to the sacrum. Prophylaxis is best achieved by using nondistracting hardware systems and fixating the lumbar spine with rods contoured to restore the normal lumbar lordosis, especially when the sacrum is incorporated into the fusion.

CONCLUSION

Advances in fixation techniques and surgical techniques have improved the outcomes of deformity correction. With a more sophisticated understanding of the biomechanical requirements of the spine, a functional spine can better be reconstructed after a disabling deformity develops. Advances in spinal biomechanics have clarified that understanding the spine from a global perspective is critical. The traditional experimental model of the spine evaluated the spinal motion segment. We now understand that restoring stability at the segmental level is only the first step in the process and that restoring global spinal balance is equally important. Complications related to adjacent level instability, adjacent level deformity, and flat-back syndrome are increasingly recognized as failures in foresight during initial surgical treatment and as shortcomings in our understanding of global spinal balance. Spinal surgeons must aggressively adopt a global perspective of patients' biomechanical needs and requirements. The use of finite element analysis models of the spine promises a more complete picture of the spinal biomechanics in the near future. Until then, a comprehensive understanding of current spinal biomechanics and the current surgical methodologies available is a prerequisite for contemporary spinal surgeons.

206 CLINICAL NEUROSURGERY

REFERENCES

1. Albee FH: Transplantation of a portion of the tibia into the spine for Pott's disease. **JAMA** 57:885–886, 1911.
2. Alberstone CD, Benzel EC: History. In Benzel E. (ed) *Spine Surgery: Techniques, Complication Avoidance, and Management.* New York: Churchill Livingstone, 1999, pp 1–21.
3. Anderson PA, Montesano PX: Morphology and treatment of occipital condyle fractures. **Spine** 13:731–736, 1988.
4. Apostolides PJ, Dickman CA, Golfinos JG, et al: Threaded Steinmann pin fusion of the craniovertebral junction. **Spine** 21:1630–1637, 1996.
5. Arai S, Ohtsuka Y, Moriya H, et al: Scoliosis associated with syringomyelia. **Spine** 18:1591–1592, 1993.
6. Beekman CE, Hall V: Variability of scoliosis measurement from spinal roentgenograms. **Phys Ther** 59:764–765, 1979.
7. Bernhardt M: Normal spinal anatomy: Normal sagittal plane alignment. In Bridwell K, DeWald R. (eds): *The Textbook of Spinal Surgery.* Philadelphia: Lippincott-Raven, 1997, pp 185–191.
8. Cantor JB, Lebwohl NH, Garvey T, et al: Nonoperative management of stable thoracolumbar burst fractures with early ambulation and bracing. **Spine** 18:971–976, 1993.
9. Chen TY, Crawford NR, Sonntag VKH, et al: Biomechanical effects of progressive anterior cervical decompression. **Spine** 26:6–14, 2001.
10. Cherny WB, Sonntag VKH, Douglas RA: Lateral mass posterior plating and facet fusion for cervical spine instability. **BNI Quarterly** 7:2–11, 1991.
11. Connor AN: Developmental anomalies and prognosis in infantile idiopathic scoliosis. **J Bone Joint Surg Br** 51:711–713, 1987.
12. Denis F: The three column spine and its significance in the classification of acute thoracolumbar spine injuries. **Spine** 8:817–831, 1983.
13. Dickman CA, Crawford NR: Biomechanics of the craniovertebral junction. In Dickman C, Spetzler R, Sonntag V. (eds): *Surgery of the Craniovertebral Junction.* New York: Thieme, 1998, pp 59–80.
14. Dickman CA, Greene KA, Sonntag VKH: Injuries involving the transverse atlantal ligament: Classification and treatment guidelines based upon experience with 39 injuries. **Neurosurgery** 38:44–50, 1996.
15. Dickman CA, Mamourian A, Sonntag VKH, et al: Magnetic resonance imaging of the transverse atlantal ligament for the evaluation of atlantoaxial instability. **J Neurosurg** 75:221–227, 1991.
16. Dickman CA, Papadopoulos SM, Sonntag VKH, et al: Traumatic occipitoatlantal dislocations. **J Spinal Disord** 6:300–313, 1993.
17. Dickman CA, Sonntag VKH: Posterior C1-C2 transarticular screw fixation for atlantoaxial arthrodesis. **Neurosurgery** 43:275–281, 1998.
18. Dubousset J, Herring JA, Shufflebarger H: The crankshaft phenomenon. **J Pediatr Orthop** 9:541–550, 1989.
19. Duffield RC, Carson WL, Chen LY, et al: Longitudinal element size effect on load sharing, internal loads, and fatigue life of tri-level spinal implant constructs. **Spine** 18:1695–1703, 1993.
20. Eleraky MA, Llanos C, Sonntag VKH: Cervical corpectomy: Report of 185 cases and review of the literature. **J Neurosurg (Spine 1)** 90:35–41, 1999.
21. Fehlings MG, Cooper PR, Errico TJ: Posterior plates in the management of cervical instability: Long-term results in 44 patients. **J Neurosurg** 81:341–349, 1994.

22. Goldstein LA, Waugh TR: Classification and terminology of scoliosis. **Clin Orthop** 93:10–22, 1973.
23. Greene KA, Dickman CA, Marciano FF, et al: Transverse atlantal ligament disruption associated with odontoid fractures. **Spine** 19:2307–2314, 1994.
24. Grubb SA, Lipscomb HJ, Coonrad RW: Degenerative adult onset scoliosis. **Spine** 13:241–245, 1988.
25. Hadley MN, Browner CM, Dickman CA, et al: Compression fractures of the thoracolumbar junction: A treatment algorithm based on 110 cases. **BNI Quarterly** 5:10–19, 1989.
26. Hadley MN, Browner CM, Sonntag VKH: Axis fractures: A comprehensive review of management and treatment in 107 cases. **Neurosurgery** 17:281–290, 1985.
27. Hadley MN, Dickman CA, Browner CM, et al: Acute traumatic atlas fractures: Management and long term outcome. **Neurosurgery** 23:31–35, 1988.
28. Hadley MN, Dickman CA, Browner CM, et al: Acute axis fractures: A review of 229 cases. **J Neurosurg** 71:642–647, 1989.
29. Hadley MN, Fitzpatrick BC, Sonntag VKH, et al: Facet fracture-dislocation injuries of the cervical spine. **Neurosurgery** 31:661–666, 1992.
30. Halliday AL, Zileli M, Stillerman CB, et al: Dorsal thoracic and lumbar screw fixation and pedicle fixation techniques. In Benzel E. (ed): *Spine Surgery: Techniques, Complication Avoidance, and Management.* New York: Churchill Livingstone, 1999, pp 1053–1064.
31. Harrington PR: Treatment of scoliosis. **J Bone Joint Surg Am** 44A:591–610, 1962.
32. Harrington PR: The history and the development of Harrington instrumentation. **Clin Orthop** 93:110–112, 1973.
33. Heller JG, Silcox DHI: Postlaminectomy instability of the cervical spine. Etiology and stabilization technique. In Frymoyer JW (ed): *The Adult Spine: Principles and Practice.* Philadelphia: Lippincott-Raven, 1997, pp 1413–1434.
34. Herman JM, Sonntag VKH: Cervical corpectomy and plate fixation for postlaminectomy kyphosis. **J Neurosurg** 80:963–970, 1994.
35. Hibbs RA: An operation for progressive spinal deformities. **NY Med J** 93:1013–1016, 1911.
36. Holdsworth FW: Fractures, dislocations, and fracture dislocations of the spine. **J Bone Joint Surg Am** 45B:6–20, 1963.
37. Holt RT, Dopf CA, Isaza JE, et al: Adult kyphosis. In Frymoyer JW (ed): *The Adult Spine: Principles and Practice.* Philadelphia: Lippincott-Raven, 1997, pp 1537–1578.
38. Jefferson G: Fracture of the atlas vertebra. Report of four cases, and a review of those previously recorded. **Br J Surg** 7:407–422, 1920.
39. Karahalios DG, Apostolides PJ, Sonntag VKH: Stabilization and fusion techniques for atlantoaxial instability. **Crit Rev Neurosurg** 6:13–19, 1996.
40. Konstantinou D, Levi ADO, Sonntag VKH, et al: Odontoid screw fixation. **BNI Quarterly** 13:14–19, 1997.
41. Korovessis P, Piperos G, Sidiropoulos P, et al: Adult idiopathic lumbar scoliosis. A formula for prediction of progression and review of the literature. **Spine** 19:1926–1932, 1994.
42. Lagrone MO, Bradford DS, Moe JH, et al: Treatment of symptomatic flatback after spinal fusion. **J Bone Joint Surg Am** 70:569–580, 1988.
43. Levi ADO, Sonntag VKH, Dickman CA: Management of postoperative infections after spinal surgery. **Technique Neurosurg** 5:274–281, 1999.
44. Lubicky JP: Congenital scoliosis. In Bridwell KH, DeWald R (eds): *The Textbook of Spinal Surgery.* Philadelphia: Lippincott-Raven, 1997, pp 345–364.
45. Machida M: Cause of idiopathic scoliosis. **Spine** 24:2576–2583, 1999.

46. Marcotte P, Dickman CA, Sonntag VKH, et al: Posterior atlantoaxial facet screw fixation. **J Neurosurg** 79:234–237, 1993.
47. Naderi S, Detwiler PW, Sonntag VKH: Degenerative spondylolisthesis: When to fuse? **Spine** 22:2807–2812, 1998.
48. Pal GP, Sherk HH: The vertical stability of the cervical spine. **J Neurosurg** 13:447–449, 1988.
49. Paramore CG, Dickman CA, Sonntag VKH: The anatomical suitability of the C1-2 complex for transarticular screw fixation. **J Neurosurg** 85:221–224, 1996.
50. Rahm MD, Hall BB: Adjacent-segment degeneration after lumbar fusion with instrumentation: A retrospective study. **J Spinal Disord** 9:392–400, 1996.
51. Raynor RB, Pugh J, Shapiro I: Cervical facetectomy and its effect on spine strength. **J Neurosurg** 63:278–282, 1985.
52. Sanders JO, Herring JA, Browne RH: Posterior arthrodesis and instrumentation in the immature (Risser-grade-0) spine in idiopathic scoliosis. **J Bone Joint Surg Am** 77A:39–45, 1995.
53. Spence KF Jr., Decker S, Sell KW: Bursting atlantal fracture associated with rupture of the transverse ligament. **J Bone Joint Surg Am** 52:543–549, 1970.
54. Terek RM, Wehner J, Lubicky JP: Crankshaft phenomenon in congenital scoliosis: A preliminary report. **J Pediatr Orthop** 11:527–532, 1991.
55. Vishteh AG, Crawford NR, Melton MS, et al: Stability of the craniovertebral junction after unilateral occipital condyle resection: A biomechanical study. **J Neurosurg (Spine 1)** 90:91–98, 1999.
56. Zdeblick TA, Bohlman HH: Cervical kyphosis and myelopathy. Treatment by anterior corpectomy and strut-grafting. **J Bone Joint Surg Am** 71:170–182, 1989.

CHAPTER

11

Biomaterials and Implantable Devices: Discoveries in the Spine Surgery Arena

EDWARD C. BENZEL, M.D., LISA A. FERRARA, M.S., SHUVO ROY, PH.D., AND AARON J. FLEISCHMAN, PH.D.

INTRODUCTION

Most research regarding biomaterials and implantable devices in the spine surgery arena has been focused in the areas of neural protection, neural recovery, and spine structural integrity. It is emphasized that there has been, in general, a failure of medicine and of surgery to manage many of the problems and pathologies facing the modern-day spine surgeon in these arenas. It is with this in mind that the future of spine medicine and surgery will depend on current and future innovations to rectify these inadequacies.

In the pages that follow, seven categories of innovations and their predicted time frame of clinical development and application are presented. Some, such as subsidence and dynamism, osteointegration, and motion preservation techniques are currently being applied clinically. Others are only in the development phase or, in some cases, in the early concept phase.

As Dorothy in *The Wizard of Oz* so poignantly stated, "Toto, we're not in Kansas any more." Things in our modern-day lives have drastically changed, and they are continuously changing. In this ever-changing world, the future of medicine, and indeed spine surgery, depends on innovation. With each innovation we reach further and further afield from "Kansas." That is the price we must pay for innovation and one of its products—progress.

INNOVATIONS

Subsidence and dynamism, osteointegration, motion preservation, monitoring devices, modulating devices, robotics, and biological interventions are the innovations that are addressed in this chapter. Although one might contend that other categories of innovations exist, they arguably will fall within the confines of the seven addressed here.

The authors chose these innovation categories, at least in part because of their biases. This must be taken into consideration when reading on. Each innovation category is presented separately with rough time frames for their preclinical development and clinical application.

Subsidence and Dynamism (1990–2010)

In the early to mid 1990s, a greater understanding of subsidence and its negative effect on surgical and non-surgical intervention for a variety of pathologies was realized. Implantable devices that 'took subsidence into account' were developed and eventually clinically employed. These, in general, were based on sound biomechanical principles. It behooves one to remember that the attainment of structural integrity is a primary or at least a strong secondary goal of all spine operations. Therefore, the definition of spine stability proposed by White and Panjabi is appropriately restated here as: "the ability of the spine under physiological loads to limit patterns of displacement so as to not damage or irritate the spinal cord or nerve roots and, in addition, to prevent incapacitating deformity or pain due to structural changes."[8] In order to achieve the goal of spinal stability, particularly in cases in which osteoporosis and subsidence may play a significant role, several principles must be adhered to. These are particularly relevant regarding ventral cervical spine surgery in the osteoporotic patient. First, there is no adequate substitute for 'good carpentry.' Care must be taken to meticulously and accurately fashion the bone graft and accepting mortise site so that excessive subsidence is not encouraged and so that surface area of contact is optimized. This brings up the second point—the maximization of the surface area of contact between the strut graft and the vertebral body. Obviously, larger (in cross sectional area) struts will subside into the vertebral body less than smaller struts. Finally, the effective employment of the "boundary effect" (the increased axial load bearing ability associated with the edge of an inhomogeneous structure that is more structurally sound at its periphery, such as an aluminum can or vertebral body) can minimize subsidence.[1] Therefore, placing an interbody strut close to the edge of a vertebral body, near the cortical wall (buttress), provides greater axial load-bearing ability than a strut placed in the center of the vertebral body.

It also behooves the spine surgeon to heed Wolff's Law; "bone is laid down where stresses require its presence, and bone is absorbed where stresses do not require it".[1] Literally translated, this law and its corollaries state that bone (e.g., interbody bone graft struts) heals best under compression. The interbody strut graft and the vertebral body margins must 'see' bone healing enhancing forces or loads (compression).

Here is where dynamism potentially plays a role. An effective dynamic implant is not loaded axially. Hence, it allows the interbody strut to be compressed (axially loaded) and to 'see' the bone healing enhancing forces of compression. Its purpose, therefore, is twofold: (1) to allow the aforementioned compression of the bone graft strut to occur and (2) to limit rotation, translation, angular motion, and deformation.

In this latter regard, it is emphasized that implants function differently under different loading conditions. A ventral cervical plate may function as a distraction device by bearing axial loads; as a tension-band fixator by resisting extension; as a cantilever; and as a three-point bending device. The latter is true only if an intermediate point of fixation into a vertebral body is provided (e.g., intermediate screws into a vertebral body). This latter mode (three-part bending fixation) significantly assists in resisting angular, rotational, and translational deformations. These factors play a significant role in the clinical success of a construct.

DiAngelo and Foley provided a scientific foundation for what should be intuitive regarding the aforementioned factors. First they observed that a rigid ventral plate causes an interbody strut graft to be significantly loaded (compressed) in extension and to be unloaded (distracted) in flexion. They also observed that this phenomenon was significantly blunted if an axially dynamic implant was used.[2] In summary, dynamic spine stabilization, along with the employment of multiple points of fixation (including and particularly the employment of intermediate points of fixation to the parent spine) is playing, and will increasingly play, a role in the surgical management of the osteoporotic cervical spine *(Fig. 11.1)*.

We will learn much more about subsidence and dynamic spine stabilization in this decade. This augmented understanding most certainly will lead to further innovations regarding the enhancement of bone healing by strategies that heed Wolff's law.

Osteointegration (1990–2020)

Surgeons have traditionally assumed that bony fusion is the ultimate method of achieving spine stability. This, however, may not be entirely so. Orthopedic advancements, predominantly in the joint replacement arena, have contributed a significant amount of knowledge regarding bone-implant interfaces. It is indeed possible for biological and non-biological surfaces to bond—i.e., osteointegrate *(Fig. 11.2)*. Interbody strategies that take this into account will most likely become increasingly clinically applied in the near future. This may open many avenues for the surgical restoration of ventral spine structural in-

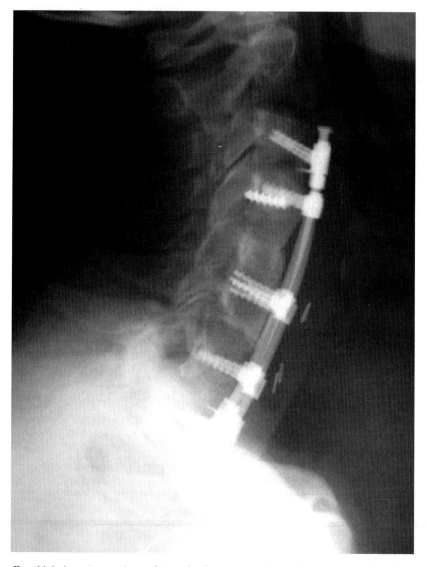

FIG. 11.1 A postoperative radiograph of a patient who underwent a complex reconstruction and deformity correction procedure utilizing multiple intermediate points of
fixation and a dynamic implant (note that the implant's upper platform has subsided).

tegrity. Kyphoplasty, vertebroplasty, and interbody strut applications
for osteointegration techniques will most likely be greatly expanded
in the next two decades, as well. It is emphasized that the concept of
osteointegration has been aggressively applied in the joint and artificial disc arenas (see below).

A

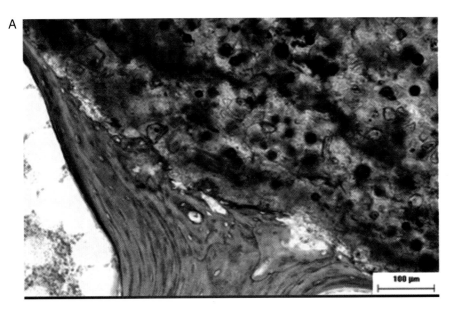

B

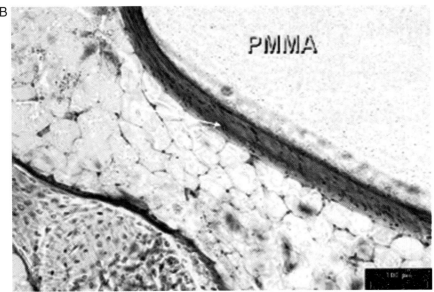

FIG. 11.2 A bioactive, self-setting bone bonding composite material that has established an intimate fit with bone and that has a calcium phosphate-rich layer within the composite material. Therefore, this material by definition has demonstrated its ability to osteointegrate (from Orthovita with permission)(A). Compare and contrast the osteointegrated interface in A with that of an interface without osteointegration (B). In the latter case, fibrous tissue (arrow) formed between the bone and polymethymethacrylate (PMMA).

Motion Preservation Strategies (2000–2030)

Motion preservation strategies for spine surgery are essentially of three types, or rather fall into one of three categories: (1) biological disc replacement, (2) nucleus pulposus replacement, and (3) mechanical disc replacement. Each has its proponents and opponents and has been developed to varying degrees.

Biological strategies involve the development of new disc interspace material (tissue). This genetic engineering process is confined by all the difficulties and complications associated with other genetic strategies. Containment, delivery, and toxicity, as well as biomechanical considerations are most certainly significant concerns.

Nucleus pulposus replacement, in the context used here, refers to the process of nucleus pulpous enucleation and replacement with a material that cushions or allows mobility of the two adjacent endplates with respect to each other. This can be accomplished with a pillow-like device (e.g., the Ray device) or with a pill-shaped structure that conforms to one degree or another with the cavity left by the enucleation portion of the procedure *(Fig. 11.3A)*. This strategy is plagued by prosthesis migration, prosthesis subsidence into the vertebral body, toxicity, and as of yet unknown biomechanical complications.

Mechanical disc replacement strategies are the most mature of the three categories regarding clinical applications. They have been clinically studied for over a decade, with many advances in the technology made during this time frame. These disc replacement devices are true disc replacements, in that the entire disc interspace is usually resected prior to the insertion of the mechanical disc. Mechanical discs usually involve either a ball-in-socket technology or a similar strategy

B

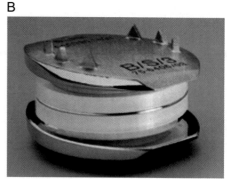

A

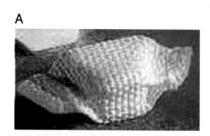

FIG. 11.3 Artificial discs. An intervertebral nucleus pulposus replacement device (PDN device from Raymedica, Inc)(A). A mechanical artificial disc (SB Charite III from Link Spine Group)

that involves a mechanical component and an interface with bone via an osteointegration process *(Fig. 11.3B)*. Hybrids that use the osteointegration interface component, and a polymer or similar material instead of the truly mechanical ball-in-socket-like strategy, have also been employed.

All disc replacement strategies have failings. They do not adequately consider that the remainder of the spine will continue to degenerate, including the dorsal facet joints at the involved motion segment. Osteophytes form, and ligaments and other supporting soft tissues may be excessively stressed by such prostheses.

The interface between the implant and the vertebral body is exposed to significant loads; thus, this interface is prone to failure with time. The mobile portion of the artificial disc (if one is used) is exposed to relentless translational, rotational, flexural, and axial loading. It is expected, therefore, that failure at this point will be common. Finally, biological approaches run the risks associated with containment, control, toxicity, and structural failure. It must be remembered that even if one can effectively apply biological technologies to the disc interspace, a physiologically and biomechanically sound and functional disc is not guaranteed.

In view of the aforementioned, it is predicted that over the next several decades artificial disc technology will become increasingly popular, but ultimately meet with failure. The realization that a fusion procedure in a well-selected patient is an effective and well-conceived operation with predictable results may, and probably will, overtake the enthusiasm currently associated with artificial disc replacement technology.

Monitoring Devices (2010–2030)

The traditional biomechanics laboratory has been the foundation and the fundamental basic science associated with the structural aspects of spine surgery. This laboratory has provided much information that has been applied clinically over the past several decades. This information, it must be realized, is often misleading. The data can, in fact, be used in an intentionally misleading manner (1). The major problem associated with the traditional biomechanics laboratory and the data that is produced are related to the assumptions that are involved with an experiment and its interpretation. These assumptions are myriad. They include assumptions regarding soft tissue contributions to stability, assumptions that the loading conditions employed in the laboratory are the same as those seen clinically, and assumptions regarding the type and quality of the specimen, etc.

For example, let's assume that a hypothetical biomechanical experiment is associated with 10 assumptions (a conservative estimate) and that each assumption is associated with a 20% error (also very conservative). This implies that the accuracy associated with each assumption is 80%. The overall accuracy of the experiment is, therefore, $0.8^{10} = 0.11 = 11\%$.

An ability to monitor the same parameters as studied in the traditional biomechanics laboratory in an *in vivo* manner would be ideal. This would virtually eliminate the vast majority of the assumptions and their associated errors. This concept was conceived and tested as early as the 1960s (3). However, the ability to measure spinal stresses through wireless transmission was not achieved (and only in a rudimentary manner) until a decade later (4–6). What is needed to make this strategy clinically practical are small inexpensive miniaturized implantable monitoring devices and a method for communicating the data derived to the external environment in a manner that is compliant with patient comfort and convenience. MEMS technology may provide a component of the solution of this problem.

MEMS is an acronym for MicroElectroMechanical Systems. It refers to the integration of mechanical (including those that are movable) components and fluidics with traditional electronics chip technology. Gears, tubes, levers, motors, and specifically textured surfaces may be combined with microchip circuitry to create sensor systems that enable the monitoring of pressure, loads, strains, and chemistries; to name only a few potential applications. Such devices can have features that are nanometer to micrometer in size. With the rapid pace of research in MEMS technologies to create complex systems, it should become possible to design systems that can be combined to perform extremely complex tasks in the near future (7). This poses a challenge to the surgeons, engineers, and scientists involved in the design and the clinical incorporation of such devices. The internal fluidic environment of the human body is harsher than seawater and can damage electronic and mechanical integrity, even at the microlevel. Biocompatibility and immune responses to a foreign body further complicate the concept of implantable technology (7).

Furthermore, such technology, although expensive on the 'front end,' is inexpensive after satisfactory products have been designed. The development and manufacture of such devices takes place in a clean room environment, thus adding to the cost of research and production. The ultimate cost-effectiveness of this technology is predominantly related to batch production strategies. The manufacture of MEMS devices involves many serially performed processes, such as photolithography, etching, and masking on silicon wafers. Once designed and prototyped, the batch manufacturing process, however, simplifies the production process, thus reducing costs significantly *(Fig. 11.4)* (7).

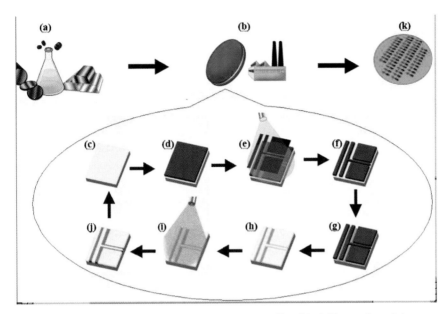

FIG. 11.4 The MEMS bulk manufacturing process. Graphical illustration of the major processing steps in microelectronics fabrication. Raw materials—silicon (Si) wafers, ultra-pure chemical reagents, and highly purified metals (a)—are gathered and processed inside cleanroom environments (b). The fabrication of microelectronics is generally based on repeated cycles of process sequences as shown in (c) though (j). Many chips of the same microelectronics circuit can be produced on one Si wafer. Typical processes include the growth of silicon dioxide (SiO_2) on the Si wafer (c), deposition of thin films of a photosensitive polymer (termed photoresist) (d), which is subsequently patterned by exposing it to ultraviolet (UV) light through a photomask (e), development of the exposed photoresist (those areas of the photoresist exposed to the light become soluble and are washed away in the developing solution reproducing the pattern from the photomask in the photoresist and selectively exposing the underlying SiO_2; (f)), etching of the exposed SiO_2 by wet chemicals or plasma in order to expose the surface of the underlying Si wafer (g), the subsequent removal of photoresist (h), and the doping of the exposed wafer surface to change electrical characteristics (dopant atoms of boron (B) or phosphorus (P) are ionized and accelerated toward the surface of the wafer and embedded to a uniform depth underneath the surface of the exposed Si wafer and SiO_2;(I)). The thickness of the SiO_2 is chosen to be thick enough so that no ions can penetrate into the Si underneath and afterwards, the SiO_2 is removed to leave behind a doped region of the wafer with the same pattern as drawn on the photomask (j). This cycle is repeated for additional photomasks until the microelectronics fabrication process is complete (k). (From Neurosurgery with permission[7])

MEMS pressure and load sensors may be housed on or within implants, thus providing information that may be extremely valuable from a research and clinical perspective *(Fig. 11.5)*. Such information may assist the surgeon in determining the status of a bony fusion by

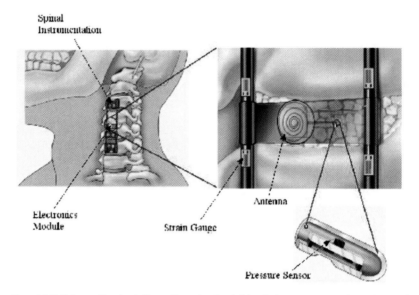

FIG. 11.5 Schematic depiction of an implantable fusion assessment system using MEMS pressure sensors and strain gauges. The strain gauges monitor loads on the instrumentation while the pressure sensor is used to assess the pressure within the bone graft. The measured pressure and load information is transmitted to an external receiver via wireless telemetry. (From Neurosurgery with permission[7])

demonstrating the characteristic loading patterns of a solid arthrodesis (versus a pseudoarthrosis; *Fig. 11.6).*

Microtools such as tweezers or ultrasharp instruments may also be produced by utilizing MEMS technologies. Such devices may play a particularly unique role in microsurgery and the cellular and subcellular manipulations associated with new genetic engineering and molecular biological clinical strategies.

Nanotechnology, the further miniaturization of sensors, tools, gears, levers, pores, and channels at nanoscale dimensions using a fabrication process similar to MEMS, is the next wave of implantable technologies. The ability to integrate biology at the molecular level with nanosized channels and pores that follow fluid dynamic laws could lead to the control and manipulation of proteins and genes that, in turn, could change the course of a disease.

Modulating Devices (2020–2050)

Micro and nanotechnologies can be further employed to both monitor and modulate surgeon actions, implanted devices, pharmacological infusions, etc. Tools that enhance intended surgeon actions, but eliminate or minimize unintended actions are nearly viable at this time. A tool, such as a micromanipulator, that enhances nonpredictable motions and eliminates predictable, repetitive motions (e.g., tremors) would be of great assistance to the surgeon. Devices that interpret pressure and load information from an implant, and in turn, enable the infusion of agents to enhance fusion (if necessary) would also be of great benefit. Detachable navigation techniques may permit the performance of duties by the surgeon that otherwise could not be performed. The realization of true detachable navigation technologies dictates that propulsion and accurate navigation capabilities and a mission are included in the 'package.' Propulsion techniques include the incorporation of MEMS actuators, shape memory metal alloys, and artificial muscles (electrically responsive membranes constructed from polymeric materials). Potential missions include chemical analysis, delivery of drugs, or remodeling of bone or soft tissues.

Smart materials (e.g., shape memory alloys) can change configuration or shape in response to temperature or electrical changes. They are alloys that are usually composed of varying fractions of nickel and titanium (TiNi). The metal is annealed at high temperatures into a pre-programmed configuration and is pliable when cooled. The mechanical properties of TiNi are similar to steel, thus further adding to the attractiveness of the material. The ability to alter the material at different temperatures or by electrical stimulation and have it return to the original programmed shape, lends credence to the prospect that

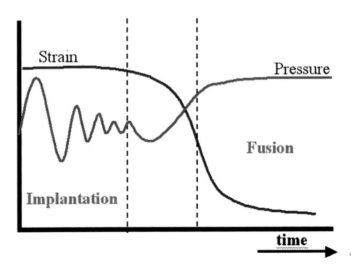

FIG. 11.6 Graph showing possible relative variations in strains on spinal implants and pressure within bone graft versus time. The dashed lines depict the phases of fusion maturation. (From Neurosurgery with permission[7])

spinal implant manipulation *in vivo*, the guidance of detached or attached navigation devices, and smart surgical tools or sutures, etc., are clinically realizable technologies.

Robotics (2000 and beyond)

Robots have been used in the automotive and aerospace industries for some time. Recently, they have been employed in selected clinical situations. Thus, the interface of man and machine is in the process of being enhanced in the surgical arena. Remote surgery, access to traditionally inaccessible body regions (thus enabling minimally invasive surgery) and the amplification of surgeon accuracy and the minimization of iatrogenic tissue injury are but a few of the advantages that robots may provide. Currently, there are still limitations to the use of robotics in surgery. The surgeon must monitor and control the robot and its application with often suboptimal haptic feedback (tactile feedback to the surgeon that is programmed into the robotic arm). The concept of "surgery by feel" is often the determining factor in a successful spinal stabilization, (i.e., the determination of the adequacy of screw purchase in bone). The advent of biomimetics and improved haptic technologies are helping bridge the gap that still exists between man and machine *(Fig. 11.7)*.

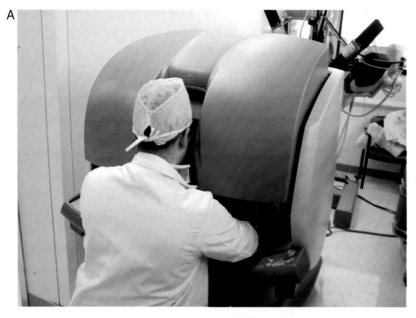

FIG. 11.7 A robotic approach to spine surgery involves the surgeon (A) accurately directing a distant operative action (B).

B

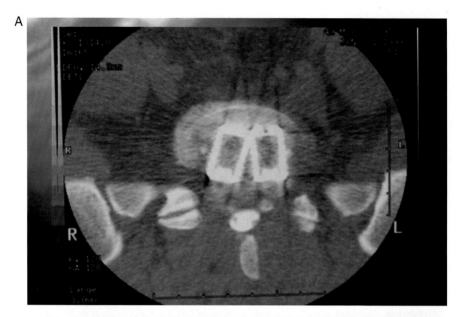

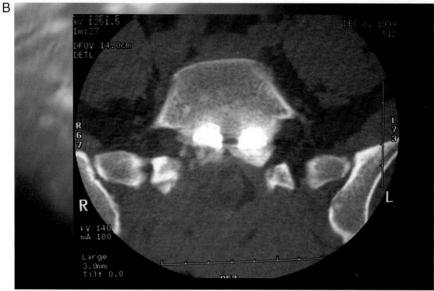

Fig. 11.8 A patient underwent cage L5-S1 fusion with a bioactive material (in lieu of bone graft). He did well for 6 weeks, but then developed recurrent leg pain. A myelogram CT demonstrated bony overgrowth that necessitated operative removal with relief of pain (A). A surgical decompression was performed that involved total removal of the offending (intracanal) portion of the mass. The pain recurred 3 months later. A subsequent myelogram CT (7 months following the second operation) demonstrated a second recurrence of bony overgrowth (B). Subsequent CT scans have demonstrated no further bony regrowth (C).

This case illustrates the problem of containment and of, as of yet, poorly defined biological processes that have been "turned on". The question remains, "can we turn them off?"

Biological Interventions (2000 and beyond)

Bone, disc (and other soft tissues) and neural regeneration or augmentation are all amenable to biological interventions. As already mentioned in this chapter, biological interventions expose the patient to the risks associated with the accuracy of the delivery of the agents, the containment of the agents in the desired space, their toxicity, and the as of yet unknown variables associated with molecular biological applications in the clinical arena. Perhaps an even greater concern is the complexity of the processes that are involved with biological interventions. This complexity makes the solution of complex clinical problems very difficult. In addition, the unpredictable, unexpected and possibly untoward effects of such interventions may be annoying or even catastrophic *(Fig. 11.8)*.

The areas in which such interventions may become clinically applicable include nuclear replacement (already mentioned), the clinical application of BMPs and related agents, and neural regeneration. With all of these strategies, cost and containment are significant issues.

Nucleus regeneration may involve the employment of semipermeable membranes that allow specific cells or humoral agents to pass into a disc space. These can spurn and nuture the regeneration process. Molecular biological strategies may also be applied.

Neural regeneration techniques must not only overcome the humoral

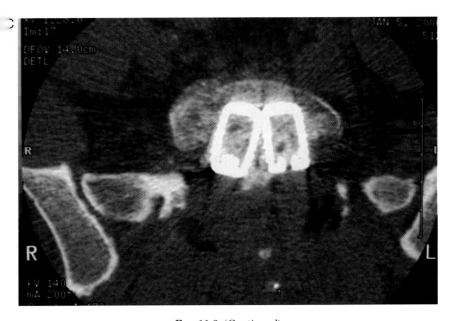

FIG. 11.8 *(Continued)*

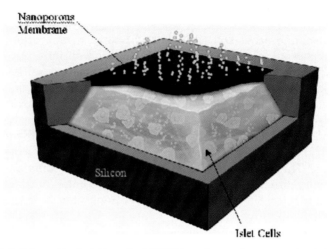

Nanoporous
Membrane

Silicon

Islet Cells

Fig. 11.9 Schematic depiction of a MEMS-based neural regeneration interface. The perforated silicon chip spatially constrains the growing ends of the nerve fibers in close proximity. The electrodes are incorporated for possible recording and stimulation (A). Schematic cut-away depiction of a micromachined biocapsule for the transplantation of pancreatic islet cells. The nanometer-sized pores in the membrane allow for nutrient and insulin transport but ensure an immunoprivileged environment for the islet cells (B). (From Neurosurgery with permission[7])

stimulation barriers required to induce regeneration, they must overcome physical barriers and the complexity of the nervous system with antegrade and retrograde growth and complex synaptic connections (that, by the way, are not well understood). MEMS, microfluidic based nanotechnology, and polymer science can be utilized to create textured surfaces that facilitate neural growth. Grids, channels, and tubes that can be electrically stimulated by fluidic passages can be used to accurately direct neuronal growth and the connection (via synapses) of these neurons to distal neurons for signal transmission *(Fig. 11.9A)*. Micromachined biocapsules that contain transplanted cells could be used for the controlled release of biologically regulated drugs without the risk of immunological complications *(Fig. 11.9B)*. The possibilities are endless.

As one can see, discoveries in the spine surgery arena are ongoing and monumental. They most likely will revolutionize spine care, while obligatorily diminishing or, at the very least, stabilizing cost. These are good things.

No Dorothy, we're not in Kansas anymore. We, however, can hopefully use technology to bring Kansas closer and to make it a better place in which to live.

REFERENCES

1. Benzel EC: *Biomechanics of Spine Stabilization.* AANS Publications. 2001, pp. 526.
2. DiAngelo DJ, Foley KT, Vossel KA, Rampersaud YR, Jansen TH: Anterior cervical plating reverses load transfer thought multilevel strut-grafts. **Spine** 25:783–795, 2000.
3. Nachemson A, Elfstrom G: Intravital wireless telemetry of axial force in Harrington distraction rods in patients with idiopathic scoliosis. **J Bone Joint Surg** 53-A: 445–465, 1971.
4. Rohlmann A, Bergmann G, Graichen F: Loads on an internal spinal fixation device during walking. **J Biomechanics** 30:41–47, 1997.
5. Rohlmann A, Bergmann G, Graichen F, Weber U: Comparison of loads on internal spinal fixation devices measured *in vitro* and *in vivo.* **Med Eng Phys** 19:539–546, 1997.
6. Rohlmann A, Calisse J, Bergmann G, Weber U: Internal spinal fixator stiffness has only a minor influence on stresses in the adjacent discs. **Spine** 24:1192–1196, 1999.
7. Roy S, Ferrara L, Fleischman A, Benzel EC: MEMS and neurosurgery: A new era in a new millennium. **Neurosurgery** 49(4)779–797, 2001.
8. White AA, Panjabi MM: *Clinical Biomechanics of the Spine,* 2nd ed. Philadelphia: Lippincott, 1990, pp 1–125.

III

General Scientific Session III Reinventing Neurosurgery: The Future of Neurovascular Surgery

CHAPTER

12

Endovascular Surgery: The Future Without Limits

ELAD I. LEVY, M.D., BERNARD R. BENDOK, M.D., ALAN S. BOULOS, M.D.,
ADNAN I. QURESHI, M.D., LEE R. GUTERMAN, Ph.D., M.D.
AND L. NELSON HOPKINS, M.D.

To improve, change is necessary. To be perfect, it is necessary to change often.

WINSTON S. CHURCHILL

INTRODUCTION

It is only within the past few years that technological advances in endovascular neurosurgery have enabled clinicians to treat various cerebrovascular and neoplastic pathologies. Many of these disease processes were considered previously untreatable by conventional surgical techniques without the risk of unacceptable morbidity. Much has been written on the history and origins of endovascular therapy. In previous articles, our group and others have chronicled the development of modern-day endovascular neurosurgery (8, 27). More than 150 years ago, the fathers of endovascular therapy began with rudimentary techniques that included electrothermic formation of thrombus and injection of fibrin into aneurysm sacs (12, 45). Perhaps one of the most interesting historical accounts of coil embolization involves that by Werner et al. (68), who described using silver wire to fill an intracerebral aneurysm, after which the wire was heated to 80°C.

Over the next two decades, investigators and clinicians implemented particles for both aneurysm and arteriovenous malformation (AVM) embolization. Luessenhop and Spence described the use of methyl methacrylate particle injection into the internal carotid artery for intracranial AVM embolization (8, 42). In 1965, Alksne and Fingerhut (2) investigated the use of carbonyl iron spheres suspended in 25% polyvinyl pyrrolidine to occlude aneurysms. More than a decade would pass until Allcock et al. attempted Gelfoam embolization of an AVM (3, 8). During this time interval, Serbinenko (61), Kerber (35), and Debrun et al. (16) pioneered endovascular inflatable-balloon technology for AVMs and fistulae (8).

Building on the pioneering work of Werner's group, Mullan's group (49, 50) used copper wire directly or stereotactically inserted into aneurysms, after which electrothrombosis was attempted within a

2-hour period. Although only one patient worsened, three others required surgical clipping for aneurysm recurrence.

As we now move further from the pioneering efforts of our endovascular forefathers and settle in to the new millennium, we must take pause. We have arrived at a critical junction where technological developments are abundant and indications seem unsupported without data from clinical trials. As former baseball player and coach Yogi Berra stated, "You got to be very careful if you don't know where you're going, because you might not get there." Most of us know that we want to arrive at a place where patients can be treated optimally, efficiently, cost-effectively, and with the least possible morbidity. As clinicians, investigators, and practicing physicians in the contemporary arena of evolving health care, the paths chosen must be carefully considered and the options weighed. We will undoubtedly come to several forks along our paths to optimal patient care. Though Mr. Berra warns us to explore all avenues with a destination in mind, he also encourages us to be ready for the serendipitous discoveries when he states, "When you come to a fork in the road, take it!"

ANEURYSM MANAGEMENT: TOWARD COMPLETE ERADICATION

Craniotomy for aneurysms may become of historical interest within the next few decades. Currently, however, the field of endovascular therapy is not sufficiently developed to provide the best treatment options for some aneurysm morphology. Giant aneurysms remain a challenge for current coil technology. Some of the reports in the early 1990s demonstrate that only 15% of wide-necked aneurysms were completely occluded (fundus-to-neck ratio of less than 2) by Guglielmi detachable coils (GDC, Target Boston Scientific, Fremont CA) (18). Additionally, follow-up angiography for coiled aneurysms demonstrated concerning recanalization rates. In a report by Byrne et al. (9) in 1995, follow-up of 42 aneurysms at 6 months demonstrated recanalization in 17% of small aneurysms, 19% of large aneurysms, and 50% of giant aneurysms. Other aneurysms that may be difficult to coil include those in the ophthalmic region. Roy et al. (58) reported their results with coil treatment of 28 ophthalmic segment aneurysms; 50% of cases were completely occluded and 39% were classified as having small residual necks. Although there were no deaths, the procedural stroke rate was 3.5%.

In the late 1990s, reports focusing on the technical aspects of coiling of wide-necked aneurysms began to emerge. Moret et al. (46) and Sanders et al. (59) published their experiences using the balloon-remodeling technique. Short-term results achieved with lesions that were previously untreatable by use of endovascular methods were excellent, and the morbidity and mortality rates in this small number of cases were similar to those for routine GDC embolization. The first prospective, randomized study comparing GDC embolization to surgery was reported by Vanninen et al. in 1999 (65). Patients who had aneurysms that were suited to either therapy were randomized to one treatment arm and matched for age, Hunt and Hess score, Fischer grade, and aneurysm site and size. Mortality rates were 4% and 2% for the surgical and endovascular groups, respectively. The 3-month angiographic studies demonstrated 37 of 39 (95%) coiled aneurysms to be 95% or more occluded (26 were completely occluded and the remaining 11 had an acceptable neck remnant). Immediate postsurgical angiograms demonstrated 74% complete ligation. In a larger series of 395 aneurysms, the results of endovascular and microsurgical aneurysm management (102 aneurysms were surgically clipped and 293 were coiled) were comparable (41). Management decisions were based on the shape of the aneurysm as follows: aneurysms with narrow necks and neck diameter-to-sac diameter ratios of less than one-third were selected for coiling.

Both our group (19) and Higashida et al. (26) were among the first to report stent-assisted coiling of fusiform basilar artery aneurysms. Stent-assisted coiling for aneurysms with wide or complex necks has become more popular, in part due to Mericle et al. (44) and Sekhon et al. (60) in 1998 and Lanzino et al. (37) in 1999, each of whom reported optimal results by use of this method. Since then, many reports have demonstrated the utility of stent-assisted coiling for complex or fusiform aneurysms (13, 32, 67). On the basis of studies conducted by Imbesi and Kerber (33, 34) using slipstreams to demonstrate blood flow from parent vessels into aneurysms sacs, in conjunction with data from Wakhloo et al. (67), Lieber et al. (40), and others, we postulate that aneurysm thrombosis and protection from hemorrhage results from dramatic reduction in the vortitional forces caused by blood flowing into the aneurysm neck. Therefore, when stents with decreasing porosity become available for use in the intracranial circulation, the future of fusiform aneurysm surgery may entail simply placing a stent across the friable, complex neck of the aneurysm. Tomorrow's intracranial stents may be asymmetric, covered only unilaterally to occlude the aneurysm neck while permitting flow through perforating vessels. This technology, however, will be dependent on higher resolution fluoroscopic imaging capabilities.

How has aneurysm surgery been improved upon since the development and integration of the microscope in Donoghy's lab in the late 1960s? How has the morbidity of aneurysm surgery been reduced since the integration of temporary clipping in the late 1970s? Although microscopes and instrumentation have improved the ability of surgeons to better define aneurysms and neighboring vital structures, patient outcomes have not appreciated dramatic improvement. Clearly, advances in endovascular technology have exploded in recent years, resulting in lower morbidity and mortality and lower total treatment cost, albeit a lower rate of complete aneurysm occlusion. Rapid advancement of endovascular technology reflects the dynamics in the field of endovascular therapy and the tremendous potential for technological improvement and modification, most of which has not yet been realized. Despite technological improvements, however, it is imperative that randomized prospective trials or epidemiological studies comparing clipping to coiling be conducted to determine if one technique is superior to the other and in which settings each technique may be optimally used. At this point, it seems that the greatest limitations are our imagination, interest from industry in constructing devices designed specifically for treatment of intracranial aneurysms, and financial support. The not-so-distant future of aneurysm surgery will involve restoring the native parent vessel lumen by endothelialization across aneurysm necks. Perhaps this will be by microcatheter delivery of gene therapies to the aneurysm or by delivery of endothelial growth factors. Current technology involves the use of liquid embolic agents for aneurysm therapy (with either stent or balloon protection of the parent vessel). Perhaps the next generation of these liquid embolics will be impregnated with factors, such as endothelial-derived growth factors, that promote neoendothelialization. Additionally, evolving computer software capable of flow pattern analysis may simulate the influence of various devices used for treatment before actual treatment is carried out. Such computer-assisted endovascular therapy could predict the device with the lowest morbidity and greatest chance for success, thus improving the patient's chances for an optimal outcome.

INTRACRANIAL STENOSIS: STENTING WITH LOCAL PHARMACOTHERAPY

Clinicians are increasingly able to negotiate the more flexible stents available today throughout the proximal tortuous vessels of the cerebral circulation. Before the development of endovascular therapies for intracranial atherosclerotic disease, technically difficult surgical revascularization procedures, such as occipital-to-posterior inferior cerebellar artery bypass, were needed. Many patients with intracranial stenosis have comorbidities that increase the risk of surgery substantially. Surgical morbidity is as high as 30 to 40% in some series (7, 28, 29, 63). The advent of balloon angioplasty for intracranial stenosis has provided clinicians and patients with another option for the treatment of medically refractory symptomatic lesions.

After the initial report of basilar artery angioplasty by Sundt et al. (64), several other clinicians began exploring the possibilities of intracranial angioplasty. Connors and Wojak (14) have reported their extensive experience with intracranial angioplasty. In a recent cohort of patients, they observed a 16% rate of significant residual stenosis and a 14% rate of dissection, without any permanent significant morbidity. Some investigators using single-photon emission computed tomographic (SPECT) studies have found improvements in, and even normalization of, cerebral blood flow with up to 40% residual stenosis on angiography following balloon angioplasty of intracranial vessels (17). According to a review of the literature regarding the evolution of coronary and intracranial angioplasty procedures conducted by Horowitz and Purdy (31), restenosis rates following angioplasty may be as high as 30% in the presence of thrombus in the coronary circulation. To achieve reduced restenosis rates and long-term vessel patency, stents are being placed for the treatment of intracranial atherosclerotic disease. Driven by the lack of satisfactory results, some groups have described intracranial stenting for intracranial stenosis. Rates of morbidity and mortality vary considerably, ranging from 0 to 30% (23, 37, 39). This variation may be a reflection of lesion selection.

Possibly, the types of lesions best suited for stent-assisted angioplasty can be inferred from the results provided by Mori et al. (47), for stenotic intracranial lesions treated with angioplasty alone. These stenotic lesions can be divided into three groups: type C lesions are tortuous, angulated, longer than 10 mm, and associated with restenosis rates of 100% at 1 year and a stroke risk of 87% at 1 year; type B lesions are 5 to 10 mm in length, eccentric, and may or may not be best suited for angioplasty, as evidenced by a 33% rate of recurrent stenosis at 1 year and with only 33% likelihood for immediate success; type A lesions are less than 5 mm in length with a concentric configuration and are associated with a 92% immediate success rate and no restenosis at 1 year. Although successful results with type A lesions have been achieved by use of angioplasty alone, type B lesions may be better suited for stent-assisted angioplasty. Type C lesions are probably high risk for both stenting and angioplasty.

Perhaps the greatest concern following stenting of intracranial stenosis is the development of restenosis, either immediately adjacent to or within the stented portion of the vessel. Several new stents not yet widely available for intracranial use are aimed at reducing thrombosis and restenosis rates. These include those that are radiated or coated with heparin, phosphorylcholine, paclitaxel, nitric oxide, or rapamycin (sirolimus). Recent clinical and experimental studies in the cardiac literature have demonstrated promising results with drug-coated stents with respect to inhibiting neointimal formation and concomitant restenosis. It is of benefit to briefly describe some of the mechanisms by which some of these drug-coated stents inhibit restenosis.

Sirolimus, or rapamycin, is an immunosuppressive agent commonly used in liver and renal transplant patients. This agent was first isolated from soil samples from Easter Island collected in 1965 (25). Although initially thought to have only antifungal capabilities, it was found to bind to the tacrolimus-binding protein (FKBP). This binding complex prevents the translation of mRNAs that encode for cell-cycle regulators. FKBP12 is involved in the control of transforming growth factor (TGF)-beta receptor I signaling. The rapamycin-FKBP complex, in turn, interacts with a kinase called the target of rapamycin (TOR). TOR is involved in the phosphorylation of proteins such as translation inhibitor 4E-BP1, eukaryotic translation initiator protein 4G1 (eIF4G1), and p70S6 kinase. Recently, Zohlnhöfer et al. (71) found that FKBP12 is upregulated at the mRNA and protein level in specimens of human neointima. The effects of rapamycin after binding to FKBP may be arrest of the cell cycle and decreased receptor signaling and protein synthesis, resulting in reduced neointimal formation and resultant restenosis.

Recent clinical trials comparing sirolimus-coated to uncoated stents have demonstrated impressive reductions in restenosis rates. Preliminary results from the RAndomized, double-blind study with the sirolimus-eluting Bx VELocity™ balloon (Cordis Neurovascular, Miami Lakes, FL) (RAVEL), a multicenter study conducted in Europe and Latin America of 220 patients with cardiac vessel stenosis, show no restenosis at 6 months (48). Additionally, there was marked reduction in neointimal formation in the sirolimus-coated stent group versus the uncoated-stent group. Other trials of smaller scale have demonstrated comparable results.

Other coated stents that have shown impressive results in coronary clinical trials include those coated with paclitaxel (Taxol). The mechanism of action is believed to be alteration of microtubule stability, in turn causing cell-cycle arrest and decreased cellular migration and signaling. Recent pilot data demonstrated no restenosis in 30 patients at follow-up (62). Early results from the ASian Paclitaxel-Eluting Stent Clinical Trial (ASPECT) showed that restenosis rates dropped from 27% in the control group to 4% in the high-dose paclitaxel group, likely due to reductions in intimal hyperplasia (6). The Taxol coating in the stents used in this trial was not designed for slow release. The use of newer, slow-release Taxol-coated stents may lead to even lower rates of restenosis. These encouraging results in the coronary vasculature provide impetus for investigations in the intracranial circulation. Localized drug delivery capable of altering the physical properties of intracranial intravascular or extravascular pathology or dysfunctions at the molecular level is the next step transcatheter therapy must take toward improvement of neurological diseases.

Radiated stents have shown much variability in inhibiting restenosis. It seems almost counterintuitive that, on one hand, we would use radiation to induce vessel fibrosis of AVMs and cavernous malformations but, on the other hand, look to radiation to prevent restenosis from neointimal and fibrovascular deposition. Results in the current literature are inconsistent and seem to depend on the model (i.e., which animal was used), radiation source, and radiation dose. Hence, it remains difficult to draw conclusions about radiated stents.

STROKE INTERVENTION

A Team Approach

Acute stroke therapy is perhaps the area where interventionists may be able to make the most significant contribution with respect to benefiting numerous treatable patients. An estimated 600,000 to 731,100 strokes occurred in 1996 in the United States, making stroke the third-leading cause of mortality (approximately 160,000 deaths) and the leading cause of severe neurological disability. The economic implications are staggering, as it is a leading cause of long-term disability (1). An estimated $3.8 billion was paid to Medicare beneficiaries with the diagnosis of stroke who were discharged from short-stay hospitals. It is clear that the number of stroke patients is far too great to be effectively cared for by neurointerventional radiologists, neurologists, and endovascular neurosurgeons. Therefore, it is imperative that other practitioners, such as cardiologists, become involved in acute therapy for these patients.

It seems intuitive that cardiologists should become familiar with recognizing, diagnosing, and treating acute-onset stroke because a significant number of strokes result from cardiogenic sources. Additionally, many stroke patients typically have cardioemboli and are followed by cardiologists for underlying cardiac diseases. In one study, 300 consecutive patients with acute focal brain ischemia underwent an examination by a cardiologist and had electrocardiography, Holter-electrocardiography, and echocardiography performed (30). Of these, 188 patients had a potential cardiac source of embolism. In another study, 29 of 50 consecutive patients with transient ischemic attack or mild stroke had clinically significant coronary artery disease (55). Patients with cardiac and atherosclerotic disease often require anticoagulation therapy. Cardiologists are intimately familiar with current antiplatelet and fibrinolytic therapies, which are essential for stroke prevention, intraprocedural management, and postoperative care.

Interventional cardiologists are quite knowledgeable about catheter-based treatment and possess the necessary catheter skills to treat stroke with endovascular therapy. As "time is brain," immediate stroke treatment following thromboembolic complications of cardiac intervention yields the greatest chance for recovery. In a study of 20,924 cardiac catheterizations, stroke rates were 0.12% for interventional procedures and 0.10% for diagnostic catheterizations. The potential for immediate treatment exists with cardiologists trained to treat stroke-related complications (53).

Clearly, the current state of cardiology training precludes stroke treatment by these clinicians. Although cardiologists are accustomed to triaging and managing emergencies, interventional cardiologists must be trained to understand and conduct a comprehensive neurological examination so that they can localize lesions to specific territories (capsule, cortex, or brainstem). Additionally, they must become familiar with anatomic and pathologic findings and interpretation of computed tomographic, magnetic resonance imaging, and angiographic studies. Should further intervention be required, such as ventricular drainage or partial lobectomy, neurosurgeons must be readily available. The future of stroke intervention relies heavily on a multidisciplinary, cross-specialty team approach consisting of endovascular-trained neurosurgeons, neurologists, radiologists, and cardiologists. To achieve maximum benefit, stroke recognition and treatment must start in the field with emergency medical technicians and personnel.

Intraarterial Pharmacologic and Mechanical Thrombolysis

Patient outcome following intra-arterial pharmacologic thrombolysis of posterior circulation stokes is intimately based on location, time to treatment, and presenting condition (38). Although intra-arterial therapy may be more effective than an intravenous approach, it is still ineffective in 35 to 40% of patients treated (22). Studies of newer agents and higher dosing may show greater effectiveness. The gold standard for pharmacological reperfusion in acute myocardial infarction is rapid infusion of the tissue-plasminogen activator alteplase, along with aspirin and heparin (69). Tenecteplase, a newer third-generation triple-combination mutant of alteplase, has been studied in the Assessment of the Safety and Efficacy of a New Thrombolytic (ASSENT-2) clinical trial and demonstrated similar 30-day mortality rates to those observed with alteplase (4). Moreover, although reteplase has shown improved reperfusion rates in the cardiac literature as compared to alteplase, a combination of glycoprotein IIB/IIIa inhibitors plus fibrinolytic therapy has shown superior results to those of alteplase alone. In a phase II trial reported by the Strategies for Patency Enhancement in the Emergency Department (SPEED) investigators, the combination of full-dose abciximab, 5 U plus 5 U bolus doses of reteplase, and 60 U/kg of heparin provided increased reperfusion in the setting of acute myocardial infarction, as compared to reteplase alone (5). Combination therapies must be tested for safety, effectiveness, and efficacy in the cerebrovascular circulation in the setting of vessel occlusion. The results from the cardiac literature, albeit a different organ system, are encouraging for improved recanalization rates following intra-arterial pharmacologic thrombolysis.

Mechanical thrombolysis provides additional options for endovascular surgeons when pharmacologic means fail. Balloon and snare devices can be used to morselize clot and establish vessel patency. Maintaining vessel patency, however, remains difficult in the setting of acute thrombosis because of release of clotting factors and initiation of the coagulation cascade by pre-existent thrombus. Additionally, sludging of flow in spastic or atherosclerotic vessels portends further clot formation. In this setting, stenting may be an option for maintaining vessel patency. We have recently inserted stents into vessels that continue to occlude following temporary recanalization in the setting of acute stroke *(Fig. 12-1)*. Angiographic results have been excellent, but patient outcomes have been suboptimal due to prolonged occlusion time. Perhaps stenting should be considered earlier in the treatment of acute stroke.

The future of mechanical stroke intervention may be in the development of small, retractable parachute devices that can be negotiated throughout the cerebral vessels to engulf clot. Similar to the distal protection devices that are being tested in clinical trials of carotid stenting, smaller versions of the devices may be passed distal to the obstruction and then retracted, thereby engulfing the thrombus.

Among the newest devices currently being investigated in the clinical setting is the AngioJet Rheolytic Thrombectomy system (Possis Medical Inc., Minneapolis, MN). By using jets of saline that create a vacuum, this system mechanically morselizes and aspirates thrombus. Recently, catheters have been developed for this system for use in vessels as small as 2 mm, thus allowing clinicians to treat acute occlusions of the distal intracranial internal carotid artery, vertebral and basilar arteries, and proximal portions of some middle cerebral arteries.

Combination medical regimens with improved recanalization potential, intracranial devices specifically designed for clot lysis and capture,

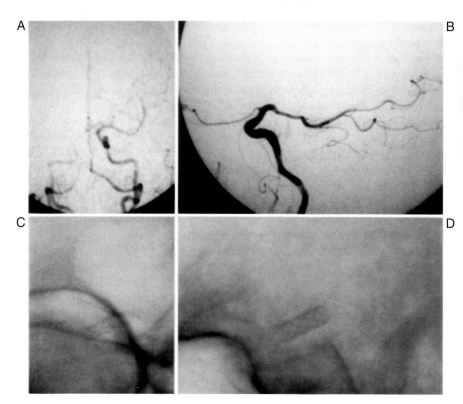

Fig. 12.1 An elderly gentleman presented with acute onset of left-sided weakness and deterioration of his mental status. (A) Digital subtraction intracranial angiogram showing right internal carotid occlusion in the supraclinoid region. The anterior communicating artery does not appreciably cross-fill to the right hemisphere. There is no significant meningeal collateralization. (B) The right internal carotid artery occlusion is at the level of the posterior communicating and ophthalmic arteries. (C) Unsubtracted fluoroscopic view of a 2.5 × 12-mm stent in the proximal portion of the middle cerebral artery. (D) Lateral view demonstrating the stent in the proximal portion of the middle cerebral artery. (E) Digital subtraction angiogram of the right internal carotid artery demonstrating filling of the middle cerebral artery and the distal branches with persistent occlusion of the anterior cerebral artery. (From Levy EI, Boulos AS, Bendok BR, Horowitz MB, Kim SH, Qureshi AI, Guterman LR, Hopkins LN: Intracranial stenting for cerebrovascular pathology. **Contemp Neurosurg** 23:1–10, 2000. Reprinted with permission.)

and more clinicians capable of treating stoke will significantly optimize the management of the ever-increasing population of stroke victims.

TUMOR THERAPIES: TARGETED TRANSARTERIAL ADMINISTRATION

Methods for the treatment of intracranial neoplastic processes continue to evolve. Only within the past few years has localized chemotherapy via bioabsorbable materials gained widespread acceptance.

E

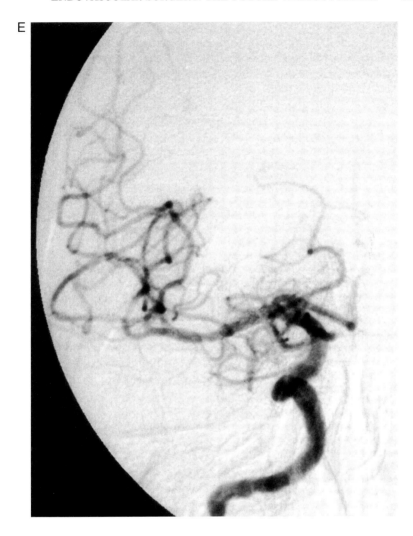

Additionally, non-invasive radiosurgery has demonstrated efficacy for both benign and metastatic disease processes (21, 36). The treatment of malignant glial tumors, however, remains problematic. Although we have made advances in the diagnosis and treatment of many brain neoplasms, only modest improvements have been gained in life expectancy rates for diseases such as glioblastoma multiforme. As approximately 150,000 to 200,000 metastatic brain neoplasms are newly diagnosed annually, potential for significant impact on national health care and this population exists (52).

Transcatheter administration may be an effective modality for introducing novel chemotherapeutic agents directly into the tumor circulation, potentially bypassing harmful systemic effects. An early report of intraarterial chemotherapy demonstrated a reduction in tumor burden with organ and bone marrow preservation from harmful side effects (35a). In one series of 100 procedures in which carboplatin was delivered intraarterially to intracranial neoplasms, only three patients (of 10 studied with magnetic resonance imaging) demonstrated reduction of tumor mass (54). Despite this modest result, further investigation of intraarterial delivery of chemotherapeutic agents is warranted.

In a novel research application aimed at targeting tumors, antitumor agents are attached to the endoglin, which is expressed predominantly on endothelial cells and is upregulated in angiogenic areas of tumors. By using antibodies to endoglin, it is possible to link virus vectors (and possible other antineoplastic agents) that target tumor vasculature (51).

Tumor embolization for preoperative management of vascular tumors such as meningiomas and hemangiopericytomas has been useful for minimizing blood loss during surgery. With current advances in material science and surface coating techniques, it is not difficult to imagine that embolic spheres coated with antineoplastic and antiangiogenesis factors could be delivered directly to the tumor vasculature. This treatment would have the combined effect of devascularization through vessel occlusion and tumor control through target specific pharmacology.

Recently, several tumor-selective radiation sensitizers have been studied in critical trials. As documented by magnetic resonance imaging, intravenously administered gadolinium texaphyrin seems to have an affinity for metastatic neoplasms to the brain (57, 66). Perhaps intraarterial administration to the vascular pedicles feeding these lesions would allow for increased dosing of radiation sensitizers, concurrent with reduced uptake by non-target tissue, thus increasing the effectiveness of either stereotactic or fractionated radiotherapy. Additionally, local delivery of radiation sensitizers to tumor vasculature at high concentration would likely eliminate systemic side effects such as renal toxicity (56).

ACCESS: TOWARD RAPID MOBILIZATION

One of the disadvantages of cerebral angiography and interventional procedures is the need for 4 to 6 hours of leg immobilization following femoral artery access. Although new groin closure devices have become available, they are fraught with complications such as delayed hemorrhage and hematoma formation, pseudoaneurysm formation, and infection. In a report by Chamberlin et al. (11), collagen plug devices (VasoSeal, Datascope, Montvale, NJ; Angio-Seal, St. Jude Medical, St. Paul, MN) were successful in 79% of patients; and percutaneous suture closure devices (Perclose, An Abbott Laboratories Subsidiary, Redwood City) were successful in 86% of patients who underwent transcatheter coronary interventions and who received abciximab, aspirin, and heparin. The failure rate for various percutaneous closure devices ranges from 6 to 12%, with 2.5% requiring surgical intervention in one study (24). The development of smaller profile stents and balloons, along with catheters with larger inner-to-outer diameter ratios has enabled the performance of diagnostic angiography and some endovascular surgery through transradial approaches.

Advantages of the transradial route, as compared to the transfemoral route, are clear. Most importantly, patients are not required to remain supine and ambulation is not limited. Additionally, because less tissue overlies the radial artery than the femoral artery, compression of the radial artery access site is more direct. Risks of massive blood loss from retroperitoneal or thigh hematomas do not exist with the radial approach. Other limitations of the transfemoral route include the risk of femoral nerve damage, pseudoaneurysms, and limb claudication in patients with iatrogenic femoral artery dissection or baseline peripheral vascular disease. Studies published in the coronary literature suggest that radial arteriography is safe and effective for assessing the coronary circulation. As demonstrated by Campeau (10), transradial coronary angiography was successful in 88 of 100 patients. Wu et al. (70) recently found no increase in complication rate, radial artery occlusion, or hand function following cannulation of the radial artery with 8-French sheaths, through which most interventions are typically feasible. Although most of the literature on transradial intervention and angiography comes from the cardiac literature, Matsumoto et al. (43) analyzed the effectiveness of the transradial approach for cerebral angiography in 70 patients. This group demonstrated a greater than 95% success rate without any major complications. A report by Fessler et al. (20) described the transradial approach for intracranial stenting in patients with limited access. As the radial artery is a smaller vessel than the femoral artery, it is more prone to spasm and iatrogenic dissection. Therefore, immediately following sheath insertion, a mixture of heparin (5000 IU/ml), verapamil (2.5 mg), lidocaine (2%, 1.0 ml), and nitroglycerine (0.1 mg) is infused through the introducer sheath to relieve or prevent vasospasm.

There is an economic incentive to using the transradial route. One randomized, single-center study reported a significantly reduced median length of stay in patients who underwent transradial catheterization as compared to those who underwent transfemoral catheterization (3.6 vs. 10.4 hours) (15). Additionally, the transradial access group described less discomfort during the first week after the procedure. In this same study, 80% of patients who had both transradial and transfemoral catheterizations strongly favored the transradial route, and an additional 7% moderately favored this route. In our own study of 132 patients who underwent transradial cerebral angiography, there was a 9% minor complication rate, and no major complications. Patients typically were discharged home after approximately 2 hours of observation.

SUMMARY

The new millennium brings with it tremendous advances in technology and information sharing. Various medical, surgical, and engineering specialties are becoming more focused, thus enabling experts in these fields to gain insight and understanding previously unappreciated by those who came before us. Economic and technologic evolution will eliminate some of the drawbacks of endovascular therapy, such as persistent neck remnants. It is likely that drug delivery systems exist that would allow maximal benefit with little or no systemic adverse effects. It is likely that devices are available that could minimize various procedural complications. We as future neurosurgeons must persist in the quest to find collaborations that will promote cross-fertilization and cross-pollination among cardiologists, neurosurgeons, physicists, radiologists, neurologists, engineers, and other scientists so that the technology can be translated to reality. It is clear that, in time, transcatheter techniques will replace many operations for the treatment of cerebrovascular pathologies. Let us not allow ourselves the luxury of time.

REFERENCES

1. AHA. Heart and stroke facts. In *1997 Statistical Supplement.* American Heart Association, 1998, Dallas, Texas.
2. Alksne J, Fingerhut A: Magnetically controlled metallic thrombosis of intracranial aneurysms: A preliminary report. **Bulletin Los Angeles Neurological Society** 3:154–155, 1965.
3. Allcock J, Drake C, Fox A, et al: Treatment of cerebral arteriovenous malformation by direct embolization into feeding vessels at craniotomy. American Society of Neuroradiology. Hamilton, Bermuda, 1977.
4. Anonymous: Single-bolus tenecteplase compared with front-loaded alteplase in acute myocardial infarction: the ASSENT-2 double-blind randomized trial. Assessment of the Safety and Efficacy of a New Thrombolytic Investigators. **Lancet** 354:716–722, 1999.

5. Anonymous: Trial of abciximab with and without low-dose reteplase for acute my-ocardial infarction. Strategies for Patency Enhancement in the Emergency De-partment (SPEED) Group. **Circulation** 101:2788–2794, 2000.
6. Anonymous: Transcatheter Therapeutics (www.tctmd.com/expert-presentations), 2001.
7. Ausman JI, Shrontz CE, Pearce JE, et al: Vertebrobasilar insufficiency. A review. **Arch Neurol** 42:803–808, 1985.
8. Bashir Q, Thornton J: Timeline: endovascular therapy for arteriovenous malforma-tions. **Surgical Neurology** 54:300–303, 2000.
9. Byrne JV, Adams CB, Kerr RS, et al: Endosaccular treatment of inoperable in-tracranial aneurysms with platinum coils. **Br J Neurosurg** 9:585–592, 1995.
10. Campeau L: Percutaneous radial artery approach for coronary angiography. **Cathet Cardiovasc Diagn**16:3–7, 1989.
11. Chamberlin J, Lardi A, McKeever L, et al: Use of vascular sealing devices (VasoSeal and Perclose) versus assisted manual compression (Femostop) in transcatheter coronary interventions requiring abciximab (ReoPro). **Catheter Cardiovasc In-terv** 47:143–147, 1999.
12. Ciniselli L: Sulla elettro-puntura nella cura degli aneurismi. **Gazz Med Ital Lomb** 6:9–14, 1847.
13. Cloft HJ, Kallmes DF, Jensen ME, et al Endovascular treatment of ruptured, pe-ripheral cerebral aneurysms: parent artery occlusion with short Guglielmi de-tachable coils. **Am J Neuroradiol** 20:308–310, 1999.
14. Connors JJ, 3rd, Wojak JC: Percutaneous transluminal angioplasty for intracranial atherosclerotic lesions: Evolution of technique and short-term results. **J Neuro-surg** 91:415–423, 1999.
15. Cooper C, El-Shiekh R, Cohen D, et al: Effect of transradial access on quality of life and cost of cardiac catheterization: A randomized comparison. **Am Heart J** 138:430–436, 1999.
16. Debrun GL, P., Caron J, Hurth M, et al: Detachable balloon and calibrated-leak bal-loon techniques in the treatment of cerebral vascular lesions. **J Neurosurg** 49:635–649, 1978.
17. Derdeyn CP, Cross DT, 3rd, Moran CJ, et al: Reversal of focal misery perfusion af-ter intracranial angioplasty: case report. **Neurosurgery** 48:436–440, 2001.
18. Fernandez Zubillaga A, Guglielmi G, Vinuela F, et al: Endovascular occlusion of in-tracranial aneurysms with electrically detachable coils: Correlation of aneurysm neck size and treatment results. **Am J Neuroradiol** 15:815–820, 1994.
19. Fessler RD, Guterman LR, Qureshi A, et al: State of neuroendovascular surgery: endoluminal reconstruction of basilar fusiform aneurysms (abstr). Transcatheter Cardiovascular Therapeutics—Eleventh Annual Symposium. Washington DC, 1999.
20. Fessler RD, Wakhloo AK, Lanzino G, et al: Transradial approach for vertebral ar-tery stenting: Technical case report. **Neurosurgery** 46:1524–1528, 2000.
21. Flickinger J, Kondziolka D, Lunsford L, et al: A multi-institutional experience with stereotactic radiosurgery for solitary brain metastasis. **Int J Radiat Oncol Biol Phys** 28:797–802, 1994.
22. Furlan A, Higashida R, Wechsler L, et al: Intra-arterial prourokinase for acute is-chemic stroke. The PROACT II study: A randomized controlled trial. Prolyse in Acute Cerebral Thromboembolism. **JAMA** 282:2003–2011, 1999.
23. Gomez CR, Misra VK, Liu MW, et al: Elective stenting of symptomatic basilar ar-tery stenosis. **Stroke** 31:95–99, 2000.
24. Gonze M, Sternbergh Wr, Salartash K, et al: Complications associated with percu-taneous closure devices. **Am J Surg** 178:209–211, 1999.

25. Halloran PF: Sirolimus and cyclosporin for renal transplantation. **Lancet** 356:179–180, 2000.
26. Higashida RT, Smith W, Gress D, et al: Intravascular stent and endovascular coil placement for a ruptured fusiform aneurysm of the basilar artery. Case report and review of the literature. **J Neurosurg** 87:944–949, 1997.
27. Hopkins L, Lanzino G, Guterman L: Treating complex nervous system vascular disorders through a "needle stick": Origins, evolution, and future of neuroendovascular therapy. **Neurosurgery** 48:463–475, 2001.
28. Hopkins LN, Budny JL: Complications of intracranial bypass for vertebrobasilar insufficiency. **J Neurosurg** 70:207–211, 1989.
29. Hopkins LN, Budny JL, Castellani D: Extracranial-intracranial arterial bypass and basilar artery ligation in the treatment of giant basilar artery aneurysms. **Neurosurgery** 13:189–194, 1983.
30. Hornig CR, Haberbosch W, Lammers C, et al: Specific cardiological evaluation after focal cerebral ischemia. **Acta Neurol Scand** 93:297–302, 1996.
31. Horowitz M, Purdy P: The use of stents in the management of neurovascular disease: a review of historical and present status. **Neurosurgery** 46:1335–1343, 2000.
32. Horowitz MB, Levy EI, Koebbe CJ, et al: Transluminal stent-assisted coil embolization of a vertebral confluence aneurysm: Technique report. **Surg Neurol** 55:291–296, 2001.
33. Imbesi SG, Kerber CW: Analysis of slipstream flow in two ruptured intracranial cerebral aneurysms. **Am J Neuroradiol** 20:1703–1705, 1999.
34. Imbesi SG, Kerber CW: Analysis of slipstream flow in a wide-necked basilar artery aneurysm: evaluation of potential treatment regimens. **Am J Neuroradiol** 22:721–724, 2001.
35. Kerber C: Balloon catheter with a calibrated leak. A new system for superselective angiography and occlusive catheter therapy. **Radiology** 120:547–550, 1976.
35a. Kerber CW, Wong WH, Howell SB, Hanchett K, Robbins KT: An organ-preserving selective arterial chemotherapy strategy for head and neck cancer. **Am J Neuroradiol** 19:935–941, 1998.
36. Kondziolka D, Levy E, Niranjan A, et al: Long-term outcomes after meningioma radiosurgery: Physician and patient perspectives. **J Neurosurg** 91:44–50, 1999.
37. Lanzino G, Wakhloo AK, Fessler RD, et al: Efficacy and current limitations of intravascular stents for intracranial internal carotid, vertebral, and basilar artery aneurysms. **J Neurosurg** 91:538–546, 1999.
38. Levy EI, Firlik AD, Wisniewski S, et al: Factors affecting survival rates for acute vertebrobasilar artery occlusions treated with intra-arterial thrombolytic therapy: a meta-analytical approach. **Neurosurgery** 45:539–548, 1999.
39. Levy EI, Horowitz MB, Koebbe CJ, et al: Transluminal stent-assisted angioplasty of the intracranial vertebrobasilar system for medically refractory, posterior circulation ischemia: Early results. **Neurosurgery** 48:1215–1223, 2001.
40. Lieber BB, Stancampiano AP, Wakhloo AK: Alteration of hemodynamics in aneurysm models by stenting: influence of stent porosity. **Ann Biomed Eng** 25:460–469, 1997.
41. Lot G, Houdart E, Cophignon J, et al: Combined management of intracranial aneurysms by surgical and endovascular treatment. Modalities and results from a series of 395 cases. **Acta Neurochir** 141:557–562, 1999.
42. Luessenhop A, Spence W: Artificial embolization of cerebral arteries: Report of use in a case of arteriovenous malformation. **JAMA** 172:1153–1155, 1960.
43. Matsumoto Y, Hokama M, Nagashima H, et al: Transradial approach for selective cerebral angiography: technical note. **Neurol Res** 22:605–608, 2000.

44. Mericle RA, Lanzino G, Wakhloo AK, et al: Stenting and secondary coiling of intracranial internal carotid artery aneurysm: Technical case report. **Neurosurgery** 43:1229–1234, 1998.
45. Moore C, Murchison C: On a new method of procuring consolidation of fibrin in certain incurable aneurysms: With the report of a case in which an aneurysm of the ascending aorta was treated by the insertion of a wire. **Proc R Med Chir Soc Lond** 4:327–335, 1864.
46. Moret J, Cognard C, Weill A, et al: Reconstruction technic in the treatment of wide-neck intracranial aneurysms. Long-term angiographic and clinical results. Apropos of 56 cases. **J Neuroradiol** 24:30–44, 1997.
47. Mori T, Kazita K, Chokyu K, et al: Short-term arteriographic and clinical outcome after cerebral angioplasty and stenting of carotid and atherosclerotic occlusive disease. **Am J Neuroradiol** 21:249–254, 2000.
48. Morice M, Serruys P, Sousa J, et al: The Ravel Trial. Transcatheter Therapeutics (www.tctmd.com/expert-presentations), 2001.
49. Mullan S, Beckman F, Vailati G: An experimental approach to the problem of cerebral aneurysms. **J Neurosurg** 21:838–845, 1964.
50. Mullan S, Raimondi A, Dobben G, et al: Electrically induced thrombosis in intracranial aneurysms. **J Neurosurg** 22:539–547, 1965.
51. Nettelbeck D, Miller D, Jerome V, et al: Targeting of adenovirus to endothelial cells by a bispecific single-chain diabody directed against the adenovirus fiber knob domain and human endoglin (CD105). **Mol Ther** 3:882–891, 2001.
52. Niranjan A, Lunsford L: Radiosurgery: where we were, are, and may be in the third millennium. **Neurosurgery** 46:531–543, 2000.
53. Plehn JF, Davis BR, Sacks FM, et al: Reduction of stroke incidence after myocardial infarction with pravastatin: The Cholesterol and Recurrent Events (CARE) study. The Care Investigators. **Circulation** 99:216–223, 1999.
54. Qureshi AI, Suri MF, Khan J, et al: Superselective intra-arterial carboplatin for treatment of intracranial neoplasms: experience in 100 procedures. **J Neurooncol** 51:151–158, 2001.
55. Rokey R, Rolak LA, Harati Y, et al: Coronary artery disease in patients with cerebrovascular disease: A prospective study. **Ann Neurol** 16:50–53, 1984.
56. Rosenthal D, Becerra C, Toto R, et al: Reversible renal toxicity resulting from high single doses of the new radiosensitizer gadolinium texaphyrin. **Am J Clin Oncol** 23:593–598, 2000.
57. Rosenthal D, Nurenberg P, Becerra C, et al: A phase I single-dose trial of gadolinium texaphyrin (Gd-Tex), a tumor selective radiation sensitizer detectable by magnetic resonance imaging. **Clin Cancer Res** 5:739–745, 1999.
58. Roy D, Raymond J, Bouthillier A, et al: Endovascular treatment of ophthalmic segment aneurysms with Guglielmi detachable coils. **Am J Neuroradiol** 18:1207–1215, 1997.
59. Sanders W, Burke T, Mehta B: Embolization of intracranial aneurysms with Guglielmi detachable coils augmented by microballoons. **Am J Neuroradiol** 917–920, 1998.
60. Sekhon LH, Morgan MK, Sorby W, et al: Combined endovascular stent implantation and endosaccular coil placement for the treatment of a wide-necked vertebral artery aneurysm: Technical case report. **Neurosurgery** 43:380–384, 1998.
61. Serbinenko FA: Balloon catheterization and occlusion of major cerebral vessels. **J Neurosurg** 41:125–145, 1974.
62. Sousa JE, Costa MA, Abizaid A, et al: Lack of neointimal proliferation after implantation of sirolimus-coated stents in human coronary arteries: a quantitative

coronary angiography and three-dimensional intravascular ultrasound study. **Circulation** 103:192–195, 2001.

63. Spetzler RF, Carter LP: Revascularization and aneurysm surgery: Current status. **Neurosurgery** 16:111–116, 1985.

64. Sundt TM, Jr., Smith HC, Campbell JK, et al: Transluminal angioplasty for basilar artery stenosis. **Mayo Clin Proc** 55:673–680, 1980.

65. Vanninen R, Koivisto T, Saari T, et al: Ruptured intracranial aneurysms: acute endovascular treatment with electrolytically detachable coils—A prospective randomized study. **Radiology** 211:325–336, 1999.

66. Viala J, Vanel D, Meingan P, et al: Phases IB and II multidose trial of gadolinium texaphyrin, a radiation sensitizer detectable at MR imaging: preliminary results in brain metastases. **Radiology** 212:755–759, 1999.

67. Wakhloo AK, Lanzino G, Lieber BB, et al: Stents for intracranial aneurysms: the beginning of a new endovascular era? **Neurosurgery** 43:377–379, 1998.

68. Werner S, Blakemoore A, King B: Aneurysm of the internal carotid artery within the skull. Wiring and electrothermic coagulation. **JAMA** 116:578–582, 1941.

69. White H, Van de Werf F: Thrombolysis for acute myocardial infarction. **Circulation** 97:1632–1646, 1998.

70. Wu SS, Galani RJ, Bahro A, et al: 8 french transradial coronary interventions: clinical outcome and late effects on the radial artery and hand function. **J Invasive Cardiol** 12:605–609, 2000.

71. Zohlnhöfer D, Klein CA, Richter T, et al: Gene expression profiling of human stent-induced neointima by cDNA array analysis of microscopic specimens retrieved by helix cutter atherectomy: detection of FK506-binding protein 12 upregulation. **Circulation** 103:1396–1402, 2001.

CHAPTER

13

Carotid Artery Stenting: Fact or Fiction

MARC R. MAYBERG, M.D.

INTRODUCTION

Angioplasty and stenting procedures for atheromatous disease affecting the craniocervical circulation have received considerable attention in recent years *(Fig. 13.1)*. Advances in endovascular techniques and stent technology have enabled the successful application of these procedures to lesions of the cervical carotid and vertebral arteries, as well as intracranial vertebral, basilar, and carotid arteries. Compared to carotid endarterectomy (CEA) the major potential advantages for carotid angioplasty and stenting (CAS) are the relative noninvasive nature of the procedure, the potential reduction or elimination of complications directly related to surgical aspects of CEA (e.g., cranial nerve injury, wound complications), and potential reduction in cost. However, it is not clear whether CAS provides any relative advantage over CEA for morbidity related to peri-procedural stroke and death, anesthetic complications, or long-term protection against subsequent stroke. This chapter will examine the extant data which exists for CAS versus CEA. These data will be reviewed in relation to the dynamic state of technology changes affecting both procedures, as well as current practice pattern trends in North America.

RATIONALE FOR CAROTID REVASCULARIZATION

In large part, the initial rationale for CEA and CAS has been based upon the concept that delivery of additional blood to the brain will be beneficial in preventing cerebral ischemia due to large vessel occlusive disease. This premise is based upon the concept of *hemodynamically significant stenosis*; i.e., that flow through a vessel remains relatively constant until there is a 70% reduction in luminal diameter (90% reduction in lumen cross-sectional area). At this point, flow through the vessel is relatively abruptly reduced *(Fig. 13.2)*. However, the brain is exceptionally well adapted to regulating cerebral blood flow (CBF) in conditions of both chronic and acute vascular occlusion.

247

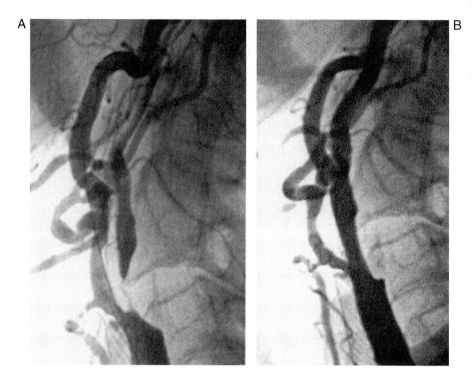

FIG. 13.1 Anteroposterior radiographs of cervical carotid arteries before (left) and after (right) carotid angioplasty and stenting.

Primarily through collateral pathways (extracranial collaterals, pial collaterals, and circle of Willis) and inherent regional autoregulation, CBF usually remains within the normal range with adequate hemodynamic reserve in the face of single or multiple large vessel stenosis or occlusion. In fact, stroke specifically due to hemodynamic insufficiency is relatively uncommon, and the great majority of strokes are embolic or thrombotic in origin. The clinical significance of this finding was supported by the EC-IC Bypass Trial (1), which showed no significant protection against ipsilateral stroke or any stroke for STA-MCA bypass among patients with carotid or middle cerebral lesions not amenable to endarterectomy. This lack of efficacy was present despite a low peri-procedural morbidity and mortality with an overall excellent technical success rate in establishing adequate bypass flow. Despite some controversy regarding the methodology of the study design (2, 3), it can be concluded that potential augmentation of CBF by EC-IC bypass for the general cohort of patients with inoperable carotid

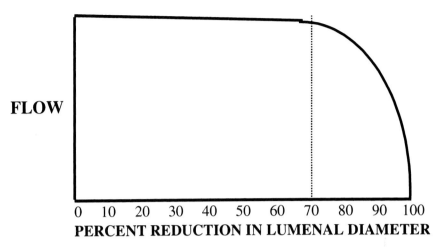

FIG. 13.2 Schematic representation of hemodynamically significant stenosis. At constant pressure, flow through a lumen in vitro is relatively constant until luminal diameter reaches 70%, above which flow is dramatically reduced.

and MCA lesions does not provide significant benefit. Whether select subgroups may benefit from this procedure remains to be shown (4).

Despite the lack of efficacy for EC-IC bypass, numerous studies have shown a high correlation between atheromatous stenosis of large craniocervical vessels and subsequent stroke in the vascular distribution of these arteries (5–9). Most likely, the relationship between degree of stenosis and stroke risk correlates to *hemodynamic factors acting at the site of stenosis*. Local turbulence, alterations in shear stress, and relative reductions in flow, in combination with the dynamic interface between blood and the atheroma, lead to the development of platelet thrombi and fibrin thrombi with subsequent distal embolization and/or thrombosis of the parent vessel, leading to ischemia and stroke. These factors are clearly apparent at the time of carotid endarterectomy, where thrombus deposition and intra plaque hemorrhage are frequent findings in the intraoperative specimen. These features of carotid plaque pathophysiology clearly have a significant impact upon the consequences of the revascularization procedure used. In CEA, the distal carotid artery is clamped prior to any manipulation, and thereby relative protection is afforded against distal embolization during the course of the procedure. For CAS, on the other hand, balloon angioplasty and stent deployment is associated with dislodgment of emboli into the intracranial circulation, as frequently demonstrated during transcranial Doppler (TCD) monitoring in CAS *(Fig. 11.3)*. The clinical significance of these

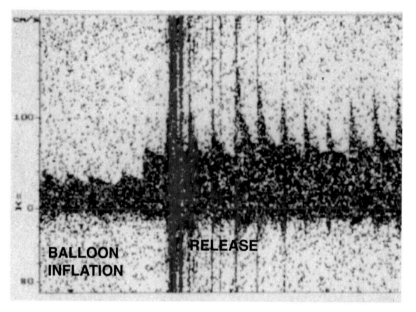

FIG. 13.3 Transcranial Doppler (TCD) signals in middle cerebral artery ipsilateral to CAS. With balloon inflation, there is a reduction in the TCD waveform. Upon release, there is a high frequency of transient signals in the MCA, which diminishes over time. These signals likely represent emboli in the MCA.

emboli during CAS is not known. Pharmacologic and mechanical strategies to mitigate the effects of embolization during CAS have been developed (see below), which may minimize their consequence.

DATA FROM TRIALS FOR CAROTID ENDARTERECTOMY

Trials for Asymptomatic Stenosis

Three major prospective randomized trials examined the efficacy of CEA in preventing stroke in patients with **asymptomatic carotid stenosis**. The **CASANOVA Study** (10) randomized patients with asymptomatic carotid stenosis (greater than 50% but less than 90%) to either immediate carotid endarterectomy (N = 206) or no immediate surgery, including some patients who underwent delayed surgery after developing ischemic symptoms, progressive severe stenosis, bilateral stenosis or contralateral stenosis (N = 204). At 3-year follow-up, using death or new stroke as primary endpoints, there was no difference in primary outcome (ipsilateral stroke or death) between the immediate surgery group and the other group of patients (10.7% versus 11.3%). However, nearly half of the patients in the "no immediate surgery" group eventually did have an endarterectomy for one of the reasons stated above. The unusual study design for this trial considerably lessens its statistical validity.

The **VA Asymptomatic Stenosis Trial** (7) randomized patients with asymptomatic carotid stenosis (greater than 50%) to operative (N = 211) or nonoperative therapy (N = 233). At a mean follow-up of 4 years, the combined outcomes encompassing ipsilateral neurological ischemic events (TIA and stroke) were reduced the incidence for the surgical group (8%) in compared to the medical group (20.6%) ($P <$ 0.001). However, the sample size was not sufficiently large enough to show a statistically significant difference in stroke alone. For the outcome measure ipsilateral stroke, the incidence for the surgical group was 4.7% (including perioperative strokes) in contrast to 9.4% in the medical group ($P = 0.056$). However, when perioperative mortality (1.9%) was included with surgical stroke rate, the difference between the two groups was not statistically significant.

The **Asymptomatic Carotid Atherosclerosis Study** (**ACAS**) trial (11) substantiated the hypothesis that carotid endarterectomy may prevent stroke in certain patients with asymptomatic carotid stenosis. Among 1662 individuals randomized with high grade carotid stenosis (>60% diameter reduction by ultrasound and/or angiography), there was a projected overall 53% relative risk reduction in the primary outcome measure ipsilateral stroke over 5 years (mean follow-up was 2.7 years) in patients receiving carotid endarterectomy (5.1%) compared to unoperated patients (11.0%). Although 9% of patients were not treated according to their randomization status, the stroke risk reduction was comparable for analysis by intent-to-treat or actual treatment. The stroke risk reduction was more prominent in men and was apparently independent of degree of stenosis or contralateral carotid artery disease. A substantial portion of the surgical risk was attributable to angiography (1.2% stroke rate), and the initial risk for surgery plus angiography was offset by a constant risk of ipsilateral stroke at approximately 2.2% per year in the non-surgical group (9). The surgical benefit was apparent by 10 months and was statistically significant at 3 years.

TRIALS FOR SYMPTOMATIC STENOSIS

The **European Carotid Surgery Trial** (**ECST**) (5) entered patients with mild (defined as less than 30%), moderate (30–69%), or severe (70–99%) carotid stenosis, who were randomized to surgical or non-surgical treatment. Interim analysis of 2200 patients (mean follow-up = 2.7

years) led to premature termination of the trial for mild and severe steno-sis groups. For mild stenosis, among 374 randomized patients there was no significant difference in ipsilateral stroke between the surgical and non-surgical groups. There were more treatment failures in the surgery group, which was attributed to the 2.3% risk of death or disabling stroke during the first 30 days after surgery. For severe stenosis, however, sur-gery was shown to be beneficial in preventing stroke. There was a 7.5% risk of ipsilateral stroke or death within 30 days of surgery. At 3 years of follow-up, there was an additional 2.8% risk of stroke in the surgery group (total = 10.3%) compared to 16.8% in the non-surgery group ($P <$ 0.0001). Importantly for the outcome measures, death or ipsilateral dis-abling stroke, the incidence was reduced from 11% in the non-surgery group to 6% in the surgery group. ECST used a different criterion for de-termining carotid stenosis than North American Symptomatic Carotid Endarterectomy Trial (NASCET), VA Symptomatic Stenosis Trial (VASST) or ACAS. When re-analyzed using NASCET criteria, patients in ECST with >70% stenosis had a stroke risk and achieved benefit from surgery at rates comparable to NASCET or VASST.

NASCET (6) prematurely stopped randomizing patients with carotid stenosis greater than 70% due to the overwhelming stroke risk reduc-tion observed in the surgical group. A total of 659 patients in this cat-egory of stenosis were randomized to surgical (N = 331) or non-surgical (N = 328) therapy. At a mean follow-up of 24 months, the primary out-come measure ipsilateral stroke was noted in 26% of non-surgical pa-tients, compared to 9% of patients with endarterectomy, for an overall risk reduction of 17% (relative risk reduction = 71%). The benefit for surgical patients was highly significant ($P < 0.001$) for a variety of out-come measures, including stroke in any territory, major strokes, and major stroke or death from any cause. A perioperative morbidity/mor-tality of 5.8% was rapidly surpassed in the non-surgical group, such that surgical benefit was apparent by 3 months. In addition, the protective effect of surgery was durable over time, with few strokes noted in the endarterectomy group beyond the perioperative period. The secondary outcome functional disability (assessed by a standardized disability scale) was significantly less in the surgery group over time ($P < 0.001$) (12). Multivariate analysis demonstrated that surgical benefit was in-dependent of a variety of concurrent demographic variables such as age, sex, or risk factors for stroke. There was a direct correlation between surgical benefit and the degree of angiographic stenosis.

Enrollment in the **V.A. Symptomatic Stenosis Trial (VASST)** was discontinued in early 1991 based upon preliminary data consis-tent with the NASCET findings. Subsequent analysis demonstrated a statistically significant reduction in the primary outcome measures ip-silateral stroke or crescendo TIA for patients with carotid stenosis

>50% (13). A total of 193 men aged 35 to 82 years (mean = 64.2 years) were randomized to surgical (N = 91) or non-surgical (N = 98) treatment. The complication rate of cerebral angiography was low, with no permanent residual deficits and transient complications in 5% (2% local vascular; 2% transient neurologic, 1% minor allergic). Two-thirds of randomized patients demonstrated angiographic internal carotid artery stenosis greater than 70%. Secondary outcome measures describing complications of surgery were relatively infrequent, including respiratory insufficiency requiring extended intensive care monitoring (5%), minor to moderate wound hematoma (5%), cranial nerve deficit (5%), myocardial infarction (2%) and pulmonary embolism (1%).

At a mean follow-up of 11.9 months, there was a significant reduction in stroke or crescendo TIA in patients receiving carotid endarterectomy (7.7%) compared to non-surgical patients (19.4%), or a risk reduction of 11.7% (relative risk reduction = 60%; P = 0.028). Among stratified subgroups, the benefit of surgery was most prominent in TIA patients compared to TMB or stroke, although these differences were not statistically significant. The benefit for surgery was apparent as early as 2 months after randomization, and persisted over the entire period of follow-up. The efficacy of carotid endarterectomy was durable with only one ipsilateral stroke beyond the 30-day perioperative period. Discounting one pre-operative stroke, a peri-operative morbidity of 2.2% and mortality of 3.3% (total = 5.5%) was achieved over multiple centers among relatively high-risk patients.

Meta-Analysis of CEA Trials

The symptomatic stenosis carotid endarterectomy trials were designed to enable a meta-analysis, which is currently in progress. The Carotid Endarterectomy Trials Collaborative Group (CETCG) is a database of approximately 7000 patients enrolled in NASCET, ECST, and the VA trials (14). The data from ECST have been corrected to determine the degree of carotid stenosis using the same calculations employed in NASCET and the VA trial. The data comprises over 35,000 patient years of follow-up including individual patients followed up to 14 years after randomization. The meta-analysis showed a high concordance of data among all three trials. For stenosis in the 70–99% category, CEA consistently provided protection against any stroke or death, any ipsilateral stroke or death, or disabling ipsilateral stroke. For stenosis from 50–69%, CEA was efficacious in reducing the risk of any stroke or death. For 30–49% stenosis, surgery provided no benefit. The beneficial effect of surgery was significant for up to 10 years of follow-up. In the cumulative analysis, operative mortality was 1.1% and the risk of peri-operative stroke or death was 7%. Subgroup analysis revealed that CEA provided additional benefit for the following cohorts: older patients, men, surgery performed sooner rather than later after the presenting effect, stroke versus transient ischemic attack (TIA). Of note, there was no benefit for surgery in patients with critical (99%) stenosis. A recent analysis of the ECST data with 14-year follow-up showed that the benefit from CEA was extremely durable, with highly significant reduction in stroke risk out to 14 years (15). The risk of ipsilateral ischemic stroke following surgery was 1% per year, and the risk of disabling ipsilateral ischemic stroke was 0.5% per year. Additional post hoc analyses of the peri-operative morbidity from the NASCET data (16, 17) demonstrated a risk of death at 1.1%, disabling stroke at 1.8%, and non-disabling stroke at 4.5%. The incidence of non-stroke/death complications, however, was higher, including wound complications (9.3%), cranial nerve deficits (8.6%), myocardial infarctions (1%), other cardiovascular complications (7.1%), and respiratory complications (0.4%). Among surgical patients in NASCET, medical complications were three times more prevalent compared to the non-surgical group and were increased in patients with pre-operative angina, myocardial infarction, or hypertension.

Cost Effectiveness of Carotid Endarterectomy

Despite the efficacy of CEA in preventing stroke among both symptomatic and asymptomatic patients with carotid stenosis, concerns remain regarding the cost-effectiveness of the procedure. For patients with high-grade (>70%) stenosis (6), the absolute risk reduction compared to best medical treatment was 17%. By these data, approximately six procedures would be required to prevent one stroke over 2 years of follow-up. On the other hand, based upon data from ACAS (18), the absolute risk reduction at 2 years provided by CEA was only 1.5%. In this regard, approximately 70 procedures would be required to prevent one stroke. By quality adjusted life year (QALY) analysis, the estimated cost for high-grade symptomatic stenosis is $45,000/QALY, whereas the estimate for asymptomatic stenosis for greater than $100,000/QALY. Based upon the estimated prevalence of asymptomatic stenosis in the U.S. population at approximately three million, it may be that wide scale CEA for this indication is not cost-effective and could conceivably be limited from a health care policy perspective.

CAROTID ANGIOPLASTY AND STENTING

Data regarding the risk and efficacy for CAS from prospective, randomized multicenter trials does not exist at present, although several retrospective series have been reported (19, 20). A retrospective registry analysis of 5,210 CAS procedures on 4,757 patients was recently

reported (21). In this analysis with self-reported outcomes from multiple centers, technical success of the procedure was 98.4%. The incidence of minor strokes was 2.7%, major strokes 1.5%, and death within
30 days 0.9%, for a total 30 day stroke and death rate of 5.1%. The
rate of restenosis in this study was low, with 2% restenosis at 6 months
and 3.5% restenosis at 12 months. A single prospective, single-center
analysis for CAS reported on 604 procedures with a mean follow-up
of 17 months (22). Technical success was nearly 100%, as above. Thirty
day stroke/death rates included minor stroke 5.5%, major stroke 1%,
fatal stroke 0.6%, and non-stroke death 1%, for a total 30 day
stroke/death rate of 7.4%. The author noted a decreasing incidence of
peri-CAS stroke over the course of the analysis with a substantial reduction in stroke rates in the later epoch compared to the initial experience. Only two risk factors were identified for peri-CAS stroke:
age > 80 years and hypertension.

Several prospective, randomized trials for CAS have been reported
or are in progress. The Schneider Trial was discontinued due to a
higher than anticipated complication rate; results of the study have
not been disseminated. The CAVATAS Trial (23) randomized 504 patients with carotid stenosis to endovascular treatment or CEA. The
endovascular patients received angioplasty alone (74%) or CAS (26%).
Stroke rates at 30 days did not differ significantly between CAS (6.4%)
or CEA (5.9%). Although recurrent high-grade stenosis was more frequent in the CAS group, there was no significant difference in ipsilateral stroke between groups at 3 years.

Two trials comparing CAS and CEA are ongoing. CREST (24) will
randomize patients meeting NASCET criteria (intermediate and high-
grade symptomatic stenosis ipsilateral to stroke, TIA, or amaurosis
fugax) to CEA versus CAS. This multi-center, multi-national trial projects to enter 2,500 patients and primary outcomes include ipsilateral
stroke, all stroke, and death. All patients will receive clopidogrel before and after procedures and neuroprotection devices will be used for
the CAS procedure. SAPPHIRE is randomizing high-risk patients with
medical or anatomical risk factors (Sundt Class III-IV) to CEA versus
CAS. Over 400 patients have been randomized to date at 25 centers
(25). Primary outcome measures are analogous to those for CREST.

FUTURE DEVELOPMENTS IN THE TREATMENT
OF CAROTID ATHEROMATOUS DISEASE

A significant problem in the design and implementation of prospective randomized trials for CAS is related to the rapidly changing technology in this field. During the trial period for NASCET, ECST, and

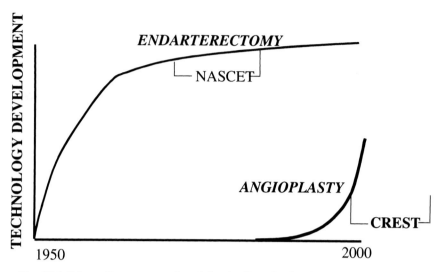

Fig. 13.4 Schematic representation of the timeline of technology development related to carotid endarterectomy versus carotid angioplasty and stenting.

the VA trial, surgical techniques, technology, and best medical therapy were relatively consistent over the interval of the studies *(Fig. 13.4)*. This enabled equivalent comparison for CEA to best medical therapy during an interval of several years. For CAS, however, it may be difficult to compare outcomes for the procedure during the multiple years required for the study, owing to the dynamic state of CAS technology. Technical and pharmacologic solutions to emboli, for example, are developing at a rapid pace. CAS patients are now routinely treated with antiplatelet agents such as clopidogrel, abciximab, and new reversible intravenous antiplatelet agents. In addition, there are numerous mechanical neuroprotection devices in use, including distal occlusion balloons (26), proximal occlusion balloons and catheters (27), and distal filters (28). Retrospective series for neuroprotection devices suggest substantial reductions in the incidence of cerebral embolization associated with these devices, which could potentially reduce the stroke risk associated with CAS. Implantation of stents with polymer-implanted antiplatelet agents (29) may provide additional benefit. In addition, angioplasty and stenting is being applied to intracranial stenoses with good reported results (30), and patients with tandem lesions are being treated in this manner *(Fig. 13.5)*. The efficacy of intraarterial thrombolysis for completed stroke was recently demonstrated (31). Intraarterial thrombolysis may enable the treatment of

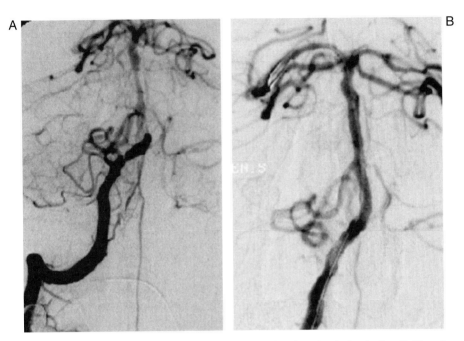

Fig. 13.5 Anteroposterior angiograms of vertebrobasilar circulation before (left) and after (right) intracranial angioplasty and stenting.

intracranial thrombi secondary to CAS, and further reduce the morbidity associated with this procedure. New techniques of mechanical thrombolysis for intracranial stenosis using the AngioJet catheter may further reduce the risk of hemorrhagic conversion by eliminating the need for pharmacologic thrombolysis; a prospective randomized trial is currently underway (TIME).

Ultimately, a major driving force in the application of CAS for the treatment of carotid stenosis will likely be the increased utilization of this procedure by physicians other than interventional neuroradiologists or neurosurgeons. At present, Medicare reimbursement for CAS is limited to those patients enrolled in Institutional Review Board-approved clinical trials. However, assuming demonstration of efficacy for CAS (or equivalence to CEA), it may be assumed that FDA approval for CAS is forthcoming. In this setting, there is high likelihood that the number of CAS procedures performed in the U.S. will increase significantly, and that neurovascular specialists may be involved in only a minority of those procedures.

CONCLUSIONS

At present, there are no scientifically valid data to support the utilization of CAS. It is clear that the procedure can be performed with excellent technical success. Based on single center prospective and multicenter retrospective analyses, the current procedural stroke/death rates are approximately equivalent to those of CEA. Experience suggests, however, that bias and imprecision inherent to such analyses typically lead to underestimation of true outcome events. It is also likely, however, that the risks of CAS will be less in the future as technological improvements occur. Little or no data exists to define the long-term risks of CAS or the durability of the procedural efficacy. It is imperative that CAS be compared to CEA in well-designed prospective, randomized trials, such as those that are currently in progress.

REFERENCES

1. The EC/IC Bypass Study Group: Failure of extracranial-intracranial arterial bypass to reduce the risk of ischemic stroke: Results of an international randomized trial. **N Engl J Med** 313:1191–1200, 1985.
2. Langfitt T, Goldring S, Zervas N: The extracranial-intracranial bypass study. A report of the committee appointed by the American Association of Neurologic Surgeons to examine the study. **N Engl J Med** 1987;316:817–820, 1987.
3. Sundt TM Jr: Was the international randomized trial of extracranial-intracranial arterial bypass representative of the population at risk? **N Engl J Med** 316:814–816, 1987.
4. Grubb RL Jr, Powers WJ: Risks of stroke and current indications for cerebral revascularization in patients with carotid occlusion. **Neurosurg Clin North Am** 12(3): 473–487, 2001.
5. European Carotid Surgery Trialists' Collaborative Group: European Carotid Surgery Trial: Interim results for symptomatic patients with severe (70–99%) or with mild (0–29%) carotid stenosis. **Lancet** 337:1235–1243, 1991.
6. North American Symptomatic Carotid Endarterectomy Trial Collaborators: Beneficial effect of carotid endarterectomy in symptomatic patients with high-grade stenosis. **N Engl J Med** 325:445–453, 1991.
7. Hobson RW II, Weiss DG, Fields WS, Goldstone J, Moore WS, Towne JB, Wright CB: Efficacy of carotid endarterectomy for asymptomatic carotid stenosis. The Veterans Affairs Cooperative Study Group. **N Engl J Med** 328(4):221–227, 1993.
8. Norris JW, Alexandrov AV, Bladin CF, Maggisano R: Progress in evaluating carotid artery stenosis. **J Vasc Surg** 22(5):637–638, 1995.
9. Mayberg MR, Winn HR: Endarterectomy for asymptomatic carotid artery stenosis. Resolving the controversy. **JAMA** 273(18):1459–1461, 1995.
10. CASANOVA Study Group: Carotid surgery versus medical therapy in asymptomatic carotid stenosis. **Stroke** 22:1229–1235, 1991.
11. Executive Committee for the Asymptomatic Carotid Atherosclerosis Study: Endarterectomy for asymptomatic carotid artery stenosis. **JAMA** 273:1421–1428, 1995.
12. Haynes RB, Taylor DW, Sackett DL, Thorpe K, Ferguson GG, Barnett HJ: Preven-

CAROTID ARTERY STENTING: FACT OR FICTION   259

tion of functional impairment by endarterectomy for symptomatic high-grade
carotid stenosis. North American Symptomatic Carotid Endarterectomy Trial Collaborators. **JAMA** 271:1256–1259, 1994.

13. Mayberg MR, Wilson SE, Yatsu F, Weiss DG, Messina L, Hershey LA, Colling C,
    Eskridge J, Deykin D, Winn HR: Carotid endarterectomy and prevention of cere-
    bral ischemia from symptomatic carotid stenosis. **JAMA** 266:3289–3294, 1991.
14. Rothwell PM, Gutnikov SA, Eliasziw M, Fox AJ, Taylor W, Mayberg MR, Barnett
    HJ, Warlow CP: Overall results of a pooled analysis of individual patient data
    from trials of endarterectomy for symptomatic carotid stenosis. 26th International
    Stroke Conference, Ft Lauderdale, Florida, February 14–16, 2001, p 12.
15. Cunningham E, Rothwell P: Personal communication, 2001.
16. Ferguson GG, Eliasziw M, Barr HW, Clagett GP, Barnes RW, Wallace MC, Taylor
    DW, Haynes RB, Finan JW, Hachinski VC, Barnett HJ: The North American
    Symptomatic Carotid Endarterectomy Trial : Surgical results in 1415 patients.
    Stroke 30(9):1751–1758, 1999.
17. Paciaroni M, Eliasziw M, Sharpe BL, Kappelle LJ, Chaturvedi S, Meldrum H, Bar-
    nett HJ: Long-term clinical and angiographic outcomes in symptomatic patients
    with 70% to 99% carotid artery stenosis. **Stroke** 31(9):2037–2042, 2000.
18. Moore WS, Kempczinski RF, Nelson JJ, Toole JF: Recurrent carotid stenosis: Re-
    sults of the asymptomatic carotid atherosclerosis study. **Stroke** 29(10):2018–2025,
    1998.
19. Dietz A, Berkefeld J, Theron JG, Schmitz-Rixen T, et al: Endovascular treatment
    of symptomatic carotid stenosis using stent placement: long-term follow-up of pa-
    tients with a balanced surgical risk/benefit ratio. **Stroke** 32(8):1855–1859, 2001.
20. Malek AM, Higashida RT, Phatouros CC, Lempert TE, et al: Stent angioplasty for
    cervical carotid artery stenosis in high-risk symptomatic NASCET-ineligible pa-
    tients. **Stroke** 31(12):3029–3033, 2000.
21. Wholey MH, Wholey M, Mathias K, Roubin GS, Diethrich EB, et al: Global experi-
    ence in cervical carotid artery stent placement. **Catheter Cardiovasc Interv**
    50(2):160–167, 2000.
22. Roubin GS, New G, Iyer SS, Vitek JJ, Al-Mubarak N, Liu MW, et al: Immediate
    and late clinical outcomes of carotid artery stenting in patients with symptomatic
    and asymptomatic carotid artery stenosis: a 5-year prospective analysis. **Circu-
    lation** 103(4):532–537, 2001.
23. Anonymous: Endovascular versus treatment in patients with carotid stenosis in the
    Carotid and Vertebral Artery Transluminal Angioplasty Study (CAVATAS): A ran-
    domized trial. **Lancet** 357(9270):1279–1237, 2001.
24. Hobson RW II. CREST (Carotid Revascularization Endarterectomy versus Stent
    Trial): background, design, and current status. **Semin Vasc Surg** 13(2):139–143,
    2000.
25. Yadav S: Personal communication, 2001.
26. Martin JB, Pache JC, Treggiari-Venzi M, Murphy KJ, Gailloud P, et al: Role of the
    distal balloon protection technique in the prevention of cerebral embolic events
    during carotid stent placement. **Stroke** 32(2):479–484, 2001.
27. Parodi JC, La Mura R, Ferreira LM, Mendez MV, Cersosimo H, et al: Initial eval-
    uation of carotid angioplasty and stenting with three different cerebral protection
    devices. **J Vasc Surg** 32(6):1127–1136, 2000.
28. Reimers B, Corvaja N, Moshiri S, Sacca S, Albiero R, DiMario C, et al: Cerebral
    protection with filter devices during carotid artery stenting. **Circulation**
    104(1):12–15, 2001
29. Fontaine AB, Borsa JJ, Dos Passos S, Hoffer EK, et al: Evaluation of local abcix-

imab delivery from the surface of a polymer-coated covered stent: in vivo canine studies. **J Vasc Interv Radiol** 12(4):487–492, 2001.

30. Rasmussen PA, Perl J II, Barr JD, Markarian GZ, Katzan I, Sila C, Krieger D, Furlan AJ, Masaryk TJ: Stent-assisted angioplasty of intracranial vertebrobasilar atherosclerosis: an initial experience. **J Neurosurg** 92(5):771–778, 2000.

31. del Zoppo GJ, Higashida RT, Furlan AJ, Pessin MS, Rowley HA, Gent M: PROACT: A phase II randomized trial of recombinant pro-urokinase by direct arterial delivery in acute middle cerebral artery stroke. PROACT Investigators. Prolyse in Acute Cerebral Thromboembolism. **Stroke** 29(1):4–11, 1998.

CHAPTER

14

Endovascular Therapy for Vasospasm

JAYASHREE SRINIVASAN, M.D., JOSEPH ESKRIDGE, M.D.,
M. SEAN GRADY, M.D., DAVID W. NEWELL, M.D.,
AND H. RICHARD WINN, M.D.

INTRODUCTION

The incidence of angiographic vasospasm following subarachnoid hemorrhage is reported to be as high as 60%–80% and the incidence of symptomatic vasospasm as high as 30% (1–3). The morbidity and mortality associated with vasospasm have had a significant negative impact on the outcome of patients with aneurysmal subarachnoid hemorrhage (3, 4). Over the past two decades, a variety of modalities have been used for the prevention of ischemia secondary to vasospasm. These include treatment with the calcium-channel blocker nimodipine, which may improve outcome both by a direct neuroprotective effect and by action on cerebral blood vessels (5, 6), and hypervolemic-hypertensive-hemodilutional (HHH) therapy (7). Despite this, a subgroup of patients may progress to develop delayed ischemic neurological deficits (DIND); endovascular therapy may be employed to reverse these deficits.

DIAGNOSIS

Subarachnoid hemorrhage may lead to a sustained contraction of smooth muscle cells of the large cerebral vessels generally between 4 and 10 days after the hemorrhage, followed by collagen deposition in the adventitia and thickening of the intima, which may persist for weeks following the resolution of clinical vasospasm (8). These morphological changes may result in a reduction in cerebral blood flow (CBF); however, although most patients may develop some degree of narrowing, the majority does not develop DINDs (9). It is only when CBF is greatly reduced, and compensatory mechanisms such as autoregulation, collateral flow, and increased oxygen extraction are exhausted, that ischemic deficits result.

The diagnosis of clinical vasospasm is made on the basis of the clinical examination and ancillary studies. The development of a new focal neurologic deficit or a deterioration in the level of consciousness may herald the onset of vasospasm (1). Other causes for clinical deterioration, such as hydrocephalus, intracranial hemorrhage or edema, seizures, and infection need also be considered; however, these may aggravate the ischemia secondary to vasospasm and should not exclude vasospasm if the index of clinical suspicion is high.

We routinely used transcranial Doppler (TCD) to detect vessel narrowing and to follow the course of vasospasm with time and treatment (10) *(Fig. 14-1)*. In the middle cerebral artery (MCA), a velocity of >120 cm/sec is considered mild vasospasm, >160 cm/sec moderate vasospasm, and >200 cm/sec severe vasospasm (11). In the vertebrobasilar distri-

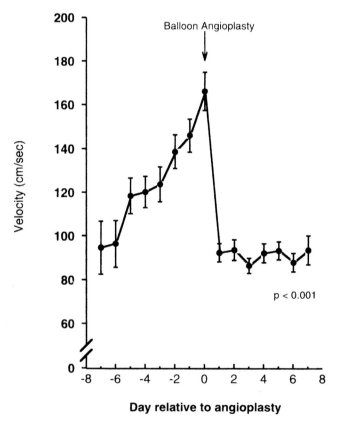

FIG. 14.1 Graph illustrating the use of transcranial Doppler (TCD) to measure velocity in the distal internal carotid or middle cerebral vessels in 39 patients to document development of vasospasm and sustained response to angioplasty. From Elliott JP, Newell DW, Lam DJ, et al.: Comparison of balloon angioplasty and papaverine infusion for treatment of vasospasm following aneurysmal subarachnoid hemorrhage. **J Neurosurg** 88:277–284, 1998, with permission.

bution, >65 cm/sec is consistent with vasospasm and >95 cm/sec consistent with severe vasospasm (12). Although TCD can accurately diagnose proximal vessel spasm, it cannot detect distal vessel vasospasm (e.g., A2 arteries) which is present in a minority of cases (13). Blood flow studies may complement TCD findings and improve the accuracy of diagnosis; these include Xenon computed tomography (XeCT) (14) and single photon emission computed tomography (SPECT) (15). Using XeCT, regions of interest with a cerebral blood flow (CBF) of <20 cc/100gm/min are considered at risk for ischemia (14).

We have found CBF studies to be particularly useful in high-grade patients in whom it may be difficult to detect clinical deterioration or responsiveness to HHH therapy. Both TCD and blood flow studies may be used after endovascular therapy to monitor the efficacy of the treatment and to diagnose recurrent vasospasm (10, 15, 16).

We treat all patients with nimodipine and utilize HHH therapy as indicated by transcranial Doppler velocities. We proceed to endovascular therapy only if the patient deteriorates clinically or develops perfusion deficits on SPECT despite maximal medical treatment. As discussed below, however, the timing of endovascular intervention is critical and should be instituted within 12 hours of onset of symptoms (17, 18).

ENDOVASCULAR TECHNIQUES

Angioplasty of cerebral arteries as a treatment for vasospasm was first described by Zubkov in 1984 (19). In their landmark paper, Zubkov et al. performed angioplasty on 105 major cerebral arteries in 33 consecutive patients without any complications, although 28 of these patients underwent angioplasty before definitive treatment of the ruptured aneurysm. Since that time, refinement in techniques and improvement in balloon catheters have confirmed the safety and angiographic efficacy of angioplasty (17, 20, 21). In addition, intraarterial papaverine infusion has been used to both as an adjunct to angioplasty and as a treatment for distal arterial vasospasm (22–24).

Endovascular therapy is performed under general anesthesia after a head CT is done to exclude a large infarct or hemorrhage. Arterial blood pressure and intracranial pressure are monitored throughout; a head CT is repeated immediately after therapy to rule out hemorrhagic transformation. Systemic anticoagulation with 5000–7000 IU heparin is instituted prior to angioplasty. Using a transfemoral approach, a low pressure (0.5 atm) silicon microballoon catheter is placed at the site of vessel narrowing and gradually inflated. The balloon is inflated only to 25% of its maximal size initially, and then deflated; the degree of inflation is the increased and repeated until vessel dilatation is complete. It is important to avoid overinflation beyond the normal diameter of the artery, as this may result in vessel rupture (17). All significantly narrowed vessels are treated with angioplasty, not just the vessel responsible for the clinical symptoms.

The mechanism of action of balloon angioplasty has been studied in animal models although the reason for its sustained effect is still not known. Electron microscopy has revealed stretched and torn collagen fibers (25), endothelial denudation, and rupture of the internal elastic lamina (8) and stretched smooth muscle fibers (8). In vitro studies on canine vasospastic vessels indicate significant impairment in vascular reactivity following angioplasty which persists for 2 to 3 weeks (8). Thus, angioplasty disrupts the ability of smooth muscle cells to contract for a period of time by mechanisms as yet unknown.

Intra-arterial papaverine is given via a superselective catheter positioned just proximal to the affected area (10, 26). A total of 300 milligrams of papaverine is infused per side gradually over 30–60 minutes, with careful monitoring of the ICP and arterial blood pressure. Papaverine is an alkaloid compound which causes smooth muscle relaxation through phosphodiesterase inhibition and possibly by decreasing the level of intracellular calcium (27, 28). Macdonald et al. found that, in a rabbit model, the efficacy of papaverine was influenced by the duration of the vasospasm and the degree of vessel narrowing (29). Conversely, Milburn et al. found no correlation between duration of vasospasm and response to papaverine (28). The limitations of papaverine treatment are still under consideration; a major drawback has been the recurrence of vasospasm following treatment (10). In vessels with severe vasospasm, papaverine may be infused first to facilitate microcatheter entry into a spastic vessel.

RESULTS OF ENDOVASCULAR THERAPY

The results of endovascular therapy for vasospasm have been reported in multiple case series with variable selection criteria, follow-up, and outcomes (10, 17, 18, 20, 30–34). To date, no controlled, prospective trial has been conducted to assess the impact of endovascular treatment on outcome; without a true untreated comparison group, any conclusions regarding this treatment modality must be interpreted with caution. The results of treatment with angioplasty have been found to be consistently better than with papaverine infusion alone (10, 34).

Balloon Angioplasty

In most series to date, balloon angioplasty has been studied with regard to its immediate effect on neurological deficit, as well as on long-term outcome. In 1992, Higashida et al. reported the clinical results of 28 patients treated with balloon angioplasty, with immediate improvement in 60.7% and favorable long-term outcomes in 60.7% (20). In two cases, vessels ruptured during the procedure with devastating consequences. In contrast, Coyne et al. in 1994 reported an immediate improvement in only 31% of their 13 patients and a favorable long-term outcome in only 38%, although they had no complications related to the procedure itself. They attributed 5/6 deaths to vasospasm (31). In analyzing their results, they felt that the poor grade of many of the patients (Grade 4–5) and the long duration (18 hours) between development of DINDs and treatment may have contributed to the worse outcomes. Since then, however, multiple series have confirmed an immediate improvement in neurologic deficit in at least 60% of patients (10, 16–18, 30, 32).

In Eskridge et al.'s series of 50 consecutive patients with symptomatic vasospasm, 61% were improved post-treatment; the complications included two vessel ruptures, with subsequent death of both patients, one branch vessel occlusion, and two aneurysmal rebleeds 4 and 12 days following treatment (17). Long-term follow-up was not reported. The authors did note a tendency towards better responsiveness in patients treated within 12 hours of onset of clinical symptoms but a worse outcome in patients with a GCS score of less than 12.

Bejjani et al. also in 1998 described 31 patients who were treated with angioplasty. Although they used different criteria for improvement post-therapy, they found that 72% of patients were better after treatment. Importantly, they too found time to be a predictor of short-term results: angioplasty performed within 24 hours of onset of neurologic symptoms resulted in 90% of patients having marked or moderate improvement, whereas angioplasty after 24 hours resulted in only 36% of patients having moderate improvement. However, this stratification did not extend to long-term outcome; 25/29 patients in follow-up had a Glasgow outcome scale (GOS) of 1 regardless of timing of angioplasty. Given the small number of patients, the actual long-term impact of timing of angioplasty is difficult to determine (30).

In 1999, Rosenwasser et al. further investigated the effect of early treatment of clinical vasospasm. In their series of 84 patients treated with cerebral angioplasty, they found a 70% early favorable outcome in 51 patients treated within 2 hours of symptom onset and a 40% good outcome in patients treated after 2 hours. At 6 month follow-up, 33/84 (39.2%) had a good outcome and 30/84 (35.7%) a fair outcome; no distinction was made as to the effect of the timing of treatment on late outcomes (18). They reported no complications related to the angioplasty procedure.

In 2000, Polin et al. summarized the results of angioplasty in patients enrolled in the tirilizad in SAH trial. Unlike the previous single center studies, these patients were treated at 15 different centers without a consistent vasospasm treatment protocol. Of these 38 patients, only 4 improved after treatment and 53% achieved a good/fair long-term outcome. When compared to a matched control group who had a 60% favorable outcome, angioplasty had no beneficial effect (33). However, there were numerous drawbacks to this study. Most importantly, no pre-treatment CT scan was reported and yet large hemispheric infarctions were seen on 22/29 late follow-up CT scans. Of the seven patients with normal CT scans, five had made a favorable outcome. Because no standardization of treatment was attempted, the maximum vasospasm was judged to be severe in only 13/38 cases; the indications for angioplasty were variable and other causes for clinical deterioration not well documented. The extent of medical treatment was also inconsistent. Fifteen of 38 patients were treated >12 hours after onset of symptoms and a high vasospasm recurrence rate was noted, contrary to other published reports. It is difficult to interpret the comparison of outcomes given the limitations of the study.

When Le Roux et al. analyzed 224 patients with a Grade I–III SAH, they found symptomatic vasospasm in 17.4% (39 patients). In the 17 patients for whom angioplasty was not used or not available, 76.5% achieved a good outcome. This is in contrast to the 22 remaining patients, who had a 96.6% good outcome. Not all of these patients were treated with angioplasty, so the improved outcome may in part be accounted for by aggressive medical therapy for vasospasm (4).

These results are summarized in *Table 14-1.*

Papaverine Infusion

Multiple small case series evaluating papaverine have been reported in the literature (10, 22, 23, 34). The results have been mixed. In 1992, Kassell et al. described 12 patients treated with intra-arterial papaverine; although 57% had marked reversal of angiographic vasospasm, only 25% had dramatic neurologic improvement (23).

Firlik et al. evaluated 15 consecutive patients treated with papaverine, alone (10 cases) or combined with angioplasty (5 cases). These patients were selected on the basis of development of a delayed neurologic deficit and XeCT documentation of ischemic regions of interest (ROI) with CBF <20 cc/100gm/min. Although 78% had some angiographic reversal of vasospasm, only 26% had clear neurologic improvement. Of the 9 patients who underwent XeCT after treatment, only 46% had augmentation of CBF; there was poor correlation between clinical change and increased CBF (34). There were several complications: one patient

TABLE 14.1
A comparison of current studies on the results of balloon angioplasty for treatment of vasospasm

Author	# of Patients	Early Outcome	Long-term Outcome	Complications
Bejjani (30) (1998)	31	72% improved PTA <24hrs: 90% improved PTA >24hrs: 36% improved	25/29 independent PTA time ns	1 death from vasospasm 2 groin/1 retroperitoneal hematoma
Coyne (31) (1994)	13	31% improved	38% independent 46% dead	5/6 deaths due to vasospasm
Eskridge (17) (1998)	50	61% improved	N/A	2 vessel ruptures 2 aneurysmal rebleeds (4 and 12 days after PTA) 1 MCA branch occlusion
Firlik (16) (1997)	14	86% improved	N/A	1 patient no PTA possible due to technical difficulty
Fujii (32) (1995)	19	63% improved	68% good-excellent at discharge	1 hemorrhagic transformation
Higashida (20) (1992)	28	60.7% improved	60.7% good-excellent	2 vessel ruptures
Polin (33) (2000)	38	11% improved	53% good or moderate disability	
Rossenwasser (18) (1999)	84	PTA <2hrs: 70.5 improved PTA>2hrs: 40% improved	39% good 36% fair 8.3% dead (no distinction made in timing of PTA)	None

had a paradoxical angiographic narrowing following papaverine infusion, with a resultant hemispheric infarction, one experienced transient brainstem depression during infusion of the vertebral artery, and one developed a seizure and hypotension with carotid artery infusion.

Elliott et al. compared the efficacy of papaverine infusion (13 patients) with balloon angioplasty (39 patients). Using serial TCD examinations, the velocities of the internal carotid arteries (ICA) and middle cerebral arteries (MCA) before and after treatment were documented. Prior to angioplasty, the mean ICA/MCA velocity increased from a baseline of 95 ± 12 cm/sec to 166 ± 9 cm/sec just prior to treatment; following angioplasty, the velocity decreased to 92 ± 4 cm/sec and remained stable (Fig. 14-1). Just prior to papaverine infusion, the mean TCD velocity increased to 158 ± 8 cm/sec and decreased to 127 ± 13 cm/sec on post treatment day 1; significantly, however, the velocities returned to pretreatment levels by day 2 (Fig. 14-2). Clinically, 67% of patients treated with angioplasty demonstrated some neurologic recovery. Although 62% of papaverine treated patients ultimately made a favorable outcome, five of these eight patients required retreatment or conversion to balloon angioplasty. The sustained effects of angioplasty were not seen with papaverine therapy. Using SPECT scanning in 37 patients, angioplasty resulted in increased perfusion in 71% of patients, whereas papaverine improved perfusion in only 31%. There were no treatment related complications in this series (10).

Fandino et al. measured jugular bulb vein oxygen saturation (SvjO2) and arteriovenous differences in lactate (AVDL) before and after papaverine infusion in 10 patients. Three patients also underwent angioplasty and endovascular therapy was instituted soon after failure of medical treatment, although the duration of neurologic deterioration was not given. All 10 patients had early neurologic improvement and no re-treatment was required. Nine of the 10 patients had an improvement in SvjO2 following papaverine, which was maintained with aggressive HHH therapy; however, there were no significant differences in AVDL before and after therapy. Overall, seven patients made a favorable outcome. The precise indications for angioplasty and the small number of patients bring into question the validity of these findings, in particular the sustained effect of papaverine infusion. Nevertheless, this study does document improved global perfusion following papaverine vasodilatation (35).

CEREBRAL BLOOD FLOW STUDIES

The diagnosis and treatment of vasospasm may be monitored by cerebral blood flow studies. Lewis et al. used SPECT scanning in 10 patients and showed a significant increase in CBF in eight patients who had neurologic improvement whereas there was no change in CBF in the two patients who had no clinical change (15).

Firlik et al. successfully used XeCT to diagnose clinical vasospasm in 14 patients. Prior to angioplasty, the mean number of ROI's at risk was 11.4 ± 4.3 with a mean CBF of 13 ± 2.1 ml/100gm/min. Angioplasty was possible in 13 patients; 12 (92%) demonstrated clinical improvement. The number of at risk regions of interest decreased to 0.9 ± 1.6 and the average CBF increased to 44 ± 13.1 ml/100gm/min, well above the ischemic threshold. One patient required repeat angioplasty in a different vessel 3 days after initial treatment; she did not respond to the second course of treatment. One patient suffered a hemorrhagic transformation and expired after angioplasty. Using specific CBF criteria, these authors were able to obtain a high response rate to endovascular treatment (16).

LONG-TERM EFFECTS OF ANGIOPLASTY

As described above, both angioplasty and papaverine infusion, although safe procedures, are associated with some immediate risks. The long-term consequences of cerebral angioplasty, unlike coronary angioplasty, are benign. We studied 28 patients an average of 44 months following angioplasty with transcranial Doppler. All patients had normal TCD examinations without evidence of intracranial vessel stenosis or occlusion. When autoregulatory function was assessed in the MCA territories, no difference was found between the previously treated and untreated territories; autoregulation was normal, indicating that no significant cerebrovascular occlusive disease had developed (36). The lower pressure used to dilate cerebral arteries (0.5 atm) compared to coronary arteries (3–4 atm) likely leads to less vessel remodeling and therefore fewer vessel occlusions.

FUTURE STUDIES

Despite advances in endovascular technology, the efficacy of treatment is dependent on appropriate and timely identification of symptomatic vasospasm. Megyesi et al. performed transluminal angioplasty on one internal carotid artery (ICA) in 12 dogs; they then exposed both ICAs to blood clot. Angiography performed after 7 days revealed that the vessels which had undergone angioplasty did not develop vasospasm, whereas the untreated vessels did (37). Thus, angioplasty prevented the development of vasospasm. The safety of prophylactic balloon angioplasty was then evaluated in a pilot study of 13 patients. In this series, Fisher grade 3 patients were treated with angioplasty

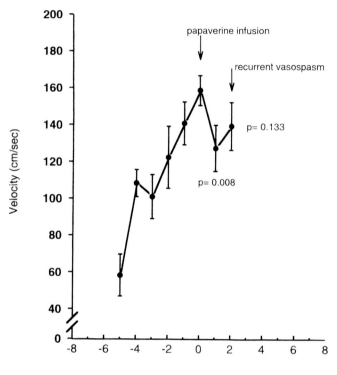

Day relative to papaverine infusion

FIG. 14.2 Graph illustrating the results of papaverine infusion as a treatment for distal ICA or MCA velocity in 13 patients. Although there was an initial decrease in velocity following treatment, the velocities failed to reach normal levels and increased again within two days after treatment. From Elliott JP, Newell DW, Lam DJ, et al.: Comparison of balloon angioplasty and papaverine infusion for treatment of vasospasm following aneurysmal subarachnoid hemorrhage. **J Neurosurg** 88:277–284, 1998, with permission.

within 3 days after bleeding and after securing of the ruptured aneurysm. One patient died secondary to a vessel rupture during angioplasty, but no patient developed a delayed neurologic deficit. Overall, eight patients made a good recovery and two a moderate recovery. The other two deaths were secondary to poor outcomes in grade 4–5 patients. Although TCD velocities did increase in some patients, none of these increases was considered severe. The role of prophylactic angioplasty in high risk patients will be assessed in a randomized, prospective study currently underway (38).

A final consideration is determination of which patients will become symptomatic from vasospasm. Although many patients have angiographic evidence of vasospasm, DINDs are less frequent. Ratsep et al. found that a significant proportion (60%) of patients have perturbed autoregulation following subarachnoid hemorrhage; however, only those who had impaired autoregulation distal to the arterial vasospasm developed ischemic deficits (39). The ability to identify at risk patients early may improve the response to endovascular therapy. It is also possible that prophylactic angioplasty may be useful in this subset of patients.

CONCLUSIONS

Over the past two decades, treatment of vasospasm following subarachnoid hemorrhage has advanced with the advent of calcium channel blockers, HHH therapy, and endovascular treatment. At the current time, balloon angioplasty appears to be the therapy of choice for symptomatic vasospasm, provided it is instituted within 12 hours of development of neurologic decline and before CT appearance of an infarct. Despite the many reports of its efficacy, no prospective trial has been conducted to date. Papaverine has more limited utility for the treatment of distal vessel vasospasm and as an adjunct to balloon angioplasty; however, its effects are frequently transient and multiple treatments may be required. As our understanding of the pathophysiology of vasospasm increases, the effectiveness of this therapy will likely improve.

REFERENCES

1. Heros RC, Zervas NT, Varsos V: Cerebral vasospasm after subarachnoid hemorrhage: an update. **Ann Neurol** 14(6):599–608, 1983.
2. Kassell NF, Sasaki T, Colohan AR, Nazar G: Cerebral vasospasm following aneurysmal subarachnoid hemorrhage. **Stroke** 16(4):562–572, 1985.
3. Kassell NF, Torner JC, Haley EC, Jr., Jane JA, Adams HP, Kongable GL: The International Cooperative Study on the Timing of Aneurysm Surgery. Part 1: Overall management results. **J Neurosurg** 73(1):18–36, 1990.
4. Le Roux PD, Elliott JP, Downey L, et al.: Improved outcome after rupture of anterior circulation aneurysms: a retrospective 10-year review of 224 good-grade patients. **J Neurosurg** 83(3):394–402, 1995.
5. Allen GS, Ahn HS, Preziosi TJ, et al.: Cerebral arterial spasm—A controlled trial of nimodipine in patients with subarachnoid hemorrhage. **N Engl J Med** 308(11):619–624, 1983.
6. Barker FG, 2nd, Ogilvy CS: Efficacy of prophylactic nimodipine for delayed ischemic deficit after subarachnoid hemorrhage: A metaanalysis. **J Neurosurg** 84(3):405–414, 1996.
7. Awad IA, Carter LP, Spetzler RF, Medina M, Williams FC, Jr: Clinical vasospasm after subarachnoid hemorrhage: Responsive to hypervolemic hemodilution and arterial hypertension. **Stroke** 18(2):365–372, 1987.

8. Chan PD, Findlay JM, Vollrath B, et al.: Pharmacological and morphological effects of in vitro transluminal balloon angioplasty on normal and vasospastic canine basilar arteries. **J Neurosurg** 83(3):522–530, 1995.
9. Seiler RW, Grolimund P, Aaslid R, Huber P, Nornes H: Cerebral vasospasm evaluated by transcranial ultrasound correlated with clinical grade and CT-visualized subarachnoid hemorrhage. **J Neurosurg** 64(4):594–600, 1986.
10. Elliott JP, Newell DW, Lam DJ, et al.: Comparison of balloon angioplasty and papaverine infusion for the treatment of vasospasm following aneurysmal subarachnoid hemorrhage. **J Neurosurg** 88(2):277–284, 1998.
11. Sloan MA, Haley EC Jr, Kassell NF, et al.: Sensitivity and specificity of transcranial Doppler ultrasonography in the diagnosis of vasospasm following subarachnoid hemorrhage. **Neurology** 39(11):1514–1518, 1989.
12. Sloan MA, Burch CM, Wozniak MA, et al.: Transcranial Doppler detection of vertebrobasilar vasospasm following subarachnoid hemorrhage. **Stroke** 25(11):2187–2197, 1994.
13. Newell DW, Grady MS, Eskridge JM, Winn HR: Distribution of angiographic vasospasm after subarachnoid hemorrhage: Implications for diagnosis by transcranial Doppler ultrasonography. **Neurosurgery** 27(4):574–577, 1990.
14. Yonas H, Sekhar L, Johnson DW, Gur D: Determination of irreversible ischemia by xenon-enhanced computed tomographic monitoring of cerebral blood flow in patients with symptomatic vasospasm. **Neurosurgery** 24(3):368–372, 1989.
15. Lewis DH, Eskridge JM, Newell DW, et al.: Brain SPECT and the effect of cerebral angioplasty in delayed ischemia due to vasospasm. **J Nucl Med** 33(10):1789–1796, 1992.
16. Firlik AD, Kaufmann AM, Jungreis CA, Yonas H: Effect of transluminal angioplasty on cerebral blood flow in the management of symptomatic vasospasm following aneurysmal subarachnoid hemorrhage. **J Neurosurg** 86(5):830–839, 1997.
17. Eskridge JM, McAuliffe W, Song JK, et al.: Balloon angioplasty for the treatment of vasospasm: results of first 50 cases. **Neurosurgery** 42(3):510–516; discussion 516–517, 1998.
18. Rosenwasser RH, Armonda RA, Thomas JE, Benitez RP, Gannon PM, Harrop J: Therapeutic modalities for the management of cerebral vasospasm: Timing of endovascular options. **Neurosurgery** 44(5):975–979; discussion 979–980, 1999.
19. Zubkov YN, Nikiforov BM, Shustin VA: Balloon catheter technique for dilatation of constricted cerebral arteries after aneurysmal SAH. **Acta Neurochir** 70(1–2):65–79, 1984.
20. Higashida RT, Halbach VV, Dowd CF, Dormandy B, Bell J, Hieshima GB: Intravascular balloon dilatation therapy for intracranial artery vasospasm: Patient selection, technique, and clinical results. **Neurosurg Rev** 15(2):89–95, 1992.
21. Newell DW, Eskridge JM, Mayberg MR, Grady MS, Winn HR: Angioplasty for the treatment of symptomatic vasospasm following subarachnoid hemorrhage. **J Neurosurg** 71(5 Pt 1):654–660, 1989.
22. Kaku Y, Yonekawa Y, Tsukahara T, Kazekawa K: Superselective intra-arterial infusion of papaverine for the treatment of cerebral vasospasm after subarachnoid hemorrhage. **J Neurosurg** 77(6):842–847, 1992.
23. Kassell NF, Helm G, Simmons N, Phillips CD, Cail WS: Treatment of cerebral vasospasm with intra-arterial papaverine. **J Neurosurg** 77(6):848–852, 1992.
24. Livingston K, Guterman LR, Hopkins LN: Intraarterial papaverine as an adjunct to transluminal angioplasty for vasospasm induced by subarachnoid hemorrhage. **Am J Neuroradiol** 14(2):346–347, 1993.
25. Yamamoto Y, Smith RR, Bernanke DH: Mechanism of action of balloon angioplasty in cerebral vasospasm. **Neurosurgery** 30(1):1–5; discussion 5–6, 1992.

26. McAuliffe W, Townsend M, Eskridge JM, Newell DW, Grady MS, Winn HR: Intracranial pressure changes induced during papaverine infusion for treatment of vasospasm. **J Neurosurg** 83(3):430–434, 1995.
27. Mathis JM, Jensen ME, Dion JE: Technical considerations on intra-arterial papaverine hydrochloride for cerebral vasospasm. **Neuroradiology** 39(2):90–98, 1997.
28. Milburn JM, Moran CJ, Cross DT 3rd, Diringer MN, Pilgram TK, Dacey RG Jr: Increase in diameters of vasospastic intracranial arteries by intraarterial papaverine administration. **J Neurosurg** 88(1):38–42, 1998.
29. Macdonald RL, Wallace MC, Montanera WJ, Glen JA: Pathological effects of angioplasty on vasospastic carotid arteries in a rabbit model. **J Neurosurg** 83(1): 111–117, 1995.
30. Bejjani GK, Bank WO, Olan WJ, Sekhar LN: The efficacy and safety of angioplasty for cerebral vasospasm after subarachnoid hemorrhage. **Neurosurgery** 42(5): 979–986; discussion 986–987, 1998.
31. Coyne TJ, Montanera WJ, Macdonald RL, Wallace MC: Percutaneous transluminal angioplasty for cerebral vasospasm after subarachnoid hemorrhage. **Can J Surg** 37(5):391–396, 1994.
32. Fujii Y, Takahashi A, Yoshimoto T: Effect of balloon angioplasty on high grade symptomatic vasospasm after subarachnoid hemorrhage. **Neurosurg Rev** 18(1):7–13, 1995.
33. Polin RS, Coenen VA, Hansen CA, et al.: Efficacy of transluminal angioplasty for the management of symptomatic cerebral vasospasm following aneurysmal subarachnoid hemorrhage. **J Neurosurg** 92(2):284–290, 2000.
34. Firlik KS, Kaufmann AM, Firlik AD, Jungreis CA, Yonas H: Intra-arterial papaverine for the treatment of cerebral vasospasm following aneurysmal subarachnoid hemorrhage. **Surg Neurol** 51(1):66–74, 1999.
35. Fandino J, Kaku Y, Schuknecht B, Valavanis A, Yonekawa Y: Improvement of cerebral oxygenation patterns and metabolic validation of superselective intraarterial infusion of papaverine for the treatment of cerebral vasospasm. **J Neurosurg** 89(1):93–100, 1998.
36. Srinivasan J, Moore A, Eskridge J, Winn HR, Newell DW: Long-term follow up of angioplasty for cerebral vasospasm. **Acta Neurochir Suppl** 77:195–197, 2001.
37. Megyesi JF, Findlay JM, Vollrath B, Cook DA, Chen MH: In vivo angioplasty prevents the development of vasospasm in canine carotid arteries. Pharmacological and morphological analyses. **Stroke** 28(6):1216–1224, 1997.
38. Muizelaar JP, Zwienenberg M, Rudisill NA, Hecht ST: The prophylactic use of transluminal balloon angioplasty in patients with Fisher Grade 3 subarachnoid hemorrhage: A pilot study. **J Neurosurg** 91(1):51–58, 1999.
39. Ratsep T, Asser T: Cerebral hemodynamic impairment after aneurysmal subarachnoid hemorrhage as evaluated using transcranial doppler ultrasonography: Relationship to delayed cerebral ischemia and clinical outcome. **J Neurosurg** 95(3): 393–401, 2001.

15

Honored Guest Presentation:
Neurorestoration and the Emergence
of Molecular and Cellular Neurosurgery

MICHAEL L.J. APUZZO, M.D., MARK A. LIKER, M.D.,
AND ARUN PAUL AMAR, M.D.

INTRODUCTION

One of the principal enterprises of civilized intellectual endeavor has been the pursuit, both in concept and practical reality, of utopia—a state of an impossible ideal. Utopian literature dates back to the 5th century BC. In his play *The Birds,* Aristophanes described an ideal city in the air to contrast to imperial Athens. Aristotle, particularly in the *Nicomachean Ethics,* alluded to ideal social situations and communities. However, it was Plato who first systematically addressed and analyzed the concept of utopia, through the voice of Socrates, and presented in *The Republic* a heightened sophistication to the organized thoughts in this regard.

Nearly two thousand years later, the influence of *The Republic* was evident in Sir Thomas More's *Utopia* (1516); the promise of "science as liberator" and universal benefactor was introduced in this work and later vigorously championed by Francis Bacon in his *New Atlantis* (1627). While envisioning landmark scientific advances, Bacon postulated that, through skillful research and subsequent discovery, society would have the means to harness nature, achieving both panacea and ultimate liberation.

The examination and expression of the theme of scientific utopias reached its peak in the 20th century with notable prophetic novels by H.G. Welles and his portrayal of the technological progress in consummate glorification with *A Modern Utopia* (1905) and *The Shape of Things to Come* (1933). Concurrently, science was seen to play a central role in Aldous Huxley's *Brave New World* (1932), but there, in contrast, it served to enslave rather than to liberate.

There is no debate regarding the immense importance of science in 21st century society, as it and the technologies it has developed form the basis of the complete spectrum of human activity: our domiciles, food, transportation, communication, entertainment, and, ultimately, provision of health care (15). In neurosurgery, we continue to strive for the ideal, at times perhaps moving to the chimeric. Our times are in many ways characterized by the perception that we can accomplish everything in this generation, particularly if we are able to apply the proper technology. Molecular biology is such a tool *(Table 15.1)* and offers immense promise for the idealized study and management of neurological disorders with great, sweeping impact envisioned for global neurodegenerative deficiencies, localized neurodegenerative disorders, neoplasms, stroke, and traumatic disorders (119). The history and observed capability of neurological surgery has been principally ablative. Now, with the amalgam of molecular biology and neurosurgery (molecular and cellular neurosurgery)—based on the tools of molecular genetics, stem cell biology, and molecular biology, and the acquired technical capabilities of endovascular access with blood-brain-barrier manipulation and the precision of image-directed stereotaxy— the capability for restoration seems to be at our immediate threshold and a new ability for neurorestoration is at hand (64, 82, 88, 119, 120).

From many aspects, the evolution of neurosurgery over the past 50 years in attitude and technology may be viewed as a march characterized by progressive minimalism in technical therapeutic approaches. The advent of new capabilities in cellular and molecular biology, when coupled with neurosurgical needs and capabilities, with an endpoint of cellular and molecular neurosurgery, would seem to offer us ultimate minimalism and a concept of medical utopia accompanied by a truly liberating Brave New World!

TABLE 15.1

Major Advances in Molecular Biology Between 1970 and 2001

Time	Molecular Technique	Investigator
1970s	Restriction endonucleases	Herbert Boyer
1970	Reverse transcriptase	David Baltimore, Howard Temin, Satoshi Mizutani
1975	Monoclonal antibodies	Cesar Milstein, Georges Kohler
1975	Discovery of introns	
1977	Automated DNA sequencing	Frederick Sanger
1985	*Human Genome Project proposal*	
1988	Polymerase chain reaction	Kary Mullis
1990	Human gene therapy protocols	
2001	*Human Genome Project completed*	Francis Collins, Craig Venter

Modified from Rutka et al. **Neurosurgery** 46:1034–1051, 2000.

HISTORICAL PERSPECTIVE

The emergence of modern cellular science of the nervous system was principally grounded in the neuron doctrine that was advanced by the brilliant Spanish anatomist Santiago Ramon Y Cajal at the turn of the century. This doctrine presented the major tenets of neurobiology and showed that the brain is composed of discrete cells called *neurons* and that these serve as elementary signaling units. He concurrently advanced the principle of *connection specificity*, which implies that neurons form highly specific connections with one another and that these are invariant and defining for each species. A third principle was termed *dynamic polarization,* according to which information flows only in one direction within the neuron, usually from the dendrites down the axon shaft. With his contemporary Charles Sherrington, he further proposed that neurons contacted one another only at specialized points called *synapses*—regions of neuronal communication.

Within these tenets, which disclosed a complex and highly refined central nervous system (CNS) architecture for each individual, was the apparently immutable barrier that adult mammalian central nervous neurons did not grow functional axons after damage and the ability for reconstitution or restoration of function was permanently lost.

However, with Tello, Cajal focused on the postulate that neurons could regenerate, regrow, and establish functional synapses if they were provided access to a permissive environment. This concept has been studied with greater enthusiasm and increasingly positive disclosure during the past quarter century as it became apparent that cell transplantation offers the possibility to circumvent apparent biological limitations (41). These disclosures have invited fuel to the concept of cellular and molecular neurosurgery with the surgeon/biologist providing neural architectural and functional restoration.

Our laboratory, one of the first CNS tumor immunology study groups, was established in 1976 and was deeply involved in the relation of the biological systems of brain, neoplasm, and general immune system. The combination of increasing biological insights and technical advances related to imaging and stereotaxy gave impetus to a flurry of activity related to grafting of dopamine-producing cells into the brains of Parkinsonian humans. The work of Eric Backlund at the Karolinska Institute and Ingacio Madrago in Mexico City was seminal in instituting adrenomedullary autografting to caudate beds in multiple centers internationally with variable clinical success. Our experiences with unilateral and bilateral stereotactically placed adrenomedullary striatal autografts was remarkably encouraging to us and indicated that, although an endpoint had not been achieved, improved cellular sources and possible environmental manipulations could effect more dramatic and sustained change (6).

ADVANCES IN MOLECULAR BIOLOGY

A remarkable escalation of our comprehension of detailed elements of cellular and molecular biology occurred during the years 1975–2001 (88), with major landmarks including:

1. Restriction endonucleases (1970s)
2. Reverse transcriptase (1970)
3. Monoclonal antibodies (1975)
4. Discovery of introns (1975)
5. Automated DNA sequencing (1977)
6. Human genome project proposal (1985)
7. Polymerase chain reaction (1988)
8. Human gene therapy (1990 to present)
9. Human genome project completed (? 2001)

The culmination of this remarkable era—the sequencing of the entire human genome—heralds an even more fertile and exciting period for cellular and molecular neurosurgery.

BACKGROUND OF THE HUMAN GENOME PROJECT (8, 19, 47, 61, 80, 91, 92, 108, 109)

The Human Genome Project (HGP), an international effort to map and sequence the 3 billion base pairs constituting the human genetic code, was officially launched in the United States in 1990—the same year that Congress inaugurated the Decade of the Brain and the year the first clinical protocol of gene therapy was approved (4). The magnitude of this project is gargantuan; if one were to print out all the information in the human genome letter by letter, it would fill a stack of books as tall as a 12-story building (26).

The goals of the HGP were to increase our understanding of how we function as healthy human beings, to identify the approximately 40,000 genes that govern our biological operations, and to reveal the chemical basis for many of the roughly 4000 genetic diseases that afflict us. In addition, it was believed that this anthropological template would undoubtedly result in tests for screening and diagnosing genetic disorders as well as provide the foundation for novel treatments.

At its outset, the HGP was expected to cost less than the Apollo project by an order of magnitude (109). Like the space initiative, however, the rapid progress of the HGP has both fueled and thrived on the development of a number of key enabling technologies and resources. Most important among these include the development of DNA host/vector systems capable of accommodating large clones of genomic DNA (such as the yeast artificial chromosome and bacterial artificial chromosome), discovery of the polymerase chain reaction (a means of amplifying small quantities of DNA for large scale analysis), computer and informatics tools capable of analyzing unfathomable amounts of data, and Internet technologies facilitating the exchange of this data (61). Because of these advances, the cost of genomic sequencing has dropped from $2–$5 per base to an order of magnitude less (19). As of January 2000, 50% of the sequence was available in the public domain (8). Milestones have been met ahead of schedule, and a "working draft" of the sequence is now available. A complete and highly accurate reference sequence is expected to be available by 2003, coinciding with the 50 year anniversary of the fundamental description of the structure of the DNA double helix (8, 47).

The project was initially proposed by the Department of Energy in 1985. Their goal was to obtain DNA sequences in order to study the genetic changes induced by ionizing radiation. Critics quickly pointed out that 95% of our DNA does not code for genes and that the project would lead to an enormous amount of expensive but not very useful information. They favored an *ad hoc* approach to identifying genes rather than a systematic national effort. Others in the scientific community were convinced that knowledge of the whole sequence would be invaluable. In order to mediate these concerns, the NIH became a joint sponsor. After 14 months of deliberation, the National Research Council (NRC) of the National Academy of Sciences unanimously agreed on the merit of this project.

The initiation of the project coincided with a number of advances that made it technically feasible to complete the program within the time and budget allotted, whereas such an ambitious plan would have been unthinkable the preceding decade. These advances were already being applied to genomic research on model organisms such as *E. coli*, yeasts, the roundworm *C. elegans*, *Drosophila*, and the mouse.

Conceptually, the project consists of two interrelated strategies. The first goal was to establish a genetic map, which is assembled by determining how frequently two markers are inherited together. These markers can include genes, classic restriction fragment length polymorphisms, and other detectable DNA sequences. Genetic maps are measured in centimorgans (two markers are 1 cM apart if they are separated 1% of the time during transmission from parent to child due to recombination events at meiosis). Genetic maps measured in cM don't give a precise assessment of physical distance along the chromosome, although 1 cM is roughly equivalent to 1 million base pairs of DNA. Thus, to create a linkage map with a resolution of 1 cM, about 3000 well-spaced markers would be needed. Each should be identified by sequence-tagged sites (STS), which are short, unique DNA sequences that serve as fingerprints for individual markers.

The next stage was creation of the physical map, which shows the location of landmarks on the DNA. Base pairs are the unit of measurement on a physical map. The lowest resolution physical map of the human genome shows the banding patterns of chromosomes, which have a resolution of about 10 million base pairs. The highest resolution map would be the complete sequence of all 3 billion base pairs. The first physical mapping goal was assembling the STS maps of all 24 chromosomes (22 paired autosomes plus X and Y). The other goal was assembling overlapping sets (contigs) of cloned DNA or closely spaced, unambiguously ordered markers with continuity over lengths of 2 million base pairs for large portions of the genome. The genetic linkage map can be used to help order these contigs. With good contig maps, the particular regions of chromosomes needed to locate genes of interest will be available.

Integrating the genetic and physical maps has provided a framework upon which to hang the sequence and the means to connect the linear DNA code of each chromosome. Integration of these two types of maps has uncovered the genetic bases of many rare diseases inherited by simple Mendelian laws. These insights can then be extended to components of relatively common but complex polygenic diseases such as diabetes, cancer, or Alzheimer's. One example is the discovery of single nucleotide polymorphisms (SNPs) in the genetic code, idiosyncratic variations that occur about once every 1000 bases. Although some of these contribute to harmless individual differences best called traits, others contribute to increased susceptibility to illness. It is estimated that most of us carry a total of four or five serious mutations (called recessives) and a larger number conveying vulnerability to various diseases (19). SNPs may thus serve as markers for identifying disease genes by linkage studies in families or from the discovery of genes involved in human diseases, leading to better screening and preventive therapies in patients with predisposing conditions.

Once the genome is decoded, the next task will be to annotate the linear sequence with gene structure and function. This can be done by many strategies, including comparative genomics (looking at differences and similarities across species), computational analysis, experimental confirmation by cDNA sequencing, detecting homology of newly discovered gene products with proteins of known function, and establishing the association of specific genes with disease phenotypes by mutation screening. Function can also be inferred from the temporal and spatial distribution of gene expression in different tissue samples. Finally, gene expression can be manipulated *in vivo*. Specific genes in murine pluripotent undifferentiated embryonic stem cells can be inactivated. These cells can then be injected into blastocysts to generate chimeric animals from which "knockouts" can be bred. These knockout mice can then be subject to experiments that clarify the functional significance of the gene in question (88). For instance, a knockout model of Canavan's disease was reported this year and may be useful to assay gene therapy approaches to this disorder.

The commercial applications of the HGP have yet to be realized. Nonetheless, because of the promised bounty of the project, industry has become increasingly involved in what has become "the race" to decode the sequence. In typical corporate style, their approach has been more parsimonious than the government's effort. They have concentrated on the fraction of the genome that is actually transcribed into mRNA and subsequently translated into proteins by constructing catalogues of short cDNA sequences (complementary DNA reverse transcribed from mRNA templates) called expression sequence tags (ESTs). While multinational pharmaceutical companies are sponsoring similar efforts, the most publicized figure in this sector is Craig Venter, founder of the for-profit Institute for Genome Research. Venter recently announced an EST map of the entire sequence, which he intends to patent and vend to other researchers. However, some are skeptical of this claim.

Although the description of the linear sequence of the human DNA code promises to be the ultimate in biological reductionism, there are implications that may not have been apparent to the early pioneers of molecular genetics. About 5% of the federally funded HGP budget has been allocated to considering the ethical, legal, and social ramifications of the project (80, 109). These include issues such as the responsible use of genetic information, fairness in the use of genetic testing by employers and insurers, and methods for protecting individual privacy. It is imperative that neurosurgeons be involved in deciding such issues.

THERAPEUTIC IMPLICATIONS OF
THE HGP FOR CNS THERAPIES

It is estimated that 80% of the new genes discovered by the HGP contribute to the unique properties of the human brain (91). In theory, this affords great potential to treat a broad array of acquired and inherited neurologic disorders. As of 1998, the genetic locus of more than 300 neurological disorders had been identified (103).

TABLE 15.2
Possibilities for Gene Therapy of Central Nervous System Disorders

CNS Disorder	Possible Mode of Gene Therapy
Global neurodegenerative enzyme deficiencies (recessive mutation in a single gene)	Viral vector-mediated gene replacement with a single normal allele
	Genetically transformed neural progenitor cells
Localized neurodegenerative disorders	Viral vector-mediated transfer of therapeutic gene
	Embryonic implants
	Transplantation of genetically modified cells
	Direct transfer of plasmid DNA-lipofectin complex
Brain tumors	Transfer of drug susceptibility "suicidal" gene
	Transduction with "toxic" genes
	Transduction with antisense cell-cycle genes
	Adoptive immunotherapy
Stroke	Introduction of therapeutic genes
	Genetic manipulations with fibrinolytic system

CNS, central nervous system; DNA, deoxyribonucleic acid
Zlokovic BV, Apuzzo MLJ: **Neurosurgery** 40:789–804, 1997.

The magnitude of these advances in molecular biology and similar expansion of the database in cellular biology allow audacious concepts to be developed regarding cellular and molecular neurosurgery. In companion papers published in 1997, we presented these concepts in detail (119, 120). Reasonable *disease targets* included global neurodegenerative deficiencies, localized neurodegenerative disorders, brain neoplasms and stroke *(Table 15.2)*. *Vector systems* for delivery of genes to the CNS included retrovirus, herpes simplex virus, adenovirus, liposomes and neuroprogenitor cells. Techniques for vector mediated *delivery* included: (1) local central nervous system stereotactic infection or infusion of viral vectors, vector-producer cells or cell replacement; (2) local cerebrospinal fluid injection or infusion (ventricle, cisterna magna, or subarachnoid routes); (3) osmotic blood-brain-barrier manipulation with intravenous or intra-arterial injection or infusion; (4) local intra-arterial infusion; or (5) blood-brain-barrier disruption by permeabilizers such as RMP-7 *(Table 15.3)*.

These concepts based on substantive developments allowed for further meaningful progress toward neurorestoration. However, it is important to consider that the nervous system, in a sense, may be represented in its fabric and complexity as a unique framework created for an individual, its refinement of structure and function coupled with defiance toward reproducibility or restoration after alteration, being unsurpassed in nature. Principles and therapeutic interventions are required to address this individuality and to take advantage while enhancing what is being increasingly shown to be a remarkable *plasticity* in the central nervous system under given conditioned circumstances.

TABLE 15.3
Vector Systems for Delivery of Genes to the Central Nervous System

Vector	Advantages	Disadvantages
Retrovirus	Target limited to mitotic cells (tumor) Delivery of toxic genes to treat tumors Delivery of genes into cells that are then grafted into the brain Not inactivated in the CSF	Cannot infect neurons and other postmitotic cells Unlikely to be useful in gene replacement therapy Low titers and low levels of viral integration Limited size of DNA insert Inactivation in plasma Transient gene expression
Herpes simplex virus	Infection of neurons, postmitotic cells No DNA insertion in host genome High titers (replication-compromised) Virus can enter latency	Lytic infection Neurotoxicity Recombination to wild type of lytic virus Transient gene expression Low titer (replication-defective, amplicon)
Adenovirus	Infection to neurons, postmitotic cells Gene expression without integration in host genome Insert capacity of 35 kilobases No oncogenicity Low level of neurotoxicity	Inflammatory response Transient gene expression
Liposomes	No toxicity inherent in viruses Easy to clone plasmid DNA Can be produced in quantity	Very transient expression No cell type specificity
Neural progenitors	Easy to clone (large supply of material for transplantation) Ideal for genetic manipulation Ability to migrate throughout the CNS	Allogeneicity Potential toxicity

CSF, cerebrospinal fluid; DNA, deoxyribonucleic acid; CNS, central nervous system
Zlokovic BV, Apuzzo MLJ: **Neurosurgery** 40:805–813, 1997.

One approach is somatic gene therapy, a technique for supplanting or complementing defective or absent genes with copies of functional ones. Two strategies of gene transfer to the CNS are currently employed (4). In the "*in situ*" approach, the transgene is directly delivered into the brain for direct transduction of the target cells. In the "ex vivo" strategy, the transgene is introduced into cells grown *in vitro*, which are then grafted into the organism. A final approach, "in vivo" gene therapy, entails injecting the genetic vector directly into the bloodstream. Clinical examples of the last category are sparse, however.

Rational drug design is another approach that has benefited from the revolution in molecular genetics partially spawned by the HGP. For instance, once a cell surface receptor is identified as a possible pharmaceutical target, scientists can clone a family of similar receptors, express them in cell lines, and test a vast array of reagents for activation or inhibition of a biological response (such as triggering calcium influx into a neuron).

The HGP and the molecular biology attendant to it are likely to result in many treatments for which neurosurgeons may play a role. Some possibilities are listed below (47, 65, 119):

Transplantation

Data obtained from the HGP will enable scientists to genetically engineer animals to have specific combinations of human antigens matching those of a transplant patient. Xenotransplantation could then be performed with less risk of rejection. Alternatively, tissue engineering with stem cells could produce opportunities for allografts and autografts. These strategies might play a role in movement disorders and other neurodegenerative conditions.

Oncology

The HGP will identify many of the genes implicated in the stages of tumor progression. These include oncogenes, tumor suppressor genes, and DNA repair genes. Understanding the structure and functions of the proteins encoded by these genes will allow their manipulation in favorable ways. Strategies for gene therapy of brain tumors include activation of prodrugs, stimulation of favorable immune responses, modulation of angiogenesis, control of apoptosis and tumor suppression, oncolytic virus therapy, and antisense therapy (24, 96, 115). However, the treatment of brain tumors is more formidable than that of genetic diseases of the CNS, since effective cancer therapy requires complete eradication of all tumor cells, whereas genetic disease therapy may require the modification of only a small percentage of cells to be effective (115).

Stroke

By understanding the genes involved in cerebrovascular accidents, the local milieu can be modulated to minimize damage to CNS tissue and promote functional repair. For instance, neuroprotection has been demonstrated against a variety of *in vitro* and *in vivo* rodent models of ischemic insults with vectors overexpressing genes that target various facets of excitotoxic injury, such as energetic components, calcium excess, accumulation of reactive oxygen species, protein malfolding, inflammation, free radical damage, and triggering of apoptosis pathways (90, 111).

Other Disorders

Based on an evolving technologies that allow the addition, alteration, or elimination of individual genes to create transgenic animal models, constitutive or conditional gene knockout and subsequent gene-transfer facilitated rescue strategies are elucidating the gene products involved in the etiology and pathophysiology of a number of diverse conditions. This information has impelled initial efforts to treat epilepsy (20), psychiatric illnesses (63), and other conditions using gene therapy approaches.

REQUISITE ELEMENTS FOR SUCCESSFUL GENE THERAPY OF THE CNS

In spite of the information that the HGP promises to deliver, the application of these insights into restorative therapies of the CNS remains a formidable obstacle. Several considerations must be addressed in order for gene therapy to achieve the following goals:

1. Efficient transfection of host cells
2. Selective, sustained, and regulated expression of foreign genes in the CNS
3. Lack of toxicity or immune excitation

The requisite elements of this process, their current impediments, and the windows of opportunity that circumvent such obstacles are summarized below.

Identification of Appropriate Candidate Diseases

Selection of ideal targets for gene therapy of the CNS must begin by considering the underlying genetic events to be overcome and their spatio-temporal distribution. These circumstances mandate the requirements for physical dispersal of the transgene product, its duration of regulated expression, and the quantity of gene product sufficient to correct the disease.

For instance, at present, there are no good approaches to treat global CNS disorders that are polygenic in origin. In contrast, inherited monogenic enzyme deficiencies represent a category of disease potentially amenable to gene therapy. Although specific recessive metabolic disorders are rare, collectively they comprise a significant proportion of the neurodegenerative disorders (119). Ideally, gene replacement with a single normal allele would be sufficient to abrogate the abnormal CNS phenotype. Global gene replacement therapy of these metabolic disorders requires a vector system that produces long-term gene expression in neurons and glia throughout the brain (119).

Conversely, stroke and vasospasm following subarachnoid hemorrhage represent disorders with more limited spatial and temporal involvement. Thus, their requirements for physical distribution and duration of transgene expression are less stringent. In fact, transient gene expression may be advantageous in diseases such as ischemia, in which normal repair processes and angiogenesis obviate the need for continuing therapeutic intervention (79, 119). It is becoming increasingly evident that processes such as apoptosis and secondary injury continue for days after a cerebrovascular accident (49, 90). Thus, although some neurons die within the first hours, others may be protected by gene therapy strategies that take hours or days for the products of viral or other vector genes to be expressed in transfected tissues (111).

Similarly, for conditions such as Parkinson's disease (PD), characterized by degeneration of discrete populations of neurons within well-circumscribed areas in the brain, successful gene transfer may employ local delivery strategies. However, because of the chronic nature of the disease, transgene expression must be long-lasting (68).

In many cases, transduction need not be ubiquitous. In lysosomal storage diseases, for instance, a low level of enzymatic activity (5–10% of that found in normal individuals) may be all that is required to achieve normal cellular function (119). Similarly, in other conditions, transgene products may be secreted by expressing cells and taken up by nonexpressing cells or transferred by direct cell contact (119). This serendipitous event accounts for the tumoricidal "bystander effect" noted in gene therapy trials of gliomas using herpes simplex virus thymidine kinase to activate gancyclovir. The bystander effect may result from transfer of toxic gancyclovir metabolites across intercellular gap junctions, or from transfer of apoptotic vesicles or local inflammatory responses against virally infected tumor cells (115). As another example, the adventitial cells of blood vessels may be transfected after injecting vector containing the nitric oxide (NO) synthase gene into the subarachnoid space (SAS). The products of that gene, such as NO and cyclic guanidine monophosphate, can then diffuse into the smooth muscle of the arterial media leading to vasodilatation, even though the muscle cells themselves are not transfected (77, 111). Similarly, while it is unknown how many neurons and how much circuitry must be restored to reconstruct a damaged system, some data suggest that less than 10% restoration may be sufficient (78). A final example of how beneficial effects on behavior can be accomplished without having to transfect every involved cell concerns "*ex vivo*" approaches to gene therapy. For instance, PD is characterized by local depletion of dopamine within the corpus striatum. Cells engineered to secrete dopamine into the extracellular milieu can be introduced locally in the striatum. Because dopamine appears to function as a paracrine, slow-acting neurotransmitter, a regional increase in dopaminergic tone is likely to improve the extrapyramidal symptoms associated with PD (39).

Viral Vector Design (4, 79, 86, 88, 103, 116, 120)

Vectors consist of vehicles for transferring exogenous DNA into target tissues. Viruses have evolved highly efficient mechanisms to deliver nucleic acids to specific cell types while evading host immunosurveillance. For these reasons, several of them have been deliberately subverted for use as carriers of recombinant genetic material. Viral vectors currently used in gene therapy research and clinical application include retroviruses (RV), adenoviruses (AV), adeno-associated viruses (AAV), recombinant herpes simplex virus (HSV), and lentiviruses (LV), among others. Selectivity is enhanced by exploiting natural differences in the biological properties of each class of virus.

For instance, RV vectors have the characteristic of integrating and expressing vector genes only in proliferating cells, because their entry into the nucleus requires breakdown of the nuclear membrane, an event that typically only occurs during cell division (11). The preferential integration of RV into replicating cells suggests a possible strategy for selective expression in CNS tumor cells, since adult neurons are mitotically quiescent. Another application that exploits this property is the use of RV to deliver genes into cells grown in tissue culture and then grafted into the brain to treat localized CNS disease. In this "*ex vivo*" approach, the gene product can influence neurons that are not directly transfected by the virus. RV vectors are typically engineered as plasmids that contain the therapeutic gene of interest flanked by viral promoter elements, polyadenlylation signals, and reverse transcription and integration sequences. The most commonly used RV backbone is the Moloney murine leukemia virus (MuLV). One advantage is that RV is not inactivated by CSF, although it is susceptible to complement-mediated inactivation in plasma. The RV vector system is limited by relatively low transduction efficiency, partially due to rapid inactivation of the viral genome. For this reason, the RV plasmid is frequently transfected into packaging cell lines to create vector-producing cells. These cells contain the genes required for viral replication (such as viral encapsidation and structural proteins) *in trans* and produce high titers of infectious, replication-defective virions (100). Unfortunately, these cells may be highly immunogenic, even in the brain. In other cases, the products necessary for replication and integration are supplied *in trans* by replication-competent but non-transforming helper viruses that later have to be completely removed from purified vector, which is often a difficult task. The broad range of cell types possessing amphotropic receptors for the MuLV limits target cell specificity and dilutes the number of viral particles reaching their target. This fact, coupled with the inability to generate high titers, limits the efficiency of *in situ* gene therapy approaches using RV (4). Furthermore, RV have a high rate of genetic variability resulting from reverse transcriptase errors that can lead to mutation rates of 5%, leading to secondary disease and unpredictable outcomes. Finally, the size of the DNA inserted into the RV is limited to about 7.5kb (79).

Despite their natural tropism for the respiratory tract, recombinant adenoviruses can express foreign transgenes in both neurons and glial cells (86). Other advantages include their ability to infect a wide variety of both dividing and nondividing cells and the availability of high titer preparations. They are neither neurotoxic nor cytolytic. Their genome consists of linear, double stranded DNA that can be engineered to be replication deficient by deletion of early regulatory genes. Unlike RV, they do not require vector-producing cells for infection. They are not associated with the hazard of insertional mutagenesis. AV can be transported in neurons by retrograde axonal transport (86). For instance, intranasal injections will transfect neurons in the olfactory pathways and in some remote brain regions (111). Among their disadvantages, adenoviral DNA generally remains episomal, leading to transient expression of the transgene. Also, AV tend to incite a significant immune reaction, and efforts to reduce their immunogenicity have resulted in decreased expression of the transgene (103). Induction of two immune responses has been observed (116). Cytotoxic T-lymphocytes produce tissue damage and may destroy the corrected cell, whereas B-cell and T-helper cell activation leads to production of antiviral antibodies that make repeat administration less effective and potentially unsafe (96). In addition, cell infection is relatively nonselective, and transgene capacity (4.5 kb) is low (86).

HSV is a large, linear, double-stranded DNA virus capable of efficiently infecting a wide host range, including postmitotic neurons. In fact, neurons are more successfully infected than glia because of natural neurotropism. For this reason, HSV vectors may become important for the treatment of neurodegenerative disorders. HSV replicates successfully only in dividing cells, and attenuated HSV viruses have been used to achieve selective cytolysis of dividing tumor cells. HSV can also establish latency in nondividing neurons. Other useful HSV vectors are replication defective except when propagated in complementing cell lines. Large transgenes up to 30 kb can be inserted. Like the adenoviruses, HSV vectors lose the transgene over time because it remains episomal and is not integrated into the host genome. Also, transcriptional regulation is difficult when non-HSV promoters are used. HSV is potentially neurotoxic and can lead to cytolytic infection, even in normal cells. It is also highly immunogenic.

Lentiviruses are a class of RVs whose genome encodes additional nonstructural proteins that function in transcriptional regulation of the viral genome. Unlike other RVs, LVs are efficiently transduced and integrated into nondividing as well as dividing cells because they can pass through pores in the intact nuclear membrane. The human immunodeficiency virus (HIV) is one example of a lentivirus being currently researched as a potential vector for CNS gene transfer (100).

The adeno-associated virus genome consists of single stranded DNA. The parental wild-type virus is a defective parvovirus that requires helper functions from other viruses to reproduce progeny, thus limiting the potential for unwanted vector spread. Although 80% of humans have antibodies directed against AAV, infection is generally not pathogenic. Other advantages of using AAV in gene therapy include the absence of neurotoxic damage and the lack of an immune response after infection. The latter results because most viral genes are deleted. AAV are also more compact than other viruses and may be more effective in traversing small pores, such as those in the blood-brain-barrier (88). They can integrate into host DNA at a specific site on the short arm of chromosome 19 in humans, leading to stable gene expression. They are able to infect nondividing and dividing cells. AAVs are resistant to many physical and chemical factors such as detergents, a wide range of pH, repeated freeze-and-thaw cycles, lyophilizing, and heat denaturing up to 60 degrees C. Transduction efficiency is generally low, however, and they do not display any inherent neurotropism. For these reasons, AAVs commonly require helper viruses such as HSV or AV, which entail attendant risks. In addition, AAVs have a low transgene capacity (4.7 kb).

Non-viral Vectors

Transfer of functional genes into cells can also be accomplished by nonviral vehicles. Plasmid DNA is safe, does not induce inflammation, does not require cell division for uptake or expression, and is easily prepared (111). However, DNA is negatively charged in water and is therefore repelled from cellular membranes, which are also negatively charged. As a result, naked DNA plasmids transfect fewer than 1% of the cells exposed to them (111). For this reason, DNA must be complexed with positively charged agents to facilitate their uptake into cells. Direct injection of plasmid DNA combined with lipofectin (a cationic lipid that attracts the negatively charged DNA) is one potential approach of transferring therapeutic genes into endogenous neural cells (119).

Another strategy for overcoming the negative charge of DNA is to enclose it in the form of cationic liposomes. The latter are small, positively charged, spherical lipid bilayers composed of amphipathic elements that spontaneously self assemble. Liposomes can fuse with cell membranes and deliver their contents into the intracellular environment. Liposomes also protect the DNA from degradation and limit toxicity and immunogenicity. There is no limitation to the size of the DNA plasmid contained within. Liposomes can be stored easily. Furthermore, they can transfect both mitotic and postmitotic cells. Targeting to specific cells may be controlled by coupling glycolipids, specific cell adhesion molecules, receptors, or human monoclonal antibodies within the liposomal vector (86). Unfortunately, compared with viral systems, the transfection efficiency is low (1–2% of exposed cells), and delivery is nonselective (111). Because there is no mechanism for the tranfected gene to be integrated into host chromosomes, gene expression is transient. Transfer across the BBB is exceptionally difficult. Liposomes are also rapidly ingested by immune phagocytic cells.

Finally, instead of using viruses to deliver genes into target cells that then produce the appropriate protein, the gene products themselves can be delivered to tissues by transplanting cells that are engineered to secrete them into the extracellular space ("*ex vivo*" gene therapy).

Selective Expression

Selective expression of transgenes by host cells in the CNS can be accomplished by designing constructs in which the gene is placed downstream of a promoter that demonstrates developmental and tissue specificity, such as the glial fibrillary acidic protein promoter found exclusively in astrocytes (88, 111). Promoters that are regulated by temperature, exposure to drugs such as tetracycline, and other environmental factors can also direct expression of transgenes and control cellular differentiation or replication.

For instance, one limitation of gene therapy for stroke is that ischemia typically inhibits protein synthesis, including that from viral

vector DNA, thus diminishing transgene expression. However, production of heat shock proteins are generally spared, and one possible
solution is to place expression of the transgene under the control of
an inducible heat shock promoter (90).

In other settings, the efficiency and specificity of transgene expression can also be enhanced by engineering vectors with appropriate localization signals that target the foreign DNA into the nucleus to interact with transcription factors unique to specific cells (96).

Physical Delivery

Delivery of the gene therapy vector into the brain presents several
unique challenges, including limited and potentially risky access
through the skull (thus precluding repeat administration), sensitivity
to volumetric changes (thus minimizing the size of the inoculum and
decreasing the reserve for inflammatory responses), and the blood-
brain-barrier (BBB) (20).

Several routes of access to the brain have been investigated (Table
15.4). The vector can be injected directly into the parenchymal space,
either stereotactically or via craniotomy. For widespread conditions
such as global neurodenerative disorders or infiltrative gliomas, however, limited diffusion of the vector represents a significant short-
coming with this strategy. For instance, following direct inoculation
with AV or HSV, transduction is mostly limited to a 2-mm radius from
the inoculation site. Even with the use of vector producing cells to increase viral titer and exposure time at the tumor site, virally infected
cells have only been detected 20 to 30 cell diameters from the transplant site following stereotactic injection in humans (115). The use of
replication-competent viruses, leading to secondary and tertiary infections, may overcome this problem (115). By applying a pressure gra-
dient during infusion, convection-enhanced delivery may also improve
the volume of distribution of viral vectors up to 200 cubic mm. In some
cases, spread of vectors to remote regions of the brain may be mediated by anterograde or retrograde transport within neurons projecting to the injection site (20).

Vectors can also be administered within the ventricles or cerebrospinal fluid cisterns of the subarachnoid space (SAS). However, the
rate of diffusion from the CSF system into the parenchymal tissue is
considerably slower than the CSF convection flow (120). Intrathecal
injection of adenovirus into the cisterna magna results in gene transfer to the leptomeningeal cells overlying major arteries, to fibroblasts
in the adventitia of large vessels, and occasionally to smooth muscle
cells of small vessels (77). This strategy may find important application in treating cerebral vasospasm, since the presence of blood within

TABLE 15.4

Techniques for Vector-mediated Delivery of Genes to the Central Nervous System

Technique	Advantages	Disadvantages
Local CNS stereotactic injection/infusion of viral vectors, vector producer cells, or cell replacement	Single small tumors Localized neurodegenerative disorders (transplantation of transfected cells)	Not applicable to treat multiple tumor metastases, neurodegenerative enzyme deficiencies, or stroke Diffusion problem for large tumors
Local CSF injection/infusion (ventricle, cisterna magna, subarachnoid space)	CSF does not inactivate retroviral vectors Meningeal metastases and stroke	Poor diffusion of vectors into CNS Not applicable for brain tumors, global CNS disorder, or brain repair
Osmotic BBB opening with I.V. or I.A. injection/infusion	Potential for parenchymal metastases and large tumors Potential for global CNS disease	Possible neurotoxicity Possible systemic toxicity
Local I.A. infusion	Potential for delivery of genetic material via liposomes Potential for stroke	May not be efficient for viral-mediated delivery for global CNS disorder, brain Tumors and brain repair
BBTB permeabilizers (e.g., RMP-7)	Potential for brain tumors (large and multiple metastases)	May not be applicable for brain repair

CNS, central nervous system; CSF, cerebrospinal fluid; BBB, blood-brain barrier; I.V., intravenous; I.A., intra-arterial; BBTB, blood-brain-tumor barrier

Zlokovic BV, Apuzzo MLJ: **Neurosurgery** 40:805–813, 1997.

the SAS does not prevent viral-mediated gene transfer to these cells after intracisternal injection (74).

Introduction of a vector into the ventricles may transfer genes to the ependymal cells and choroid plexus, thus providing a source of secreted products that enter the CSF and then penetrate the brain. Expression by the ependyma also results in considerable extracellular secretion and diffusion, which is useful for overexpressing proteins that exert their effect extracellularly but not effective for delivering genes with intracellular mechanisms of action (90).

Endovascular intra-arterial delivery, preceded by blood-brain-barrier (BBB) disruption, is the strategy with the highest likelihood of global transgene distribution. Potential problems include transport across the BBB, thromboembolic complications resulting from extended flow interruption not tolerated by CNS tissue, and inactivation by plasma components. In addition, nonselective BBB disruption may produce neurotoxic effects in regions of the brain not intended for gene replacement strategies (121).

Regardless of the route of entry into the brain, the need for subsequent permeation throughout the interstitial space of the parenchyma remains another significant limitation. Cells with inherent migratory ability may prove to be the best vectors in this regard. Various classes of progenitor cells, including embryonic and adult neural stem cells and glial precursors, have been efficiently transfected before engrafting; they have been found to migrate widely and integrate into the existing cellular architecture. In this way, cells can be engineered to produce deficient enzymes, neurotransmitters, or neurotrophic factors (discussed below).

Integration and Regulation of Long-term, Stable Expression

Vectors must convey the therapeutic gene into the nucleus for transcription into mRNA and subsequent translation into protein. The requirements for the duration and regulation of this process depend on the disorder being treated. In most cases, integration into the cellular genome is desirable.

However, as stated, for acute ischemic brain insults in which long-term stable expression of therapeutic genes may not be necessary, in vivo plasmid DNA transfer strategies may be sufficient.

Lack of Toxicity

Principal limitations of some viral vectors include insertional mutagenesis (e.g. the random integration of virus into host chromosome leading to activation of proto-oncogenes or inactivation of tumor suppressor genes), provocation of cytotoxic T-cell response to cells expressing viral proteins (viral capsid proteins appear to be particularly immunogenic), and the cytopathic effects of some viruses on the host cell (103). Reversion to the wild-type, infectious phenotype remains a concern with some viral vectors. Germ-line transmission from integration of viral sequences into gametes is another potential concern (96). Also, recombination of the defective virus with a wild-type strain may give rise to a hypervirulent strain and possible immunologic problems as well (86).

CELL REPLACEMENT AND GENE THERAPY FOR NEURORESTORATION

As we begin the 10th decade of modern exploration into neural regeneration, following Tello's 1911 description of regrowth of adult CNS neurons within a conditioned environment, mastery of neural stem cell properties holds promise for exciting new avenues of intervention for a variety of CNS diseases. The following year, in 1912, Allen identified mitotic cells in the adult rat brain in a region analogous to the embryonic subventricular zone (2). During this period, the immutability of the adult central nervous system had been established as a fundamental tenet of neuroscience, and a nihilistic approach to neural injury had been the mainstay of clinical neuroscience until recent events provoked a reevaluation of these theories. During the last decade, spurred by the development of advanced microbiological techniques applied to the field of embryology, vertebrate multipotential cells with the ability to differentiate into both neuronal and glial subtypes have been identified both through in vivo fate mapping and in vitro lineage studies, and their properties have been gradually defined (29, 106, 110). Fundamental and important contributions have been made with regard to vertebrate/non-human stem cells in terms of isolation, growth fates, passaging and plasticity, confirming the multipotential, functional traits of stem cells and their progeny and factors needed to enhance replication (83, 84). The promise of human neural regeneration and CNS plasticity came closer to reality in 1998 when two groups reported isolating and growing cultures of self-renewing human pluripotential stem cells, one group using cells from *in-vitro* fertilization and the other from aborted fetuses (94, 104). Neural stem cells derived from the adult brain have also been investigated to identify the breadth of plasticity but results thus far have been equivocal. In general, research has primarily focused on specific properties of the human neural stem cells such as proliferative capabilities, functional characteristics, and *in vivo* incorporation with regard to their restorative potential.

Strategies for CNS restoration have embraced three avenues of exploration:

1. *Replacing affected cell populations* and connections by neural grafts
2. Providing *trophic support* by introducing neurotrophins and/or cytokines to diminish or prevent progressive neurodegeneration, stimulate neurite outgrowth, guide growing axons, and promote establishment of functional synapses
3. Replacing missing *neuroactive molecules* such as enzymes and transmitters

Initial practical entry to accomplish elements of these goals has been attempted through the employment of fetal grafts to replace cellular elements, act as tissue bridges, prevent degeneration, and to evoke robust restorative mechanisms for surprisingly unusually well-modeled cytoarchitecture. Interestingly, although early investigations of fetal neural tissue transplantation were pursued in order to investigate the development and restorative potential of the nervous system, it was discovered that functional improvement subsequently resulted following tissue engraftment. Further animal studies confirmed that grafted fetal tissue could integrate in the host brain and improve functional deficits following acute injury in animal models of Huntington's and Alzheimer's diseases and other neurodegenerative pathologies (43, 89, 95). In addition, over the past decade a number of studies have demonstrated sustained grafted cell viability, incorporation and modestly positive clinical improvements in Parkinson's disease *(Fig. 15.1)* (6, 14, 30–38, 55–57, 76, 113). The most recent notable work from the University of Colorado and Columbia University in a prospective double-blinded study of fetal dopamine neural grafting demonstrated graft survival, function and modest clinical benefit in patients under sixty years of age (36). However, unexpected and untoward responses potentially relating to dopamine overdose have dampened enthusiasm for fetal-cell transplantation in humans, calling into question support for further human experimentation until basic science research has been completed. Nonetheless, a second double-blinded study is underway and may provide insight into difficulties encountered in the first.

Problems exist limiting further development of this therapeutic modality. These include ethical concerns and the need for six fetuses per patient for treatment. There is a cellular loss of 90–95%, and standardization is difficult with major issues of the quality and purity of grafted materials always present. The heterogeneous nature of the graft substrate is not well suited for what has become a primary therapeutic consideration—the *genetic engineering* of implanted cells.

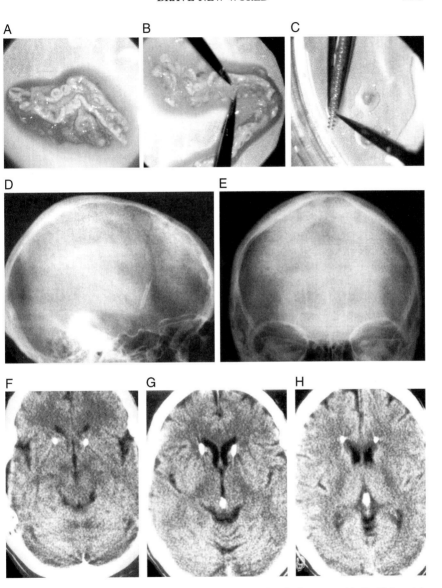

FIG. 15.1 Dissection of adrenal medullary tissue and coil placement (*A, B, C*) for striatal implantation (*D,* lateral, and *E,* anterior/posterior plain roentgenograms) in a Parkinsonian patient (*F, G, H,* axial computed tomography scans). From Apuzzo MLJ, et al.: **Neurosurgery** 26:746–757, 1990.

However, in spite of these imperfect elements, the overall experience has clearly demonstrated that cell replacement actually works! Although specific fetal cell grafting is not promising as a therapeutic mode for routine use, over the past two decades it has become evident that the both developing and, surprisingly, adult mammalian central nervous system retains a population of undifferentiated, multipotent cell precursor, neural *stem cells,* the plastic properties of which offer advantage for the design of more practical and effective therapies for many neurological disorders. With the identification and isolation of neural stem cells, the natural progression of research turned to methods of stem cell incorporation in experimental models of injury. Numerous studies have revealed engraftment and functional plasticity of transplanted cells, reversing both the neurochemical changes and functional deficits associated with these models *(Fig. 15.2)* (1, 22, 27, 48, 60, 98, 99, 118).

Strategies for CNS regeneration via stem cell technology must originate from a perspective treating properties of the microenvironment and the implanted stem cells as separate but interacting entities, keep-

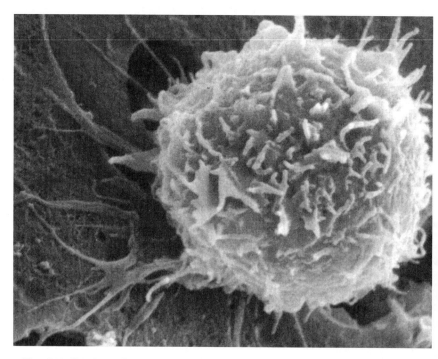

FIG. 15.2 Scanning electron micrograph of stem cell adherent to porous membrane in tissue culture.

ing in mind that the failure of CNS neurons to regenerate is not only a function of the neuron but of the inhibitory features of the damaged environment (85). The presence of gliosis, locally released factors, alterations in extracellular proteins, incipient plasticity, immune responses, and other factors following local or global injury must be considered in the equation of the transplanted cell's functional survival. Simultaneously, the intrinsic properties of the stem cell must be facilitated to allow for adequate engraftment in the desired location and appropriate phenotypic expression. The multitude of relational permutations is complicated by the fundamental "intelligence" of the stem cell, which is as yet poorly understood.

STEM CELLS (GENERAL BIOLOGY)

Although elements of debate continue, it currently appears that stem cells possess the capacity of unlimited or prolonged self-renewal and can differentiate into a multitude of tissues, recently assessed as approximately half of the 220 human tissue types, including neurons, astrocytes, and oligodendrocytes. A *totipotent* stem cell can give rise to an entire organism or regenerate any portion of the organism. A *pluripotent* cell is restricted in that it cannot produce trophoblasts and placenta (broad definition) and can differentiate into more than one alternative type of mature cell (restricted definition). This is the same as the so-called embryonic stem cell (ES). Stem cells are alternatively defined as multipotential. Between the stem cell and its terminally differentiated cell there is an intermediate population of committed progenitor cells with incrementally more limited proliferative capacity and restricted differentiation potential, sometimes known as transit amplifying cells.

There are two general strategies by which stem cells generate differentiated progeny (110). There are invariant mechanisms in which stem cells give rise through asymmetric cell division to one daughter stem cell with identical differentiation potential and a progenitor cell with more restricted potential. These latter cells serve to directly amplify the population of available fully differentiated cells. Second, there are highly complex regulative mechanisms in which a stem cell gives rise to daughter cells that have a finite probability of being stem cells or committed progenitors. The majority of mammalian self-renewing tissues fall into this latter group. Although mechanistically very different, the two strategies involve multiple extrinsic and intrinsic feedback controls and reciprocal intercellular interactions.

To consider therapy related to the nervous system specifically requires direction to the issue of neural stem cells. This term is employed to describe cells that can generate neural tissues or are derived from the nervous system. They have some capacity for self-renewal and can give rise to cells other then themselves (asymmetric cell division). They can also be derived from more primitive cells that have the capacity to generate neural stem cells and stem cells of other tissues. Their repertoire may vary and depends on both extrinsic and intrinsic factors to determine the direction of differentiation (41, 42).

Stem cell populations have been isolated from a number of sources including embryonic and adult brain tissue, spinal cord, muscle cells, hematopoietic cells, and oligodendrocyte precursor cells (1, 52–54, 99). Sources of stem cells for research have been primarily from aborted human fetuses and "spare" embryos from *in vitro* fertilization; however, attempts are being made at characterizing the properties of adult stem cells that may offer an abundant renewable source for these striking cells, of particular importance given the present U.S. political environment (73). There is increasing evidence that stem cell populations isolated from *adult* tissues may demonstrate remarkable plasticity upon transplantation into recipients, generating blood lineage progeny or skeletal muscles (10, 44). Some of the studies with adult stem cells have not been replicated despite attempts, perhaps indicating the differentiation limits of the adult variety (72, 105).

Evidence suggests that progenitor cells from some stages of embryonic development will not possess a broad differentiation potential, and that during the course of the embryological period, progenitor cells become restricted and may not be able to differentiate even into all varieties of neural cells (21, 23, 28, 66). In addition, factors present at the time of stem cell propagation play a large role in the determination of cell type. Epidermal growth factor (EGF) and fibroblast growth factor (FGF) facilitate differentiation of stem cells after implantation into the postnatal CNS. However, evidence suggested that particular cells within the germinal matrix zone are sensitive to either of the two factors giving rise to a particular cell lineage and may arise at different times during embryonic development (69, 117).

Until a more profound understanding of neural stem cell properties is achieved, functional reversal of CNS injuries resulting from stroke, trauma or tumor cannot be attained. In these situations, a global loss of cytoarchitecture and functional neuronal network is too complex an entity to benefit from stem cell therapies in the near future. Requirements for functional recovery would include cellular replacement, axonal guidance and disinhibition of growth, manipulation of intracellular signaling and neurotrophic factor delivery, and bridging and synapse formation in a functionally coherent fashion. Progress in identifying and understanding factors and molecules important in axon growth and guidance has brought this goal closer to reality. These substrates include netrins, important in neuronal and axonal migration in the developing CNS, semaphorins/collapsins that act as chemorepellants or attractants for growth cones, extracellular matrix molecules, and a variety of neurotrophic and growth factors, neurotransmitters and cytokines (51). A near-term goal may be the facilitated recovery of neuronal cells entering the apoptosis cascade through stem cell transplantation, or implantation at specific sites prior to planned injury from surgical intervention or immediately following injury in the course of surgery. The presence of stem cells in sites of acute injury may provide a buffer to neuronal loss from ischemia or hypoxemia.

CONTROL OF CELL FATE (SIGNALS)

Intrinsic

Order within a stem cell compartment depends on cell autonomous regulators modulated by external signals. These intrinsic regulators include the proteins responsible for establishing asymmetric cell division, transcription factors, nuclear factors controlling gene expression and chromosomal modifications in stem and non-stem daughters, and clocks that may set the number of rounds of division within the transit amplifying population. Transcription factor control has been widely identified in tumor and mutation models of disease (45, 58). Intracellular clocks control changes in the level of cell cycle promotors or inhibitors (62). Progressive shortening of telomeres may act as a mitotic clock in most human tissues, as the cells multiply toward senescence. This is described in telomerase-null mice in which long-term renewal of hematopoietic stem cells is compromised by the sixth generation of progeny. However, stem cells may not be subject to senescence because of constitutive telomerase activity (62, 87, 110).

Alteration of the intracellular signals that a cell uses to transduce response to injury or inhibition may be useful in preventing stem cell death and promoting regeneration. For example in the apoptosis cascade, there exist a variety of identified transcription factors (fas, p53, c-Jun, bax, bcl-2) that are involved and may represent opportunities to intervene (13, 51).

Extrinsic

External signals that control stem cell fate collectively make up the stem cell microenvironment. These involve a complex interplay of short and long-range signals between stem cells, daughter cells and long-range cells. They include *secreted factors, cell-cell interactions* mediated by integral membrane proteins, and *integrins* and *extracellular matrix factors*. Stem cell numbers are regulated by positive and negative feedback loops that have been conserved during evolution. Secreted factors that are highly conserved both between species and between tissues and that appear to regulate stem cell proliferation and fate include TGFβ and Wnts (67, 81, 93, 110). As opposed to hematopoietic cell models in which secreted factors may act in a *selective* role, to prevent the death of lineage-committed progenitors, these secreted factors may play an *instructive* role in the differentiation of neural crest stem cells (25, 67, 71, 93). Secreted factors can potentially act over many cell diameters. Conversely, cell-cell interactions, integrins, and the local extracellular matrix act over a close distances.

However, concerns exist regarding application of signaling molecules in vivo. There are a variety of cell types in the CNS, each of which responds differently to injury. In addition, some factors may be facilitory to a particular cell type but depending on concentration may have adverse systemic effects. In addition, timing the application of the signaling molecules may be critical as a recent study has shown that once a sprouting axon has encountered inhibitory factors, it loses its ability to respond to neurotrophins and their intracellular mediators (17).

Plasticity

It is important to distinguish between potentiality and plasticity. The former defines the total array of cell types an individual cell or cell line can develop if placed in the appropriate environment. The latter describes the ability of a cell to differentiate into a variety of fates in response to environmental cues.

Migrational and engraftment capabilities of stem cells enable discrete or global localization of the cells or of their protein products irrespective of site of transplantation (40, 60, 101, 118). Numerous studies have exhibited the property of tropism for regions of CNS injury, in models of stroke, tumor, degenerative disease and trauma (1, 22, 27, 48, 99, 118). This provides a homogeneous distribution of the differentiated cell product in the region of interest and robust incorporation of the cells. In this regard, conditioning techniques, site preparation and targeted implantation therefore appear to be factors unimportant in engraftment. The inherent quality of the stem cell to accommodate to regions of engraftment and to differentiate into an array of phenotypes points to the highly plastic nature of the cell. These properties obviate the need to acquire donor cells from particular sites and to involve tissue-specific promoters. They may also minimize the need for significant cell transduction maneuvers and may permit greater engraftment using xenografts. By possessing the capability to differentiate along all cell lines, the stem cells may promote functional restoration by replacing the range of cell varieties injured in addition to reconstructing the premorbid neural architecture. Furthermore, undesired deposition of desired protein products can be minimized without the use of promoters or conditioning techniques.

It had been believed that the stem cell derived from a specific organ could produce only that organ. However, this concept is currently being challenged. A recent study supports the notion that neural stem cells have a wide potential for differentiation. Clarke et. al. implanted β-galactosidase-labelled cultured adult neural stem cells into chick or mouse embryos in the early stages of development (18). The cells were allowed to develop in the growing embryo. In later embryonic stages, β-galactosidase cells were identified in many cell types, including non-neural derivatives. It is also intriguing that the cells were not identified in the blood lineage and that only six out of 600 embryos expressed this chimeric phenotype, perhaps indicating that a few rare stem cells types were collected in the batch and participated in the majority of the findings presented. Another potential basis for these types of rare findings is that perhaps the CNS contains a small number of highly pluripotent cells, perhaps misdirected germ cells or pluripotential, non-neural stem cells that were collected in the adult tissue and implanted (3, 9, 102, 112). The latter presumption is supported by two recent investigations using bone marrow stem cells injected into newborn mice or irradiated adults the cells emerge and are able to be isolated in brain tissue (12, 70).

FUTURISTIC SCENARIO

It has been envisioned that a cell biopsy taken from a patient and the nucleus of somatic cell could be transferred into an enucleated donor oocyte with nuclear transfer techniques pioneered in mice and sheep. The resulting embryo would be allowed to develop until the blastocyst stage. Then the inner cell mass of the blastocyst would be recovered by immunosurgery and cultured with subsequent harvest of embryonic stem cells (ES). The ES cells could then be directed to differentiate into a particular cell type required and then transferred to the patient. For many reasons we are currently quite far from this stage, but with the progress that has been made up to the present time, realization of this ideal may not be as far away as believed. Techniques of nuclear transfer are being perfected, as are the techniques of molecular biology for genetic manipulation of stem cells. By using the patient's somatic cell, immune responses would be limited. In addition, genetic errors found to cause the primary disease process may be altered or erased using modern technology prior to reestablishment of the genetic material with stem cells as a vector.

Combining a variety of current and developing technologies, we may broaden the therapeutic umbrella of stem cells. Stem cell technology has provided a platform for advances in genetic engineering. Genetic engineering may be useful in transducing stem cells with genes for particular protein products, either for diseases with known deficiencies or to alter the microenvironment to enhance stem cell engraftment. The cells can be easily transduced *ex vivo* by a variety of genetic transfer methods and by multiple transgenes. The gene products, in turn, enjoy a substantial and sustained rise in levels in a rapid fashion. Due to the chimerical nature of the stem cell, it may survive below the "radar" of normal immunological responses and maintain transgene expression for long periods (5, 7, 16, 114). This in part relates to its low-level production of normal neuronal products (lysosomal enzymes, myelin, cell-surface molecules). In addition, the stem cells may serve to amplify distribution of viral-mediated genes to large CNS regions by acting as producer cells for viral vectors. Although elements of debate continue, it currently appears that stem cells possess the capacity of unlimited or prolonged self-renewal and can differentiate into neurons, astrocytes, and oligodendrocytes.

Use of endovascular microcatheter technology may provide a more rapid targeted implantation of progenitor cells to a specific vascular region either in anticipation of or following injury. Stereotactic and microtransplantation/micropump techniques are developing which can provide targeted placement of cells into deep brain structures to enhance the volume of engraftment and may provide a continuous injection or cells or factors over a period of time in an open- or closed-loop feedback mechanism. Stereotactic radiosurgery may be a useful adjunct by using the stem cells as producer cells for viral vector-mediated transfection and radiosensitization of CNS tumor cells. Combining the application of microelectrode implantation and stem cell engraftment may enhance the therapeutic value of these two independent technologies in the treatment of Parkinson's disease, pain syndromes, and epilepsy due to the intrinsic plastic nature of the cells to environmental clues.

IN-VITRO STUDIES

The study of these cells documents the problems and complexity of modern cellular and molecular biology. Standard methodology for source tissue development requires dissection of a fertile region of an adult or fetal brain that has shown to contain dividing cells, such as the subventricular zone or the hippocampus. The tissues are disaggregrated and the dissociated cells are exposed to a high concentration of mitogens such as fibroblast or epidermal growth factor in a defined or supplemental medium on a binding matrix. After proliferation, the cells are induced to differentiate by withdrawing mitogens and exposing them to factors that may induce development into certain lineages. Cellular fates are then determined by antibody staining. Retrovirus tagging to identify clones is also employed.

However, in spite of a concerted effort to effect standardization, different laboratories have reached a variety of differing results. There have been inherent problems in defining a population of cells especially when attempting to demonstrate the capacity that cells have the ability to develop into all of the mature fates described. There is a need to specifically define signaling cascades that control development and differentiation.

Transplantation studies of characterized stem cells *in vivo* have been undertaken. Investigators have grafted cell populations expanded with mitogens and/or genetically marked cells back to the brain. In certain studies, the fetus-derived cells were grafted into developing brain to determine the range of cell types developing through differentiation. The range was greater than expected as the cells were observed to migrate broadly through central and peripheral nervous tissue but also were observed to differentiate into neurons and glia in adult brain. The fate of grafted cells appeared to be dictated by the environment rather than by the cell itself. In damaged developing brain tissue, cells have been shown to migrate to areas of damage and effect repair of architecture that is indistinguishable from normal host cells.

Plasticity is apparently not limited to the developing brain, as stem cells derived from adult hippocampus can be expanded *in vitro* and grafted back to adult hosts where they have been demonstrated to generate new neurons and glia in architectural patterns appropriate to the environmental settings. In addition, there are indications that this potential may extend beyond neural tissue.

In spite of some remarkable observations, reality has dealt a number of clear caveats that create difficulties that require resolution. One key issue is that at the time of expansion to a population size adequate to track, only a small percentage retains stem cell properties. To a certain extent, this may be mitigated by serial grafting. In addition, studies that have claimed to show multipotentiality of cells *in vitro* may be contaminated by differentiation or other genetic modification due to modifications associated with extended mitogen exposure.

Also, the identity of a stem cell is inferred from procedures. To date, only one study proposes to have isolated clonogenic human CNS stem cells by using antibodies to identified cell-surface markers and fluorescence-activated cell sorting methods (107). Other researchers have circumvented the problem by immortalizing neural precursor cells (97). However, difficulties relating to the identification and isolation of individual CNS stem cells persist. Markers are required to identify them in their most primitive state. However, for their most primitive state, cells are quiescent and do not produce antigen.

In vivo stem cells have been detected by employing retrovirus, thymidine and bromodeoxyuridine. Retrovirus can be employed to track a cell lineage but the procedure in generally inefficient. However, widespread cell proliferation has been documented, accompanied by differentiation and physiological functional units of appropriate type in the rat and songbird.

It is apparent that stem cell biology represents a complex process of proliferation, migration, differentiation and survival, each stage of which is governed by complex factors both intrinsic and extrinsic, each of which require definition for us to effect controlled regulation for therapeutic purposes. We will need to consider specific cells in specific microenvironments that will require our ability to nurture, modulate and regulate these intrinsic and extrinsic processes. An example of the benefit of such knowledge of regulatory capability has recently been provided by Kondo and Raff (54). During animal development cells become more restricted in the cell types that they may produce. In the central nervous system multipotential stem cells produce precursors that divide a limited number of times before they terminally differentiate into either neurons or glial cells. They demonstrated that certain extracellular signals could induce oligodendrocyte precursor cells to *revert* to multipotential neural stem cells which could self renew and differentiate to produce neurons, astrocytes and oligodendrocytes.

The potential therapeutic endpoints for stem cell technology appear to be limitless due to the diverse plasticity of the cells. However, targeted diseases must be carefully chosen based on current understanding of stem cell properties and tested first in non-human disease models due to the substrate's underlying profound complexity. Two types of injuries can be defined as endpoints in the application of stem cells: defined loss of specific protein product and global loss of cytoarchitecture.

At this time, the only disease model effectively cured by stem cell technology is a rodent model of myelin deficiency (118). In the model of a dysmyelinated shiverer mouse, oligodendroglial cells are globally dysfunctional as they lack myelin basic protein. A particular line of viral-gene transfected/immortalized neural stem cells was implanted in the ventricular compartment at birth. The donor cells differentiated into oligodendroglia with resultant myelination and reduction in symptom expression. Despite the global nature of the disease, but due to the defined protein product absent, this was a perfect venue for application of the stem cells. They responded to the absence of a particular product and migrated to regions where myelin was needed. Other disease entities where a particular gene product is absent or deficient are candidates for research. In another study, retroviruses encoding the human beta-hexosaminidase alpha-subunit, the deficiency of which results in Tay-Sachs disease, were used to transduce multipotent neural cell lines (60). At various times following transplantation in fetal and neonatal mouse brains, high levels of the transcript and protein were identified.

Identification of the particular substrate absent in human disease is primary in developing the model followed by creation of a genetic mutant or application of a particular toxin to create the CNS injury. Parkinson's disease is an excellent model for stem cell application. Diminution of a specific protein product, dopamine, is known to result in Parkinsonian features and rodent and non-human primate models have been developed based on MPTP or 6-OHDA administration. In addition, quantification of other related protein products such as dopamine transporter (DAT) and tyrosine hydroxylase (TH) has been performed and behavioral scales have been developed for both rat and non-human primate models. Following stem cell transplantation, specific protein levels and cytoarchitectural changes can be assessed and quantified and alterations made to enhance functional recovery.

GENETIC ENGINEERING STRATEGIES COMBINING GENE THERAPY AND CELLULAR TRANSPLANTATION

Because of the limitations of viral vectors delineated above, extensive efforts have been directed to using cellular elements as the vehicles expressing exogenous genes of interest (41, 49, 78, 82). These cells can be engineered to serve as "biological pumps," providing sources of proteins such as metabolic enzymes, neurotransmitters, or neurotrophic factors (100). In other cases, they may serve to replete populations of absent or degenerating cells, or remyelinate damaged axons. These three simultaneous capacities—cell replacement, remyelination, and *ex vivo* gene therapy—hold great promise for restorative neurosurgery.

Among the many advantages CNS therapy using genetically engineered cells is their migratory ability, which enhances physical dissemination of the transgene product. In some circumstances, ubiquitous expression throughout the brain has been achieved (118). It is unlikely that the radial glia found in the developing brain persist in the adult mammalian CNS. However, neural progenitor cells may use a novel cellular process called "chain migration," which involves homotypic interactions between the migrating cells and tube-like structures formed by specialized astrocytes, mediated by highly polysialated glycoprotein neural cell adhesion molecules (NCAMs) (42).

Another advantage is that engrafted cells undergo differentiation in response to cues from the local microenvironment and structural integration with the existing cytoarchitecture (46). Morphological maturation, physiological development, synaptogenesis, and reconstitution of functional circuitry have all been documented.

Candidate cells for transfection and subsequent transplantation include neural precursors from fetal, neonatal, and adult human tissue, differentiated and cultured tumor cells, immortalized cell lines, and xenografts. Cryopreservation enhances the stability, reproducibility, and transportability of such cells. Only a few studies have used primary neurons as transgene carriers because they are difficult to obtain and maintain in culture and are not easily transfected by classical methods (86). Astrocytes have also been used with minimal success. Autologous fibroblasts and myoblasts have the advantage of minimal potential for rejection, but they cannot establish synaptic contact with host tissue, thus limiting their role in cell replacement therapy (86). Fetal cells, owing to their plasticity and lack of immune excitation, have been suggested as solutions to the latter problem. However, due to its heterogeneity, primary fetal tissue is not well suited for the genetic engineering required for gene therapy (78). Also, ethical limitations have curtailed its use.

Recently, neural precursor cells have been clonally expanded in cell culture, leading to a renewable supply of material available for transplantation. These cultured progenitor cells can be readily modified *ex vivo* by transfection with viral vectors *in vitro* and then reimplanted into the brain parenchyma, cerebral vasculature, or CSF. This approach circumvents some of the limitations of *in situ* gene therapy. For instance, the latter strategies depend on relaying new genetic information through established endogenous neural populations and circuits that may have already degenerated or failed to develop, while the *ex vivo* approach does not (78).

Subsequent expression of the therapeutic gene can be regulated by coupling it to a repressible or inducible promoter. Alternatively, cells may be selected prior to transplantation using fluorescence-activated cell sorting (FACS) based on the presence of fluorescent transgenes placed under the control of specific promoters, leading to populations of cells enriched with a certain phenotype (82). It seems clear that cellular transplantation therapies must be complemented by appropriate neurotrophic factors (e.g., brain derived neurotrophic factor, nerve growth factor, glial cell line-derived neurotrophic factor) and mediators such as retinoic acid that induce differentiation along the desired paths (88, 103).

Current challenges to the feasibility of transplanting neural precursor cells involve identifying the various diffusible factors (autocrine, paracrine, or endocrine) and contact-mediated interactions that induce their development along certain lineages, regulate their proliferation, and form the substrates of their migration.

Risks of immortalized cell lines (e.g., cultured neurons genetically altered with a retrovirus to continuously divide) include oncogenic transformation. Other generic limitations of allogeneic and xenogeneic cellular transplantation include immunologic rejection.

Finally, the *ex vivo* approach using cells genetically engineered with viral DNA suffer some of the same technical difficulties inherent to the *in situ* approach, such as potential expression of viral genes, initiation of an antiviral immune response, reversion of the viral vector to a replication-competent state, and inactivation of transcription and/or expression of foreign genes (78).

PROSPECTS FOR ENDOVASCULAR DELIVERY OF CELLULAR AND MOLECULAR THERAPEUTICS TO THE CNS

Intra-arterial delivery of gene therapeutic agents, either using viral vectors or genetically modified cells, circumvents some of the limitations inherent to other delivery routes. For instance, this strategy can be used to treat infiltrative tumors or global CNS disorders not amenable to strategies with limited diffusion potential.

The BBB remains an impediment to endovascular delivery strategies and has been labeled the "Achilles heel of CNS therapeutics" (75). Transport across the BBB includes both transcellular and pericellular routes. The BBB limits particles based on electrical charge, lipid solubility, and molecular weight (59).

The BBB can be transiently opened by brief infusions of mannitol over 15–30 seconds. This produces osmotic shrinkage of the endothelial cells and opening of their tight junctions, as well as activation of intracellular signaling pathways and release of biologically active compounds (59, 121). Permeability is effectively increased 5 to 15 minutes postinfusion and normalizes within 2 hours. Viral vectors up to 70 nm in size can cross the BBB after osmotic disruption (120). Delivery of inactivated HSV increased 4-fold in the ipsilateral hemisphere following intracarotid administration preceded by BBB disruption (59). Following intracarotid infusion of HSV or AV preceded by osmotic disruption, transgene expression has been demonstrated throughout the basal ganglia and cerebral cortex. Astrocytes may be selectively targeted because their foot processes help cuff the endothelial cells and integrate the BBB (59).

Several vasoactive compounds, including histamine, leukotriene C4, bradykinin, interferon beta, and tumor necrosis factor-alpha, have been shown to be effective in permeabilizing the BBB (59, 121). RMP-7 is a selective bradykinin B2 agonist with increased half-life. It has been shown to be 100-fold more potent than bradykinin in mice and is resistant to enzymatic degradation (59). At low concentrations, both bradykinin and RMP-7 preferentially open the blood-brain-tumor-barrier while having little effect on permeability around the tumor (59, 120). Uptake of chemotherapy or other agents after bradykin and RMP-7 infusion can be increased by up to 10-fold.

Endovascular approaches to gene therapy are limited by the requirement of prolonged contact between the vector and the luminal surface or increased intraluminal pressure (74). Although this is generally accomplished by arresting blood flow, such a technique is not practical in the brain (111). Newer endovascular devices may overcome this problem by permitting distal perfusion while promoting prolonged contact of the vector with the endothelium (50).

When injected intraluminally, RV vectors transfect less than 1% of cells in the arterial wall, but those that are transfected achieve long term expression (e.g., years). AV have 10 to 100 times greater transfection efficiency but can only achieve short term expression (e.g., days (111). One strategy to overcome this conflict to harvest endothelial or smooth muscle cells from blood vessels, transfect them with RV *ex vivo* (while they are replicating in tissue culture), and then seed them back into blood vessels after the endothelium of the recipient vessel is removed (111).

Although several barriers exist between the intravascular compartment and the brain parenchyma, the communication between these regions has been demonstrated by several physiologic experiments. In fact, some have even speculated that "neural stem cells" isolated from various regions of the brain may actually originate from the blood (42). These observations suggest the potential feasibility of endovascular delivery of cellular and molecular therapeutics to the CNS.

CONCLUSIONS

The transfer of a transgene or a gene product is a concept frequently employed in an attempt to correct a central nervous system disorders. This may be effected by either mechanical delivery of DNA into cells in vitro and viral vector delivery into various mammalian cells or in situ introduction. Viral vector delivery offers the advantages of relative ease of employment, efficiency and stability of the preparation. Stem cells are ideal messengers of in vitro infection and subsequent delivery. This methodology of combined therapy offers opportunity to reestablish and maintain microenvironmental factors that are favorable to recreate specific neuroarchitecture, thus promoting favorable plasticity. Therefore, stem cells engineered to express appropriate factors may potentially play actual role in the restoration process.

Cajal foresaw this moment in neuroscience provided by discovery of the CNS stem cell: "once the development was ended, the founts of growth and regeneration of the axons and dendrites dried up irrevocably. In the adult centres the nerve paths are something fixed, ended and immutable. Everything may die, nothing may be regenerated. It is for the science of the future to change, if possible, this harsh decree."

REFERENCES

1. Aboody KS, Brown A, Rainov NG, Bower KA, Liu S, Yang W, Small JE, Herrlinger U, Ourednik V, Black PM, Breakefield XO, Snyder EY: Neural stem cells display extensive tropism for pathology in adult brain: Evidence from intracranial gliomas. **Proc Natl Acad Sci** 97:12846–12851, 2000.
2. Allen E: The cessation of mitosis in the central nervous system of the albino rat. **J Comp Neurol** 22:547–568, 1912.
3. Anderson DJ, Gage FH, Weissman IL: Can stem cells cross lineage boundaries? **Nat Med** 7:393–395, 2001.
4. Anderson WF: Human gene therapy. **Nature** 392 (Suppl):25–30, 1998.
5. Ansari AA, Mayne A, Freed CR, Breeze RE, Schneck SA, O'Brien CF, Kriek EH, Zhang YB, Mazziotta JC, Hutchinson M: Lack of a detectable systemic humoral/cellular allogeneic response in human and nonhuman primate recipients of embryonic mesencephalic allografts for the therapy of Parkinson's disease. **Transplant Proc** 27:1401–1405, 1995.
6. Apuzzo MLJ, Neal JH, Waters CH, Appley AJ, Boyd SD, Couldwell WT, Wheelock VH, Weiner LP: Utilization of unilateral and bilateral stereotactically placed adrenomedullary-striatal autografts in Parkinsonian humans: Rationale, techniques, and observations. **Neurosurgery** 26:746–757, 1990.
7. Bakay RAE, Boyer KL, Freed CR, Ansari AA: Immunological responses to injury and grafting in the central nervous system of nonhuman primates. **Cell Transplant** xx:109–120, 1998.
8. Bentley DR: The human genome project—An overview. **Med Res Rev** 20:189–196, 2000.
9. Bjorklund A, Svendsen CN: Chimeric stem cells. **Trends Molec Med** 7:144–146, 2001.
10. Bjornson CR, Rietze RL, Reynolds BA, Magli MC, Vescovi AL: Turning brain into blood: a hematopoietic fate adopted by adult neural stem cells *in vivo*. **Science** 283:534–537, 1999.
11. Blomer U, Naldini L, Verma IM, Trono D, Gage FH: Applications of gene therapy to the CNS. **Hum Molec Genet** 5:1397–1404, 1996.

12. Brazelton TR, Rossi FM, Keshet GI, Blau HM: From marrow to brain: expression of neuronal phenotypes in adult mice. **Science** 290:1775–1779, 2000.

13. Bredesen DE: Neural apoptosis. **Ann Neurol** 38:839–851, 1995.

14. Breeze RE, Wells TH, Jr., Freed CR: Implantation of fetal tissue for the management of Parkinson's disease: a technical note. **Neurosurgery** 36:1044–1047, 1995.

15. Brenner S: The impact of science on society. **Science** 282:1411–1412, 1998.

16. Brevig T, Holgersson J, Widner H: Xenotransplantation for CNS repair: immunological barriers and strategies to overcome them. **Trends Neurosci** 23:337–344, 2000.

17. Cai D, Shen Y, De Bellard M, Tang S, Filbin MT: Prior exposure to neurotrophins blocks inhibition of axonal regeneration by MAG and myelin via a cAMP-dependent mechanism. **Neuron** 22:89–101, 1999.

18. Clarke DL, Johansson CB, Wilbertz J, Veress B, Nilsson E, Karlstrom H, Lendahl U, Frisen J: Generalized potential of adult neural stem cells. **Science** 288:1660–1663, 2000.

19. Collins FS: Sequencing the human genome. **Hosp Pract**:35–54, 1997.

20. Costantini LC, Bakowska JC, Breakefield XO, Isacson O: Gene therapy in the CNS. **Gene Ther** 7:93–109, 2000.

21. Desai AR, McConnell SK: Progressive restriction in neural progenitors during cerebral cortical development. **Development** 127:2863–2872, 2000.

22. Doering LC, Snyder EY: Cholinergic expression by a neural stem cell line grafted to the adult medial septum/diagonal band complex. **J Neurosci Res** 61:597–604, 2000.

23. Dunnett SB, Nathwani F, Bjorklund A: The integration and function of striatal grafts. **Prog Brain Res** 127:345–380, 2000.

24. Engelhard HH: Gene therapy for brain tumors: The fundamentals. **Surg Neurol** 54:3–9, 2000.

25. Enver T, Greaves M: Loops, lineage, and leukemia. **Cell** 94:9–12, 1998.

26. Fink L, Collins FS: The human genome project: View from the National Institutes of Health. **J Am Med Wom Assoc** 52:4–7, 1997.

27. Flax JD, Aurora S, Yang C, Simonin C, Wills AM, Billinghurst LL, Jendoubi M, Sidman RL, Wolfe JH, Kim SU, Snyder EY: Engraftable human neural stem cells respond to developmental cues, replace neurons, and express foreign genes. **Nat Biotech** 16:1033–1039, 1998.

28. Frantz GD, McConnell SK: Restriction of late cerebral cortical progenitors to an upper-layer site. **Neuron** 17:55–61, 1996.

29. Fredriksen K, McKay RDG: Proliferation and differentiation of rat neuroepithelial precursor cells in vivo. **J Neurosci** 8:1144–1151, 1988.

30. Freed CR, Breeze RE, Fahn S: Placebo surgery in trials of therapy for Parkinson's disease. **N Engl J Med** 342:353–354, 2000.

31. Freed CR, Breeze RE, Rosenberg NL, Schneck SA: Embryonic dopamine cell implants as a treatment for the second phase of Parkinson's disease. Replacing failed nerve terminals. **Adv Neurol** 60:721–728, 1993.

32. Freed CR, Breeze RE, Rosenberg NL, Schneck SA, Kriek E, Qi JX, Lone T, Zhang YB, Snyder JA, Wells TH: Survival of implanted fetal dopamine cells and neurologic improvement 12 to 46 months after transplantation for Parkinson's disease. **N Engl J Med** 327:1549–55, 1992.

33. Freed CR, Breeze RE, Rosenberg NL, Schneck SA, Wells TH, Barrett JN, Grafton ST, Huang SC, Eidelberg D, Rottenberg DA: Transplantation of human fetal dopamine cells for Parkinson's disease. Results at 1 year. **Arch Neurol** 47:505–512, 1990.

34. Freed CR, Breeze RE, Rosenberg NL, Schneck SA, Wells TH, Barrett JN, Grafton ST, Mazziotta JC, Eidelberg D, Rottenberg DA: Therapeutic effects of human fetal dopamine cells transplanted in a patient with Parkinson's disease. **Prog Brain Res** 82:715–721, 1990.

35. Freed CR, Breeze RE, Schneck SA: Transplantation of fetal mesencephalic tissue in Parkinson's disease. **N Engl J Med** 333:730–1, 1995.

36. Freed CR, Greene PE, Breeze RE, Tsai WY, DuMouchel W, Kao R, Dillon S, Winfield H, Culver S, Trojanowski JQ, Eidelberg D, Fahn S: Transplantation of embryonic dopamine neurons for severe Parkinson's disease. **N Engl J Med** 344:710–719, 2001.

37. Freed CR, Rosenberg NL, Schneck SA, Breeze RE: Improved drug responsiveness following fetal tissue implant for Parkinson's disease. **Neurochem Internat** 20 (Suppl):321S–327S, 1992.

38. Freeman TB, Olanow CW, Hauser RA, Nauert GM, Smith DA, Borlongan CV, Sanberg PR, Holt DA, Kordower JH, Vingerhoets FJ: Bilateral fetal nigral transplantation into the postcommissural putamen in Parkinson's disease. **Ann Neurol** 38:379–88, 1995.

39. Freese A: Restorative gene therapy approaches to Parkinson's disease. **Med Clin N Amer** 83:537–548, 1999.

40. Fricker RA, Carpenter MK, Winkler C, Greco C, Gates MA, Bjorkland A: Site-specific migration and neuronal differentiation of human neural progenitor cells after transplantation in the adult rat brain. **J Neurosci** 19:5990–6005, 1999.

41. Gage FH: Cell therapy. **Nature** 392 (Suppl):18–24, 1998.

42. Gage FH: Mammalian neural stem cells. **Science** 287:1433–1438, 2000.

43. Gage FH, Bjorklund A: Cholinergic septal grafts into the hippocampal formation improve spacial learning and memory in aged rats by an atropine-sensitive mechanism. **J Neurosci** 6:2837–2847, 1986.

44. Galli R, Borello U, Gritti A, Minasi MG, Bjornson C, Coletta M, Mora M, De Angelis MG, Fiocco R, Cossu G, Vescovi A: Skeletal myogenic potential of human and mouse neural stem cells. **Nat Neurosci** 3:986–991, 2000.

45. Gat U, DasGupta R, Degenstein L, Fuchs E: De Novo hair follicle morphogenesis and hair tumors in mice expressing a truncated beta-catenin in skin. **Cell** 95:605–614, 1998.

46. Han SS, Fischer I: Neural stem cells and gene therapy: Prospects for repairing the injured spinal cord. **JAMA** 283:2300–2301, 2000.

47. Hernandez A, Evers BM: Functional genomics: Clinical effect and the evolving role of the surgeon. **Arch Surg** 134:1209–1215, 1999.

48. Herrlinger U, Woiciechowski C, Sena-Esteves M, Aboody KS, Jacobs AH, Rainov NG, Snyder EY, Breakefield XO: Neural precursor cells for delivery of replication-conditional HSV-1 vectors to intracerebral gliomas. **Molec Ther** 1:347–357, 2000.

49. Hodge CJ, Boakye M: Biological plasticity: The future of science in neurosurgery. **Neurosurgery** 48:2–16, 2001.

50. Hopkins LN, Lanzino G, Guterman LR: Treating complex nervous system vascular disorders through a "needle stick": Origins, evolution, and future of neuroendovascular therapy. **Neurosurgery** 48:463–475, 2001.

51. Horner PJ, Gage FH: Regenerating the damaged central nervous system. **Nature** 407:963–970, 2000.

52. Horner PJ, Power AE, Kuhn HG, Palmer TD, Winkler J, Thal LJ, Gage FH: Proliferation and differentiation of progenitor cells throughout the intact adult rat spinal cord. **J Neurosci** 20:2218–2228, 2000.

53. Johansson CB, Momma S, Clarke DL, Risling M, Lendahl U, Frisen J: Identifica-

tion of a neural stem cell in the adult mammalian central nervous system. **Cell** 96:25–34, 1999.

54. Kondo T, Raff M: Oligodendrocyte precursor cells reprogramed to become multi-potential CNS stem cells. **Science** 289:1754–1756, 2000.

55. Kordower JH, Freeman TB, Chen EY, Mufson EJ, Sanberg PR, Hauser RA, Snow B, Olanow CW: Fetal nigral grafts survive and mediate clinical benefit in a patient with Parkinson's disease. **Movement Disord** 13:383–93, 1998.

56. Kordower JH, Freeman TB, Snow BJ, Vingerhoets FJ, Mufson EJ, Sanberg PR, Hauser RA, Smith DA, Nauert GM, Perl DP: Neuropathological evidence of graft survival and striatal reinnervation after the transplantation of fetal mesencephalic tissue in a patient with Parkinson's disease. **N Engl J Med** 332:1118–1124, 1995.

57. Kordower JH, Styren S, Clarke M, DeKosky ST, Olanow CW, Freeman TB: Fetal grafting for Parkinson's disease: expression of immune markers in two patients with functional fetal nigral implants. **Cell Transplant** 6:213–9, 1997.

58. Korinek V, Barker N, Moerer P, Van Donselaar E, Huls G, Peters PJ, Clevers H: Depletion of epithelial stem-cell compartments in the small intestine of mice lacking Tcf-4. **Nat Genet** 19:379–383, 1998.

59. Kroll RA, Neuwelt EA: Outwitting the blood-brain barrier for therapeutic purposes: Osmotic opening and other means. **Neurosurgery** 42:1083–1100, 1998.

60. Lacorazza HD, Flax JD, Snyder EY, Jendoubi M: Expression of human beta-hexosaminidase alpha-subunit gene (the gene defect of Tay-Sachs disease) in mouse brains upon engraftment of transduced progenitor cells. **Nat Med** 2:424–9, 1996.

61. Lanchbury JS: The human genome project. **Br J Rheumatol** 37:119–125, 1998.

62. Lee HW, Blasco MA, Gottlieb GJ, Horner JW, Greider CW, DePinho RA: Essential role of mouse telomerase in highly proliferative organs. **Nature** 392:569–74, 1998.

63. Lesch KP: Gene therapy to the brain: Emerging therapeutic strategy in psychiatry? **Biol Psychiatry** 45:247–253, 1999.

64. Levy ML, Tung H, Couldwell WT, Hinton DR, Apuzzo MLJ. Neurosurgery, molecular medicine, and the Pandora panacea continuum: Future implications for glioma therapy. In Selman W (ed.): *Clinical Neurosurgery*. Vol. 39. Baltimore: Williams & Wilkins, pp. 421–462, 1992.

65. Lewis ME: Crossing the blood-brain barrier to central nervous system gene therapy. **Clin Genet** 56:10, 1999.

66. Lim DA, Fishell GJ, Alvarez-Buylla A: Postnatal mouse subventricular zone neuronal precursors can migrate and differentiate within multiple levels of the developing neuraxis. **Proc Natl Acad Sci** 94:14832–14836, 1997.

67. Lo L, Sommer L, Anderson DJ: MASH1 maintains competence for BMP2-induced neuronal differentiation in post-migratory neural crest cells. **Curr Biol** 7:440–50, 1997.

68. Mandel RJ, Rendahl KG, Snyder RO, Leff SE: Progress in direct striatal delivery of L-Dopa via gene therapy for treatment of Parkinson's disease using recombinant adeno-associated viral vectors. **Exp Neurol** 159:47–64, 1999.

69. Martens DJ, Tropepe V, Van der Kooy D: Separate proliferation kinetics of fibroblast growth factor-responsive and epidermal growth factors-responsive neural stem cells within the embryonic forebrain germinal zones. **J Neurosci** 20:1085–1095, 2000.

70. Mezey E, Chandross KJ, Harta G, Maki RA, McKercher SR: Turning blood into brain: Cells bearing neuronal antigens generated *in vivo* from bone marrow. **Science** 290:1779–1782, 2000.

71. Morrison SJ, Shah NM, Anderson DJ: Regulatory mechanisms in stem cell biology. **Cell** 88:287–98, 1997.
72. Morshead CM, Tropepe V, Iscove N, Van der Kooy D: The potential role of neural stem cell transformation in turning brain into blood in irradiated recipients. **Neurosci Abstr** 26:827, 2000.
73. Morshead CM, Van der Kooy D: A new 'spin' on neural stem cells. **Curr Opin Neurobiol** 11:59–65, 2001.
74. Muhonen MG, Ooboshi H, Welsh MJ, Davidson BL, Heistad DD: Gene transfer to cerebral blood vessels after subarachnoid hemorrhage. **Stroke** 28:822–828, 1997.
75. Neuwelt EA, Abbott NJ, Drewes L, Smith QR, Couraud PO, Chiocca EA, Audus KL, Greig NH, Doolittle ND: Cerebrovascular biology and the various neural barriers: Challenges and future directions. **Neurosurgery** 44:604–609, 1999.
76. Olanow CW, Freeman TB, Kordower JH: Neural transplantation as a therapy for Parkinson's disease. **Adv Neurol** 74:249–269, 1997.
77. Ooboshi H, Welsh MJ, Rios CD, Davidson BL, Heistad DD: Adenovirus-mediated gene transfer in vivo to cerebral blood vessels and perivascular tissue. **Circ Res** 77:7–13, 1995.
78. Ourednik V, Ourednik J, Park K, Snyder EY: Neural stem cells: A versatile tool for cell replacement and gene therapy in the central nervous system. **Clin Genet** 56:267–278, 1999.
79. Papadopoulos MC, Giffard RG, Bell BA: Principles of gene therapy: Potential applications in the treatment of cerebral ischemia. **Br J Neurosurg** 14:407–414, 2000.
80. Patrinos A, Drell DW: The human genome project: View from the Department of Energy. **J Am Med Wom Assoc** 52:8–10, 1997.
81. Peifer M: Signal transduction: Neither straight nor narrow. **Nature** 400:213–215, 1999.
82. Pincus DW, R R, Goodman, Frasier RA, Nedergaard M, Goldman SA: Neural stem and progenitor cells: A strategy for gene therapy and brain repair. **Neurosurgery** 42:858–868, 1998.
83. Reynolds BA, Weiss S: Clonal and population analyses demonstrate that an EGF-responsive mammalian embryonic precursor is a stem cell. **Develop Biol** 175:1–13, 1996.
84. Reynolds BA, Weiss S: Generation of neurons and astrocytes from isolated cells of the adult mammalian nervous system. **Science** 255:1707–1710, 1992.
85. Richardson PM, McGuinness UM, Aguayo AJ: Axons from CNS neurons regenerate into PNS grafts. **Nature** 284:264–265, 1980.
86. Ridet JL, Privat A: Gene therapy in the central nervous system: Direct versus indirect gene delivery. **J Neurosci Res** 42:287–293, 1995.
87. Rudolph KL, Chang S, Lee HW, Blasco M, Gottlieb GJ, Greider C, DePinho RA: Longevity, stress response, and cancer in aging telomerase-deficient mice. **Cell** 96:701–12, 1999.
88. Rutka JT, Taylor M, Mainprize T, Langlois A, Ivanchuk S, Mondal S, Dirks P: Molecular biology and neurosurgery in the third millennium. **Neurosurgery** 46:1034–1051, 2000.
89. Sanberg PR, Giordano M, Henault MA, Nash DR, Ragozzino ME, Hagenmeyer-Houser SH: Intraparenchymal striatal transplants required for maintenance of behavioral recovery in an animal model of Huntington's disease. **J Neurotransplant** 1:23–31, 1989.
90. Sapolsky RM, Steinberg GK: Gene therapy using viral vectors for acute neurologic insults. **Neurology** 53:1922–1931, 1999.

91. Savill J: Science, medicine, and the future: Prospecting for gold in the human genome. **Br Med J** 314:43–45, 1997.
92. Schuler GD: A gene map of the human genome. **Science** 274:540–546, 1996.
93. Shah NM, Goves AK, Anderson DJ: Alternative neural crest cell fates are instructively promoted by TGFbeta superfamily members. **Cell** 85:331–343, 1996.
94. Shamblott MJ, Axelman J, Wang S, Bugg EM, Littlefield JW, Donovan PJ, Blumenthal PD, Huggins GR, Gearhart JD: Derivation of pluripotent stem cells from cultured human primordial germ cells. **Proc Natl Acad Sci** 95:13726–13731, 1998.
95. Sladek JR, Redmond DE, Collier TJ, Bount JP, Elsworth JR, Taylor JR, Roth RH: Fetal dopamine neural grafts: Extended reversal of methylphenyltetrahydropyridine-induced parkinsonism in monkeys. **Prog Brain Res** 78:497–506, 1988.
96. Smith AE: Gene therapy: Where are we? **Lancet** 354:S1–S4, 1999.
97. Snyder EY: Immortalized neural stem cells: Insights into development; prospects for gene therapy and repair. **Proc Assoc Amer Physic** 107:195–204, 1995.
98. Snyder EY, Taylor RM, Wolfe JH: Neural progenitor cell engraftment corrects lysosomal storage throughout the MPS VII mouse brain. **Nature** 374:367–70, 1995.
99. Snyder EY, Yoon C, Flax JD, Macklis JD: Multipotent neural precursors can differentiate toward replacement of neurons undergoing targeted apoptotic degeneration in adult mouse neocortex. **Proc Natl Acad Sci** 94:11663–8, 1997.
100. Suhr ST, Gage FH: Gene therapy in the central nervous system: The use of recombinant retroviruses. **Arch Neurol** 56:287–292, 1999.
101. Taylor RM, Snyder EY: Widespread engraftment of neural progenitor and stemlike cells throughout the mouse brain. **Transplant Proc** 29:845–7, 1997.
102. Temple S: Stem cell plasticity-building the brain of our dreams. **Nat Rev** 2:513–520, 2001.
103. Thompson TP, Lunsford LD, Kondziolka D: Restorative neurosurgery: Opportunities for restoration of function in acquired, degenerative, and idiopathic neurologic diseases. **Neurosurgery** 45:741–752, 1999.
104. Thomson JA, Itskovitz-Eldor J, Shapiro SS, Waknitz MA, Swiergiel JJ, Marshall VS, Jones JM: Embryonic stem cell lines derived from human blastocysts. **Science** 282:1145–1147, 1998.
105. Tropepe V, Hitoshi S, Sirard C, Mak TW, Rossant J, Van der Kooy D: Direct neural fate specification from embryonic stem cells: A primitive mammalian neural stem cell stage acquired through a default mechanism. **Neuron** 30:65–78, 2001.
106. Turner DL, Cepko CL: A common progenitor for neurons and glia persists in rat retina late in development. **Nature** 328:131–136, 1987.
107. Uchida N, Buck DW, He D, Reitsma MJ, Masek M, Phan TV, Tsukamoto AS, Gage FH, Weissman IL: Direct isolation of human central nervous system stem cells. **Proc Natl Acad Sci** 97:14720–14725, 2000.
108. van Ommen GJB, Bakker E, den Dunnen JT: The human genome project and the future of diagnostics, treatment, and prevention. **Lancet** 354:S5–S10, 1999.
109. Watson JD: The human genome project: A statement of need. **Hosp Pract** 26:69–73, 1991.
110. Watt F, Hogan B: Out of Eden: Stem cells and their niches. **Science** 287:1427–1433, 2000.
111. Weihl C, Macdonald RL, Stoodley M, Luders J, Lin G: Gene therapy for cerebrovascular disorders. **Neurosurgery** 44:239–253, 1999.
112. Weissman IL: Stem cells, units of development, units of regeneration, and units in evolution. **Cell** 100:157–168, 2000.
113. Widner H: The case for neural tissue transplantation as a treatment for Parkinson's disease. **Adv Neurol** 80:641–9, 1999.

114. Widner H, Brundin P: Immunological aspects of grafting in the mammalian central nervous system: A review and speculative synthesis. **Brain Res** 13:287–324, 1998.
115. Wildner O: In situ use of suicide genes for therapy of brain tumors. **Ann Med** 31:421–429, 1999.
116. Wilson JM: Vectors: Shuttle vehicles for gene therapy. **Clin Exp Immunol** 107:31–32, 1997.
117. Winkler C, Fricker RA, Gates MA, Olsson M, Hammang JP, Carpenter MK, Bjorklund A: Incorporation and glial differentiation of mouse EGF-responsive neural progenitor cells after transplantation into the embryonic rat brain. **Molec Cell Neurosci** 11:99–116, 1998.
118. Yandava BD, Billinghurst LL, Snyder EY: Global cell replacement is feasible via neural stem cell transplantation: Evidence from the dysmyelinated shiverer mouse brain. **Proc Natl Acad Sci** 96:7029–7034, 1999.
119. Zlokovic BV, Apuzzo MLJ: Cellular and molecular neurosurgery: Pathways from concept to reality—Part 1: Target disorders and concept approaches to gene therapy of the central nervous system. **Neurosurgery** 40:789–804, 1997.
120. Zlokovic BV, Apuzzo MLJ: Cellular and molecular neurosurgery: Pathways from concept to reality—Part II: Vector systems and delivery methodologies for gene therapy to the central nervous system. **Neurosurgery** 40:805–813, 1997.
121. Zlokovic BV, Apuzzo MLJ: Strategies to circumvent vascular barriers of the central nervous system. **Neurosurgery** 43:877–878, 1998.

IV

General Scientific Session IV
Reinventing Neurosurgery: Sports and Spinal Injury

16

The Evaluation of Athletes with Cerebal Concussion

JOSEPH C. MAROON, M.D., MEL FIELD, M.D., MARK LOVELL, PH.D., ABPN,
MICHAEL COLLINS, PH.D., AND JEFFREY BOST, P.A.-C

THE EVALUATION OF ATHLETES WITH CEREBRAL CONCUSSION

The national publicity given to the career-ending or damaging effects of cerebral concussion in professional athletes like Steve Young, Troy Aikman, Eric Lindros, Merrill Hodge, Al Toon, and many others, has dramatized the significance of this injury to parents, coaches, trainers, players, and all those involved with athletics at all levels. What is the significance of a concussion? How many are too many? Does it cause permanent brain damage? And finally, when can an athlete safely return to contact sports? These are all questions asked each time one of the hundreds of thousands athletes each year in the United States experiences a cerebral concussion.

To assist in this dilemma, particularly with the return-to-play question, various individuals as well as organizations have formulated and espoused guidelines to assist with decision making in athletes. These guidelines have evolved over the last 20 years based on clinical impression, anecdotal experiences, and medical consensus—not on hard scientific data.

The purpose of this work is to review the various guidelines used in the management of athletes with cerebral concussion, describe innovations in computerized neuropsychological testing that greatly facilitate decision making in athletes with minimal traumatic brain injury (MTBI), and identify novel approaches that may dramatically impact the management of cerebral concussion in the future.

THE INCIDENCE OF CEREBRAL CONCUSSION IN SPORTS

Until the early 1970s little attention was given to the incidence of cerebral concussion in sports. In 1983 Gerberich published his results of a survey of head coaches and players of 103 secondary school football teams in the state of Minnesota (1). His figures astounded the sports world when he reported an incidence of 19 per 100 participants experienced a cerebral concussion from football. This translated to over 200,000 concussions per season at the high school level.

More recently Powell and Barber-Foss published their results of a survey of 246 certified athletic trainers who were asked to report injury and exposure data for high school varsity athletes at 235 high schools in the United States during the years 1995 through 1997 (2). This survey included both girls' and boys' sports at the high school level. Powell and Barber-Foss determined that cerebral concussions occurred in all the major sports including wrestling, baseball, field hockey, girls' volleyball, softball, and boys' and girls' basketball and soccer. They found, however, that the incidence was markedly reduced from that reported by Gerberich (1). Instead of 200,000 concussions per year, they determined an incidence of approximately 40,000 per 1.1 million in high school football participants (Table 16.1).

McCrea et al. in 1997 found an incidence of 4.3% of cerebral concussions in a group of 353 high school and 215 college football players (3). This number is comparable to the 3.7% reported by Powell and Barber-Foss (2). The conclusion is at this time that approximately 4% to 5% of high school football players will experience cerebral concussion during each season. This translates to approximately 30,000 to 50,000 concussions from football at the high school level on an annual basis. In other sports, the incidence is substantially lower (Table 16.1).

GUIDELINES FOR CONCUSSION MANAGEMENT

In 1963 the Congress of Neurological Surgeons established an ad hoc committee to study head injury nomenclature with an emphasis on sports-related concussion (4). This committee drew up the first set of guidelines based on the definition that "a cerebral concussion is a clinical syndrome characterized by immediate and transient post-traumatic impairment in neural function, such as alteration of consciousness, a disturbance of vision, equilibrium, etc., due to brain stem involvement." Concurrently this definition was divided into three separate levels—mild, moderate, and severe—and management recommendations were appended to each level of injury (Table 16.2).

It became apparent that post-traumatic amnesia could markedly alter the function of an athlete as well as return-to-play decisions. In 1986 therefore, Cantu modified the definition espoused by the Congress of Neurological Surgeons and incorporated post-traumatic amnesia to better define "a transient neurological disturbance" (5) (Table 16.3).

In 1991 national interest was raised regarding the management of

TABLE 16.1
National Estimates of Mild Traumatic Brain Injury Frequency for Selected High School Sports. 1995–1997

Male Sports

	Baseball	Basketball	Football	Soccer	Wrestling
# of Players	501,356	612,016	1,081,054	333,258	253,908
Estimated # of Injuries	1,153	4,590	39,566	3,068	4,012
Expected # of Injuries per Team*	0.05	0.13	1.93	0.22	0.39

Female Sports

	Basketball	Field Hockey	Softball	Soccer	Volleyball
# of Players	504,836	63,383	336,628	333,258	412,641
Estimated # of Injuries	5,250	292	1,548	3,799	578
Expected # of Injuries per Team*	0.16	0.10	0.08	0.26	0.02

Reprinted with permission from Powell JW, Barber-Foss KD: Traumatic brain injury in high school athletes. **JAMA** 282: 958–964, 1999 (2)

Copyright © 1999, American Medical Association

*Calculated as the injury rate per athlete exposures multiplied by the average number of exposures per school.

TABLE 16.2

Congress of Neurological Surgeons Guidelines for Cerebral Concussion

Level	Definition	Management Recommendations
I.	Mild, No loss of consciousness, Transient neurological disturbance	Athlete removed from contest but may return to play after completely normal neurologically
II.	Moderate, Loss of consciousness, with complete recovery occurring in <5 minutes	Athlete removed from contest and not permitted to resume contact during that game: may return in 1 week contingent upon neurological and neuropsychological findings
III.	Severe, Unconsciousness lasting >5 minutes	Managed as a severe head injury, with possible hospitalization and appropriate diagnostic testing

concussion in an article by Kelly et al. published in JAMA describing new guidelines for the prevention of catastrophic outcome from concussion in sports (6). These guidelines were developed through the sports medicine committee of the Colorado Medical Society. The major difference between the Colorado guidelines and the Congress of Neurological Surgeons and Cantu guidelines was that loss of consciousness was not required for their grade II concussion designation, rather confusion with amnesia for 15 minutes defined a grade II concussion. The authors emphasized the importance of a mental status evaluation and described various neurological and exertional tests that physicians and trainers might use on the sidelines for evaluating athletes before return to competition.

The next set of guidelines was that introduced through the Quality Standards Subcommittee of the American Academy of Neurology (7). This subcommittee again emphasized the importance of alteration in mental status without loss of consciousness and the importance of confusion and amnesia as the hallmarks of concussion *(Table 16.4)*.

The most recent proposed guidelines are those from Cantu in 2001 (8). In an effort to better define the pathophysiology using post-traumatic amnesia and loss of consciousness, he modified his previ-

TABLE 16.3

Guidelines Proposed by Cantu

Grade	Definition	Posttraumatic Amnesia
1	Mild, No loss of consciousness	<30 minutes
2	Moderate, Loss of consciousness <5 minutes	>30 minutes
3	Severe, Loss of consciousness >5 minutes	>24 hours

TABLE 16.4
American Academy of Neurology Guidelines

Grade	Definition	Management Recommendations
1	Transient confusion, No loss of consciousness, Symptoms resolve in <15 minutes	May return to play the same day if normal sideline assessments at rest and with exertion
2	Transient confusion, No loss of consciousness, Symptoms last > 15 Minutes	Defer contact until 1 full week without symptoms at rest and with exertion
3	Any loss of consciousness (brief or prolonged)	If brief (seconds), defer contact for 1 week without symptoms; If prolonged (minutes), defer contact for a minimum of 2 weeks without symptoms

ous guidelines as shown in *Table 16.5*. The most significant differentiation from the American Academy of Neurology guidelines is that a grade II concession is considered if there is loss of consciousness for less than a minute or post-traumatic amnesia or post-concussion symptoms and signs for less than 30 minutes. The American Academy of Neurology guidelines considers any loss of consciousness a grade III or severe concussion. Also Cantu considers a post-traumatic amnesia lasting 24 hours or more or post-concussion signs and symptoms greater than 7 days as representing a grade III or severe concussion. The importance of grading the concussions is that management decisions follow the grade of concussion *(Table 16.6)*. The time to return to play for a grade II concussion may be substantially less than that for the athlete who has experienced a grade III concussion. Although all the definitions were constructed with return-to-play guidelines,

TABLE 16.5
Evidence Based Cantu Revised Concussion Grading Guidelines

Grade	Definition	Post Traumatic Amnesia/Post Concussion Signs and Symptoms
1	Mild, No loss of consciousness	<30 minutes
2	Moderate, Loss of consciousness <1 minute	>30 minutes
3	Severe, Loss of	PTA = 24 hours / PCSS > 7 days

From Cantu RC: Post-traumatic (retrograde and anterograde) amnesia. Pathophysiology and implication of grading and safe return to play. **J Athletic Training** 36 (3), 2001.

TABLE 16.6
Clinical/Management Recommendations for Grading Scales

Guideline	Severity of Grade		
	1	2	3
Cantu	Athlete may return to play that day in select situations if clinical examination results are normal at rest and with exertion; if symptomatic, athlete may return to play in 7 days	Athlete may return to play in 2 weeks if asymptomatic at rest and with exertion for 7 days	Athlete may return to play in 1 month if asymptomatic at rest and exertion for 7 days
Colorado	Remove athlete from contest and evaluate immediately and every 5 minutes; permit athlete to return if amnesia or symptoms do not appear for 20 minutes	Remove athlete from contest and disallow athlete to return; examine athlete next day; permit athlete to return to practice after 1 week if asymptomatic	Transport patient to hospital: perform neurological examination and observe overnight; permit athlete to return to play after 2 weeks if asymptomatic
Practice parameter, American Academy of Neurology	Examine athlete immediately for mental status changes; athlete can return to contest if no symptoms or mental status changes at 15 minutes	Remove athlete from contest and disallow athlete to return; examine athlete on site for symptoms or mental status changes; athlete can return to play in 1 week if asymptomatic	Remove athlete from contest and transport to hospital; perform neurological examination and and observe overnight; permit athlete to return to play if asymptomatic after 1 week (if loss of consciousness was brief) or 2 weeks (if loss of consciousness was prolonged)

Reprinted with permission from, Collins MW, Lovell MR, McKeag DB: Current issues in managing sports-related concussion. **JAMA** 282:2283–2285, 1999. Copyright © 1999, American Medical Association.

none of these guidelines was developed on the basis of specific scientific knowledge regarding the process of recovery from concussion. The American Academy of Neurology guidelines and practice options were based on a review of the literature and the deliberation of a panel of experts (7), not on empirical data. Some of the problems with the existing guidelines are the following:

1. Too much importance has been assigned to loss of consciousness.
2. They are not based on scientific criteria or data.
3. There is considerable variability in the grading systems.
4. Do not take into account pre-existing cognitive abilities of athletes.

The emphasis on loss of consciousness as the most significant marker of concussion is now seriously questioned. In the past it has been assumed that injuries that result in traumatic loss of consciousness require a greater degree of force than do blows to the head that result in confusion or post-traumatic amnesia. Recently Lovell et al. specifically evaluated the importance of concussion in patients with MTBI (9). He and his associates could find no support for weighing loss of consciousness more heavily than other markers, such as amnesia or confusion, in decision making regarding return to previous activities. Loss of consciousness did not result in greater neuropsychological impairment compared with concussion patients who did not experience loss of consciousness.

NEUROPSYCHOLOGICAL TESTING

The vagaries of using the various arbitrary guidelines for return-to-play decisions was seriously called into question by none other than Coach Chuck Noll, four-time Super Bowl coach of the Pittsburgh Steelers. In 1990 a confrontation of sorts occurred when I, as senior author and team physician for the Pittsburgh Steelers, informed Coach Noll that his starting quarterback, who had experienced a grade II concussion a week before, could not play the following week against the Dallas Cowboys. Coach Noll was informed that the guidelines indicated a 2-week removal from contact sports. Well familiar with the guidelines himself, he informed the senior author that he also examined the player who had absolutely no symptoms of a post-concussion syndrome or residual amnesia, and he performed flawlessly in practice. He challenged the physician to provide more objective scientific based criteria for eliminating professional athletes from their job.

Stunned by this criticism, Coach Noll's challenge was taken. Collaboration was then begun with Dr. Mark Lovell, a neuropsychologist interested in sports-related concussion, who subsequently with other neuropsychologists and trainers was part of a collaborative effort to develop neurocognitive tests that would eliminate the subjective component of decision making in return-to-play activities.

The authors initially reviewed the previous work of Rimel et al., Yarnell and Lynch, Barth et al., Macciocchi et al., and others who had evaluated athletes with neurocognitive tests (10–14). It was determined on the basis of these studies that neuro-psychological testing provided a sensitive guide to ongoing and even cumulative problems following athletic MTBIs.

We then set out to develop a specific series of neuropsychological tests that we subsequently called "The Pittsburgh Steelers Neuropsychological Test Battery" *(Table 16.7)*. The characteristics of this test battery included the ability to evaluate a large number of athletes in a limited period of time—approximately 20–30 minutes per player. The tests had to be administered by paramedical personnel, such as trainers, speech pathologists, or others. The data had to be valid, reliable, and repeatable.

With this pen-and-pencil test battery, we again approached Coach Noll and also Steelers president and owner Dan Rooney. They allowed us to attain baseline testing on all members of the Pittsburgh Steelers football organization. Upon experiencing a concussion, an athlete was re-tested within 24–48 hours and then again if symptoms persisted for 5–7 days. The data was so convincing from these studies that subsequently 30 out of 31 teams in the National Football League (NFL) and all the teams in the National Hockey League (NHL) accepted this test battery and methodology as the standard for evaluating and managing professional athletes with cerebral concussion.

TABLE 16.7
The Pittsburgh Steelers Neuropsychological Test Battery

Test	Ability Evaluated
Orientation questionnaire	Orientation, posttraumatic amnesia
Hopkins Verbal Learning Test	Memory for words (verbal memory)
Trail-making Test	Visual scanning, mental flexibility
Stroop Test	Mental flexibility, attention
Controlled Oral Word Association Test	Word fluency, word retrieval
Digit Span (from Wechsler Memory Scale-Revised)	Attention span
Symbol Digit Modalities	Visual Scanning, attention
Grooved-pegboard Test	Motor speed and coordination
Delayed Recall from Hopkins Verbal Learning Test	Delayed memory from previously learned word list

IMPACT

After several years of experience and data gathering, it became apparent that pen-and-paper method of evaluating large groups of athletes was very inefficient. To test an entire athletic team was very time and labor intensive, and many schools outside the professional teams were reluctant to accept these tests because of limited financial resources and the costs involved for personnel and interpretation.

Because of these limitations and with athletes in mind, we recently developed a fully computer-based software program entitled "IMPACT" or Immediate Post-Athletic Concussion Cognitive Testing. Ten specific test modules *(Table 16.8)* plus a post-concussion symptom scale *(Table 16.9)* were incorporated into a software program that could be completed by the average athlete in approximately 20–25 minutes on a personal computer. The test battery evaluates multiple aspects of neuropsychological function including attention span, sustained and selective attention, reaction time to 1/1,000 of a second, and several dimensions of memory. It can be administered with minimal supervision by a technician, trainer, or anyone even slightly familiar with the software. The test battery currently consists of three forms which can be easily expanded to an almost infinite number by randomly varying the stimulus array. This feature minimizes the practice effects that have limited the usefulness of many paper-and-pencil procedures. The modules can be administered as a complete test battery or chosen separately on the selection of inter-stimulus intervals, for each module is easily adjusted.

TABLE 16.8
Computerized Neuropsychological Testing for Athletic Concussion Test Modules

Test Module	Cognitive Process Measured
Continuous Performance Test	Sustained Attention, Reaction Time
Verbal Working Memory	Memory for Words, Working Memory
Symbol Memory	Immediate Visual Memory
Sequential Digit Tracking	Sustained Attention, Reaction Time
Number/Symbol Matching	Processing Speed, Visual Motor Speed
Symbol-matching Memory Condition	Visual Memory
Visual Span	Visual Attention, Immediate Memory
Work/Color Tracking	Focused Attention, Response Inhibition
Visual Symbol Search	Visual Scanning, Reaction Time
Post-concussion Symptom Scale	Concussion Symptoms, as reported by the Athlete
Concussion History Form	History of Concussion, as reported by the Athlete

TABLE 16.9
Pittsburgh Steelers Postconcussion Scale

Player Name: _____
Date of Concussion: _____
Position: _____

Symptom	None		Moderate			Severe	
Headache	0	1	2	3	4	5	6
Nausea	0	1	2	3	4	5	6
Emesis	0	1	2	3	4	5	6
Balance Problems	0	1	2	3	4	5	6
Fatigue	0	1	2	3	4	5	6
Trouble Falling Asleep	0	1	2	3	4	5	6
Sleeping More Than Usual	0	1	2	3	4	5	6
Drowsiness	0	1	2	3	4	5	6
Sensitivity to light/noise	0	1	2	3	4	5	6
Irritability	0	1	2	3	4	5	6
Sadness, Sense of Depression	0	1	2	3	4	5	6
Nervousness	0	1	2	3	4	5	6
Numbness or Tingling	0	1	2	3	4	5	6
Feeling Slowed Down	0	1	2	3	4	5	6
Sensation of Being "in a fog"	0	1	2	3	4	5	6
Difficulty with Concentration	0	1	2	3	4	5	6
Difficulty with Memory	0	1	2	3	4	5	6
Total Score							

All test data are stored in the format that facilitates comparison of post-concussion test performance with baseline performance for each athlete. For each of the 10 modules data are provided regarding correct or incorrect performance as well as processing speed and reaction time. Changes in reaction time after concussion were previously identified as highly sensitive indicators of brain malfunction. The validity, reliability, and ease of administration have now been confirmed in a major study of high school and college students (to be published.) We have now substituted IMPACT for the pen-and-pencil tests with the Pittsburgh Steelers, the Philadelphia Eagles, and other professional teams, and we anticipate that a conversion will take place completely within the next year or two. Most importantly, however, the program was designed to provide to high school and college students the same level of quality of neurocognitive testing that is available to the professional athlete. Accordingly, we now have eight teams in the Big Ten, several in the Pack Twelve, and other major conferences, as well as many smaller colleges utilizing IMPACT this football season. In addition, over 100 high schools have now attained baseline testing on their athletes with the goal of utilizing this in all contact sports.

FUTURE DIRECTIONS

Although numerous scales and tests are used to measure cerebral concussion severity, the pathophysiological processes resulting in neurocognitive deficits after a concussion are poorly understood. Most theories related to MTBI in athletes are derived from in-vivo animal models and human studies of severe traumatic brain injury utilizing cerebral blood flow (CBF) measurements, MR spectroscopy, positron emission tomography (PET), or microdialysis. Most experts do agree that the symptoms associated with a concussive injury are somehow related to a metabolic dysfunction that occurs in the brain after the initial traumatic event (15). Decreased CBF, hyperglycolysis, glutamate induced excitotoxicity, and cellular ionic fluxes occurring after head injury have all been implicated as the causes for this dysfunction (15–23). However, conventional methods of localizing the dysfunction in the brain, such as CT, MRI, or EEG, have failed to consistently recognize areas of injury after cerebral concussion.

Recently, functional magnetic resonance imaging (fMR), a fairly new technology that measures differential brain metabolism and blood flow in response to a stimulus, has been used to study aspects of memory and behavior in patients with certain psychiatric disorders or brain lesions with encouraging results. However, fMR has not been used to study athletes with MTBI. To date, only one study has evaluated the use of fMR with brain injury (24). In that study, brain activation patterns in response to a working memory test were compared in MTBI patients within 1 month of their injury to healthy individuals. The authors found a significant difference between the two groups in activation patterns of working memory circuitry in response to different processing loads but similar task performances. Interestingly, Fontaine et al. studied severe TBI patients without focal structural lesions by MRI in 1999 (25). Each patient underwent a neuropsychological evaluation to test memory, attention, executive function, and global neurobehavioral assessment. Regional cerebral glucose metabolism was measured by PET. A close link was found between cognitive and behavioral disorders and decreased cortical metabolism in prefrontal and cingulate cortex. Tests of memory and executive function correlated with regional metabolism in the mesial and lateral prefrontal cortex and the cingulate gyrus. Behavioral disorders correlated with mesial prefrontal and cingulate metabolisms. Based on these and other studies, a strong argument can be made for the development of better tech-

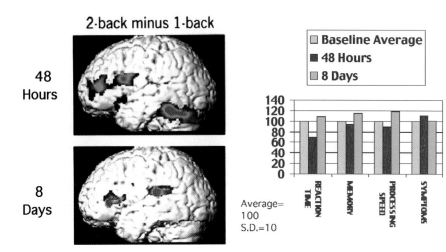

FIG. 16.1 ƒMRI and neuropsychological testing in a female high school basketball athlete who suffered a concussion without loss of consciousness. The patient had classic post-concussive complaints at 48 hours post-injury. These complaints had resolved by post-injury day 8.

niques to identify athletes at risk for permanent deficits following cerebral concussion.

Using the powerful combination of ƒMR and IMPACT we are now beginning to systematically examine cognitive recovery in athletes following concussion. Pilot data has shown dramatic differences in ƒMR brain activation during various stages of recovery after cerebral concussion (*Fig. 16.1*). Furthermore, these changes in brain activation appear to follow a trend similar to that seen with neurocognitive testing. Given these early results we suspect that the combination of computerized neuropsychological testing and ƒMR may represent a potentially useful tool for correlating the neurocognitive and neurobehavioral deficits following cerebral concussion with the anatomic and physiological abnormalities that ensue after MTBI. Results of such work will likely redefine the way athletes are evaluated for a concussive injury, provide an objective and sensitive means to measure postconcussive recovery, and determine risk of returning to play based on neurocognitive and physiological data.

ACKNOWLEDGMENT

This work was supported by the Dennis and Rose Heindl Neuroscience Research Fund.

REFERENCES

1. Gerberich SG, Priest JD, Boen JR, Straub CP, Maxwell RE: Concussion incidences and severity in secondary school varsity football players. **Am J Public Health** 73:1370–1375, 1985.
2. Powell JW, Barber-Foss KD: Traumatic brain injury in high school athletes. **JAMA** 282:958–963, 1999.
3. McCrea M, Kelly JP, Kluge J, Ackley B, Randolph C: Standardized assessment of concussion in football players. **Neurology** 48:586–588, 1997.
4. Ad Hoc Committee to Study Head Injury Nomenclature: Proceedings of the Congress of Neurological Surgeons in 1964. **Clin Neurosurg** 46:386–394, 1996.
5. Cantu RC: Guidelines for return to contact sports after a cerebral concussion. **Physician Sports Med** 14:755–783, 1986.
6. Kelly J, Nichols JS, Filley C, Lillehel K, Rubinstein D, Kleinschmidt-DeMasters B: Concussion in sports: Guidelines for the prevention of catastrophic outcome. **JAMA** 266:2867–2869, 1991.
7. Quality Standards Subcommittee, American Academy of Neurology: Practice parameter: The management of concussion in sports (summary statement). **Neurology** 48:581–585, 1997.
8. Cantu RC: Post-traumatic (retrograde and anterograde) amnesia. Pathophysiology and implication of grading and safe return to play. **J Athletic Training** 2001 (In Press).
9. Lovell MR, Iverson GL, Collins MW, McKeag D, Maroon JC: Does loss of consciousness predict neuropsychological decrements after concussion? **Clin J Sport Med** 9:193–198, 1999.
10. Rimel RW, Giordani B, Barth JT, Boll TJ, Jane JA: Disability caused by minor head injury. **Neurosurgery** 9:221–228, 1981.
11. Yarnell PR, Lynch S: Retrograde memory immediately after concussion. **Lancet** 1:863–864, 1970.
12. Barth JT, Alves WA, Ryan TV, Macciocchi SN, Rimel RW, Jane JA, Nelson WE: Mild head injury in sports: Neuropsychological sequelae and recovery of function. In Levin HS, Eisenberg HM, Benton AL (eds): *Mild Head Injury*. New York: Oxford University Press. 1989, pp 257–275.
13. Macciocchi S, Barth JT, Alves W, Rimel RW, Jane JA: Neuropsychological functioning and recovery after mild head injury in collegiate athletes. **Neurosurgery** 39:510–514, 1996.
14. Matser BJT, Kessels AG, Lezak MD, Jordan BD, Troost J: Neuropsychological impairment in amateur soccer players. **JAMA** 282:971–973, 1999.
15. Hovda DA, Prins M, Becker D, Lee S, Bergsneider M, Martin NA: Neurobiology of concussion. In Bailes JE, Lovell MR, Maroon JC (eds): *Sports-related Concussion*. St. Louis: Quality Medical Publishers. 1999, pp 12–51.
16. Kawamata T, Katayama Y, Hovda DA, Yoshino A, Becker DP: Administration of excitatory amino acid antagonists via microdialysis attenuates the increase in glucose utilization seen following concussive brain injury. **J Cereb Blood Flow Metab** 12:12–24, 1992.
17. Katayama Y, Becker DP, Tamura T, Hovda DA: Massive increases in extracellular potassium and the indiscriminate release of glutamate following concussive brain injury. **J Neurosurg** 73:889–900, 1990.
18. McIntosh TK, Faden AL, Bendall MR, Vink R: Traumatic brain injury in the rat: Alterations in brain lactate and pH as characterized by ^{1}H and ^{31}P nuclear magnetic resonance: **J Neurochem** 49:1530–1540, 1987.

19. McIntosh TK, Faden AL, Yamakami I, Vink R: Magnesium deficiency exacerbates and pretreatment improves outcome following traumatic brain injury in rats: ^{31}P magnetic resonance spectroscopy and behavioral studies. **J Neurotrauma** 5:17–31, 1988.

20. Vink R, Faden AL, McIntosh TK: Changes in cellular bioenergetic state following graded traumatic brain injury in rats: Determination by phosphorus 31 magnetic resonance spectroscopy. **J Neurotrauma** 5:315–330, 1988.

21. Yamakami I, McIntosh TK: Effects of traumatic brain injury on regional cerebral blood flow in rats as measured with radiolabeled microspheres. **J Cereb Blood Flow Metab** 9:117–124, 1989.

22. Yamakami I, McIntosh TK: Alterations in regional cerebral blood flow following brain injury in rat. **J Cereb Blood Flow Metab** 11:655–660, 1991.

23. Yuan X, Prough DS, Smith TL, Dewitt DS: The effects of traumatic brain injury on regional cerebral blood flow in rats. **J Neurotrauma** 5:289–301, 1988.

24. McAllister TW, Saykin AJ, Flashman LA, Sparling MB, Johnson SC, Guerin SJ, Mamourian AC, Weaver JB, Yanofsky N: Brain activation during working memory 1 month after mild traumatic brain injury. **Neurol** 53:1300–1308, 1999.

25. Fontaine A, Azovi P, Remy P, Bussel B, Samson Y: Functional anatomy of neuropsychological deficits after severe traumatic brain injury. **Neurol** 53:1963–1968, 1999.

17

Honored Guest Presentation:
The Legacy of Galen of Pergamon
The Neurosurgeon in the Arena of Sport

MICHAEL L.J. APUZZO, M.D., MICHAEL Y. WANG, M.D., BYRON HANSEN, M.S., JOSEPH SKIBA, CHERISSE BERRY, B.S., AND MICHAEL L. LEVY, M.D.

Organized sport represents a global pandemic of focus and activity. Modern society has embraced the athlete, athleticism, and its representation of robust health, personal achievement, and individual accomplishment. It is certainly debatable whether or not this is justified; however, attendant to these matters issues of care of the amateur, collegiate, and professional athlete frequently assume significant importance for a variety of reasons and demand the attention and personal involvement of the neurosurgeon. Issues are often complex and surpass the scope of care in the "usual patient" and circumstance. This discussion will consider a number of points related to the problems of the neurosurgeon as a consultant and team surgeon at high school, collegiate, and professional levels with particular focus on the sport of football.

All physicians and surgeons owe a great depth of gratitude to *Galen of Pergamon*, and the contemporary sports physician and surgeon represents in many ways the modern personification of Galen—the "physician to the gladiators."

GALEN OF PERGAMON

Born in the Roman territory of Pergamon in AD 129, Galen was the son of the noted architect Nicon. Pergamon had been a Greek colony 15 miles from the sea on the Northeastern coast of Ionia (Turkey). It was legendary for the physical beauty of its landscape, the complexity of its temple complex, and its wealth as a financial hub.

According to myth Nicon was instructed by Aesculapius to persuade his son to study medicine. In his teen years Galen was unusually precocious from the intellectual point of view producing works on philosophy, ethics, and other learned topics. At the age of seventeen he entered the city's famed *aesculapion*, an elaborate center of religious activity and healing. Because of its enormous importance within the Roman Empire, the Aesculapion of Pergamon drew a college of famed individuals representing a variety of medical sects and professional orientations. During this period, Galen was most attracted to approaches towards healing based on a comprehension of anatomy and physiology. Subsequently, during a decade of study and travel, he observed aspects of philosophy, life sciences, and medicine in the prominent intellectual centers of Corinth, Smyrna, and Alexandria where he enjoyed a protracted period of study (3).

At the age of twenty-eight, Galen returned to Pergamon to enter into the more formal practice of medicine, and it was there that he attended to the gladiators at the spectator amphitheater from AD 159 to 168.

The first recorded gladiatorial games took place in the Roman Forum in 264 BC. In the earliest times gladiators fought only in pairs, but with the passage of time public demand called for greater spectacle and gladiators fought in the hundreds, supplied by slaves, prisoners of war, criminals and mercenaries. As the complexity of the spectacles grew, variety shows emerged featuring the hunting of tigers, leopards, crocodiles, giraffes, rhinoceroses, panthers, and elephants. Later combat was staged pitting the gladiators against animals. These events created opportunities for the study of anatomy, physiology, and therapeutic measures in both man and beast *(Fig. 17.1)* (9).

Galen was a keen observer and analytical thinker. During his seven successive appointments as physician to the gladiators he focused his intellect on the anatomy, physiology, and treatment of the wounded, observing the sick and dead of both human and animal species. His experiences in the arena led to many human medical and anatomical concepts while initiating and feeding an interest in the importance of animal experimentation.

Galen went on to Rome to make more observations in the Coliseum related to both human and animal participants, subsequently developing more than five hundred treatises dealing with philosophy, science, and medicine. Written in Attic Greek, they totaled more than four million words. His effect was to initiate a transition away from the medical theories of Hippocrates and to *establish medicine as an applied science deeply rooted in observation, experimentation, and dissection methods.* His work emerged as a guiding force in science and medicine for over thirteen hundred years *(Fig. 17.2)* (17).

Today in many figurative as well as practical ways individuals engaged in American football, particularly at its higher levels, represent modernity's gladiators incarnate and thus the parallel exists in numerous dimensions on Saturdays and Sundays each fall. Likewise, opportunities exist for therapeutic advancement, injury prevention, and

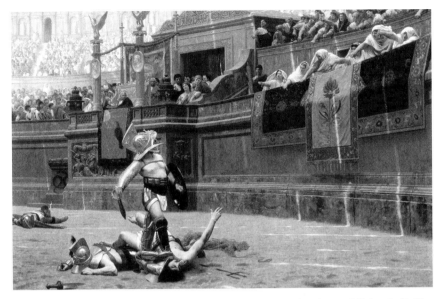

FIG. 17.1 The Gladiatorial Arena of Sport representing the times of Galen in *Pollice Verso* by Jean-Léon Gérome (1872). (Reprinted courtesy of the Phoenix Art Museum.)

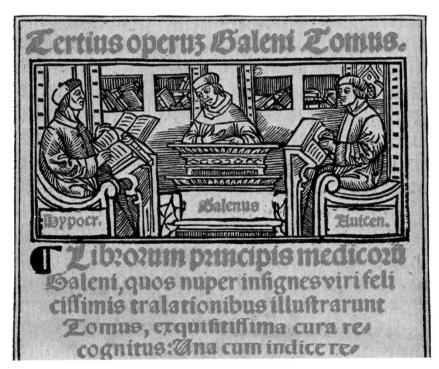

FIG. 17.2 Manuscript (1528) representing the icons of Medicine over a period of more than 1600 years. Galen spans the times from Hippocrates to Avicenna. (National Library of Medicine, Bethesda, Maryland.)

novel comprehension related to both minor and major neural injuries. Our modern "Coliseums" do in fact represent massive clinical laboratories for enhancing the state of knowledge regarding neural function and the complete spectrum of injury. The neurosurgeon is uniquely qualified to observe, participate, and elicit proper knowledge for the benefit of the athlete and mankind in general through active and appropriate involvement in these events and the issues attendant to them.

Although numerous key issues are attendant to this topic, the following discussion will focus upon three topics:

1. Minor brain injury, the neuropathology and neurobiology of cerebral concussion
2. Head protection, helmet development
3. Practical issues attendant to the neurosurgeon in the arena of sport

CEREBRAL CONCUSSION

Introduction

Historically, concussion has been described in terms of the transient nature of altered neurologic function, and this entity was defined largely by the *absence* of demonstrable central nervous system pathology in the setting of a neurological deficit. However, over the past several decades the realization that repeated concussive injuries lead to permanent structural neurological changes has emerged. This has been especially true in the setting of sports-related head injury. Research in both animals and humans has now demonstrated disruptions in metabolic homeostasis at the cellular and molecular level that are not grossly evident (45). In addition, modern functional imaging modalities now have the ability to detect certain elements of these changes radiographically. Based upon these advances an improved understanding of the effects of repeated head trauma in the arena of sport has been synthesized.

Pathologic Changes

In the immediate postinjury period, structural pathologic changes following concussion occur at the cellular and subcellular level and are difficult to detect. Changes in the *microglia* are a sensitive marker for head trauma. In animal models of concussion where injury patterns are mild and without cell death or local hemorrhage, increases in astrocytic activity and intermediate filament formation occur at the site of injury in the cerebral cortex, and microscopic foci of neuronal shearing and microglial proliferation occur (5, 46). These changes occur in the absence of astrocytic proliferation and are most prominent 2 to 4 days after contusion.

With more severe injuries, changes are seen in the *neurons* themselves. Jane et al., in a primate deceleration model of concussion with loss of consciousness, demonstrated axonal disruption in the brainstem and reticular formation (26). Injury to axons in these regions could account for lapses in consciousness in this model and in humans, and the degree of pathologic change correlates with known electrophysiologic changes after head injury.

Povlishock et al., in an electron microscopy study of cat brains subjected to concussive injury, demonstrated reversible subcellular changes in the neuronal pool coincident with lapses in consciousness (51). In that study, *reticular* and *raphe neurons* suffered membrane perturbations as demonstrated by the cellular uptake of horseradish peroxidase administered intravenously. This abnormal intracellular flooding was seen at 3 and 30 minutes after injury. At 2 and 6 hours cell membrane integrity was restored, and at 12 to 24 hours the peroxidase was sequestered in vacuoles. The neurons otherwise appeared ultrastructurally normal, suggesting that transient disruptions in the reticular formation may be the result of subcellular structural perturbations unassociated with apoptosis.

This mechanical disruption of the cell membranes from trauma leads to the leakage of ions and macromolecules (19, 49). This increased membrane permeability further disrupts cellular homeostasis, leading to the loss of ionic potentials and cellular dysfunction. Increased cellular permeability may also expose the intracellular milieu to the locally elevated levels of excitotoxic amino acids.

Percussion injuries above two atmospheres of pressure also cause pathologic damage to *vascular structures* in the brain. Under these conditions, the blood brain barrier may become compromised, allowing the passive movement of macromolecules directly from the blood to the brain (15). This increased permeability further impairs the nutrient supply to damaged tissues and contributes to local edema.

Metabolic Effects

Following mild head injury, derangements in homeostasis may occur at the subcellular level that are not apparent structurally on gross pathological examination or imaging studies. The cascade of events occurring after mild trauma has been elaborated largely in animal models. These models bear relevance to the clinical setting of athletic-related head trauma as they produce alterations in the level of consciousness without overt cellular death or tissue destruction. In the rat model of concussive brain injury, a fluid percussion technique is the most frequently utilized, allowing accurate regulation of force, acceleration, and injury focus. Periods of unconsciousness relate to the amount of kinetic energy transmitted to neural tissues in these models.

The initial effect of mild head trauma is *potassium ion efflux*. In the rat model, impact producing lapses of consciousness 200–250 seconds were associated with a five-fold increase in extracellular potassium as detected by microdialysis (32, 61). Elevations in potassium disrupt neural transmission and may be responsible for the loss of consciousness associated with concussion (39). Potassium efflux may be due to neuronal membrane disruption (49, 51), axonal stretching (29), or the opening of voltage and ligand-gated ion channels (32). In addition, excitatory amino acids activate kainite, AMPA, and NMDA receptors locally, allowing both potassium and sodium to follow ionic gradients (32). The administration of kynurenic acid, which interferes with this pathway, results in decreased potassium ion efflux following trauma in animal models.

The surrounding glial cells respond to this increase in extracellular potassium by reuptake of excess ions (48). However, as this buffering capacity is exceeded, the extracellular potassium levels may rise abruptly and lead to further depolarization. This results in the further *release of excitatory amino acids* that exacerbate the already deranged homeostasis. This cascade of events may eventually result in a compensatory hyperpolarization with quiescent neuronal activity. Because the effects of this phase often involve brain regions unaffected by the primary insult, it has been characterized as a "spreading depression." (20).

In order to restore membrane potentials, *local increases in glucose utilization* occur after the injury and persist for up to four hours (10, 35, 36, 58). This glucose demand will frequently exceed the capacity for aerobic metabolism, resulting *in glycolysis and lactate accumulation* (42), and in studies where the energy consuming ionic pumps were blocked with ouabain prior to injury, these increases in glucose demand were not seen, and no lactate accumulation occurred.

Bioenergetic deterioration at the cellular level also plays a role in exacerbating neuronal dysfunction. Excitatory amino acid accumulation has also been demonstrated in vivo through analysis of cerebrospinal and extracellular fluids in trauma patients. These macromolecules open NMDA channels, allowing an influx of calcium ions and intracellular hypercalcemia (14), which can persist for up to 4 days. Mitochondria are able to buffer small rises in intracellular calcium, but once this capacity has been exceeded perturbations in energy production occur (68). *Reductions in intracellular magnesium* may also contribute to a reduced capacity for cellular energy production (65).

Excitotoxic cholinergic activation also contributes to cellular dysfunction. Trauma induces a *biphasic response of acute cholinergic hyperfunction followed by hypofunction at several days* (37). Immediately following injury, extracellular acetylcholine levels as measured by microdialysis exceeds two times the normal levels and can persist for several days (54). The resulting stimulation of muscarinic (M1 and M3) receptors may contribute to alterations in consciousness and lower seizure thresholds (44). Cholinergic activation also potentiates glutamate toxicity by sensitizing NMDA receptors and *increasing intracellular calcium* through IP_3 (53).

These metabolic changes from mild trauma are largely transient. Sodium hemostasis is restored in several hours, intracellular calcium normalization may take up to several days, and clearance of excitotoxic neurotransmitter receptors occurs from several days to two weeks. These time intervals represent periods of neuronal susceptibility to further insults and additional minor trauma results in cellular swelling, membrane disruption and apoptosis (61).

Cerebral Perfusion

Cerebral blood flow and brain glucose demand are closely coupled in the normal brain. However, following even mild trauma, derangements can occur in the vascular milieu. While mild trauma does not cause the large-scale effects on the blood vessels that major head injury produces, *local derangements in cerebral perfusion do occur*. Increases and decreases in blood flow vary depending upon the time interval after trauma.

In the first few hours following mild or moderate trauma there is a global decrease in cerebral blood flow. In animal models, reductions in blood flow of up to 50% have been demonstrated (69, 70). The effect of this decreased perfusion is compounded by the increased metabolic demands in the injured tissue, rendering the neuronal pool especially vulnerable to damage. These vascular effects are presumably the result of local controllers of vasomotor tone such as angiotensin II, prostacyclins, nitric oxide, and endothelium-dependent relaxing factor (EDRF), but the exact mechanism remains unproven.

Following the acute phase, a period of cerebral hyperemia peaks at 24 hours postinjury (52) and may occur for up to 14 days (55). These blood flow changes have been demonstrated experimentally in animal models and in humans by SPECT, PET, and xenon CT imaging. *Blood flow derangements are found not only at cortical injury sites but also within what appears to be normal white and gray matter as demonstrated by conventional CT and MRI.*

These abnormalities may represent a response to the increased metabolic demands of injured tissues or an uncoupling of local metabolism and perfusion. While this "dissociated vasoparalysis" is transient, it is likely a contributor to the increased susceptibility of the brain to additional mild insults, and the temporal pattern of the blood flow changes may be correlated with clinical findings such as headache and altered psychomotor abilities.

Gross disruption of cerebral autoregulation has also been demonstrated in some human studies following mild brain injury. In one study comparing patients with mild head injury and normal subjects, dynamic alterations of systemic blood pressure and transcranial doppler measurements were used to assess autoregulation. The compensatory response in the cerebral vasculature was shown to be abnormal in 28% of trauma patients, as opposed to 0% in normal volunteers (30).

In the chronic state following repeated minor trauma, areas of cerebral hypoperfusion can occur. In a SPECT study of patients with postconcussive symptoms, 44% were shown to have areas of decreased blood flow in what appeared to be normal brain tissue on CT and MRI. These lesions were found predominantly in the frontal and temporal lobes (31) and may explain long-term disturbances in memory and cognition following mild head injury.

Imaging Studies

The vast majority of sports-related concussions show no pathologic changes on standard MRI and CT images. However, the implementation of sophisticated MRI techniques has allowed the detection of radiographic changes following mild head injury. The use of FLAIR (fluid attenuation inversion recovery), diffusion weighted, and magnetization transfer protocols increases the yield of a positive study from 9% to 33% (27, 40). Most of these abnormalities are attributed to cerebral edema or axonal shearing and are found in the deep white matter, frontal lobes, and corpus callosum. Functional MRI has also demonstrated task-dependent alterations of blood flow in the frontal lobes of concussion victims.

PET and SPECT studies have also enhanced the detection of pathologic changes after mild head injury. These imaging modalities have the ability to detect alterations in cerebral metabolism in the absence of structural changes. PET and SPECT may be particularly useful in evaluating patients with persistent deficits or chronic subjective complaints.

In a study of 67 patients with mild or moderate brain injury, SPECT was predictive of post-concussive symptoms in 95% of cases, and the negative predictive value of SPECT was 97% (25). The most common abnormality in patients with post-concussive symptoms was hypoperfusion of the basal ganglia (50%) or frontal lobes (46%) (1). Studies of asymptomatic boxers have also demonstrate reduced cerebral perfusion in the frontal and temporal lobes on SPECT scanning (33). However, SPECT imaging has been poorly correlated with performance in neuropsychiatric tests (21, 67).

Electrophysiological Studies

Animal models of concussion show a disruption of the EEG at the time of loss of consciousness followed by a period of reversible depression and then complete recovery (59). With increasing traumatic force the tracing becomes temporarily isoelectric followed by complete recovery. However, conventional cortical EEG recordings have been poorly predictive of post-concussive symptoms (66). Quantitative EEG, with its higher sensitivity for localizing frequency abnormalities, has demonstrated some potential for detecting reduced alpha rhythms in post-concussive patients (24, 43).

Event-related potentials designed to assess for attentional-cognitive abnormalities demonstrate decreases in the P300 wave for 1 week to 6 months after concussive injury. The degree of impairment was related to ratings on the Concussion Symptoms Scale (16).

Latencies in the auditory, visual, and trigeminal evoked responses (BAER, VEP, BTER) are the most sensitive electrophysiologic alteration in patients who suffered a concussion and 11% to 17% of mild head injury victims have abnormal studies. In studies of pugilists, increased inter-peak intervals and reduced amplitudes were identified with visual evoked responses showing latencies in the P3 wave (18). Middle latency responses correlate with long-term neuropsychological outcome, suggesting a persistent dysfunction of the diencephalic and paraventricular structures (60).

Selective Areas of Vulnerability

Based upon clinical observations and animal studies a number of areas in the brain appear particularly susceptible to injury from repetitive mild head trauma. These areas may suffer from neuronal dysfunction or apoptosis even if the injury focus occurred in other regions of the brain. The concepts of diaschisis and transneuronal degeneration postulate that interconnecting neurons exert trans-synaptic effects. Apoptosis or axotomy of a neuron can thus cause the dysfunction of distant retrograde and anterograde cells (47). This may explain how these changes occur distant from focal injury sites.

Experimental studies show that metabolic changes after cortical injury occur in the hippocampi bilaterally. Hippocampal changes include the elevation of heat shock proteins, cholinergic dysfunction, and increased glucose utilization which may be directed at the restoration of ionic homeostasis (35). In animal models of concussion the CA1 and CA3 areas of the hippocampus are especially vulnerable to combinations of impact and hypoxia (41), and even in the mild head injury model these is selective neuronal loss in the hippocampi (22) with associated cognitive deficits (34).

The frontal and temporal lobes show degeneration after repeated concussive injuries, and these cortical regions demonstrate gross pathologic changes of atrophy on conventional imaging modalities such as CT and MRI. SPECT studies in humans are able to demonstrate reduced metabolism in these cortical regions as well as the basal ganglia. Magnetization transfer techniques demonstrate signal changes in the corpus callosum (40). These lesions may represent areas of demyelination or edema undetectable through conventional MRI techniques.

Second Impact Syndrome

The description of fatalities occurring after successive minor head injuries, coined the second impact syndrome, has created great concern among physicians and trainers caring for athletes at risk for head trauma. Since the original report by Schneider in 1973, 26 deaths have been attributed to the second impact syndrome (39, 57).

Second impact fatalities occur following a concussion which had produced some alteration in the baseline neurologic status. The most frequent symptoms are headache, dizziness, visual or sensory phenomena, and memory disturbances (11). A second, trivial head injury occurring prior to the resolution of symptoms then results in massive cerebral edema and death. Frequently the victim will be awake but have an altered level of consciousness for 15 seconds to several minutes before papillary dilatation and respiratory failure. This second impact may be as slight as a blow to the torso causing accelerative forces and not even directly involve the head.

Second impact syndrome is believed to be due to the *loss of cerebral autoregulation*. Hyperemia as demonstrated on SPECT and PET scanning has been associated with the acute postinjury phase and is believed to be the cause of post-concussive symptoms such as confusion and headaches. This vascular engorgement causes cerebral edema with increased intracranial pressure. The second impact results in additional injury precipitating central herniation with loss of papillary and respiratory function.

Long-Term Effects

Repeated head trauma is an occupational hazard of participation in many contact sports. Even in the absence of clear episodes of injury, *repetitive mild trauma leads to deterioration of cognitive function.* This has been demonstrated clearly in boxers who develop dementia but is also seen to varying degrees in professional American football, soccer, and hockey players.

Cholinergic insufficiency has been implicated in the pathogenesis of long-term neurological sequelae following trauma. These systems have a significant representation in the *limbic cortex, basal nucleus of Meynert, hippocampus,* and *rostral pons,* and play an important role in the maintenance of consciousness. Following the acute period of cholinergic hyperfunction, delayed hypofunction occurs starting at several days postinjury (37). This temporal dysfunction is supported by experimental studies showing attenuation of deficits by pre-trauma administration of scopolamine and post-trauma treatment with cholinergic agonists (50). *Decreases in the synthesis, storage, and release of neurotransmitter may occur in the absence of cell death.* Following repeated traumatic episodes, the *loss of forebrain cholinergic neurons* may be a causative factor in the development of long-term cognitive dysfunction and memory problems. Pharmacologic supplementation with cholinergic agonists in the chronic setting is promising but remains experimental.

The *apolipoproteins* also appear to have a role in the long-term effects of mild head injury. Cognitive dysfunction in older football players and boxers, particularly in attention and memory, have been found to be associated with the apolipoprotein $\epsilon4$ allele (28, 36). The association of the apolipoprotein $\epsilon4$ allele with Alzheimer's disease is intriguing, and it has been postulated that this genotype may represent a defect in neural reparative processes.

In consideration of these issues and disclosures, factors related to head protection deserve attention.

HEAD PROTECTION AND FOOTBALL INJURIES
Historical Background

From 1869 to 1905, football claimed 18 deaths and 159 serious injuries. To address this rising problem, helmets were first introduced in 1896. Even with the first single bar face mask appearing in 1951 and the first double bar face masks/cages appearing in 1958, both tackling drill fatalities and head injuries increased while spine injuries decreased between 1955 and 1964. The increases in football-related injuries sparked an injury data collection initiation in 1967, which documented 36 fatalities by the end of the 1968 season. As a result of head and spine injuries markedly increasing between 1965 and 1974, the rules of football began to change. The *National Operating Committee on Sports Athletic Equipment* (NOCSAE), founded in 1969, ini-

tiated research efforts for head protection and implemented safety
standards for helmets in 1973 (6, 13, 62).

The *Standard Method of Impact Test and Performance Requirements
for Football Helmets* published in 1973 requires the use of a head model
that more closely simulates the response of the human head to impact. Standards are based on the helmet falling in a guided free fall.
In each case, the helmet is positioned on a head form. The head form
is human-like and complex in function and is constructed to provide
a measure of the helmet's ability to attenuate the kinetic energy released during the test. The energy is based on the drop velocity and
the mass of the head form. The goal of NOCSAE was to develop a standard that would measure the ability of the football helmet to withstand repeated blows of various magnitudes under a wide variety of
circumstances without any sacrifice in protective quality. These circumstances include the following: players ranging in age from 14 to
experienced professionals; environmental conditions (freezing cold,
driving rain, heavy snow or high heat and humidity); and playing surfaces (hard-packed dirt, thick mud, deep grass, or artificial turf). In
addition, the helmet must be worn for multiple seasons without any
reconditioning.

In 1975, Joseph S. Torg, then Director of Sports Medicine at Temple University, observed the need for a central registry for the collection, documentation and analysis of severe neck injuries occurring in
the game of football (12, 63). During the 18 years preceding his report,
Dr. Torg found that a change had occurred in the frequency of severe
head and neck injuries. Although the incidence of head injury had decreased, the reported incidence of cervical spine injuries with frac-
ture/dislocations and with permanent quadriplegia had increased (7).
Torg attributed this increase to the implementation of playing techniques that used the top or crown of the helmet as the primary point
of contact in a high-impact situation. At the end of the 1975 season,
both the *NCAA* and the *National Alliance Football Rules Committee*
(NAFRC) enacted rules designed to prevent the use of the head as the
initial point of contact in playing techniques:

1. No player shall intentionally strike a runner with the crown or top
   of the helmet.
2. Spearing is the deliberate use of the helmet in an attempt to pun-
   ish an opponent.
3. No player shall deliberately use his helmet to butt or ram an opponent.

The NAFRC provision prohibited any technique involving a blow
with the face mask, frontal area, or top of the helmet driven directly

into an opponent as the primary point of contact either in close line play or in the open field. As a result of the prohibition of headfirst contact, there was a significant decrease in head and neck injuries.

In 1977, NCAA funded the initial *National Survey of Catastrophic Football Injuries* (NSCFI). NOCSAE established helmet safety standards in 1978 for college football and in 1980 for high school football. Currently, it is mandatory for all high school and college players to wear helmets meeting NOCSAE standards (23).

In testing helmets in 1977, Elwyn Gooding, then a Research Associate at the University of Michigan with Richard Schneider, simulated the forces present during the production of both acute subdural hematomas and cervical spine injuries with tetraplegia and compared the effectiveness of various types of protective football headgear in attenuating these forces. In this series of impact testing, Gooding used a bare headform against a rigid anvil as a signal to record specific types of impacts. These tests were repeated with different types of helmets of varying construction and under various conditions. Gooding found that in simulating impacts to both the occipital region of the head, known to produce subdural hematomas, and to the vertex of the head, known to produce cervical fractures with tetraplegia, a severe brainstem contusion, or hemorrhage, all types of helmets attenuated the blow considerably when compared to blows sustained by the bare head form against a plain anvil. After testing all types of web and foam suspension systems and combined web and foam systems, Gooding found that the better helmet is one that has a small initial rise and a distribution of force at a lower peak for a longer time. The comparison revealed that the double crown pneumatic helmet provided the best protection.

Although value exists in determining compatibility to known standards, performance in the established test methods and comparisons of various helmet designs must not be used to predict the likelihood of any headgear's capability to limit certain injuries. *There is no helmet that can prevent all head injuries.*

Current Helmet Design Assessment

The current NOCSAE standard involves a series of publications titled and numbered as follows:

1. Standard drop test method and equipment used in evaluating the performance characteristics of protective headgear- NOCSAE DOC.001-98
2. Standard Performance Specifications for newly manufactured football helmets- NOCSAE DOC.002-96

3. Laboratory procedural guide for certifying newly manufactured football helmets-NOCSAE DOC.003-96
4. Equipment calibration procedures-NOCSAE DOC.101-96

Examples of some of the NOCSAE standards include the following:

SAMPLE SIZE

1. At least 2 of each model and size must be tested. Helmets of a given model with a size smaller than 6 5/8 may not fit the smallest NOCSAE head form. In that event, testing of that size is waived so long as the other sizes of that model have been tested and meet all requirements;
2. To obtain a reasonable fit for testing purposes, helmets larger than size 7 5/8 may require "shim" pads to be inserted between the largest NOCSAE head form and the interior of the helmet, opposite from the impact site.

HELMET PREPARATION

1. Face Guards- Helmets must be tested without face guards or face guard specific hardware.

IMPACT ATTENUATION TESTS

1. The peak severity index of any impact shall not exceed 1200 SI.
2. Helmet fit must be maintained without intervention throughout the entire series of impacts. Any structural changes or other changes that take place during impact testing which result in loosening the fit to the head form shall be cause for failure. Helmet repositioning during testing is anticipated. However, additional, un-restorable, loosening of the fit is not allowed (see Section 20, NOCSAE DOC.001-98). It should be stressed that these tests offer at best limited assessment of a helmet's protective capabilities. No evaluation of rotational forces or repetitive endurance has been performed.

Helmets

The American football helmet was and is designed to protect the areas of the player's head directly covered by the helmet from direct linear impact only. The helmet was not designed, and cannot be designed, to prevent injury to or protect the cervical spine or spinal column on those areas of the neck not covered by the helmet or to prevent injuries to the brain that result from rotational acceleration. As a result of NOCSAE, critical changes became apparent in the protective qualities of football helmets beginning in the early 1970s. According to Schneider et al. *(Fig. 17.3)*, football helmets should be constructed

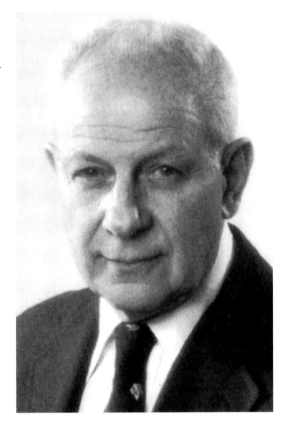

FIG. 17.3 Neurosurgeon Richard Coy Schneider, MD, a keen student and observer in the arena of sport. His contributions to the reduction of injury by rule changes and protective equipment development remain unmatched by any single individual. (Courtesy of The Society of Neurological Surgeons.)

specifically on the basis of an anatomical knowledge of the skull and brain with an understanding of the mechanical principles involved in head injuries. Schneider stated that the outer shell of the helmet should be constructed to cover either the fragile areas of the skull, which might fracture, or to cover specific portions of the intracranial contents, which are most frequently vulnerable to head injuries and may result in concussion. The firm posterior margin of the outer shell of the helmet should be cut high to avoid the "chopping effect" of this part of the helmet during cervical hyperextension injuries that may result in cervical fractures or spinal cord damage. The inner suspension system is developed to *distribute forces generated by impact uniformly over the head*. This system consists of two crowns, one within the other. Each crown is a hemisphere of hollow plastic material with arches extending from the apex to the base or circumference of the crown. Air or gas injected through valves into these structures diffuses throughout all parts of each individual crown. In the completed helmet the two crowns are injection-molded and electrically sealed together as a single piece using a high frequency sound wave. An inner crown is inflated pneumatically to fit the individual player but the outer crown lining the helmet's outer shell is inflated to the same pressure for all wearers. The presence of the two separate, pneumatically sealed systems avoids the problems of the headgear bouncing on the head. The helmet is maintained in position on the head with a four-point attached chin strap *(Fig. 17.4)*.

Helmet material must allow for more deformation and gradual de-

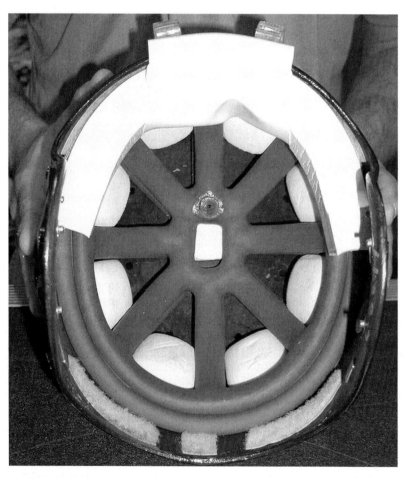

FIG. 17.4 Inner compartment of a double chamber pneumatic crown system: the outer crown is fully inflated; the inner crown is inflated to fit; shell and foam inserts may be varied in relation to cranial contour need. (Courtesy of the National Football League and the New York Football Giants.)

celeration of the head. The face guard should be flattened and the chin straps should easily release. The posterior rim of the shell should be advanced and shoulder rolls must be used. Web suspensions absorb force at fixation points; however, isolated fluid or air pockets should avoid supraorbital and occipital nerves. Helmet shell material must allow for more protection of fragile regions of the skull and areas prone to concussive injury. The initial rise must *be decreased and the lower force distributed over longer periods of time.*

Although the characteristics of energy absorption and attenuation of blows to the helmet are of critical importance in helmet design, many researchers feel that there are many other requirements and considerations which should not be overlooked. *Position maintenance* so that no slippage occurs during wear, good ventilation, good vision so that there is no restriction of peripheral vision, light weight, a smooth, hard exterior surface, good fit to the player's head, continued functional use after repeated blows, comfort, economics, appearance, ability to withstand the effects of sun, temperature, paints or cleansers on the shell or components, and durability are all essential characteristics to helmet design. Helmet designers have attempted to incorporate all of these characteristics in designing protective headgear while at the same time maximizing the helmet's linear impact absorption and attenuation capabilities.

Position maintenance and individual contour fitting are essential goals of any helmet. Helmet systems and design elements vary considerably in their ability to satisfactorily meet the requirements of the large variability of cranial contour and volume *(Fig. 17.5).*

Three companies currently provide football headgear at the NFL level. All have hard plastic shells, foams of various densities to attenuate linear impacts and a fit system that inflates. The three different types of helmets are described as follows:

1. Helmet 1 has an inflatable airliner that is a continuous tube-like design. When inflated these tubes expand to aid in the fit. The air system is nested into a foam system that is comprised of two different densities and is molded to shape. The two layers are ethyl vinyl acetate (EVA) and polyvinyl chloride nitrile rubber (vinyl nitrile). The front and rear pad of similar design and the air inflation system are used for fitting;
2. Helmet 2 uses similar foam but instead of molding the foam, die cut pieces are placed in a molded case that holds the resulting blocks of foam layers in place. Air is introduced into the same molded case causing the case to expand and fit the head. In this design, the front pad is a molded urethane that fits into a sleeve;

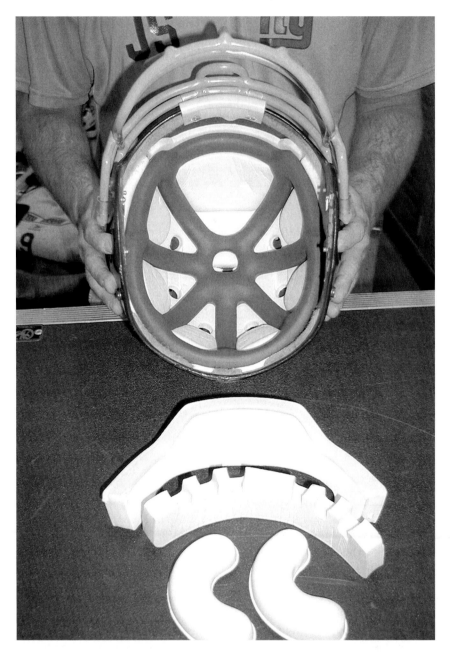

FIG. 17.5 Foam components and size variables related to a single crown air system helmet. Little opportunity for customization of fitting is available with this system. (Courtesy of the National Football League and the New York Football Giants.)

3. Helmet 3 uses a different approach. The shell is ventilated and lighter than the previous two. The air liner is similar to helmet 2 in construction but is different in shape and does not serve as a holder for the primary foam components. A unique inner liner of expanded polypropylene (EPP) increases the inner shell. A foam molded EVA component with vinyl nitrile inserts similar to helmet 1 and serves as a cover to the EPP and holder of the air fit system. A vinyl nitrile front pad is provided but is not changed for fitting.

All three helmet models utilize the same jaw pads, chin straps, and faceguards.

As an example of a new system, the designers of the new Pro-Edition helmet from Bike Athletic have developed a lightweight helmet. This new helmet has the following description: an anthropometric outer shell that better conforms to the head contours, improving the fit and comfort and creating a means of deflection. The venting system allows air to circulate and dissipate quickly. A unique, stiff skeletal sub-structure effectively supports the shell construction and assists in attenuating impacts. An inertial cushioning pad serves as the next level of energy management, and the adjustable air liner provides a custom fit. The front stabilizer pad cushions the forehead, and a permanently attached, patent-pending chin strap and cup anchor the helmet to the player's head. The new Pro-Edition helmet has passed all NOCSAE tests and standards.

Along with these elements any system must allow satisfactory flexibility to fit and maintain stability on the individual athlete. A second new system designed by Schutt offers apparent improvements *(Figs. 17.6, 17.7, and 17.8)*.

Despite the stringent efforts set forth over the last 30 years to improve safety and over 51 injury prevention rules implemented, football-related fatalities and injuries such as concussion continue to occur.

Cerebral Concussions: Clinical Issues

As noted, concussions are a frequent occurrence in the sport of American football. Concussions are characterized by an alteration in cerebral function caused by a direct or indirect (rotation) force transmitted to the head followed by a brief loss of consciousness, light-headedness, vertigo, and cognitive and memory dysfunction. Concussions may be associated with variable periods of tinnitus, blurred vision, difficulty concentrating, amnesia, headache, nausea, vomiting, photophobia, balance disturbance, delayed sleep disturbance, fatigue, personality changes, inability to perform, depression, or lethargy. Although most concussions appear to be minor, they can carry serious long-term consequences.

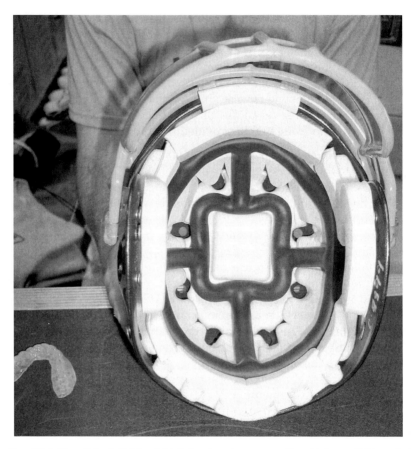

FIG. 17.6 New Schutt lightweight helmet system currently widely available only in professional level competition: innovative air crown system, with multi-sectional foam components offer complete contour fitting to multivariable cranial contour and proportion. Combined with a titanium base frame mask there is a 30+% reduction in helmet weight. (Courtesy of the National Football League and the New York Football Giants.)

Specifically, the second impact syndrome and the cumulative effects of repeated trauma can be devastating. Thus, as previously stressed, a comprehensive understanding of the pathobiology and clinical consequences of concussion is imperative (4).

Football Associated Fatalities 1945–1984

From 1945 to 1984, head injuries represented 67% of football-associated fatalities while cervical spine injuries represented 17.3% (N = 643) (8). 73.7% of the total number of head injuries and 64% of the total number of cervical spine injuries occurred during high school play;

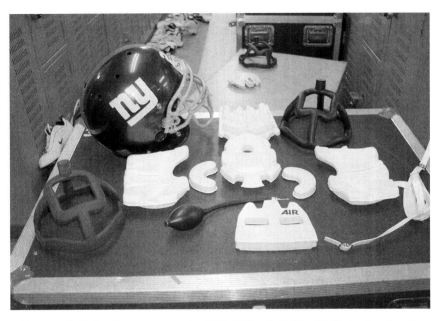

FIG. 17.7 Individual base components of Schutt Novelle lightweight helmet system from Fig. 17.6. (Courtesy of the National Football League and the New York Football Giants.)

whereas professional play accounted for 3% of head injuries and 10.8% of cervical spine injuries. During this time period, 337 subdural hematomas (SDH) and 18 skull fractures resulted. Of the head injuries, 80% occurred with SDH and of the cervical spine injuries, 81% occurred with fractures. In addition, 47% of the head injuries occurred with tackling and 72% of the cervical spine injuries occurred with tackling (64).

Incidence of Concussion in Football

Gerberich reported in 1983 that 19/100 high school players experienced concussions. According to both McCrea in 1997 and Powell in 1999, this number decreased to 4/100 high school players. However, in 2000, Delaney reported that 48/100 CFL players experienced concussions. During the 1997 CFL season, players succumbing to concussions (N = 67–69) experienced the following symptoms: confusion (69.6%), headache (61.8%), dizziness (44.9%), blurred/abnormal vision (32.8%), nausea (14.5%), memory difficulties (11.6%), and loss of consciousness (2.9%). The duration of the symptoms ranged from <5 sec (6.1%) to <60 min (56.1%) to <2 weeks (100%). The number of concussions among concussed players varied: 30.4% of concussed players experienced 1 concussion; 20.3% of concussed players experienced 2 concussions; 21.7%

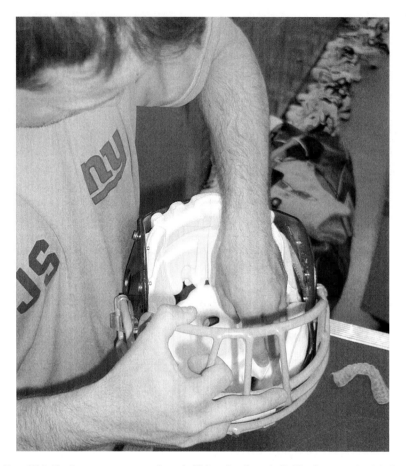

F<small>IG</small>. 17.8 Equipment manager Joseph Skiba develops individual customized helmet composites. An amalgam of proper design, fit and maintenance is essential to optimize the protective capability of the helmet construct. It, however, represents only one of many factors for establishing minimal opportunity for concussive injury. (Courtesy of the National Football League and the New York Football Giants.)

experienced 3 concussions; 5.8% experienced 4 concussions; 7.2% experienced 5 concussions; 8.65 experienced 6–10 concussions; 1.4% experienced 11–20 concussions; and 4.3% of concussed players experienced >20 concussions during the 1997 CFL season. This study found that during the 1997 CFL season, players with a previous LOC in football were 6.15 times as likely to experience a concussion than players without a previous LOC ($p < 0.05$). Players with a previous concussion in football were 5.10 times as likely to experience a concussion than players without a previous concussion ($p = 0.0001$). Players with an extra season game were 1.13 times as likely to experience a concussion ($p = 0001$) and players with more years played in football were 1.11 times as likely to experience a concussion ($p < 0.05$). Players most at risk for experiencing a concussion are quarterbacks (71.4%), running backs (58.3%), defensive linemen (54.2%), linebackers (47.6%), wide receivers (47.1%), cornerbacks/safeties (42.9%), offensive linesmen (34.6%), special teams (28.6%), punters/kickers (25.0%), and tight ends (0.0%).

The use of the head as the initial point of contact increases the potential for injury. With the implementation of NOCSAE Standards, fatalities decreased by 74% and serious head injuries decreased from 4.25/100,000 to 0.68/100,000. In fact, there were no head fatalities in 1990.

Factors to Consider in Head and Neck Injuries

From the neurosurgeon's standpoint a number of factors are important in creating a higher potential risk of head or neck injury. These factors include (1) *player position*, (2) *game speed*, (3) *field surface composition and condition*, (4) *helmet and protective equipment*, (5) *variability's in player anatomy*, (6) *previous player injuries*, (7) *weather*, and (8) *individual style of play*.

Because of their unique roles in the game of football, certain positions are at higher risk for central nervous system injury. Defensive backs, arguably the best athletes on the field, are at the greatest risk given their repetitive tackling movements at high speed. Receivers and running backs are also subjected to high-speed collisions with other players. The quarterback is frequently the focus of tackling maneuvers from various angles. He is vulnerable to open "blind side" collisions while stationary.

Progression of the game of football through various levels of organization carries an accompanying escalation in the speed of the athletes and the collective events of play in total. While skill level increases so does the mass and acceleration of individual players. In general as the speed of the player increases, so does the risk of a devastating injury.

The play surface, natural or synthetic, affects player acceleration. In general, synthetic surfaces are harder and faster. Natural surfaces make injury less likely as they are "slower." Crowning of the central field also allows for increased acceleration toward the sidelines.

Helmets are designed to be properly fit and maintained. Appropriate shoulder pads and nuchal support systems are also essential. This is generally the charge of the individual athlete, equipment managers, and trainers. However, occasionally lapses in optimization occur, particularly with under inflation of the bladder which has been found to frequently accompany concussive events. In addition, proper fitting and maintenance of head protective devices is essential.

Variations in player anatomy also affect the risk for injury. Players focus on developing protective shoulder and nuchal musculature through weight-training programs. These regions are critical in maintaining head and neck alignment during tackling maneuvers and prevent hyperflexion and hyperextension of the cervical spine. Unfortunately, many of the players particularly in so-called "skilled positions" are not focused on this preventative measure.

Previous injuries are predictive of future traumatic events. This may be the end point result of other factors discussed above. Individual styles of play that are hazardous and inattention to matters of equipment optimization make certain players prone to injury. In addition, previous injuries will independently affect player cognition and performance and affect his ability to avoid dangerous collisions.

Weather impacts the game as well. Rain, snow and other inclemencies generally reduce the game speed and the force of impact. Heat and humidity have a frequent undermining role in the athletes' energy, creating fatigue and potential vulnerability (2).

Finally, while players can adopt a protective attitude towards gameplay, certain individuals will exercise inadequate caution and add to the increased on-field risk. Strict rule statements prohibiting deliberate spearing and helmet-to-helmet contact reduce but do not eliminate these risks.

Concussion Assessment and Treatment

Anticipation, awareness, and preparation for the onset of a concussion are the best methods for treatment. Establishing a routine protocol whereby team physicians and trainers conduct a review in the pre-season is critical for treating players at risk for injury. This would include an awareness of each player's capabilities. Trainers and players must understand the mechanisms of injury: direct contact, sudden rotational or sheer forces, and rapid acceleration and/or deceleration. In evaluating injured players on the field, team physicians and trainers must first observe the posture of the athlete and note any spontaneous motion or verbalization. Second, in the event of a significant injury trainers must commence with the ABCs: checking for obstructed *airways*, spontaneous *breathing*, *pulse*, and the level of *consciousness* to rule significant associated injuries, especially to the cervical spine. In the absence of a pulse and adequate respiration, the neck should be stabilized and Glasgow Coma Scale determined.

Player Examination and Evaluation

Orientation to time, place, and person should be determined. Retrograde amnesia, dizziness, visual blurring, and head or neck pain should be evaluated. Until symptoms improve and the athlete has adequate strength, coordination, and orientation to follow instructions, the patient should remain in the sitting position, standing position, or in the cart if the player is unsteady. Once on the bench, a brief neurologic and neuropsychological examination should be performed. Particular attention should be paid to the symptoms of dizziness, light-headedness, vertigo, visual problems, photophobia, tinnitus, head-aches, and nausea/vomiting. The head, neck, scalp, skull, and facial bones should be inspected and palpated. The peri-orbital, mandibular, and maxillary areas are especially prone to injury. Trainers should assess for malocclusion or pain secondary to a mandibular fracture. Because a direct blow to the face can result in a unilateral dilatation of the pupil (3% rate of anisocoria can occur) as well as 3rd cranial nerve palsy, a careful eye exam including a check for both visual acuity and visual fields should be performed next. Extraocular motion, altitudinal asymmetry of the globes (from infra-orbital blowout fractures), and the presence of nystagmus should be assessed. Any facial asymmetry should then be evaluated. Signs of a basilar skull fracture including a middle ear exam should then be performed. The cervical spinous processes and the brachial plexus should also be palpated. Extremity strength and sensation should be symmetrical and a brief test for pathological reflexes such as a Hoffman's sign should be assessed. Lower extremity strength and coordination can be evaluated by observing the athlete while standing, squatting and walking heel-to-toe. Coordination should be tested with the finger-to-nose test, tandem walking, and the Romberg test. Detailed concentration can be evaluated by asking the individual to repeat three, four, and five digits backwards or with "serial 7's." Trainers should observe the player for a minimum of 15 minutes, reevaluating as needed. Any symptomatic players should not be allowed to return to the game. Repeat evaluations should be performed by the same individual to increase the sensitivity of detecting any changes in clinical status (38).

Standardized Assessment of Concussion (SAC)

Close observation and reliable clinical assessment can prevent more serious or catastrophic brain injury, the second impact syndrome, and cumulative neuropsychological impairment. It can, however, be difficult to note subtle concussive symptoms given the tendency on the part of players to deny symptoms. The American Academy of Neurology has developed a formal Practice Parameter for the Management of Concussion in Sports to create a valid, standardized, and systematic sideline evaluation tool for the immediate assessment of concussion in athletes by physicians and trainers. In addition, a neurologic screening examination should be performed to assess recall, strength, sensation, and coordination. Exertional maneuvers such as a 40 sec sprint, sit-ups, push ups, and knee bends can supplement this evaluation. Although the SAC

TABLE 17.1

The American Academy of Neurology Grading Guideline Practice Parameters

Grade 1

Transient confusion

No loss of consciousness

Concussion symptoms or mental status abnormalities on examination resolve in less than 15 minutes.

Grade 2

Transient confusion

No loss of consciousness

Concussion symptoms or mental status abnormalities on examination last more than 15 minutes

Grade 3

Any loss of consciousness, either brief (seconds) or prolonged (minutes)

From Jeffrey T. Barth: Future directions in sports related concussion. In Bailes JE, Lovell MR, Maroon JC (eds): *Sports-Related Concussion*. St. Louis: Quality Medical Publishing, 1999.

provides immediate information, it is not a substitute for formal clinical or neuropsychological evaluation *(Table 17.1)* (4).

In one study comparing 33 concussed high school college players with 568 normal players, the SAC score in concussed players was statistically lower than both normals and their own normal baseline. Concussed players scored on average 3.5 points (1.48 standard deviations) lower than their pre-injury baseline. Scores fell 1.58 standard deviations below the normal mean for the control group. These attempts to quantitate the effects of concussion are also useful for tracking recovery from injury. Follow-up testing of these 33 players showed that 28 had returned to their baseline within 48 hours.

Research is required to identify which SAC domain scores are most sensitive to change during injury and to characterize how orientation, concentration, and memory are affected in more severe forms of concussion. We have found that age and educational level have had a negligible impact on performance. In addition, we have found that the emotional changes attendant with athletic competition do not significantly confound test performance. The SAC, in combination with a thorough clinical examination, may represent the most sensitive and informative approach to the sideline assessment of concussion.

Return-to-Play Recommendations

In summary, a number of other rudimentary guidelines have been generated to deal with the issue of cerebral concussion in the athlete *(Tables 17.2 and 17.3)* (4). After a player suffers a concussion, he should be removed from play, evaluated, and observed. If the player is totally

TABLE 17.2
The Colorado Medical Society Guidelines for the Management of Concussion

Grade	Signs and Symptoms	1st Concussion	2nd Concussion	3rd Concussion
1 (mild)	Confusion without amnesia; no loss of consciousness	May return to play if without symptoms for at least 20 minutes	Terminate contest or practice; may return to play if without symptoms for at least 1 week	Terminate season; or may return to play in 3 months if without symptoms
2 (moderate)	Confusion with amnesia; no loss of consciousness	Terminate contest or practice; may return to play if without symptoms for at least 1 week	Consider terminating season; may return to play in 1 month if without symptoms	Terminate season; may return to play next season if without symptoms
3 (severe)	Loss of consciousness	Terminate contest or practice and transport to hospital; may return to play in 1 month after 2 consecutive weeks without symptoms	Terminate season; may return to play next season if without symptoms	Terminate season; strongly discourage return to contact or collision

From Jeffrey T. Barth: Future directions in sports related concussion. In Bailes JE, Lovell MR, Maroon JC (eds): *Sports-Related Concussion*. St. Louis: Quality Medical Publishing, 1999.

359

TABLE 17.3
The Cantu Grading System for Concussion and Guidelines for Return to Competition

Grade	Symptoms	1st Concussion	2nd Concussion	3rd Concussion
1 (mild)	No loss of consciousness, posttraumatic amnesia less than 30 minutes in duration	May return to play if asymptomatic for 1 week	Return to play in 2 weeks if asymptomatic at the time for 1 week	Terminate season; may return to play next season if asymptomatic
2 (moderate)	Loss of consciousness less than 5 minutes in duration or posttraumatic amnesia longer than 30 minutes but less than 24 hours in duration	Return to play after asymptomatic for 1 week	Minimum of 1 month; may return to play then if asymptomatic for 1 week; consider terminating season	Terminate season; may return to play next season if asymptomatic
3 (severe)	Loss of consciousness for more than 5 minutes or posttraumatic amnesia for more than 24 hours	Minimum of 1 month; may then return to play if asymptomatic for 1 week	Terminate season; may return to play next season if asymptomatic	

From Jeffrey T. Barth: Future directions in sports related concussion. In Bailes JE, Lovell MR, Maroon JC (eds): *Sports-Related Concussion.* St. Louis: Quality Medical Publishing, 1999.

asymptomatic, passes memory and concentration tests, and exhibits no symptoms with provocative testing, he can return to play.

We have employed rapid response testing of game condition commands administered by teammates and position coaches as a final level of assessment before returning to play. Finally, close observation of on field responses for a number of series is undertaken. Any observed period of unconsciousness, regardless of how brief, should preclude return to play. A player exhibiting any post-concussive symptoms should not be allowed to continue play until further evaluation by a physician. If these symptoms do not abate during the initial 15 minutes then the player should be disqualified for the rest of the game. Serial neurological evaluations should be performed as long as symptoms are present. Any deterioration of neurologic function mandates immediate transport to a medical facility where neurosurgical consultation and imaging are available.

If a player's symptoms have not cleared within 15 minutes or if he had a documented loss of consciousness, he should not return to play that same day. Any headaches in the first 48 to 72 hours following injury should preclude play indefinitely until further medical evaluation. Dizziness, slowness in responding to questions, difficulty concentrating, physical sluggishness, memory problems, and persistent retrograde amnesia should also preclude play. For the high school level athlete who experienced symptoms for longer than 15 minutes, we automatically recommend a minimum of 5 to 7 days of rest.

When symptoms are prolonged greater than 15 minutes after a concussion, great care must be exercised before returning even asymptomatic athletes to practice or competition. Our current state of knowledge regarding the neurobiology of concussion cannot specify a safe firm timetable for return to play in most circumstances. Therefore, athletes with prolonged symptoms must be individually evaluated and reevaluated. New technologies such as balance testing are promising but currently are not useful for guiding return-to-play decisions at this time.

The role of imaging studies to assess structural or physiologic alterations is particularly important in the symptomatic athlete. Additionally neuropsychological assessment with comparison to established baselines are both valuable and important. The role of electrophysiological assessment requires further definition.

THE ROLE OF THE NEUROSURGEON: TEAM INVOLVEMENT

The role of the neurosurgeon is complex and variable in the arena of sport. The neurosurgeon's principle function relates to his or her fund of knowledge in relation to neurological disease and surgery.

However, this basis must be augmented, refined, and enhanced according to elements of the individual athlete, sport, and situation. As previously stated these comments are directed to football, but by in large may be extrapolated to the realm of sport endeavor.

American football is the principal and most popular of all American spectator sports. Virtually unmatched for spectacle and pageantry, it is perhaps modern civilization's closest rival to the gladiatorial combat of Rome and its empire. The principle venues of organization are at the high school, college, and professional levels. Each level and domain within the level presents challenges and requirements that vary in complexity as the perceived importance of participation and its apparent, practical and real rewards increase for all individuals who participate. The fact that each situation within a level, and that each level is unique must be the first appreciation. However, in spite of these refinements, generalizations related to involvement and focus are possible and may be universally applied.

From a practical viewpoint, to optimize effective participation there needs to be a serious dedication to the task on the part of the individual neurosurgeon. The charge requires acting as counselor to the individual athlete, coaches, and team personnel. In addition, it necessitates functioning as a team-related coaching advisor, and a protective equipment advisor to trainers, equipment managers, and coaches as well as the individual athletes. These levels of interaction clearly extrapolate to involve families, business agents, and other interested parties. There is a distinct "ripple effect" within these parlance secondary to the celebrated status of sport at each level, producing not only new opportunities for neurosurgical and medical problem solving but also unique demands and challenges in the interpersonal sphere.

All of these individual planes of interaction are played against time frames in the "life" of a team and the athlete's involvement in it. Therefore, the neurosurgeon is an evaluator and counselor in multiple venues and these include the *"off season"* time of preparation—a period when most elective surgeries are undertaken and rehabilitation is most intense. The players active season begins with *"pre-season"* camp when the true active life and chemistry of the team are born and when protracted physical and mental strain are most intense—the "two a day" period when double on-field practices are marked by physical demands and are when positional depth status is usually established. The *practice field* is rapidly established as an arduous and routine setting of "necessary evil" where fear of injury is balanced against a need to prepare for game conditions and establish optimum skills and mental preparedness. *Game conditions* during seasonal and post-season settings provide both mental and physical challenges for all individuals. Periods of *rehabilitation* and issues of *transition to retirement* are particularly problematical periods within the professional levels requiring special situational comprehension on the part of the neurosurgeon.

In consideration of the complexities of issue, individual, venue and communal setting it is imperative that the neurosurgeon follow a number of relatively simple actions and activities to optimize his opportunity to properly and effectively employ his scientific and professional knowledge for the optimal benefit of all concerned and for his own personal satisfaction.

It is important to establish lines of communication to effectively *develop respect and trust at multiple levels*. This effort and professional activity is required to establish credibility in multiple planes of involvement. These include first and most importantly with the athletic training staff, followed by the individual athletes, coaches, equipment managers, team managers, and administration. It is very important to comprehend individuals and personalities particularly within the various niches of team environments and to comprehend team, as well as individual, goals as these in particular will play an important role in neurological assessments in very real terms. In doing this the neurosurgeon should work to understand the game of football as it is approached within his own particular environment and study individual athletic football personalities and styles of play as these elements will have definite bearing on clinical evaluation as well as in predicting risk of injury.

The neurosurgeon should begin immediately to attain a general grasp of the team situation within the ordered time frames and activity venues—off season, pre-season practice, post-practice periods, pre-game settings—all demand his presence, study, and involvement if he is to establish the presence and trust that will allow either *open communication* with the athletes trainer and coaches or allow him to be aided by a true perception of the individual situation and athlete needs.

From an intellectual and stylistic viewpoint it is important *to be serious about one's involvement*, working closely with all colleagues, particularly the orthopedists, comprehending their problems and approaches. Special respect and focus must be given to the athletic trainers whose depth of knowledge related to evaluation of musculoskeletal injury and its rehabilitation and sequela is enormous. This is particularly true at the professional level. Concurrently, comprehending issues related to head, neck, and shoulder protective equipment is essential. The combined expertise of trainers, equipment man-

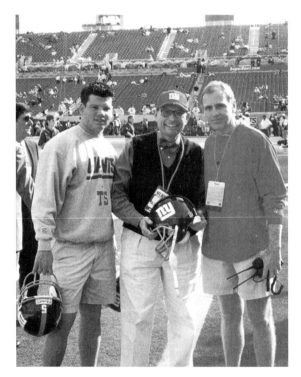

FIG. 17.9 Senior author with Giants equipment manager Ed Wagner, Jr. (R) and assistant equipment manager Tim Slaman (L) before Super Bowl XXXV, Tampa, Florida. Neurosurgeons involvement with helmet selection and design is an important facet of contribution to the level of safety in the sport. (Courtesy of the National Football League and the New York Football Giants.)

ager, and orthopedists supplements the neurosurgeons knowledge and perception of need *(Fig. 17.9)*.

Succinctly stated, it is critical to be present in the life of the team, to be involved, and to work to comprehend psyches and appreciate that issues change with situations in the metamorphose and life winds of the team.

THE TEAM ATHLETIC TRAINER'S PERSPECTIVE

The most common head injury in sports is the concussion, estimated to occur at a rate of 250,000 per year in contact sports. The risks of serious short- and long-term consequences from a minor head injury can be prevented by careful attention to the athlete's post-traumatic complaints and symptoms. If these complaints and symptoms fail to resolve, then a more complete evaluation by a neurosurgeon is recommended. The potential long-term consequences of minor head injuries remain to be elucidated; however, the available data suggest that neuropsychological impairment following a single concussion may have long-lasting residual effects. It is imperative that teams participating in contact sports, particularly at the college and professional level, have a neurosurgeon available should the need arise.

Despite this, neurosurgeons remain one of the most underutilized specialties in athletics today. Neurosurgeons integrated as part of the sports medicine team are commonly looked upon as a luxury, not a necessity, until a serious neurological injury or illness arises. The medical staff's ability to utilize the neurosurgeon's expertise can be invaluable to the athlete and the team as a whole. Unlike the orthopedist and other team physicians, whose services are needed on a regular basis, the neurosurgeon's role may be more limited, but should still be considered a critical component to the sports medicine team.

Like all those involved in the medical care of athletes, neurosurgeons need to develop treatment guidelines. Neurosurgeons should collect a current body of knowledge of the sport for which they are assuming responsibility. They should be familiar with the most common types of neurological injuries specific to their sport and the most effective management of those injuries. In addition, it is recommended that the neurosurgeon discuss equipment safety issues with the athletic trainers and equipment managers. For example, the brand and sizing of a helmet and the most effective locations for cervical collars should both be discussed in detail.

Accessibility to the neurosurgeon by the athletic trainer and head team physician in a timely manner is critical to providing effective medical care for an injured patient. It is imperative that the neurosurgeon is responsive when on call for a team. The neurosurgeon must be prepared to participate in emergencies both during practice and competition. It is always assumed that the unconscious athlete on the football field has a cervical fracture until proven otherwise and should be treated and transported accordingly; proper management of these injuries may be the responsibility of the neurosurgeon. The neurosurgeon can coordinate the rehabilitation and will help to determine, along with the athletic trainer and head team physician, when it is safe to return the player to practice and competition.

Neurosurgeons can play a significant role in educating athletes, parents, spouses, coaches, administrators, and agents regarding the risks and methods to prevent injuries of the head and neck. They should establish relationships with other team physicians and know the medical chain of command within their sports medicine team. They should never offer coaching advice on or off the field and must be professional at all times. It is important that all team physicians understand their boundaries and limitations within the team. The head coach should communicate directly with the athletic trainer; the neurosurgeon and other team physicians should maintain a distance away from the coaches unless addressed directly. Failure to adhere to these rules may result in a misunderstanding between the coaching and medical staffs and may compromise the care of an injured athlete in an emergency situation.

Collegiate and professional athletic teams should make neurosurgeons an integral part of their medical staff. In so doing, teams can improve the medical management of head and neck injuries and thereby prevent the potential long-term consequences of these injuries. At the same time, neurosurgeons who assume the responsibilities of being a team physician must be available in order to be a contributing member of a sports medicine team. By utilizing a number of different medical specialists, teams can deliver the most effective and comprehensive medical care to ensure the safety of their players.

MAJOR ISSUES FOR CLARIFICATION

Although the day-to-day issues attendant to the practical care of the athlete are the principle charges requiring the attention of the neurosurgeon, in a much larger sense, the specialty and its resources are required to resolve problems of the comprehension of "minor" head injuries. The principle physiology of molecular issues attendant to minor head injuries, as well as their sequela, require elucidation.

Issues of prevention or reduction of head and spinal injuries in all sports are in the realm of neurosurgical expertise and authority.

Neurosurgeons deserve a role in helmet design, bench testing and ultimate clinical appraisal. From the purely clinical view, several issues demand neurosurgical attention. These include involvement in determining the true incidence of "significant head injury" (i.e., brain injury) in organized sport and the true sequela of repetitious trauma in the individual athlete. Genetic profiling such as that reported by Kutner et al. related to APOE4 would seem to be an area of important study (36). Additionally, the role of imaging assessment as baseline or postinjury assay requires definition. What is the role of SPECT, functional MRI, and variation in structural MRI study in the athlete? Does the electrophysiological study of evoked responses add a useful clinical parameter of assessment in directing therapy or clinical management? How can protective devices applied to the head, neck, and shoulder regions be improved? What is the optimum role of strength and agility training in these matters? Should rules of play be altered to provide protection regarding certain events? How can information be obtained in view of apparent conflicting interests of involved parties at various levels *(Table 17.4)*? These are only a small number of important questions in the arena of sport that require neurosurgical

TABLE 17.4
Potential Reception for Participation in Neuropsychological Assessment

Players	A, +/−	Z, +/−
Players' families	A, ++/−	A, ++/−
Coaches	A, +/−	A, +/− −
Team trainers/M.D.s	A, +	A, +/−
College administration or owners	A, +/−	Z, +/− −
Fans	A, +/−	A, +/−
Insurance companies	A, +	A, +
Players' advisors or agents	Z, +/−	Z, +/− −

From Jeffrey T. Barth: Future directions in sports related concussion. In Bailes JE, Lovell MR, Maroon JC (eds): *Sports-Related Concussion*. St. Louis: Quality Medical Publishing, 1999.
A = receptive; Z = nonreceptive; + = positive implications; − = negative implications; +/− = positive and negative implications; ++/− = more positive than negative implications; +/− − = more negative than positive implications.

expertise and energies. As noted this area provides a laboratory for progress just as the ancient Coliseum provided knowledge and answers to the inquisitive and perceptive Galen of Pergamon.

ACKNOWLEDGMENTS

The senior author is indebted to the following individuals for important counsel and information: Ed Wagner, Jr., Equipment and Locker Room Manager, New York Giants Football Club; Ronnie Barnes, Head Athletic Trainer, New York Giants Football Club; Sid Brooks, Director of Equipment Operations, University of Southern California Athletic Department.

REFERENCES

1. Abdel-Dayem H, Abu-Judeh H, Kumar M, Atay S, Naddaf S, El-Zeftawy H, Luo J: SPECT brain perfusion abnormalities in mild or moderate traumatic brain injury. **Clin Nucl Med** 23:309–317, 1998.
2. Andresen B, Hoffman M, Barton L: High School Football Injuries: field conditions and other factors. **Wisconsin Med J** 88:28–31, 1989.
3. Apuzzo M: The Legacy of Galen of Pergamon. **Neurosurg** 47:545, 2000.
4. Bailes J, Lovell M, Maroon J: *Sports-Related Concussion*. St Louis: Quality Medical Publishing, 1999.
5. Baldwin S: Intermediate filament change in astrocytes following mild cortical contusion. **Glia**, 1996.
6. Bennet, Boss, Campbell, Siwoff, Smith, Wiebusch: *The NFL's Official Encyclopedic History of Professional Football*, 1977.
7. Blyth C, Mueller F: When and where players get hurt: football injury survey, part 1. **Phys Sportsmedicine** 2:42–52, 1974.

8. Blythe C, Mueller F: An Epidemiologic Study of High School Football Injuries in North Carolina, 1968–1972, Final Report, in

9. Broggi G: The Colosseum: From an amphitheater for bloody entertainment to a monument of human endurance. **Neurosurg** 47:786–790, 2000.

10. Bull R, Cummins J: Influence of potassium on the steady-state redox potential of the electron transport chain in slices of rat cerebral cortex and the effect of ouabain. **J Neurochem** 21:923–937, 1973.

11. Cantu R: Second impact syndrome. **Clin Sports Med** 17:37–44, 1998.

12. Clarke K: An Epidemiological View of the Problem. In Torg J (ed): *Athlete Injuries to the Head, Neck, and Face*. Lea & Febiger, 1981.

13. Clarke K, Powell J: Football Helmets and Neurotrauma—An Epidemiological Overview of Three Seasons. **Medicine and Science in Sports** 11, 1979.

14. Cortez S, McIntosh T, Noble L: Experimental fluid percussion brain injury: Vascular disruption and neuronal and glial alterations. **Brain Res** 482:271–282, 1989.

15. DeKosky S, Kochanek P, Clark R, Ciallella J, Dixon C: Secondary injury after brain trauma: Subacute and long-term mechanisms. **Sem Neuropsychiatry** 3:176–185, 1998.

16. Dupuis F, Johnston K, Lavoie M, Lepore F, Lassonde M: Concussions in athletes produce brain dysfunction as revealed by event-related potentials. **Neuroreport** 11:4087–4092, 2000.

17. Finger S: Galen: The birth of experimentation. In *Minds Behind the Brain: A History of the Pioneers and Their Discoveries*. New York: Oxford University Press, 2000, pp 39–51.

18. Gaetz M: Electrophysiological indices of persistent post-concussion symptoms. **Brain Inj** 14:815–832, 2000.

19. Gennarelli T, Graham D: Neuropathology of head injuries. **Sem Neuropsychiatry** 3:160–175, 1998.

20. Giza C, Hovda D: Ionic and metabolic consequences of concussion. In Cantu R (ed): *Neurologic Athletic Head and Spine Injuries*. Philadelphia: WB Saunders, 2000, pp 80–100.

21. Goldenberg G, Oder W, Spatt J, Podreka I: Cerebral corrlates of disturbed executive function and memory in survivors of severe closed head injury: A SPECT study. **J Neurol Neurosurg Psych** 55:362–368, 1992.

22. Hicks R, Smith D, Lwenstein D: Mild experimental brain injury in the rat induces cognitive deficits associated with regional neuronal loss in the hippocampus. **J Neurotrauma** 10:405–414, 1993.

23. Hodgson V: National Operating Committee on Standards for Athletic Equipment football helmet certification program. **Med Sci Sports** 7:225–232, 1975.

24. Hofman D: Limitations of the American Academy of Neurology and American Clinical Neurophysiology Society Paper on QEEG. **J Neuropsychiatry Clin Neurosci** 11:401–405, 1999.

25. Jacobs A, Put E, Ingels M, Bossuyt A: A prospective evaluation of technetium-99m-HMPAO SPECT in mild and moderate traumatic brain injury. **J Nucl Med** 35:1891–1895, 1994.

26. Jane J, Steward O, Gennarelli T: Axonal degeneration induced by experimental noninvasive minor head injury. **J Neurosurg** 62:96–100, 1985.

27. Johnston K: A contemporary neurosurgical approach to sports-related head injury. **J Am Coll Surg** 192:515–524, 2001.

28. Jordan B: Apolipoprotein e4 associated with chronic traumatic brain injury in boxing. **J Am Med Soc** 278:136–140, 1997.

29. Julian F, Goldman D: The effects of mechanical stimulation on some electrical properties of axons. **J Gen Physiol** 46:297–313, 1962.

30. Junger E, Newell D, Grant G, Avellino AG, S, Douville C, Lam A, Aaslid R, Wihh H: Cerebral autoregulation following minor head injury. **J Neurosurg** 86:425–432, 1997.
31. Kant R: TcHMPAO SPECT in persistent post-concussion syndrome after mild head injury: comparison with MRI/CT. **Brain Inj** 11:115–124, 1997.
32. Katayama Y, Becker D, Tamura T, Hovda D: Massive increases in extracellular potassium and the indiscriminate release of glutamate following concussive brain injury. **J Neurosurg** 73:889–900, 1990.
33. Kemp P, Houston A, MacLeod M, Pethybridge R: Cerebral perfusion and psychometric testing in military amateur boxers and controls. **J Neurol Neurosurg Psychiatr** 59:368–374, 1995.
34. Kotapka M, Gennarelli T, Graham D: Selective vulnerability of hippocampal neurons in acceleration-induced experimental head injury. **J Neurotrauma** 8:247–258, 1991.
35. Kuroda Y, Inglis F, Miller J, McCulloch J, Graham D, Bullock R: Transient glucose hypermetabolism after acute subdural hematoma in the rat. **J Neurosurg** 76:471–477, 1992.
36. Kutner K, Erlanger D, Tsai J, Jordan B, Relkin N: Lower cognitive performance of older football players possessing apolipoprotein e4. **Neurosurg** 47:651–658, 2000.
37. Lyeth B: Cholinergic receptors in head trauma, in Miller L, Hayes R (eds): *Head Trauma*. New York: Wiley, 2001, pp 115–139.
38. Maddocks D, Dicker G, Saling M: The Assessment of orientation following concussion in athletes. **Clin J Sports Med** 5:32–35, 1995.
39. Maroon J, Lovell M, Norwig J, Podell K, Powell J, Hartl R: Cerebral concussion in athletes: Evaluation and neuropsychological testing. **Neurosurg** 47:659–672, 2000.
40. McGowan J: Magnetization transfer imaging in the detection of injury associated with mild head trauma. **AJNR** 21:875–880, 2000.
41. Nawashiro H, Shima K, Chigasaki H: Selective vulnerability of hippocampal CA3 neurons to hypoxia after mild concussion in the rat. **Neurol Res** 17:455–460, 1995.
42. Nilsson B, Nordstrom C: Experimental head injury in the rat. Part 2: Regional brain energy metabolism in concussive trauma. **J Neurosurg** 47:252–261, 1977.
43. Nuwer M: Assessment of digital EEG, quantitative EEG, and EEG brain mapping. **Neurology** 49:277–292, 1997.
44. Olney J, de Gubareff T, Labruyere J: Seizure-related brain amage induced by cholinergic agents. **Nature** 301:520–522, 1983.
45. Omaya A: Head injury mechanisms and the concept of preventative management: A review and critical synthesis. **J Neurotrauma** 12:527–546, 1996.
46. Oppenheimer D: Microscopic lesions in the brain following head injury. **J Neurol Neurosurg Psych** 31:299–306, 1968.
47. Parker R: *Concussive Brain Trauma*. Boca Raton: CRC Press, 2001.
48. Paulson O, Newman E: Does the release of potassium from astrocyte endfeet regulate cerebral blood flow? **Science** 237:896–898, 1987.
49. Pettus E, Christman C, Giebel M, Povlishock J: Traumatically induced altered membrane permeability: Its relationship to traumatically induced reactive axonal change. **J Neurotrauma** 11:507–522, 1994.
50. Phillips L, Lyeth B, Hamm R, Jiang J, Povlishock J, Reeves T: Effect of prior receptor antagonism on behavioral morbidity produced by combined fluid percussion injury and entorhinal cortical lesion. **J Neurosci Res** 49:197–206, 1997.
51. Povlishock J, Becker D, Miller J, Jenkins L, Dietrich W: The morphologic substrates of concussion? **Acta Neuropathol** 47:1–11, 1979.

370   CLINICAL NEUROSURGERY

52. Povlishock J, Christman C: The pathobiology of traumatic brain injury. In Salzman S, Faden A (eds): *The Neurobiology of Central Nervous System Trauma.* New York: Oxford University Press, 1994, Vol 108–120.
53. Prasad M, Dhillon H, Carbary T, Dempsey R, Scheff S: Enhanced phosphodiesteric breakdown of phosphatidylinositol biphosphate after xperimental brain injury. **J Neurochem** 63:773–776, 1994.
54. Robinson S, Martin R, Davis T, Gyenes C, Ryland J, Enters E: The effect of M1 muscarinic blockade on behavior and physiological responses following traumatic brain injury in the rat. **Brain Res** 511:141–148, 1990.
55. Sakas D: Focal cerebral hyperemia after focal head injury in humans: a benign phenomenon? **J Neurosurg** 83:277–284, 1995.
56. Samii A, Hovda D: Delayed increases in glucose utilization following cortical impact injury (abstract). **Society for Neuroscience** 12 (Suppl 1)24: 738, 1998.
57. Saunders R, Harbaugh R: The second impact syndrome in catastrophic contact-sports head trauma. **JAMA** 252:538–539, 1984.
58. Shah K, West M: The effect of concussion on cerebral uptake of 2-deoxy-D-glucose in rat. **Neurosci Lett** 40:287–291, 1983.
59. Shetter A, Damakas J: The pathophysiology of concussion: A review. In Thompson R, Green J (eds): *Advances in Neurology.* New York: Raven, 1979, Vol 22, pp 5–14.
60. Soustiel J: Trigeminal and auditory evoked responses in minor head injuries and post-concussion syndrome. **Brain Inj** 9:805–813, 1995.
61. Takahashi H, Manaka S, Sano K: Changes in extracellular potassium concentration in cortex and brain stem during the acute phase of experimental closed head injury. **J Neurosurg** 55:708–717, 1981.
62. Thompson N, Halpern B, Curl W, Andrews J, Hunter S, Boring J: High school football injuries: evaluation. **Am J Sports Med** 15:117–124, 1987.
63. Torg J, Quedenfeld T, Burstein A, Spealman A, Nichols CI: The National Football Head and Neck Injury Registry: Report on Cervical Quadriplegia. **Am J Sports Med** 7, 1979.
64. Torg J, Truex RJ, Quedenfeld T, Burstein A, Spealman A, Nichols C, III: The National Football Head and Neck Injury Registry, Report and Concussions 1978. **JAMA** 241, 1979.
65. Vink R, McIntosh T: Pharmacological and physiological effects of magnesium on experimental traumatic brain injury. **Magnes Res** 3:163–169, 1990.
66. Voller B: Neuropsychological, MRI, and EEG findings after very mild traumatic brain injury. **Brain Inj** 13:821–827, 1999.
67. Wiedman K, Wilson J, Wyper D: SPECT, cerebral blood flow, MR imaging, and neuropsychological findings in traumatic head injury. **Neuropsychology** 3:267–281, 1989.
68. Xiong Y, Gu Q, Peterson P, Muizelaar J, Lee C: Mitochondrial dysfunction and calcium perturbation induced by traumatic brain injury. **J Neurotrauma** 14:23–34, 1997.
69. Yamakami I, MacIntosh T: Effects of traumatic brain injury on regional cerebral blood flow in rats as measured with radiolabeled microspheres. **J Cereb Blood Flow Metab** 9:117–124, 1989.
70. Yuan X, Prough D, Smith T, Dewitt D: The effects of traumatic brain injury on regional cerebral blood flow in rats. **J Neurotrauma** 5:289–301, 1988.

CHAPTER

18

Kids and Sports: Frequently Asked Questions

P. DAVID ADELSON, M.D., F.A.C.S., F.A.A.P., AND KEVIN L. STEVENSON, M.D.

INTRODUCTION

Sports-related head injuries remain common in children when one considers that over 36 million children between the ages of 6 and 21 years participate in organized athletics each year (20) and countless others in nonorganized sports and recreation. Even though only a relatively small percentage of all head injuries are related to athletics (35), head injuries account for a significant percentage of the morbidity and mortality in the pediatric population. Mortality as a result of head and neck injuries has been frequent in young athletes. Upwards of 70% of traumatic deaths and 20% of permanent disabilities that occur in athletic or recreational pursuits are due to injuries to the head (17). There were 36 fatalities from football in 1968, and even with rule changes there were still 26 fatalities reported between 1985 and 1994 among high school football players alone (43). It has been reported that upwards of 5 to 20% of high school athletes will suffer a concussion each football season either in games or in practice (25).

Obviously the vast majority of participating children do not die from a head injury, but a significant number still go on to have long-term cognitive and other permanent deficits. Since neurosurgeons actively participate in the care of these injured children, it becomes obvious that the proper recognition, treatment, and prevention of head injury can impact on these young athletes. Of concern is that upwards of 100% of children with a concussive head injury were given improper discharge instructions with regard to care and return to activity (24). Regardless of age, while the majority of athletic head injuries are not life threatening and do not require hospitalization, it is important for the physician, and the allied care givers (trainers and coaches) to these young athletes to recognize the potential short- and long-term effects of head injury in children so that they can be accurately diagnosed and properly treated. This chapter will review the most frequently asked questions by parents and the child athlete that we receive in the clinic, highlighted by the mechanisms, pathophysiology (including secondary sequelae), acute management, and return-to-play guidelines for the head-injured child.

FREQUENTLY ASKED QUESTION #1

A 15-year-old male gets leveled while playing football, hit in the chest while coming through the line. He does not lose consciousness but complains of getting his "bell rung."

"Did I Suffer a Concussion?"

Concussion is the most common sequela of athletic head injury with upwards of 250,000 new concussions each year. When one considers that over 1.3 million high school students participate in organized football (44), the number and percentage of adolescents sustaining concussions is staggering. Commonly described as "getting your bell rung," concussion is often treated as a minor consequence of athletics. While considerable disagreement exists regarding the definition of a concussion, a frequently cited definition is that of the Committee of Head Injury Nomenclature of the Congress of Neurological Surgeons (1966). They defined concussion as "a clinical syndrome characterized by immediate and transient post-traumatic impairment of neural functions, such as alteration of consciousness, disturbance of vision, equilibrium, etc. due to brainstem involvement" (19). Since that time, numerous other descriptions and definitions have been put forth, but despite any differences in wording, the cardinal feature of every concussion is *an alteration in mental status with or without loss of consciousness*. A concussion in the athlete is almost universally characterized by confusion and amnesia to some degree, which may require close examination to detect in the mildest of cases. A simple rule is that any athlete who has lost consciousness, no matter how brief, has suffered a concussion (52). Other potential and cardinal features of a concussion include headache, disorientation, a blank stare, slurred speech, delayed verbal responses to questions, slow and uncoordinated motor function, dizziness, emotional lability, and short-term memory deficits.

To better understand the pathophysiologic sequelae of concussive injury, experimental models have been used to show that neuronal dysfunction in the brainstem reticular activating system, cerebral ischemia, edema, neuronal depolarization with widespread acetylcholine release, neuronal disruption, and brainstem capillary damage (26, 52) may contribute to the clinical symptomatology. Further work has shown that on a cellular/biochemical level, increased neurotransmitter release resulting in significant extracellular glutamate leads to increased extracellular potassium via ligand-gated potassium channels

(33), which can have diffuse effects with what has been termed "spreading depression." At the same time, intracellular calcium rises (22), which with the increased potassium flux leads to membrane destabilization and a subsequent rise in the energy demands (hypermetabolism) of the cell in an attempt to restore homeostasis. These energy demands are initially dependent on anaerobic glycolysis with a resultant lactic acidosis (55), but within 24 hours the brain enters a phase of metabolic depression lasting upwards of 10 days (56). During this period, protein synthesis is also diminished, leading to an overall state of cerebral depression (1). These cellular post-concussive derangements likely contribute to the clinical findings in post-concussive syndrome, including altered mental status, concentration difficulties, neuropsychological deficits, and the potential for a second-impact syndrome (9). It is important to stress that there is no such thing as a minor head injury, and a concussion, no matter how "minor," is a head injury with potential long-term consequences.

FREQUENTLY ASKED QUESTION #2
"How Can I Suffer a Concussion Without Hitting My Head?"

The acute brain injury or concussion generally results from forces applied either directly to the head, or indirectly to the head and/or body leading to deformation or disruption of the neural functions and/or tissue. These forces are categorized as focal impact, linear (translational) acceleration, angular (rotational) acceleration, or a combination of these forces to cause injury. The extent of the injury is not just dependent on the amount of the force but the degrees or angles of the transmitted force and the duration of the impact.

FOCAL IMPACT

Focal impact is a force that results in the maximal stress being applied at the point of contact. This type of force usually leads to skull fractures and injury to the structures (brain parenchyma, blood vessels, dura) directly underlying the point of applied force. Although the focal injury can be severe, distant neural structures are commonly spared due to the CSF cushioning effect and the dissipation of the force by the skull.

LINEAR ACCELERATION

Linear acceleration injury occurs when force is applied in a vector perpendicular to the skull (e.g., a direct blow/jab to the face during a boxing match) (1). The applied force is transmitted to the brain causing tensile and compressive forces within the brain. Because the brain is "floating" in cerebrospinal fluid (CSF), the brain can accelerate and/or decelerate relative to the skull resulting in impact with the skull at the site of impact (coup) and/or opposite the site of impact (contre-coup). In addition, as the brain accelerates or decelerates within the skull, the rough surface of the skull base can impart injury to the parenchyma as it moves across these bony structures. Most vulnerable to skull base injury are the frontal lobes in the anterior fossa and the temporal lobes in the middle fossa. The brain, in part due to the cushioning effect of CSF, better tolerates this type of force.

ANGULAR ACCELERATION

Angular acceleration injury is caused from rapid turning of the head, resulting in a shearing force that can be transmitted deep within the brain parenchyma and brainstem (e.g., a blow to the jaw crossing punch during a boxing match). This type of force is poorly tolerated by the brain and is maximal where rotation is impaired by dural attachments to the skull: the falx cerebri and tentorium cerebelli. Impaired rotation at these structures leads to increased shearing forces being imparted to the adjacent brainstem and corpus callosum. Depending on the magnitude of the applied force, angular acceleration can lead to a variety of injuries ranging from mild concussion to death.

Two points should be kept in mind regarding the effects of forces applied to the brain. First, injury due to brain acceleration (angular or linear) does not require direct head impact (38). For example, a force applied to the chest or body can generate brain acceleration through a whiplash effect of the cervical spine. Second, acceleration of the brain is lessened if the athlete is prepared for the oncoming force by contracting the cervical musculature. This occurs because the contracted cervical musculature renders the mass of the head essentially that of the entire body and lessens the potential acceleration imparted directly or indirectly to the head (13).

FREQUENTLY ASKED QUESTION #3

A 13-year-old girl gets hit in the head with a line drive. She is knocked out for about 30 seconds and then comes around.

"How Bad a Concussion Did I Get?"

In an attempt to stratify the severity of concussions, multiple grading schemes have been developed (3, 15, 18, 51). Although no one grading system is universally accepted, they all provide the physician, trainer, and coach with a reproducible means of identifying a concussion and advising a young athlete when it is safe to return to play. Most use a 3 grade scale of mild, moderate, and severe with different criteria for severity. We will refer to the Cantu Concussion Grading Scale for convention for this chapter (12, 13, 14, 15) *(Table 18.1)*.

The vast majority of concussions (>90%) are Grade 1 or mild concussions (14, 15) and result in no loss of consciousness (LOC) and less than 30 minutes of post-traumatic amnesia (PTA). Despite their relative frequency, Grade 1 concussions are often the most difficult to detect. The young athlete, often unaware of the serious nature of such an injury, may only be momentarily stunned, take a moment, and then continue playing, at times not even leaving the contest. In these situations, it is often a teammate that notices the subtle changes or alteration in concentration in the injured athlete such as forgetting the snap count or not leaving the ice expeditiously for a line change. Coaches and/or trainers may discount this behavior as a consequence of a "good hit" and keep the child in the contest. Of concern, discounting the mildest of mental status changes that can occur following a minor head injury, is that there can be lethal consequences in these situations.

A Grade 2 or moderate concussion occurs when the injury results in a (LOC) of less than 5 minutes or PTA that lasts longer than 5 minutes but less than 24 hours. Because Grade 2 concussions involve a

TABLE 18.1
Concussion Grading Scales

	Grade 1 (Mild)	Grade 1a	Grade 2 (Moderate)	Grade 3 (Severe)	Grade 4
Cantu (13)	No LOC or PTA <30 min		LOC <5 mins, PTA 30 min–24 hrs	LOC >5 mins, PTA >24 hrs	
Colorado (18)	No LOC, confusion without amnesia		No LOC, confusion with amnesia	LOC	
AAN (3)	No LOC, symptoms <15 mins		No LOC, symptoms >15 mins	LOC	
Torg (51)	No LOC/amnesia (PTA allowed) [Grade I–II]		LOC < few mins, PTA or retrograde amnesia [Grade III–IV]	LOC with coma, confusion, amnesia [Grade V–VI]	

LOC = Loss of consciousness,
PTA = Post-traumatic amnesia,
GCS = Glasgow coma scale score

definite LOC, they are most often easier to detect than the Grade 1 concussion. A Grade 3 or severe concussion is one in which the LOC is for more than 5 minutes or PTA persists beyond 24 hours.

ACUTE INJURY ASSESSMENT

The first step in assessing the potentially head-injured athlete is recognizing that a head injury has occurred. This process is relatively easy in the unconscious athlete; it is the child that walks off the field under his or her own power that presents the larger challenge. It has been reported that 70% of football players who are "knocked out" during play, return to the game the same day (2), possibly due, in part, to lack of recognition of the head injury.

Given the often subtle nature of Grade 1 concussions, a high index of suspicion is required to correctly evaluate and manage these injuries. Any player who is slow to get up after impact, shows any gait change, shows impaired judgment or cognitive function, or "just doesn't seem right" should be examined in detail. It is critical to recognize these subtle changes as soon as possible as the PTA is commonly short-lived and objective memory testing may fail to reveal the true nature of the injury even minutes after injury.

FREQUENTLY ASKED QUESTION #4

*"How Do I Assess How Badly Injured the Child Is
Who Is Awake and Seemingly Alert?"*

The single most important acute assessment to be made in the head injured athlete is the level of consciousness. The Glasgow Coma Scale (GCS) is a rapid, reproducible means of determining the severity of central nervous system (CNS) dysfunction (50). In addition to providing an immediate post-injury gauge of consciousness, the GCS score allows the athlete's neurologic status to be followed in a standardized manner. The GCS is a scale scored on a 3 to 15 scale with 3 being the worst injured and 15 being normal based on best motor, verbal, and eye functions at the time of testing. A GCS of 8 or less denotes a severe brain injury and should prompt rapid transport to a neurosurgical center. GCS 9–12 denotes a moderate injury, and a GCS of 13–15 denotes a mild brain injury. A GCS of 13–15 indicates an arouseable though potentially confused individual. Prognostically, a GCS of 12 or greater is associated with a more than 90% chance of complete recovery while a score of 4 or less predicts an 80% chance of death or persistent vegetative state (13).

As mentioned, confusion and amnesia are common features of even the most mild of head injuries, and should be accurately assessed and should include orientation to person, place, time, and situation. This is often referred in the record as "Alert and oriented x 4". In the head-injured athlete, two distinct forms of amnesia are commonly seen and may coexist. *Anterograde* amnesia is manifested as a difficulty with memory consolidation with or without preserved immediate registration and recall. Answers to questions such as, "Who helped you off the field?" or "How did you get off the ice?" are more useful for the assessment of anterograde amnesia than digit recall or reverse spelling. *Retrograde* amnesia is present when the athlete loses memory for events occurring prior to the injury, most commonly in the immediate period prior to injury. To test for retrograde amnesia, questions such as, "What is the score?" or "Who are you guarding?" should be utilized.

Every head-injured athlete should be assumed to have a co-existing cervical spine injury until proven otherwise, particularly since they may have an altered level of consciousness and not participate in the assessment. If the child has no neck pain while relaxed, an exam of cervical range of motion attempts to elicit any dynamic pain. In addition and obviously, a rapid, but thorough, neurologic exam should be performed when there is a suspicion of head injury as soon after the injury as possible. Although a comprehensive neurologic examination on the sidelines is impossible, and unnecessary, a global assessment of neurologic function can be determined in 1 to 2 minutes without the need for any specific equipment. It is again worth stressing that the level of consciousness is the most critical component of the brief neurologic exam. Following are some simple tests to assess neurologic function that can be performed in the field.

Cranial nerve (CN) deficits can occur in conjunction with basilar skull fracture, intracranial mass lesions, and upper cervical spine injury, and while it is unnecessary to perform an in-depth cranial nerve examination in the field, a screen of key cranial nerves is critical and can be performed rapidly in the conscious athlete. Vision (CN II) is assessed by asking to count fingers. Diplopia and dysconjugate gaze often follow fractures of the skull base and/or orbit and anomalies of eye movement (CN III, IV, VI) are tested by moving the fingers throughout the field of vision. Facial nerve (CN VII) function is particularly vulnerable to trauma at several points along its course through the temporal bone and face and can be assessed by asking the athlete to smile and to forcibly close his eyes. A peripheral (outside the CNS) CN VII injury will affect both the upper and lower face ipsilateral to the injury, while a central CN VII injury will cause weakness of the lower face only. CN VIII is tested by whispering a simple word or number into each ear and asking the child to repeat what he/she hears. Temporal bone fractures causing hearing loss are also commonly associated with an ipsilateral facial nerve deficit. CN XI has both an intra- and extracranial course and injury to the accessory nerve can follow either head or upper cervical spine injury. CN XI is assessed by asking the athlete to shrug his/her shoulders against resistance. The other cranial nerves that are difficult to assess in the field include CN I (olfactory) which commonly is injured following anterior skull base fractures. CN V, IX, X, and XII are less commonly involved in minor injuries.

A brief motor examination can be performed by testing for pronator drift (upper motor neuron injury), biceps strength (C5–6), triceps (C7–8), iliopsoas (L2–3), quadriceps (L3–4), ankle dorsiflexion and toe extension (L4–5), and ankle plantar flexion (S1). Head injury leading to objective motor deficits typically manifests as a contralateral mono- or hemiparesis rather than weakness of an isolated muscle group. Isolated biceps paresis with intact triceps motor power, for example, should lead the examiner to investigate the cervical spine as the source of the pathology rather than the brain. A brief sensory examination can easily be performed by stroking key dermatomes bilaterally with the fingers. In a cursory examination, key areas to test include the shoulders (C4), thumbs (C6), anterior thorax at the level of the nipples (T5), abdomen at the level of the umbilicus (T9–10), medial knee (L4), great toe (L5), and lateral foot (S1). Similar to motor findings, sensory deficits secondary to head injury typically manifest as crossed mono- or hemihypesthesia, isolated sensory loss in a purely dermatomal pattern is more indicative of nerve root injury, sensory loss across several dermatomes may be seen in peripheral nerve injury, and a sensory level (hypesthesia beginning at a dermatomal level and extending caudally) suggests a spinal cord injury. In the acute setting, pinprick, temperature, vibration, and proprioception testing are rarely necessary.

Gait testing as an assessment of cerebellar function can be performed by having the athlete walk off the field and observing his/her gait. Any deviation from normal gait should alert trainers and physicians to the possibility of head injury. A more thorough and global assessment of cerebellar function can be obtained by finger to nose testing using the fingertip of the examiner and the tip of the athlete's nose rapidly alternating between fingertip and nose looking for dysmetria.

Obviously, a significant injury has occurred if there is neurologic dysfunction. For the majority of concussive injuries, it is simple observation of the athlete that provides the most insight into the extent of injury. Slurred speech, difficulty finding words or word substitutions, and fluent speech devoid of meaning are all signs of CNS dysfunction. Asymmetry in the spontaneous use of the extremities may indicate injury to the contralateral motor cortex, while inattention to sound on one side of the body may be seen following temporal bone fracture involving the middle ear structures or cochlear nerve. In short, any finding that deviates from normal is due to head injury until proven otherwise.

FREQUENTLY ASKED QUESTION #5

A 17-year-old football player goes head first into the line and suffers a helmet-to-helmet contact. When everyone has gotten up, he is found still down unconscious.

"How Should the Unconscious Athlete Be Treated?"

It is not uncommon for the initially unconscious athlete to rapidly regain consciousness. It should be kept in mind that the unconscious athlete may have only suffered a mild concussion, while the child who walks off of the field awake may be developing a life-threatening intracranial hematoma (41). As with the conscious athlete, anyone rendered unconscious *has a cervical spine injury until proven otherwise.* Until the cervical spine can be cleared, neck immobilization and stabilization must be maintained. As with any traumatic injury, the first priorities are the ABCs: Airway, Breathing, and Circulation. If the athlete is wearing a helmet, *it should be left on until the spine is clinically and/or radiographically cleared.* If it necessary to gain access to the athletes face to secure the airway, leave the helmet in place and remove the face mask (with bolt cutters, if necessary). In the rare situation where the helmet must be removed, it is done with extreme caution and in-line stabilization with removal of shoulder pads at the same time. Helmet removal without removal of shoulder pads leaves the cervical spine in extension, which can lead to cervical cord injury (49). The use of ammonia inhalants is strongly discouraged as the severe irritation of the nasal mucosa may cause the athlete to rapidly extend his or her neck. All unconscious athletes must be expeditiously transported to a medical facility with neurosurgical and neuroradiologic capability. It is best to coordinate a plan for the transport of a head-injured athlete prior to the event. Once the ABCs have been assessed and stabilized, the athlete should be log-rolled onto a spine board, secured, and taken to the predetermined facility, ideally with physician escort.

FREQUENTLY ASKED QUESTION #6

A 14-year-old hockey player loses consciousness after a check into the boards. He is transported to the hospital where he regains consciousness but is found to have a small subdural hematoma on CT scan.

"How Serious Is It When There Is Blood in the Head?"

SUBDURAL HEMATOMA

Acute subdural hematomas are the leading cause of death in athletes (44), with an approximate incidence three times that of acute epidural hematoma (52). Between 1945 and 1994, 352 football players died from acute subdural hematomas, the majority of them at the high school level (43). Acute subdural hematomas result (most commonly) from laceration of a vein traversing the space between the dura and cortex, and less commonly from a dural sinus or cortical artery laceration. As such, the hematoma forms directly on the brain surface. Because of the force necessary to produce a subdural hematoma, the underlying brain is often injured. As the hematoma enlarges, often rapidly, a mass lesion forms compressing and further injuring the underlying brain. Untreated, acute subdural hematomas can lead to coma and death from herniation-induced brainstem dysfunction with a mortality rate of 30 to 40% even with expert neurosurgical treatment (16). The athlete with an acute subdural hematoma is typically unconscious after injury, and usually does not regain consciousness. Focal neurologic signs, if not present immediately, may appear rapidly in the form of hemiparesis, aphasia, unilateral pupillary dilatation, or other focal finding. In the comatose athlete, a "blown pupil" may be the first finding suggestive of the intracranial mass lesion. In many athletes, the symptoms of acute subdural hematoma are due to the underlying brain injury rather than the compressive effects of the hematoma (11). Given the lethal nature of subdural hematomas, an unconscious athlete should be transported to a neurosurgical center for CT imaging and emergent craniotomy for the evacuation of the subdural hematoma as needed. Even if the mass lesion is emergently evacuated, the morbidity and mortality of subdural hematomas are high due to the associated brain injury.

Chronic subdural hematomas can develop in athletes who incur a subdural hematoma that is not recognized and/or surgically evacuated. In these instances the injury to the underlying brain is minimal and the athlete did not have significant symptoms at the time of injury. Over a period of weeks, the clot is broken down into a viscous "motor oil" fluid that expands and compresses the underlying brain. Any athlete suffering a "minor" head injury that did not require imaging who complains of persistent headache, nausea, or lethargy and/or develops a delayed focal neurologic finding (pronator drift, aphasia, etc.) should undergo CT scanning despite the length of time following the injury.

EPIDURAL HEMATOMA

Classically associated with skull fractures, epidural hematomas are the most rapidly progressing intracranial hemorrhage. The meningeal arteries lie just under, and often partially imbedded within, the inner table of the skull. A skull fracture can tear one or more of these vessels and lead to formation of a hematoma in the extradural space. The most common scenario involves a temporal bone fracture lacerating the middle meningeal artery, but epidural hematomas can occur in any location and can on occasion be secondary to venous bleeding. In younger children, epidural hematomas can even occur from bleeding from the skull itself without laceration of a meningeal vessel (52). The classically described presentation of an epidural hematoma is an immediate loss of consciousness after traumatic impact due to concussion, followed by consciousness being regained (the so-called "lucid interval"). After a period of consciousness lasting minutes to hours, the patient lapses into coma and suffers a herniation syndrome with an ipsilateral pupillary dilatation and contralateral hemiparesis or posturing due to the expanded hematoma and cerebral shift. This classic scenario is present in only 33% of patients, however (11). As previously mentioned, the epidural hematoma accumulates rapidly, producing lethal consequences in as little as 15 to 30 minutes (14, 15). The emergent need for neurosurgical intervention cannot be overstated, and a high index of suspicion is required to correctly diagnose and treat this mass lesion. Although epidural hematomas can be rapidly fatal, a good outcome can be expected if craniotomy and evacuation is performed expeditiously as the injury to the brain itself is generally minimal or altogether absent (11).

SUBARACHNOID HEMORRHAGE

Trauma is the most common cause of subarachnoid hemorrhage (SAH) which is the most common type of intracranial hemorrhage (53). The majority of instances of SAH are due to a laceration of small cortical surface vessels. Depending of the severity of the impact, consciousness may or may not be lost but the child will often complain of severe headache with a finding of nuchal rigidity secondary to meningeal irritation. Traumatic SAH, in and of itself, does not cause mass effect, and surgical intervention is not required unless the hemorrhage extends into the ventricular system causing hydrocephalus. A SAH secondary to an intracranial aneurysm or arteriovenous malformation rupture should be considered in the differential diagnosis of this form of intracranial hemorrhage, even in the setting of athletic trauma, particularly if the amount of blood is out of proportion to the injury or is the pattern of blood is fairly focal to a circle of Willis location. Any suspicion of a vascular anomaly should prompt angiography to exclude their presence.

CEREBRAL CONTUSION

Cerebral contusions can be thought of as a "bruise" of the brain parenchyma. Contusions can occur in the setting of skull fracture, especially a depressed fracture, whereby the bone is forced inward making focal impact with the cortical surface. Because the brain, floating in CSF, has the ability to move independently within the cranium, acceleration/deceleration forces can cause the brain to impact the inner table of the skull without fracture. Sudden deceleration of the head, as when a falling athlete's head makes impact with the playing surface causes the brain to impact the skull directly under the point of impact. The most common locations of contusions are the frontal, temporal, and occipital poles. Although resolution without surgical intervention is the typical course, cerebral contusions can enlarge and coalesce ("blossom") over the first 24 to 48 hours, leading to focal mass effect and sudden neurologic decline, particularly if located in the temporal lobe or cerebellum. Prompt neurosurgical evaluation and observation is mandatory for all athletes suffering a contusion.

DIFFUSE AXONAL INJURY

Diffuse axonal injury (DAI) is a primary injury produced by rotational acceleration/deceleration of the brain (23). Rotational forces cause shearing of multiple axons, widespread white matter axonal damage, and discrete focal hemorrhagic lesions in the corpus callosum and rostral brainstem. Most commonly associated with severe head injury during motor vehicle accidents, DAI is occasionally seen in athletic head injury. DAI renders the athlete immediately comatose following injury, with an absence of focal neurologic deficits (assuming there is no associated intracranial mass lesion). Immediate CT imaging is indicated, and typically fails to show any major abnormality, though occasionally petechial hemorrhages can be appreciated in the subcortical areas. MRI is confirmatory in these instances, often showing discrete lesions in the corpus callosum and brainstem.

SKULL FRACTURE

Common in the pediatric population, a skull fracture may lessen or prevent significant injury to the underlying brain by dissipating the force of impact. Skull fractures can be divided into four general categories: linear, depressed, basilar, and open. Linear fractures, the most common skull fracture in children (27), require no immediate treatment. Most are found incidentally during imaging directed at discovering intracranial mass lesions. Basilar skull fractures are linear fractures occurring or involving the skull base. Basilar fractures differ from calvarial fractures in that they often involve the numerous vascular and nervous structures that are intimately involved with the skull base. Some common associated injuries include carotid artery injury (dissection, carotid-cavernous sinus fistula, etc.), cranial nerve palsy/injury (especially CN I, II, VI, VII, and VIII), CSF leak (CSF otorrhea, rhinorrhea), and meningitis (from fracture through an air sinus). Signs, which may take hours to develop, include CSF rhinorrhea and/or otorrhea, postauricular ecchymoses (Battle's sign), periorbital ecchymoses (raccoon's eyes), hemotympanum, anosmia, facial palsy, deafness, and extraocular muscle palsy.

Depressed skull fractures involve displacement of the skull or skull fragments inward. Although most depressed skull fractures will heal spontaneously, immediate neurosurgical evaluation is required to determine if the fracture should be elevated. Indications to elevate a depressed skull fracture include an open laceration, depression greater than or equal to 10 mm, neurologic deficit related to underlying brain, CSF leak due to dural laceration, or depression in a cosmetically obvious location (i.e., forehead). Open skull fractures, by definition, involve interruption of the scalp overlying the fracture. Surgical debridement and irrigation is often required if the wound or brain is contaminated and all patients will undergo a period of antibiotic therapy.

FREQUENTLY ASKED QUESTION #7

A 15-year-old rugby player loses consciousness after taking an elbow to the head, suffering a Grade 2 concussion. Ten minutes later on the sideline, he is neurologically intact, awake, and alert.

"Why Is Not a Good Idea for Him to Return to the Match?"

The majority of children who suffer a sports-related head injury will recover without permanent morbidity. With adequate time away from contact sports, and understanding on the part of parents, coaches, and educators, the concussion resolves. Even the mildest of concussions, however, carries with it the risk of post-traumatic complications, including death. The potential life-threatening complications are either due to second-impact syndrome (SIS) or malignant cerebral swelling (MCS). The onset is often rapid with little warning and there is often little that can be done. While SIS is a devastating condition that for the most part is preventable, MCS is believed not to be preventable since it can occur even following a seemingly minor primary head injury.

SECOND IMPACT SYNDROME

First described in 1973 (47), the term "second-impact syndrome" was coined by Saunders and Harbaugh in 1984 (46) and occurs when an athlete suffers an initial head injury, followed by a second, often trivial, head injury prior to the resolution of the first. The second injury need not even involve a blow to the head, but only sufficient force to cause a secondary head acceleration/deceleration that rapidly leads to a sequence of events that can lead to sudden death (16). Following the second injury, the player typically remains conscious, but may appear initially dazed, as if suffering from a Grade 1 concussion. Within seconds to minutes, the player collapses and becomes rapidly comatose with a progression of brainstem signs including pupillary dilation, posturing, and respiratory arrest. Often prior to even being removed from the playing field, the player is moribund or dead. The feature that differentiates SIS from an intracranial hematoma is the rapidity in which the player deteriorates, often within minutes.

The mechanism of SIS is not completely understood, but is thought to occur due to loss of cerebral autoregulation (16). In SIS, the autoregulatory mechanisms of the cerebral vasculature fail and an abnormally high blood volume enters the cerebral vasculature leading to a rise in intracranial pressure and an often fatal herniation syndrome. Management of SIS requires rapid transport of the athlete to a neurosurgical center where a head CT usually shows a tremendously edematous brain and usually little more. Measures to control increased ICP are often futile, and 50% of athletes with SIS die secondary to brainstem compromise (16). Survivors have a nearly 100% certainty of severe neurologic morbidity (16). Due to the grave prognosis, and the often inefficacy of treatment, the best management scheme for SIS is prevention. Under no circumstance should an athlete return to play or practice until he or she is absolutely symptom-free and even then, serious consideration should be given to sitting out for a period of time to ensure resolution. Because SIS is preventable, educating coaches, players, and parents about this catastrophic complication of head injury should be an integral part of organized athletics.

MALIGNANT CEREBRAL SWELLING

Unique to the pediatric population, malignant cerebral swelling (MCS) is a secondary phenomenon of head injury and is often delayed in presentation. The primary pathophysiology of MCS is likely similar to that of SIS: intracerebral vascular engorgement. But what differentiates this syndrome from SIS is that MCS can occur after the first head injury. Typically, the child athlete sustains a head injury, such as a Grade 2 concussion that seemingly resolves. Within minutes to several hours, the initially awake and alert athlete undergoes rapid progressive neurologic deterioration that can culminate in coma and death due to herniation (16). Diffuse cerebral hyperemia and/ or cerebral edema, rather than a focal intracranial mass lesion, is believed responsible for the potentially lethal rise in ICP (37, 42). Although uncommon (48), this phenomenon can be rapidly fatal if not properly identified. Any young athlete who sustains any head injury, no matter how minor, must be observed by a responsible adult for the remainder of the day and/or evening, as immediate neurosurgical intervention aimed at lowering ICP is required as soon as neurologic deterioration is first detected (1).

FREQUENTLY ASKED QUESTION #8

A 12-year-old linebacker suffers a Grade I concussion after tackling an opponent. He is taken out of the game and 5 minutes later on the sideline, he is neurologically intact, awake, and alert on testing at rest and on exertion.

"Can He Return to the Game?"

Following a concussive injury, the question arises and is a concern for the physician, trainer, and/or coach is whether to allow the child to return to competition. The reality is that most young athletes do not have a financial or vocational stake in their ability to return to the playing field, either immediately to an ongoing match or to future contests. Although there are a few types and severities of injury that would be a contraindication to a return to contact sports, most children can expect to be able to return to athletics in some capacity after a period of recovery. The timing of a return to athletics is based on several factors. These include the severity of the injury and the existence of persistent symptoms.

IMMEDIATE RETURN TO ACTIVITY

The athlete suspected of having a Grade 1 concussion should be immediately removed from the contest and closely observed on the bench. If, after a brief period of time and at rest, the athlete should be questioned for headache, dizziness, impaired cognition and an accurate recall of the events without retrograde amnesia. If the child is neurologically cleared and symptom-free at rest, they should then be tested under exertion performing several sprints and a series of push-ups in an attempt to elicit neurologic symptoms of the concussion and to evaluate motor control, speed, and dexterity. If exertion fails to bring about any change in the neurologic exam, a return to the contest can be considered though as noted above, not recommended (15, 40). The decision to send an athlete back in to the contest is best made by a physician and is probably ill advised below the college level. If neurologic symptoms persist, either at rest or with exertion, the athlete is forbidden to play in the remainder of the contest but can be observed temporarily on the bench. Frequent neurologic exams should be performed during this time until symptoms disappear or 1 hour has passed. If at neurologic baseline within the hour, less frequent intervals of observation should be performed by a parent or responsible adult for several additional hours. In most cases, minimally persistent symptoms for less than an hour do not require evaluation or admission to the hospital. Any athlete who continues to have symptoms beyond 1 hour, or who develops any decline in exam should be immediately transferred to a medical center for neurosurgical evaluation and imaging.

Young athletes meeting criteria for either a Grade 2 or 3 concussion should be treated in addition to their head injury as though they have an unstable cervical spine. For that reason precautions of care and management need to be considered. Assuming an adequate airway, the neck is immobilized and the child should be removed from the playing field on a spine board with any helmet or headgear *left in place*. Airway concerns should be managed as discussed earlier. If the athlete regains consciousness and their sensorium is such that a reliable spine exam can be accomplished to clear the spine, the degree of immobilization may be lessened though in most cases, the injured player's mental status prohibits such actions. Every athlete sustaining a Grade 2 or 3 concussion should be transferred to a trauma center for evaluation and imaging of the head and cervical spine even if consciousness is quickly regained. In most cases close observation in the acute period will elicit the possible delayed presentation of intracranial hemorrhage and/or contusion (31). If the child has a negative radiologic exam, is a GCS 14—15, has easy access back to the emergency department, and will be under the care of a responsible adult, then discharge home for observation can be considered. Any questions though, and the child should be admitted overnight to ensure clearance. With very few exceptions, all athletes with a Grade 3 concussion should be admitted for neurologic observation overnight. Any patient with persistent headache, nausea, vomiting, or confusion, or any decline in exam should prompt a second CT scan, as microhemorrhages can coalesce with time, forming a symptomatic contusion (15).

FREQUENTLY ASKED QUESTION #9

A 15-year-old field hockey player gets hit in the head with a stick and is knocked out. She is taken to the local emergency department and awakens. She tests out neurologically intact, awake, and alert. She returns for follow-up 10 days later, asymptomatic.

"When Can She Return to Practice and Competition?"

While there is no such thing as a minor head injury, the major risk associated with returning to competition too early after concussion is death from second-impact syndrome, a risk that can be essentially prevented with proper time away from athletics. As such, no athlete with any symptoms following head injury should participate in any form of athletics, no matter how mild the injury. It is also known that concussions are "cumulative" in nature (28, 29), stressing the importance of prevention. It is important to accurately grade the concussion at the time of injury, as return-to-play guidelines are based on this grade.

Unlike lacerations, bruises, and fractures, head injuries related to sports often leave no external reminder to the young athlete that they have been injured. Very often athletes feel "normal" within days of their injury, and this is when many young athletes will attempt to return to their sport. With the potential for severe morbidity and mortality from a second head injury in the recovery period, it is critical to educate young athletes and their parents about the consequences of returning to play too early. In addition, physicians, coaches, trainers, and educators need to be educated about athletic head injury so as not to allow a head-injured athlete to participate in sports before it is safe to do so. Unfortunately, when a child is hospitalized for concussion, guidelines for return to athletics are often incorrect or not given. In one study, only 30.3% of young athletes hospitalized with a Grade 1 concussion received appropriate discharge instruction for return to play, Grade 2 patients received the correct guidelines only 20% of the time, and no patient with a Grade 3 concussion received appropriate instructions (24).

Return-to-Play Guidelines After Concussion (See Table 18.2)

GRADE 1 CONCUSSION

With a persistently symptomatic Grade 1 concussion, including head-ache, disequilibrium, lightheadedness, or other symptom, the athlete should not practice or compete, regardless of how he or she feels. If there was normal radiologic imaging, the child can be followed until symptoms clear. Once the athlete is asymptomatic at rest and with exertion for a minimum of 7 days, return to practice is permis-

TABLE 18.2

Concussion Return-to-Play Guidelines *(modified for the young athlete from Bailes and Cantu (6))*

	First Concussion	Second Concussion	Third Concussion
Grade 1	No activity 7 days, RTP if asymptomatic, No activity if MR positive for abnormality	No activity 4 weeks, RTP if asymptomatic last 7 days	Terminate current season, no activity in next season, RTP after following season if asymptomatic
Grade 2	No activity 4 weeks, RTP if asymptomatic last 7 days	Terminate season, no activity in next season, RTP after following season	No activity 1 year, recommend/ban contact sports) after 1 year
Grade 3	No activity 4 weeks, RTP if asymptomatic last 7 days	Terminate season, Recommend/ban contact sports, RTP (non-contact sports) after following season	Terminate season, ban contact sports, RTP (non-contact sports) after 1 year

RTP = return to play.

Authors' Note: These guidelines for return to play are more conservative than the recommendations through the referenced article, again taking into account the young athlete whose financial and vocational future are not dependent on his/ her participation.

sible. It is recommended that the player return in a practice situation for a further 7 days rather than competition to allow closer individual observation and to eliminate the potential for the child to neglect, or not report, neurologic symptoms. A second Grade 1 concussion during the same season removes the athlete from practice and competition for a minimum of 4 weeks. Return to play can only occur if the child has been absolutely asymptomatic for the final 7 days of their time off. During this time off, in-depth examination of the factors surrounding the concussions should take place, with problems identified and corrected. For example, poor neck strength may have contributed to the concussions, and a program of isometric neck strengthening can be implemented. Equipment inspection may reveal an improperly fitted helmet or the need for a neck roll. Finally, review of game films may reveal improper technique such as spearing during tackling. A third Grade 1 concussion during the same season removes the athlete from all athletics for the remainder of that season, as well as the following season. If, after two seasons, the player is asymptomatic, a return to sports is allowed. Note that two seasons does not mean 2 years; a third concussion during the fall football season would end the football season and the athlete would not be allowed to compete in the winter hockey season, but could participate in spring baseball if asymptomatic. Again, an in-depth analysis of the circumstances surrounding the concussions should take place.

GRADE 2 CONCUSSION

The young athlete with a Grade 2 concussion should not be allowed to participate in athletics for a period of 4 weeks. If, during the final week, the athlete is asymptomatic at both rest and with exertion, a return to practice is permitted, with a return to competition allowed if the athlete has no symptoms or difficulties during practice. A second Grade 2 concussion during the same season postpones a return to play until the next season. If the decision is made to allow the child to return to competition, the athlete must be free of symptoms for the 7 days preceding a return. Although some controversy exists regarding a same-season return to play after a second Grade 2 concussion, it is highly recommended (mandatory by the authors) to terminate the season. A third Grade 2 concussion in the same year (not just season) terminates sports for 1 year, and the athlete is not allowed future participation in contact sports. In addition, an athlete who has a history of several (three or more) Grade 2 concussions over two or more seasons should also be prohibited from contact sports. A ban from contact sports does not preclude athletic participation; track, tennis, golf, chess team, or other non-contact sports should be encouraged.

GRADE 3 CONCUSSION

After sustaining a Grade 3 concussion, the young athlete is prohibited from athletic practice and competition for a minimum of 1 month. A return can be considered if the athlete has been absolutely asymptomatic, both at rest and with exertion, for the 7 days prior to return after 1 month. A second Grade 3 concussion terminates the season, and should, in most cases, preclude future participation in contact athletics. In some circumstances, a return to contact sports can be considered after sitting out the current and following season, but a ban on contact sports is recommended. If allowed to return to contact sports in the future, a third concussion of any grade should place an absolute ban on future contact athletics.

Return-to-Play Guidelines After Moderate to Severe Head/ Brain Injury

Due to the residual effects commonly seen after severe head injury (spasticity, paresis, cognitive deficits, etc.), a return to athletics is often impossible. This holds especially true following DAI, MCS, and SIS where permanent neurologic disability is the norm. It is common practice to prevent any athlete who has had intracranial surgery for a head injury from returning to contact sports (34). Two possible exceptions include epidural hematomas and depressed skull fractures requiring surgical elevation. In these cases, with complete neurological recovery a return to contact sports can be considered after 1 year. Careful consideration should be given, however, since the bone at the area of surgery is not full thickness and it is recommended that all but select special cases not return to contact athletics.

There are five conditions that directly contraindicate a return to contact sports (15):

1. The presence of any postconcussion symptom
2. Permanent neurologic deficit following head injury
3. Hydrocephalus
4. Spontaneous subarachnoid hemorrhage from any cause
5. Symptomatic abnormality at the foramen magnum

In addition, any young athlete sustaining a cerebral contusion or nonsurgical intracerebral hemorrhage should also be banned from returning to contact athletics. While these last two conditions are not absolute contraindications to contact athletics, serious deliberation should take place prior to considering allowing the athlete to return to competition. It is unlikely that a pediatric athlete's future rests on his ability to compete in a contact sport, and it is difficult to imagine a scenario where the benefits of contact sports would outweigh the risks of further brain injury in this setting.

Due to the emotionality of the situation for some families, the physician may need to remind the child and his family that a ban on contact sports does not mean a ban on athletics. The young athlete who recovers from a sports-related epidural hematoma can be allowed to participate in sports where contact is at a minimum. Not only should these athletes be allowed to participate, even at the competitive level, they should be encouraged, particularly after a full recovery. The physical and psychological benefit of athletics is especially important in children after head injury, and initial trepidation often turns to enthusiasm for new endeavors with supportive encouragement.

FREQUENTLY ASKED QUESTION #10

A 16-year-old running back returns to your office 4 weeks following his second Grade 1 concussion and is complaining of persistent headaches. While he is neurologically intact, awake, and alert, he reports problems focusing at school and sleeping a lot.

"Why Am I Still Feeling So Lousy a Month After My Injury?"

Most instances of persistent symptoms are grouped into the category of "post-concussion syndrome" and include headache, irritability, minor personality changes, decreased concentration and memory, fatigue, and dizziness. Postconcussion syndrome can occur after any grade of concussion and may persist for several months. Several reports have shown that approximately 20% of patients who have suffered a concussion will report some, or all, symptoms of the post-concussion syndrome (4, 32, 54). The symptoms exhibited are believed secondary to alterations in neurotransmitter function (31) and/or metabolic derangements (55, 56), and is not associated with intracranial imaging abnormalities.

Especially common among adolescents, are persistent headaches which are often attributed to post-traumatic migraine headaches especially when associated with aura, nausea, and vomiting. They can occur soon after athletic head injury or have a delayed onset, persisting for variable periods of time (8, 30). Although the exact mechanism of trauma-induced migraine is not completely understood, cerebral vasospasm (36), and spreading depression (45) have been implicated. Like classic migraine, post-traumatic migraines can be preceded by an aura involving a focal neurologic deficit, raising concern of an intracranial mass lesion. Symptoms that persist beyond several weeks, are progressive, or are focal on exam should prompt further imaging with MR or CT to rule out intracranial pathology such as a chronic subdural hematoma though it is rare to find anything on the imaging that will change management. Once the diagnosis of post-traumatic migraine or post-concussive syndrome has been established, medical management is usually adequate. Non-narcotic analgesics such as ibuprofen or Naprosyn are often helpful in relieving headache, but for the most part the treatment of the post-concussive syndrome is largely based on rest and time. Irritability, minor personality change, and poor concentration can impact negatively upon scholastic performance, and time away from school may prove beneficial in the long term if the symptoms are particularly severe. Athletics of any kind are strictly prohibited if any symptoms of the post-concussive syndrome are present.

Neuropsychological Impairment

Although most young athletes appear asymptomatic relatively soon after most head injuries, in-depth neuropsychological testing often reveals some degree of impairment following even the most minor of injuries (7, 21, 39). Poor performance in tasks requiring auditory concentration, eye-hand coordination, short-term memory, and other cognitive function can be found in nearly every athlete who sustains a concussion or other head injury. In most athletes, neuropsychological functions return to baseline within 5 days (39), but a small percentage of players will experience cognitive difficulty for months after injury. It is well known that a player who has suffered a concussion is 4 to 6 times more likely to suffer a second concussion than a previously non-concussed athlete (25), and one possible explanation is the neurocognitive deficits uniformly present after the first concussion placing the athlete at higher risk.

Post-Traumatic Seizures

Immediate post-traumatic seizures are a concern, occurring in 2.6% of all children suffering head injury (5). Fortunately, when they do occur, post-traumatic seizures tend to be relatively short-lived and self-limited (13). Immediate management of the young athlete having a seizure involves ensuring an adequate airway and protecting the athlete from harming himself. If a mouthguard is in place and can be removed, it should be done without placing a finger into the player's mouth to avoid severe injury to the finger. Because seizures are more common after focal brain injury (contusion, subdural hematoma, etc.), an emergent CT scan should be obtained in every child who has a seizure after trauma. Chronic epilepsy requiring long-term antiepileptic medication will develop in 7.4% of severely head-injured children.

In moderately and mildly head-injured children, epilepsy will develop in 1.6% and 0.2%, respectively, a frequency that does not differ significantly from the non-injured pediatric population (5).

CONCLUSION

Head injury remains a significant contributor to athletic morbidity and mortality. In the child athlete, the importance of identification, evaluation, and appropriate management of a concussive injury are paramount to ensure the safety and avoidance of long term complications. While treatment of the head-injured young athlete varies depending on the nature and severity of the injury, unless there is an expanding mass or diffuse pathophysiologic process, time away from participation will likely result in a good and positive outcome. For all instances of head injury, the cervical spine should also be considered injured until cleared. With the exception of Grade 1 concussions, it is the very rare child who will be considered for a return to competition the day of head injury. Return-to-play guidelines are well established and should be strictly adhered to in order to prevent a catastrophic neurologic injury or long-term problems. Despite recent advances in the neurosurgical management of head injury, the single most important aspect of head injury management is prevention. With proper supervision, training, and equipment, the young athlete can have a productive, enjoyable, and safe athletic experience.

REFERENCES

1. Adelson PD, Thomas S, Hovda DA, et al: Boxing fatalities and brain injury. **Perspect Neurolog Surg** 2:167–186, 1991.
2. Alves WM, Polin RS: Sports-related head injury. In Narayan RK, Wilberger JE, Povlishock JT (eds): *Neurotrauma.* New York: McGraw-Hill, 1996, p 913.
3. American Academy of Neurology: Practice parameters: The management of concussion in sports. **Neurology** 48:581–585, 1997.
4. Anderson DW, McLaurin RL (eds): Report on the national head and spinal cord injury survey. **J Neurosurg** 53:S1–S43, 1980.
5. Annegers JF, Grabow JD, Groover RJ, et al: Seizures after head trauma: A population study. **Neurology** 30:683–689, 1980.
6. Bailes JE, Cantu RC: Head injury in athletics **Neurosurgery**. 48:26–46, 2001.
7. Barth JT, Macciocchi SN, Giordani B, et al: Neuropsychological sequelae of minor head injury. **Neurosurgery** 13:529–533, 1983.
8. Bennett DR, Fuenning SI, Sullivan G, et al: Migraine precipitated by head trauma in athletes. **Am J Sports Med** 8:202–205, 1980.
9. Bergsneider M, Hovda D, Shalmon E et al: Cerebral hyperglycolysis following severe traumatic brain injury in humans: A position emission tomography study. **J Neurosurgery** 86:241–251, 1997.
10. Bruce DA, Alavi A, Bilaniuk L, et al: Diffuse cerebral swelling following head in-

juries in children: The syndrome of "malignant brain edema". **J Neurosurg** 54:170–178, 1981.

11. Bruno LA, Gennarelli TA, Torg JS: Management guidelines for head injuries in athletics. **Clin Sports Med** 6:17–29, 1987.

12. Cantu RC: When to return to contact sports after a cerebral concussion. **Sports Medicine Digest** 10:1–2, 1988.

13. Cantu RC: Head injuries in sport. **Br J Sports Med** 30:289–296, 1996.

14. Cantu RC: Epilepsy and athletics. **Clin Sports Med** 17:61–69, 1998.

15. Cantu RC: Return to play guidelines after a head injury. **Clin Sports Med** 17:45–60, 1998.

16. Cantu RC: Second-impact syndrome. **Clin Sports Med** 17:37–44, 1998.

17. Chorley JN: Sports-related head injuries. **Curr Opin Pediatr** 10:350–355, 1998.

18. Colorado Medical Society: Report of the sports medicine committee: guideline for the management of concussion in sports. Denver: Colorado Medical Society, 1991.

19. Committee on Head Injury Nomenclature of the Congress of Neurological Surgeons: Glossary of head injury, including some definitions of injury to the cervical spine. **Clin Neurosurg** 12:386–394, 1966.

20. Committee on Sports Medicine and Fitness: *Sports Medicine: Health Care for Young Athletes* (ed 2). Elk Grove Village, IL: American Academy of Pediatrics, 1991.

21. Dikmen S, McLean A, Temkin N: Neuropsychological and psychosocial consequences of mild head injury. **J Neurol Neurosurg Psychiatry** 49:227–232, 1986.

22. Fineman I, Hovda DA, Smith M, et al: Concussive brain injury is associated with a prolonged accumulation of calcium: A 45Ca autoradiographic study. **Brain Res** 624:94–102, 1993.

23. Gennarelli TA, Thibault LE, Adams JH, et al: Diffuse axonal injury and traumatic coma in the primate. **Ann Neurol** 12:564–574, 1982.

24. Genuardi FJ, King WD: Inappropriate discharge instructions for youth athletes hospitalized for concussion. **Pediatrics** 95:216–218, 1995.

25. Gerberich SG, Priest JD, Boen JR, et al: Concussion incidences and severity in secondary school varsity football players. **Am J Publ Health** 73:1370–1375, 1983.

26. Graham DI: Neuropathology of head injury. In Narayan RK, Wilberger JEJ, Povlishock JT (eds): *Neurotrauma*. New York: McGraw-Hill, 1996, pp 46–47.

27. Greenberg MS: *Handbook of Neurosurgery* (ed 3). Lakeland, FL: Greenberg Graphics, 1994.

28. Gronwall D, Wrightson P: Delayed recovery of intellectual function after minor head injury. **Lancet** ii:605–609, 1974.

29. Gronwall D, Wrightson P: Cumulative effect of concussion. **Lancet** ii:995–997, 1975.

30. Haas DC, Pineda GS, Lourie H: Juvenile head trauma syndromes and their relationship to migraine. **Arch Neurol** 32:727–730, 1975.

31. Hugen Holtz H, Richard MT: Return to athletic competition following concussion. **Can Med Assoc J** 127:827–829, 1982.

32. Jones JH, Viola SL, LaBan MM, et al: The incidence of post minor traumatic brain injury syndrome: a retrospective survey of treating physicians. **Arch Phys Med Rehabil** 73:145–146, 1992.

33. Katayama Y, Becker DP, Tamura T, et al: Massive increases in extracellular potassium and the indiscriminate release of glutamate following concussive brain injury. **J Neurosurg** 73:889–900, 1990.

34. Kelly JP, Rosenberg JH: Diagnosis and management of concussion in sports. **Neurology** 48:575–580, 1997.

35. Kraus JF, Fife D, Cox P, et al: Incidence, severity and external causes of pediatric head injury. **Am J Dis Child** 140:687–693, 1986.

36. Lance JW: *Mechanism and Management of Headache*, vol. 10. London: Butterworths, 1978.
37. Langfitt TW, Tannenbaum HM, Kassell NF: The etiology of acute brain swelling following experimental head injury. **J Neurosurg** 24:47–56, 1966.
38. Lindberg R, Freytag E: Brainstem lesion characteristics of traumatic hyperextension of the head. **Arch Pathol** 90:509–515, 1970.
39. Macciocchi SN, Barth JT, Alves W, et al: Neuropsychological functioning and recovery after mild head injury in collegiate athletes. **Neurosurgery** 39:510–514, 1996.
40. Maroon JC, Steele PB, Berlin R: Football head and neck injuries: An update. **Clin Neurosurg** 27:414–429, 1980.
41. McLatchie G, Jennett B: Head injury in sport. **Br Med J** 308:1624–1627, 1994.
42. McQuillen JB, McQuillen EN, Morrow P: Trauma, sport, and malignant cerebral edema. **Am J Forensic Med Pathol** 9:12–15, 1988.
43. Mueller FO: Fatalities from head and cervical spine injuries occurring in tackle football: 50 years' experience. **Clin Sports Med** 17:169–182, 1998.
44. Mueller FO, Blythe CS: Can we continue to improve injury statistics in football? **Phys Sports Med** 12:79–84, 1984.
45. Oka H, Kako M, Matsushima M, et al: Traumatic spreading depression syndrome. Review of a particular type of head injury in 37 patients. **Brain** 100:287–298, 1977.
46. Saunders RL, Harbaugh RE: Second impact in catastrophic contact-sports head trauma. **JAMA** 252:538–539, 1984.
47. Schneider RC: *Head and Neck Injuries in Football*. Baltimore: Williams & Wilkins, 1973.
48. Snoek JW, Minderhoud JM, Wilmink JT: Delayed deterioration following mild head injury in children. **Brain** 107:15–36, 1984.
49. Swenson T, Lauerman W, Blanc R: Cervical spine alignment in the immobilized football player: radiographic analysis before and after helmet removal. **Am J Sports Med** 25:226–230, 1997.
50. Teasdale G, Jennett B: Assessment of coma and impaired consciousness. A practical scale. **Lancet** 2:81–84, 1974.
51. Torg JS: *Athletic Injuries to the Head, Neck, and Face*. Philadelphia: Lea & Febiger, 1982.
52. Warren WL, Bailes JE: On the field evaluation of athletic head injuries. **Clin Sports Med** 17:13–26, 1998.
53. Wirth FP: Surgical treatment of incidental intracranial aneurysms. **Clin Neurosurg** 33:125–135, 1986.
54. Wrightson P, Gronwall D: Time off work and symptoms after minor head injury. **Injury** 12:445–454, 1981.
55. Yang MS, Dewitt DS, Becker DP, et al: Regional brain metabolite levels following mild experimental head injury in the cat. **J Neurosurg** 63:617–621, 1985.

19

Boxing and the Neurosurgeon

VINCENT J. MIELE, M.D., JULIAN E. BAILES, M.D.,
AND JOSEPH L. VOELKER, M.D.

INTRODUCTION

Boxing has been described as both a brutal business and the purest of sports. Its elimination has been suggested by several prominent medical organizations and it has been banned in three countries (6). Opponents site its identification with betting and organized crime, as well as its violent nature. It has also been linked to acute neurological injury and chronic brain damage. Proponents claim that the risks of participation are no greater than other sports, especially the "extreme sports" that are gaining popularity. As physicians often involved in the treatment of acute boxing injuries, the neurosurgical community has yet to make a public statement on the activity. This article is intended as a first step in such a statement, with analysis of the acute injuries that a boxer can incur and recommendations to reduce the risk of such injuries in participants.

History of the Sport

While boxing as an unorganized form of hand-to-hand combat practice surely dates back to prehistoric man and "sparring" activity can be observed in most animals, the first record of an organized sport occurred in ancient Greece. The champion of the 23rd Olympian games, known as Onomastos from Smyrna, is given credit for first defining the rules of the game. He set these rules for his own bouts, which had no time limits or pauses in competition unless both fighters decided to take a rest, utilized no ring, and the participant won by disabling his opponent. Matches were open to all comers and participants were not matched by weight.

The sport became more brutal during the Roman Empire, which is attested to by early changes in handgear. From Homeric times to the end of the fifth century B.C., handgear known as "soft thongs" were utilized. They were made of oxhide that covered the knuckles, wrist, and lower forearm of participants with the fingers free and had a primary function of protecting the participant's hands. These evolved into the "sharp thong" in the fourth century B.C. to the time of the Roman Empire. These were essentially a glove with a hard leather ring encircling the knuckles and were more of an offensive weapon. These evolved into the Roman caestus in the second century A.D., which had metal spikes projecting out from the knuckles, designed to severely injure an opponent. This equipment essentially turned the boxer as an athlete into a gladiator with participants fighting for their lives.

Great Britain can be given credit for transforming boxing into the sport as we know it today. Several aspects of the modern game were introduced by James Figg, the heavyweight champion from 1719 through 1730. His matches were held in rings created by wooden rails and elevated on a stage. Although most of his fights resembled street brawls, referees were introduced who officiated the bouts from outside of the match area. Jack Broughton, known as the Father of British Boxing, held the English heavyweight championship after Figg. He developed rules for his own fights that were recognized in 1743 and are considered the first formal set of modern boxing rules. Broughton's Rules did not allow hitting below the belt line, gouging opponents' eyes, or hitting a fallen opponent. A squared-off ring was utilized and padded handgear known as mufflers were worn during practice to protect the participant's face—the first modern boxing glove. These rules were utilized for nearly a century in what is known as the "bareknuckle era."

The London Prize Ring Rules were first created in 1839 and were utilized through 1892 in most matches. They consisted of a set of 29 rules that elaborated on Broughton's rules eliminating biting, kicking, butting, wrestling, and low blows. They also required the use of a 24-foot square ring and created "rounds" with rest periods. A round was considered over when a participant was knocked off his feet and a new round would start after a 30-second rest period. The Queensberry Rules *(Table 19.1)* were published in 1867, and are considered the basis of modern boxing rules. They were named after the Marques of Queensberry, who gave his support to the conventions. This system made the use of gloves mandatory during matches and established 3-minute rounds with 1-minute intermissions. They also eliminated both eye gouging and wrestling during the match, and established the "10-count."

Today boxing has grown in popularity to such an extent that championship fights are viewed by millions, and promoters and casinos compete for the opportunity to host matches. Thousands of youth and adults participate at amateur and professional levels. When suggesting changes to the current system, the financial consequences as well as popular opinion must be well considered.

TABLE 19.1
Queensberry Rules

Twenty-four foot ring	No wrestling/hugging
Three-min rounds / 1-min intermission	Boxing gloves
Downed boxer must rise unassisted within 10 s	Participant hanging on ropes in helpless state, with toes off the ground, shall be considered down
No seconds or any other person to be is allowed in the ring during rounds	If contest stopped, referee names the time/place for finishing contest
Should a glove burst or come off, it must be replaced	A man on one knee is considered down
No shoes or boots with springs allowed	Contest in all other aspects to be governed by the revised rules of the London Prize Ring

ACUTE NEUROLOGICAL INJURIES (ANI)

Boxers exchange dozens of blows each round. Because the head is one of two primary targets, along with the abdomen, participants are at risk for both acute and chronic neurological injury. Acute neurological injuries (ANI) range from mild concussions and cerebral contusions to intracranial hemorrhage, diffuse axonal injury, and death *(Table 19.2)*.

It has been calculated that boxers' punches have a force equivalent to a 10 pound hammer traveling at 20 mph. These impacts produce both linear and rotational acceleration of the head. If the skull accelerates at a rate significantly faster than the brain, impact or shifts causing vacuum phenomena and microhemorrhage may result in a cerebral contusion. This type of injury is common when the brain contacts the irregularities of the skull base. Additional trauma to the head is incurred when the boxer falls and strikes his head. This can generate significant force secondary to rapid deceleration, which typically results in contrecoup contusions. All of these acute changes may be followed rapidly by cerebral edema.

Intracerebral and subdural hematomas are the most frequent form of serious and lethal boxing brain injuries. In review of boxing matches with catastrophic outcomes, these clots have been most commonly associated with repetitive blows to the head, instead of a single major

TABLE 19.2
Acute Neurologic Injuries (ANI) Associated with Boxing

Concussion	Brain Contusions
Acute Subdural / Epidural Hematoma	Subarachnoid Hemorrhage
Diffuse Axonal Injury	Cerebral Edema
Carotid/Vertebral Artery Dissection	Death

punch. A less localized but more severe type of ANI occurs when parts of the brain with different physical properties, such as the cortex and the white matter, accelerate at different speeds resulting in shearing diffuse axonal injuries. Rotational acceleration of the head can result in a swirling motion of the brain, with blood vessels acting as pivot points. These actions can result in punctate hemorrhages in the brain from small vessel tears and tearing of fiber tracts resulting in diffuse white matter injury.

Second impact syndrome (SIS) has been described in a number of contact sports including boxing (9). It occurs when an athlete returns to competition following an ANI such as a cerebral concussion and receives a second seemingly minor trauma to the head, which results in massive cerebral edema. The syndrome was first characterized in 1981, and is believed to result from dysfunction of vascular autoregulation of the brain secondary to the first trauma (2). Victims characteristically return to competition before they are completely asymptomatic from the first insult. Although rare, sports-related SIS has a high mortality rate and morbidity approaching 100%.

An additional cause of ANI to the boxer that must be considered is carotid or vertebral artery dissection. Blows to the head that cause sudden flexion of the neck can tear the intima of one or both arteries. These tears usually extend near the skull base, and result in internal carotid or middle cerebral artery occlusion, ischemia, and hemispheric infarction.

Several groups of boxers have a theoretically higher risk of sustaining ANIs. Subpopulations believed to be at higher risk include boxers that are fatigued, older, dehydrated, or those boxing "on auto." A large number of brain injuries in boxing occur as a result of fatigue. Early in the bout, the fresh participant has an increased ability to maintain good balance, block and slip punches, and move with a punch when struck (decreasing the amount of force transmitted to the brain). The ability of a participant to box "on auto," while considered to be a characteristic of a champion, also puts the individual at risk for ANI. This phrase is used to describe boxers who seem to be oblivious to the punishment they are taking and are performing instinctively. This ability to ignore physical and mental punishment is a trait that results in a participant receiving an abnormal amount of brain trauma and is frequently observed in boxing fatalities.

As the match progresses, the fatigued fighter loses this defensive ability and is more vulnerable to head trauma. Older fighters may be at increased risk of ANI secondary to the natural atrophy of the brain that occurs with age. This atrophy both magnifies the force of blows to the head (since the brain is free to travel a greater distance before striking the bony skull) and creates a potential space that increases the boxer's propensity for fluid collections such as subdural hematomas.

Dehydration in boxers can occur secondary to the loss of fluids from perspiration as a match progresses or intentionally before the fight in an effort to meet a weight requirement. This can increase the participants' vulnerability to ANI by several mechanisms. First, it can increase the fighter's fatigue and decrease defensive ability. It can also decrease the amount of cerebrospinal fluid (CSF) surrounding and buffering the brain from trauma, as well as enlarging the potential space between the brain and skull, increasing the likelihood of hemorrhages such as subdural hematoma.

BOXING FATALITIES

Up until the middle of the 20th century, the majority of boxing fatalities were unrelated to neurological injury, with many athletes dying from heart conditions and infections from sports-related injuries such as impacted teeth. Following the development of antibiotics such as penicillin, the major cause of ring fatalities shifted to acute neurological injury. Many of these fatalities initially involved the boxer striking his head on objects such as unpadded turnbuckles and concrete floors.

The number of modern fatalities associated with the sport was estimated in 1957 by a British neurosurgeon, Macdonald Critchley (3), to be 207 before the year 1957. One of the most respected repositories of boxing data, the *Ring Record Book and Boxing Encyclopedia*, reported 164 fatalities between 1918 and 1950, and 269 fatalities between 1951 and 1980. While the accuracy of data on the number of fatalities associated with the sport is questionable, the actual number of deaths related to participation is likely over 1,300 since 1880.

In 1994, the American Medical Association Council on Medical Affairs reported an annual mortality rate of 1.3 per 100,000 participants (7). This figure has been roughly translated into one death for every 7,692 fights. These reports may fall significantly short of the actual number of fatalities due to underreporting. Since many deaths related to the sport have occurred in amateur fighters in prisons or the military (4, 10), these organizations/institutions may have intentionally covered up fatalities to prevent negative attention. Additionally, for various amateur or socioeconomic reasons, some deaths may not have been considered as newsworthy. All these factors translate into an incomplete tabulation of actual catastrophic injuries from boxing.

It appears that the rate of boxing fatalities has declined in the 1980s and 1990s. This is attributed to four factors: medical advances improving both the diagnosis and treatment of the acutely injured fighter, a decrease in military drafts and the elimination by many organizations of mandatory boxing in recruits, and the increasing popularity of Asian martial arts, which have absorbed a significant percentage of potential boxers.

The fatality rate in boxing actually compares favorably to many other sports that receive less attention with respect to participant safety. The death rate per 100,000 participants has been reported to be 128 in jockeys, 123 in sky diving, 55 in hang gliding, 51 in mountaineering, 11 in scuba diving, and 7 in motorcycle racing (13). Several studies have suggested that boxers have a lower risk of fatality than many other sports participants, and this risk is continuing to decline (5, 11, 12). Moderate-to-high incidences of ANI are commonly reported in many sports such as American football, soccer, basketball, baseball, rugby, martial arts, and ice hockey (1).

CHRONIC NEUROLOGICAL INJURIES (CNI)

While chronic neurological injuries (CNI) have not garnered the same amount of attention as acute injuries until recently, they affect a much larger proportion of participants. Several studies have demonstrated that even relatively minor head injuries are often associated with measurable long-term consequences. This has also been reported in retired professional football players (Jordan B, Bailes JE, Schlosser J: Concussion history and current neurological symptoms among retired professional football players. In preparation). The risk of CNI increases with every punch absorbed; therefore professional boxers, apparently those that have been in the game for over 10 years, are particularly at risk. Blows to the head may be subclinical and result in axonal damage and destruction. While a small number of severed axons may not produce symptoms, as the quantity rises so does the incidence of clinical abnormalities. The spectrum of these abnormalities ranges from mild subclinical dysfunction to chronic traumatic encephalopathy, more commonly known as dementia pugilistica or a punch drunk state (8). These injuries have been the subject of numerous articles and chapters, and are outside of the scope of this text.

ARGUMENTS TO BAN BOXING

The sport of boxing has been banned in three countries. Notably, these prohibitions resulted more as a reaction to corruption and illegal acts than concerns over the boxers' medical safety. The sport was banned in Sweden in 1970 and in Norway in 1982, both secondary to concerns of fraud in the sport. It was banned in Iceland in 1956, following criminal acts perpetrated by several professional boxers.

Whether the goal of boxing is to incapacitate the opponent by blows to the head, or to score points by striking designated "target" areas of the body, is often debated. Proponents of the sport site the fact that the vast majority of matches are won on points, not by knockout, although a boxer attempts to knock out his opponent if possible. Boxers also score points and win matches based on a combination of offense, defense, accuracy, and generalship of the ring. This is especially true in the amateur ranks, where the strength of the blow is not taken into consideration during judging.

WHY NOT BAN BOXING

When presented with the significant acute and chronic neurological risks to which the boxer is subjected, the question is raised—can a physician in good conscience condone the sport and not recommend its elimination? The authors of this article believe this is possible, and would be in the best interest of the participants. If it were to be banned, our influence would be minimized in the matches that would still occur in the American underground or in other countries. We would cause participants to lose the advantages of prefight physicals, medical supervision during fights, and immediate access to emergency personal. There would also be the loss of our cooperation and collaboration with the leaders/regulators of the sport in an effort to minimize the risk to the participant's brain. The neurosurgery community would better serve boxers by working to make the sport safer for its participants.

It is also important to remember that all sports involve some risk. There has been no outcry to ban soccer following reports that collisions and heading the ball cause ANI and decrease the participants' IQ. We have known for years that the sport of automobile racing entails significant risk to the life of the participant, yet it flourishes. The now popular extreme sports are another example of recreational activity that has significant risk of bodily injury.

The medical community has a vocal history in the debate over the future of boxing. Over the years, several prestigious medical organizations, including the American Medical Association, the American Academy of Neurology, and the American Academy of Pediatrics have called for a ban on the sport (Table 19.3) (6). In 1994, the AMA House of Delegates passed a resolution encouraging the elimination of the sport (7).

Organized neurosurgery has not released a position statement or

TABLE 19.3
Medical Groups that Have Supported Banning Boxing (1)

American Academy of Pediatrics	American Academy of Neurology	American Medical Association
California State Medical Association	National Medical Association of Australia	National Medical Association of Canada
National Medical Association of the United Kingdom	New York State Medical Association	World Medical Association

suggested safety guidelines for the sport. Whether such a statement is overdue from a group responsible for caring for the acutely injured participants of this activity is open to debate.

GUIDELINES TO INCREASE PARTICIPANT SAFETY

Boxing is a well-recognized sport and its banning is unlikely in the foreseeable future. As neurosurgeons, we will be called upon to treat the acutely injured participants of this sport, and may suggest guidelines to increase safety. The following guidelines are suggestions to decrease the risk of neurological injury in the sport. Some have been proposed and implemented by other organizations. Unfortunately, several have the potential to significantly increase the cost of participation.

During the Contest

RINGSIDE PHYSICIAN

At least one licensed physician must be in attendance at all boxing contests and be prepared to deal with acute injuries. These physicians must have special training in the early recognition of neurological dysfunction, and have the authority to terminate a bout at the first sign of such dysfunction. They must have adequate training in cervical spine injury stabilization, and have up-to-date certifications in ATLS/ACLS. Current resuscitation equipment must be available at the ringside. Dehydration in a boxer has been theorized to increase risk of acute neurological injury. Weigh-ins for matches must occur at least 24 hours before the match to ensure boxers do not dehydrate to meet the weight requirements. Contestants should receive a neurological examination immediately before and after each bout by the ringside physician. This examination should include cranial nerves, mini-mental status, sensory and motor, and prevocational testing.

EVACUATION / NEUROSURGICAL ACCESS

No contest should be allowed unless neurosurgical and resuscitative facilities are readily available and adequate for the emergency treatment of an injured boxer. Before any contest, the nearest hospital with full trauma services should be notified that a boxing match is being held and request that trauma services be available in the event of an acute injury. Emergency medical services must be available from the first bout until the final post-bout neurological examination is completed to ensure rapid emergency evacuation of an injured boxer. The possibility of excited or disruptive large crowds necessitates a comprehensive evacuation procedure for the removal of any injured boxer to medical facilities. This plan must be in place and rehearsed prior to each boxing contest.

Athlete Licensing

Participants must obtain a permit prior to training for competitive fights in a boxing gym. To receive this authorization, a participant must undergo a neurological examination, neuropsychological testing, an electroencephalogram (EEG) and a computerized tomographic (CT) scan of the brain. Permits to participate should have an expiration date of 1 year, and following expiration, formal reassessment should be performed. The boxer's permit to participate should be designed along the lines of a passport, as has been suggested by other organizations. It should include, along with a photograph and other identification information, the participant's medical record and boxing history, including the outcomes of all bouts and all medical suspensions. The boxer at each match must present this passport or participation will not be allowed. Boxers who are placed on medical suspension must surrender their passport to the appropriate governing body, which would hold the permit until the boxer's privileges are reinstated. The passport system, along with the development of a nationwide computer network, would afford a mechanism for the medical surveillance of professional boxers.

Associated Personal Licensing / Training

National certification of individuals affiliated with boxing, including trainers, referees, judges, and ringside physicians, needs to be mandatory. An identification system or qualification similar to that suggested for the boxer should be initiated. In addition to identification information, these passports should include information on any involvement in matches resulting in knockouts, technical knockouts, and serious injuries or fatalities. Individual boxing jurisdictions should conduct on-going health education and first-aid training for all ring personnel.

Gym Licensing

Gyms dedicating the majority of their time to boxing should undergo periodic inspections and require licensing. The rationale for this intercession is to reduce the potential for medical injury during training. The majority of boxing injuries occur during training. Therefore, it is advisable that sparring be conducted under the safest conditions. The routine inspection of boxing gyms would increase the safety of participants by ensuring equipment such as headgear and turnbuckles are in good repair, and would aid in enforcing adherence to safety precautions and prohibition of boxers that are medically suspended from sparring and risking further injury. The strict regulation of boxing gyms would also provide a mechanism to enforce the recommendation that no individual be allowed to begin training without first having a complete physical examination.

Medical Suspensions

Any boxer sustaining a knockout (KO) or technical knockout (TKO) has by definition suffered a concussion and must be medically suspended from boxing for a minimum of 45 days. These individuals must also be required to undergo and have a normal neurological examination. This examination should be thorough and include exertional/prevocational testing. These individuals must also obtain both an EEG and MRI scan before reinstatement. The mandatory revocation of the boxer's license must occur if they suffer three consecutive TKOs or KOs. This would aid in the elimination of boxers that are no longer competitive who are just staying in the game as easy targets for others trying to improve their record. The requirement of MRI scanning in this population has drawbacks. The tests are costly and could conceivably cause trainers to delay "throwing in the towel" to avoid the expense. Likewise, referees aware of the expense to the fighter or his gym might delay calling a KO or TKO. Hopefully, these individuals will put the safety of the boxer first. The passport system mentioned above for affiliated personnel could help to track this problem.

Athlete Advocacy / Research Recommendations

Research into the causes of boxing-related injuries is encouraged. Jurisdictions should be required to demonstrate efforts to this end in the form of on-going research projects and educational programs. The development of a nationwide computer network to track activities of amateur and professional boxers, and collect, store, and retrieve medical information and boxing histories of boxers should be initiated. This is especially true for coordinating boxers' medical and fight experiences across state lines and between state boxing commissions. For professional boxers, the establishment of mandatory life and health insurance funds could be beneficial.

CONCLUSION

Boxing is a well-recognized sport with a long history and tradition. It is often the center of controversy since one of its goals is to strike an opponent with a force sufficient to cause unconsciousness, and it has been linked to both acute and chronic neurological injury. While banning the sport has been recommended by several medical societies, its elimination is unlikely in the near future. As neurosurgeons, we will be called upon to treat the acutely injured participants of this sport, and have a duty to suggest methods for increasing the safety of the sport. This article is meant to be a starting point for debate and the establishment of such guidelines. The views expressed are the authors' opinions and are based also upon their own personal experiences in the sport.

REFERENCES

1. Bailes JE: The management of head injuries in athletes. In Bailes JE, Day AL (eds): *Neurological Sports Medicine.* Rolling Meadows, IL: AANS, 2001, pp 1–24.
2. Bruce D, Alavi A, Bilaniul L: Diffuse cerebral swelling following head injuries in children: the syndrome of "malignant brain edema." **Neurosurgery** 54:170–178, 1981.
3. Critchley M: Medical aspects of boxing, particularly from a neurological standpoint. **Br J Med** 1:357–362, 1957
4. Enzenauer RW, Montrey JS, Enzenauer RJ, Mauldin WM: Boxing related injuries in the U.S. Army, 1980 through 1985. **JAMA** 261:1463, 1989.
5. Gonzales TA: Fatal injuries in competitive sports. **JAMA** 146:1506–1511, 1951.
6. Lundberg G: Medical arguments for nonparticipation in boxing. In Jordan B (ed): *Medical Aspects of Boxing.* Boca Raton: CRC Press; 1992. p. 11–15.
7. Lundberg GD: Boxing should be banned in civilized countries- round 2. **JAMA** 251:2696–2697,1984.
8. Martland HS: Punch drunk. **JAMA** 91:1103–1107, 1928.
9. Miele VJ, Bailes JE: Head, spine, and peripheral nerve injuries in sports and dance: an encyclopedic reference. In Bailes JE, Day AL (eds): *Neurological Sports Medicine.* Rolling Meadows, IL: AANS, 2001, pp 181–252.
10. Oelman BJ, Rose CME, Arlow KJ: Boxing injuries in the army. **J Army Med Corps** 129:32, 1983.
11. Refshauge JGH: The medical aspects of boxing. **Med J Aust** 1:611–613, 1963.
12. Ryan AJ: Intracranial injuries resulting from boxing. In Mosby T (ed): *Athletic Injuries to the Head, Face, and Neck.* Chicago: Year Book Inc, 1991, pp 31–40.
13. Some high risk sports. **Sporting News** Aug 16, 1980.

CHAPTER

20

Guidelines for the Management of Acute Cervical Spine and Spinal Cord Injuries

MARK N. HADLEY, M.D., F.A.C.S., BEVERLY C. WALTERS, M.D.,
PAUL A. GRABB, M.D., NELSON M. OYESIKU, M.D.,
GREGORY J. PRZYBYLSKI, M.D., DANIEL K. RESNICK, M.D.,
TIMOTHY C. RYKEN, M.D., AND DEBBIE H. MIELKE

INTRODUCTION

Spinal cord injuries occur approximately 14,000 times per year in North America, the majority involving the cervical spinal region. Most injuries, although not all, will include cervical spinal fracture-dislocations. Patients who sustain cervical spinal cord injuries usually have lasting, often devastating neurological deficits and disability. In addition, tens of thousands of patients per year will sustain traumatic cervical spinal injuries without spinal cord injury. The management of these patients and their injuries, cord and vertebral column, has not been standardized or consistent within a single institution, from one center to another or among centers within geographic regions. Treatment strategies are usually based on institutional or personal provider experiences, physician training and the resources available at the treatment facility. Management can affect outcome in these patients; therefore, clinicians worldwide strive to provide the "best and most timely care." Many times we may not be fully aware of what the "best care" may be or whether "timeliness" matters. In many circumstances "best care" likely encompasses a variety of treatment strategies, all with acceptable success rates and reasonable inherent risks.

The Section on Disorders of the Spine and Peripheral Nerves of the American Association of Neurological Surgeons and the Congress of Neurological Surgeons has long been interested in seeking answers to the key management issues associated with acute spine and spinal cord injuries. Identification of "best care" strategies is desired for all aspects of the care of acute cervical injury patients including pre-hospital care and transport, neurological and radiographic assessment, medical management of spinal cord injury, closed reduction of cervical fracture-dislocations and specific treatment options, both operative and non-operative, for each specific cervical injury type known to occur from the occiput through the first thoracic level. The leadership of the Spine Section charged this author group to generate guideline documents on the management of patients with acute cervical spine and cervical spinal cord injuries. This effort was initiated in May 2000. Twenty-two topics were identified and multiple questions were generated around which recommendations would be formed. A meticulous process founded in evidence-based medicine was followed. Published scientific evidence was searched for and relied upon rather than expert opinion or traditional practices. In the course of developing these recommendations, new methodology had to be created for classifying evidence on clinical assessment, resulting in a substantial contribution to the guidelines literature as a whole. The author group first convened in September 2000. One year later the task was completed.

It is the hope of the author group and the Joint Section on Disorders of the Spine and Peripheral Nerves that these guidelines will define the variety of assessment or treatment options available to a clinician in the management of an individual patient, provide direction within the broad scope of clinical practice derived from medical evidence, highlight what is known about specific issues and importantly, define what is not known, stimulating additional research.

At the time of this presentation (October 4, 2001), these Guidelines have been approved by the Section on Disorders of the Spine and Peripheral Nerves and the Congress of Neurological Surgeons. They are under review by the Section on Trauma and Critical Care, the Section on Pediatric Neurosurgery, and the American Association of Neurological Surgeons. They are being prepared for publication, as a supplement to *NEUROSURGERY*, expected to be available in March 2002. At this time, reproduction of the entire Guidelines document in Clinical Neurosurgery is neither practical (much too much text), nor appropriate (not yet approved by the above cited neurosurgical organizations). We reproduce in this chapter the Methodology of Guideline Development, specific recommendations on each of the twenty-two topics (including the rationale and summary for each) and our comprehensive master bibliography. We hope you find them of interest and value.

METHODOLOGY OF GUIDELINE DEVELOPMENT

Introduction

The evolution of medical evidence has occurred rapidly over the last fifty years. From initial reports, anecdotal in nature, to large-scale randomized controlled trials, medical evidence is variable. From the evidence, and influenced by personal experience, clinicians choose paths of disease management. The medical specialties have pioneered the use of evidence produced from experimental trials to support clinical practice decisions. The surgical specialties have lagged behind the development of large-scale studies of surgical procedures and perioperative management. However, the high cost of medical care along with practice variation from region to region has given rise to an interest in developing strategies for linking practice to underlying evidence. In the course of this endeavor it has become clear that the variability of the evidence must somehow be reflected in any recommendations derived from it.

In the 1980s, criteria to be used in selecting evidence for developing treatment recommendations were developed. In a formal document, *Clinical Practice Guidelines: Directions for a New Program*, the Institute of Medicine addressed such guideline issues as "definition of terms, specification of key attributes of good guidelines, and certain aspects of planning for implementation and evaluation." (1) The key intent of the document is to promote standardization and consistency in guideline development. In the course of the document, several key concepts in guideline development were espoused. They include:

1. A thorough review of the scientific literature should precede guideline development.
2. The available scientific literature should be searched using appropriate and comprehensive search terminology.
3. The evidence should be evaluated and weighted, reflecting the scientific validity of the methodology used to generate the evidence.
4. There should be a link between the available evidence and the recommendations with the strength of the evidence being reflected in the strength of the recommendations, reflecting scientific certainty (or lack thereof).
5. Empirical evidence should take precedence over expert judgment in the development of guidelines.
6. Expert judgment should be used to evaluate the quality of the literature and to formulate guidelines when the evidence is weak or non-existent.
7. Guideline development should be a multidisciplinary process, involving key groups affected by the recommendations.

The Guidelines for the Management of Acute Cervical Spine and Spinal Cord Injuries were developed using the evidence-based approach reflected in the above recommendations, rather than a consensus-based approach using the input of experts in a given field who make recommendations based upon a literature review and their personal experience. The author group involved in the development of these guidelines for treatment of patients with acute cervical spinal injury employed a strict process of literature review, ranking the published papers by strength of study design. Every effort was made to avoid influence by personal or professional bias by being objective in following a methodology defined in advance. The methodology chosen for this Guideline is evidence-based and follows the recommendations of the Institute of Medicine (IOM) Committee to Advise the Public Health Service on Clinical Practice Guidelines (1) as outlined in detail in the development process description below.

GUIDELINE DEVELOPMENT METHODOLOGY
Literature Search

Extensive literature searches were undertaken for each clinical question addressed. The searches involved the available English-language literature for the past 25 years, using the computerized database of the National Library of Medicine. Human studies were looked for, and the search terms employed reflected the clinical question in as much detail as relevant, as described in the individual sections. Abstracts were reviewed and clearly relevant articles were selected for evaluation.

Evaluating Strength of the Therapy Literature

Each paper found by the above-mentioned techniques was evaluated as to study type (e.g., therapy, diagnosis, clinical assessment). For therapy, evidence can be generated by any number of study designs. The strongest study protocol, when well designed and executed, is by far the randomized controlled trial (RCT). The prospectivity, presence of contemporaneous comparison groups, and adherence to strict protocols observed in the RCT diminish sources of systematic error (called *bias*). The randomization process reduces the influence of unknown aspects of the patient population that might affect the outcome (*random error*).

The next strongest study designs are the non-randomized cohort study and the case-control study, also comparing groups who received specific treatments, but in a non-randomized fashion. In the former study design, an established protocol for patient treatment is followed and groups are compared in a prospective manner, providing their allocation to treatment is not determined by characteristics that would not allow them to receive either treatment being studied. These groups would have a disorder of interest, e.g., spinal cord injury, and receive different interventions, and then the differences in outcome would be studied. In the case-control study, the study is designed with the patients divided by outcome (e.g., functional ability) and their treatment (e.g., surgery vs. no surgery) would be evaluated for a relationship. These studies are more open to systematic and random error and thus are less compelling than an RCT. However, the RCT with significant design flaws that threaten its validity loses its strength and may be classified as a weaker study.

Least strong evidence is generated by published series of patients all with the same or similar disorder followed for outcome, but not compared as to treatment. In this same category is the case report, expert opinion, and the RCT so significantly flawed that the conclusions are uncertain. All of these statements regarding study strength refer to studies on treatment. But patient management includes not only treatment, but also diagnosis and clinical assessment. These aspects of patient care require clinical studies that are different in design, generating evidence regarding choices of diagnostic tests and clinical measurement.

Evaluating Strength of the Diagnostic Test Literature

To be useful, diagnostic tests have to be reliable and valid. Reliability refers to the test's stability in repeated use, in the same circumstance. Validity describes the extent to which the test reflects the "true" state of affairs, as measured by some "gold standard" reference test. Accuracy reflects the test's ability to determine who does and does not have the suspected or potential disorder. Overall, the test must be accurate in picking out the true positives and true negatives, with the lowest possible false positive and false negative rate. These attributes are represented by sensitivity, specificity, positive predictive value, and negative predictive value. These may be calculated using a Bayesian 2 × 2 table as shown in *Table 20.1*.

Using the *Table 20.1,* the components of accuracy can be expressed and calculated as shown in *Table 20.2.*

It is the characteristic of diagnostic tests that these attributes do not always rise together, but generally speaking, these numbers should be greater than 70% to consider the test useful. The issue of reliability of the test will be discussed below when describing patient assessment.

Evaluating Strength of the Patient Assessment Literature

There are two points when patient assessment is key in the patient management paradigm. There is initial assessment, e.g., patient's condition in the trauma room, and the ultimate, or outcome, assessment. All patient assessment tools, whether they are radiographic, laboratory, or clinical, require that the measurement be reliable. In the case of stud-

TABLE 20.1

		GOLD STANDARD		
		Patient has injury	Patient has no injury	
TEST RESULT	Positive: Appears to have injury	TRUE POSITIVE (a) FALSE	FALSE POSITIVE (b) TRUE	(a) + (b)
C-SPINE FILM	Negative: Appears to have no injury	NEGATIVE (c) (a) + (c)	NEGATIVE (d) (b) + (d)	(c) + (d) (a) + (b) + (c) + (d)

ies carried out by mechanical or electronic equipment, these devices must be calibrated regularly to assure reliability. In the instance of assessments carried out by observers, reliability is assured by verifying agreement between various observers carrying out the same assessment, and also by the same observer at different times. Because a certain amount of agreement between observers or observations could be expected to occur by chance alone, a statistic has been developed to measure the agreement between observations or observers beyond chance. This is known as an index of concordance and is called the *kappa* statistic, or simply *kappa* (3). Once again, the Bayesian 2 × 2 table can be utilized to understand and to calculate kappa *(Table 20.3)*.

Using these numbers, the formula for calculating kappa is:

$$k = N(a + d) - (n_1f_1 + n_2f_2) \div N^2 - (n_1f_1 + n_2f_2) \text{ or}$$
$$k = 2(ad - bc) \div n_1f_2 + n_2f_1$$

Translating the numbers generated using these formulas to meaningful interpretations of the strength of the agreement between ob-

TABLE 20.2

Sensitivity	a/a + c	If a patient has a positive X-ray, how likely is he to have a C-spine injury?
Specificity	d/b + d	If a patient has a negative X-ray, how likely is he to not have a C-spine injury?
Positive predictive value	a/a + b	If a patient has a C-spine injury, how likely is he to have a positive test?
Negative predictive value	d/c + d	If a patient does not have a C-spine injury, how likely is he to have a negative test?
Accuracy	a + d/a + b + c + d	

TABLE 20.3

		OBSERVER #1		
		YES	NO	
OBSERVER	YES	AGREE (a)	DISAGREE (b)	$(a) + (b) = f_1$
#2	NO	DISAGREE (c)	AGREE (d)	$(c) + (d) = f_2$
		$(a) + (c) = n_1$	$(b) + (d) = n_2$	$(a) + (b) + (c) + (d) = N$

servers or observations is accomplished using the guidelines shown in *Table 20.4* (5):

Each paper on clinical assessment was examined for its adherence to the rules of reliability and the exact kappa was noted and linked to the strength of recommendations, as described below.

Linking Evidence to Guidelines

The concept of linking evidence to recommendations has been further formalized by the American Medical Association (AMA) and many specialty societies, including the Congress of Neurological Surgeons (CNS), American Association of Neurological Surgeons (AANS) and the American Academy of Neurology (AAN) (1, 2, 6, 7). This formalization involves the designation of specific relationships between the strength of evidence and the strength of recommendations, avoiding ambiguity. In the paradigm for therapeutic maneuvers, evidence is classified into that derived from the strongest clinical studies (well-designed, randomized, controlled trials), generating **Class I** evidence. **Class I** evidence is used to support recommendations of the strongest type, called practice **Standards,** indicating a *high degree of clinical certainty*. Non-randomized cohort studies, randomized controlled trials with design flaws, and case-control studies (comparative studies with less strength) are designated **Class II** evidence. These are used

TABLE 20.4

Value of k	Strength of Agreement
0	Poor
0–.20	Slight
.21–.40	Fair
.41–.60	Moderate
.61–.80	Substantial
.81–1.00	Almost perfect

TABLE 20.5

Classification of Evidence on Therapeutic Effectiveness

Class I	Evidence from one or more well-designed, randomized controlled clinical trials, including overviews of such trials.
Class II	Evidence from one or more well-designed comparative clinical studies, such as nonrandomized cohort studies, case-control studies, and other comparable studies, including less well designed randomized controlled trials.
Class III	Evidence from case series, comparative studies with historical controls, case reports, and expert opinion, as well as significantly flawed randomized controlled trials.

to support recommendations called **Guidelines,** reflecting *a moderate degree of clinical certainty.* Other sources of information, including observational studies such as case series and expert opinion, as well as randomized controlled trials with flaws so serious that the conclusions of the study are truly in doubt (**Class III** evidence), support practice **Options** reflecting *unclear clinical certainty.* These categories of evidence are summarized in the *Table 20.5.*

The general term for all of the recommendations is **Practice Parameters**. Because so few practice Standards exist, the term more commonly used to describe the whole body of recommendations is practice guidelines. Thus, we have named this document *Guidelines for the Management of Acute Cervical Spine and Spinal Cord Injuries*.

One of the practical difficulties encountered in implementing this methodology is that a poorly designed randomized controlled trial might take precedence over a well-designed case-control or nonrandomized cohort study. The authors of this document have attempted to avoid this pitfall by carefully evaluating the quality of the study as well as its type. All of these criteria apply to practice guidelines (parameters) for *treatment*. To assess literature pertaining to *prognosis*, *diagnosis*, and *clinical assessment*, completely different criteria must be used.

Criteria for prognosis have been developed and were widely used in the publications of Prognostic Indicators in Severe Traumatic Brain Injury (Walters, Chesnut). No issues of prognosis were addressed in the current document.

For diagnosis, papers are evaluated differently yet again. The issues addressed by papers on diagnosis are related to the ability of the diagnostic test to successfully distinguish between patients who have and do not have a disease or pertinent finding. This speaks to the validity of the test and is illustrated in *Table 20.6.*

For clinical assessment, there needs to be both reliability and va-

TABLE 20.6
Classification of Evidence on Diagnosis

Class I	Evidence provided by one or more well-designed clinical studies of a diverse population using a "gold standard" reference test in a blinded evaluation appropriate for the diagnostic applications and enabling the assessment of sensitivity, specificity, positive and negative predictive values, and, where applicable, likelihood ratios.
Class II	Evidence provided by one or more well-designed clinical studies of a restricted population using a "gold standard" reference test in a blinded evaluation appropriate for the diagnostic applications and enabling the assessment of sensitivity, specificity, positive and negative predictive values, and, where applicable, likelihood ratios.
Class III	Evidence provided by expert opinion, studies that do no meet the criteria for the delineation of sensitivity, specificity, positive and negative predictive values, and, where applicable, likelihood ratios.

lidity in the measure. This means that the assessment is done reliably between observers and by the same observer at a different time. For validity, the clinical assessment, like diagnostic tests described above, need to adequately represent the true condition of the patient. This latter aspect is difficult to measure, so most clinical assessments are graded according to their reliability *(Table 20.7)*.

For each question addressed in these guidelines, articles were examine and the study type was assessed and assigned a classification according to the scheme outlined above. These designations are listed in the evidentiary tables of each of the chapters.

GUIDELINES DEVELOPMENT PROCESS

A group of individuals with interest and expertise in the treatment of cervical spinal injured patients and/or guideline practice parameter development was assembled under the auspices of and with the

TABLE 20.7
Classification of Evidence on Clinical Assessment

Class I	Evidence provided by one or more well-designed clinical studies in which interobserver and intraobserver reliability is represented by a Kappa statistic of .80 or greater.
Class II	Evidence provided by one or more well-designed clinical studies in which interobserver and intraobserver reliability is represented by a Kappa statistic of .60 or greater.
Class III	Evidence provided by one or more well-designed clinical studies in which interobserver and intraobserver reliability is represented by a Kappa statistic of less than .60.

support of the Joint Section on Disorders of the Spine and Peripheral Nerves of the AANS/CNS. The group reflected expertise in spinal neurosurgery, neurotrauma, and clinical epidemiology. The issues chosen for inclusion in the document were those considered pertinent to the acute management of patients with cervical spine and/or spinal cord injury (e.g., transport, medical management, treatment of specific fracture/dislocation patterns, vascular injury, and prophylaxis for thromboembolic events).

A Medline search from January 1966 to January 2001 was carried out using the search terms described in each individual section. The search was limited to human subjects and included English language literature only for all but one of the sections. Additional papers were found through the reference lists in the articles found, as well as from other sources known to the author group. Papers were rejected on the basis of irrelevance to the clinical question at hand. Case reports were included if there was insufficient material from case series. Individuals then brought additional articles of relevance from other sources. All articles were evaluated according to the medical evidence-based scheme outlined above. For therapy, diagnosis, and clinical assessment, recommendations were derived. The drafts were revised and members of the author group different from the primary authors rewrote the drafts and the final product was agreed upon by consensus. On occasion, the assessed quality of the study design may have been so contentious and the conclusions so uncertain, that the author group designated a lower classification than might have been expected without such detailed review.

In every way, the author group attempted to adhere to the Institute of Medicine criteria for searching, assembling, evaluating, and weighting the available medical evidence and linking it to the strength of the recommendations presented in this document.

TOPIC 1: PRE-HOSPITAL CERVICAL SPINAL IMMOBILIZATION FOLLOWING TRAUMA

Recommendations

Standards: There is insufficient evidence to support treatment standards.

Guidelines: There is insufficient evidence to support treatment guidelines.

Options:
- It is suggested that all trauma patients with a cervical spinal column injury or with a mechanism of injury having the potential to cause cervical spinal injury should be immobilized at the scene and dur-

ing transport using one of several available methods.

- A combination of a rigid cervical collar and supportive blocks on a backboard with straps is very effective in limiting motion of the cervical spine and is recommended. The long-standing practice of attempted cervical spinal immobilization using sandbags and tape alone is not recommended.

Rationale

The early management of the patient with a potential cervical spinal cord injury begins at the scene of the accident. The chief concern during the initial management of patients with potential cervical spinal injuries is that neurologic function may be impaired due to pathologic motion of the injured vertebrae. It is estimated that 3% to 25% of spinal cord injuries occur after the initial traumatic insult, either during transit or early in the course of management. Multiple cases of poor outcome from mishandling of cervical spinal injuries have been reported. As many as 20% of spinal column injuries involve multiple non-continuous vertebral levels, therefore the entire spinal column is potentially at risk. Consequently, complete spinal immobilization has been used in pre-hospital spinal care to limit motion until injury has been ruled out. Over the last 30 years there has been a dramatic improvement in the neurologic status of spinal cord injured patients arriving in emergency departments. During the 1970s the majority (55%) of patients referred to Regional Spinal Cord Injury Centers arrived with complete neurological lesions. In the 1980s, however, the majority (61%) of spinal cord injured patients arrived with incomplete lesions. This improvement in the neurologic status of patients has been attributed to the development of Emergency Medical Services (EMS) initiated in 1971, and the pre-hospital care (including spinal immobilization) rendered by EMS personnel. Spinal immobilization is now an integral part of pre-hospital management and is advocated for all patients with potential spinal injury following trauma by EMS programs nationwide and by the American College of Surgeons.

Recently, the use of spinal immobilization for *all* trauma patients, particularly those with a low likelihood of traumatic cervical spinal injury has been questioned. It is unlikely that all patients rescued from the scene of an accident or site of traumatic injury require spinal immobilization. Some authors have developed and advocate a triage system based on clinical criteria to select patients for pre-hospital spinal immobilization. Several devices are available for pre-hospital immobilization of the potential spine injured patient. However, the optimal device has not yet been identified by careful comparative analysis. The recommendations of the American College of Surgeons consist of a hard backboard, a rigid cervical collar, lateral support devices, and tape or straps to secure the patient, the collar and the lateral support devices to the backboard. A more uniform, universally accepted method for pre-hospital spinal immobilization for patients with potential spinal injury following trauma may reduce the cost and improve the efficiency of pre-hospital spinal injury management. While spinal immobilization is typically effective in limiting motion, it has been associated with morbidity in a small percentage of cases.

These issues are the subject of this review on the use and effectiveness of pre-hospital spinal immobilization.

Summary

Spinal immobilization can reduce untoward movement of the cervical spine and can reduce the likelihood of neurological deterioration in patients with unstable cervical spinal injuries following trauma. Immobilization of the entire spinal column is necessary in these patients until a spinal column injury (or multiple injuries) or a spinal cord injury has been excluded or until appropriate treatment has been initiated. While not supported by Class I or Class II medical evidence, this effective, time-tested practice is based on anatomic and mechanical considerations in attempt to prevent spinal cord injury and is supported by years of cumulative trauma and triage clinical experience.

It is unclear whether the spines of all trauma victims must be immobilized during pre-hospital transport. Many patients do not have spinal injuries and therefore do not require such intervention. The development of specific selection criteria for those patients for whom immobilization is indicated remains an area of investigation.

The variety of techniques employed and the lack of definitive evidence to advocate a uniform device for spinal immobilization, make immobilization technique and device recommendations difficult. It appears that a combination of rigid cervical collar with supportive blocks on a rigid backboard with straps is effective at achieving safe, effective spinal immobilization for transport. The long-standing practice of attempted cervical spinal immobilization using sandbags and tape alone is not recommended.

Cervical spine immobilization devices are effective but can result in patient morbidity. Spinal immobilization devices should be used to achieve the goals of spinal stability for safe extrication and transport. They should be removed as soon as definitive evaluation is accomplished and/or definitive management is initiated.

TOPIC 2: TRANSPORTATION OF PATIENTS WITH ACUTE TRAUMATIC CERVICAL SPINE INJURIES

Recommendations

Standards: There is insufficient evidence to support treatment standards.

Guidelines: There is insufficient evidence to support treatment guidelines.

Options: Expeditious and careful transport of patients with acute cervical spine or spinal cord injuries is recommended from the site of injury using the most appropriate mode of transportation available to the nearest capable definitive care medical facility.

Rationale

Definitive assessment, resuscitation, and care for the patient with an acute traumatic cervical spinal injury cannot be rendered at the accident scene. Optimal care for patients with spinal injury includes initial resuscitation, immobilization, extrication and early transport of the patient to a medical center with the capability for diagnosis and treatment. Delay in transportation to a definitive treatment center is associated with less favorable outcome, longer hospitalizations, and increased costs.

Several modes of transportation are available to transport the spinal injury patient, primarily land (ambulance) and air (helicopter or fixed wing plane). Selection of the ideal mode of transportation for an individual patient depends on the patient's clinical circumstances, distance, geography, and availability. The goal is to expedite efficient, safe, and effective transportation, without an unfavorable impact on patient outcome. These issues provide the rationale to establish guidelines for transportation of patients with acute traumatic cervical spine and spinal cord injuries.

Summary

The patient with an acute cervical spinal or spinal cord injury should be expeditiously and carefully transported from the site of injury to the nearest capable definitive care medical facility. The mode of transportation chosen should be based upon the patient's clinical circumstances, distance from target facility, geography to be traveled, and should be the most rapid means available. Patients with cervical spinal cord injuries have a high incidence of airway compromise and pulmonary dysfunction, therefore respiratory support measures should be available during transport. Several studies cited suggest improved morbidity and mortality of spinal cord injured patients after the advent of sophisticated transport systems to dedicated SCI centers. These studies all provide Class III medical evidence on this issue.

TOPIC 3: CLINCAL ASSESSMENT FOLLOWING ACUTE CERVICAL SPINAL CORD INJURY
Recommendations

NEUROLOGICAL EXAMINATION

Standards: There is insufficient evidence to support neurological examination standards.

Guidelines: There is insufficient evidence to support neurological examination guidelines.

Options: The ASIA international standards for neurological and functional classification of spinal cord injury is recommended as the preferred neurological examination tool for clinicians involved in the assessment and care of acute spinal cord injury patients.

FUNCTIONAL OUTCOME ASSESSMENT

Standards: There is insufficient evidence to support functional outcome assessment standards.

Guidelines: The Functional Independence Measure (FIM) is recommended as the functional outcome assessment tool for clinicians involved in the assessment and care of acute spinal cord injury patients.

Options: The modified Barthel Index (MBI) is recommended as a functional outcome assessment tool for clinicians involved in the assessment and care of acute spinal cord injury patients.

Rationale

Acute traumatic spinal cord injury affects 12,000 to 14,000 people in North America each year. The functional consequences of an acute spinal cord injury (ASCI) are variable, therefore the initial clinical presentation of patients with ASCI is a key factor in determining triage and therapy and predicting prognosis. Consistent and reproducible neurological assessment scales are necessary to define the acute injury patient's neurological deficits and to facilitate communication about patient status to caregivers. Prognostic information provided by comparing injury victims to the outcomes of historical patients with similar injuries is of value to patients and families. The evaluation of new therapies proposed for the treatment of ASCI requires the use of accurate, reproducible neurological assessment scales and reliable functional outcome measurement tools, not only to measure potential improvement following therapy, but to determine its functional significance. For these reasons, the clinical neurological assessment and the determination of functional abilities are important aspects of the care of patients with ASCI. The purpose of this review of the medical literature is to determine which neurological assessment scales and which functional impairment tools have the greatest utility in the care of patients with acute spinal cord injuries.

Summary

A variety of injury classification schemes have been utilized to describe patients who have sustained spinal cord injuries. There are two general types of assessment scales, neurological examination scales and functional outcome scales. The most accurate and meaningful description of spinal cord injury patients, in the acute setting and in follow-up, appears to be that accomplished by using a neurological scale in conjunction with a functional outcome scale. At present, the most utilized and studied neurological assessment scales are the ASIA scores including the motor index scores, sensory scores and the ASIA Impairment scale. After multiple revisions and several refinements these scales are easy to apply, and are reliable.

The 1996 ASIA recommendations for international standards of neurological and functional classification of spinal cord injury include the ASIA scales, as noted, and the Functional Independence Measure (FIM). FIM as a functional outcome tool has been studied extensively. It appears to be the best functional outcome scale used to describe disability among SCI patients, both early and late after injury. It is easy to administer and is valid and reliable. Interrater agreement with FIM has been high in several studies with reported Kappa values of 0.53 to 0.76.

TOPIC 4: RADIOGRAPHIC ASSESSMENT OF THE CERVICAL SPINE IN ASYMPTOMATIC TRAUMA PATIENTS

Recommendations

Standards: Radiographic assessment of the cervical spine is not recommended in trauma patients who are awake, alert, and not intoxicated, who are without neck pain or tenderness, and who do not have significant associated injuries that detract from their general evaluation.

Guidelines: None
Options: None

Rationale

Spinal cord injury is a potentially devastating consequence of acute trauma and can occur with improper immobilization of an unstable cervical spine fracture. Immobilization of an injury victim's cervical spine following trauma is now standard care in the vast majority of Emergency Medical Services (EMS) systems. Immobilization of the cervical spine is maintained until spinal cord or spinal column injury is ruled out by clinical assessment and/or radiographic survey. Radiographic study of the cervical spine of every trauma patient is costly and results in significant radiation exposure to a large number of patients, very few of whom will have a spinal column injury. The purpose of this review is to define which radiographic studies are necessary in the assessment of the cervical spine in asymptomatic patients following trauma.

Summary

Clinical investigations which provide Class I evidence involving nearly 40,000 patients, plus Class II and III evidence studies involving over 5000 patients, convincingly demonstrate that asymptomatic patients do not require radiographic assessment of the cervical spine following trauma. The combined negative predictive value of cervical spine x-ray assessment of "asymptomatic" patients for a significant cervical spine injury is virtually 100%.

In contrast, the reported incidence of cervical spine injuries in the symptomatic patient ranged from 1.9% to 6.2% in these Class I evidence studies. Symptomatic patients require radiographic study to rule out the presence of a traumatic cervical spinal injury prior to the discontinuation of cervical spine immobilization. The type and extent of radiographic assessment of symptomatic patients following trauma is the topic of a separate review.

TOPIC 5: RADIOGRAPHIC ASSESSMENT OF THE CERVICAL SPINE IN SYMPTOMATIC TRAUMA PATIENTS

Recommendations

Standards: A three view cervical spine series (AP, lateral, and odontoid views) is recommended for radiographic evaluation of the cervical spine in patients who are symptomatic following traumatic injury. This should be supplemented with computed tomography to further define areas that are suspicious or not well visualized on the plain cervical x-rays.

Guidelines: There is insufficient evidence to support treatment guidelines.

Options: • It is recommended that cervical spine immobilization in awake patients with neck pain or tenderness and normal cervical spine x-rays (including supplemental CT as necessary) be discontinued following either:

 a) Normal and adequate dynamic flexion/extension radiographs; or

 b) Normal MRI study obtained within 48 hours of injury.

• Cervical spine immobilization of obtunded patients with normal cervical spine x-rays (including supplemental CT as necessary) may be discontinued:

 a) Following dynamic flexion/extension studies performed under fluoroscopic guidance; or

 b) Following a normal MRI study obtained within 48 hours of injury; or

 c) At the discretion of the treating physician.

Rationale

Trauma patients who are symptomatic, that is, complain of neck pain, have cervical spine tenderness, or have symptoms or signs of a neurological deficit associated with the cervical spine, and trauma patients who cannot be assessed for symptoms or signs (those who are unconscious, uncooperative or incoherent, intoxicated, or who have associated traumatic injuries that distract from their assessment) require radiographic study of the cervical spine prior to the discontinuation of cervical spine immobilization. Many authors have proposed strategies and imaging techniques to accomplish x-ray clearance of the cervical spine after trauma, particularly in the symptomatic or the obtunded patient. One, three, and five view static cervical spine x-rays, computed tomography (CT), magnetic resonance imaging (MRI), bone scans, flexion/extension radiographs, dynamic fluoroscopy with or without somatosensory evoked potential monitoring, and other studies have all been described as useful for the determination of spinal injury and potential spinal instability following traumatic injury. The purpose of this review is to determine the optimal radiographic assessment strategy necessary and sufficient to exclude a significant cervical spine injury in the symptomatic trauma patient.

Summary

In summary, no single radiographic study can adequately rule out cervical spinal injury in all symptomatic patients. A three-view spine cervical spine series supplemented with CT through areas difficult to visualize and "suspicious" areas will detect the vast majority of spinal injuries. This combination of studies represents the minimum required for clearance of the cervical spine in the symptomatic patient. The negative predictive value of this combination of studies is reported to be between 99% and 100% in several Class II and III evidence studies.

In the awake patient, dynamic flexion/extension views (with at least 30° excursion in each direction) are safe and effective for detecting the majority of "occult" cervical spine injuries not identified on plain x-rays. The negative predictive value of a normal three view series and flexion/extension views exceeds 99%. Patients who are unable to cooperate with active flexion/extension radiographs due to pain or muscle spasm may be maintained in a cervical collar until they are able to cooperate, or may be studied with MRI. A negative MRI within the first 48 hours of injury in addition to normal radiographs and supplemental CT appear to be sufficient for the clearance of the cervical spine. The significance of a positive MR study is currently unclear. It is suggested that cervical immobilization be continued in these patients until delayed flexion/extension views can be obtained.

In the obtunded patient with a normal three-view x-ray series and appropriate CT of the cervical spine, the incidence of significant spine injury is less than 1%. Based upon mechanism of injury and clinical judgment, the cervical spine in selected patients may be considered cleared without further study. In the remainder of cases, flexion/extension performed under fluoroscopic visualization appears to be safe and effective for ruling out significant ligamentous injury, with a reported negative predictive value of over 99%. Because the incidence of occult injury diagnosed with dynamic flexion/extension fluoroscopy in the setting of normal plain cervical spine x-rays and CT images is low, it is probably most efficient for these procedures to be performed by staff in the department of radiology, although variances in local experience should be respected. MRI represents another option for clearance of the spine in this patient population, and a negative MRI within 48 hours of injury appears to effectively eliminate the likelihood of a significant ligamentous injury. However, MRI evaluation will result in a large number of false positive examinations, and the consequences of prolonged unnecessary immobilization in the obtunded patient are not insignificant.

TOPIC 6: INITIAL CLOSED REDUCTION OF CERVICAL SPINAL FRACTURE-DISLOCATION INJURIES

Recommendations

Standards: There is insufficient evidence to support treatment standards.

Guidelines: There is insufficient evidence to support treatment guidelines.

Options:
- Early closed reduction of cervical spinal fracture-dislocation injuries with craniocervical traction is recommended for the restoration of anatomic alignment of the cervical spine in awake patients.
- Closed reduction in patients with an additional rostral injury is not recommended.
- Patients with cervical spinal fracture dislocation injuries who are not able to be examined during attempted closed reduction, or prior to open posterior reduction, should undergo MRI prior to attempted reduction. The presence of a significant disc herniation in this setting is a relative indication for a ventral decompression prior to reduction.
- MRI study of patients who fail attempts at closed reduction is recommended.
- Pre-reduction MRI performed in patients with cervical fracture dislocation injury will demonstrate disrupted or herniated intervertebral discs in one third to one half of patients with facet subluxation. These findings do not appear to significantly influence outcome following closed reduction in awake patients and therefore the utility of pre-reduction MRI in this circumstance is uncertain.

Rationale

Spinal cord injury is frequently associated with traumatic cervical spine fractures and cervical facet dislocation injuries because of the narrowing of the spinal canal caused by displacement of fracture fragments or subluxation of one vertebra over another. Reduction of the deformity helps to restore the diameter of the bony canal and eliminates bony compression of the spinal cord due to the vertebral fracture and/or subluxation. Theoretically, early decompression of the spinal cord after injury may lead to improved neurological outcome. Several large series of patients describe excellent results with closed reduction of cervical fractures and facet subluxations. However, descriptive series using pre-reduction MRI have reported a high incidence of cervical disc herniation in the facet dislocation patient population. Furthermore, case reports and small series of patients who worsened neurologically following closed cervical spinal reduction exist. Several of these reports implicate ventral compression of the spinal cord by displaced disc material. The purpose of this qualitative review is to address the following issues:

1. Is closed reduction safe and effective for reducing cervical spinal deformity in patients with cervical fractures or unilateral or bilateral facet dislocation injuries?
2. Is a pre-reduction MRI essential for the management of these patients?

Summary

Closed reduction of fracture-dislocation injuries of the cervical spine by traction-reduction appears to be safe and effective for the reduction of spinal deformity in awake patients. Approximately 80% of patients will have their injuries reduced with this technique. The overall permanent neurological complication rate of closed reduction is approximately 1%. The associated risk of a transient injury with closed reduction appears to be 2% to 4%. Closed traction-reduction appears to be safer than manipulation under anesthesia.

There are numerous causes of neurological deterioration in patients with unstable cervical spinal injuries. These include inadequate immobilization, unrecognized rostral injuries, over-distraction, loss of reduction, and cardiac, respiratory and hemodynamic instability. Therefore, the treatment of cervical spine fracture-dislocation injuries must be supervised by an appropriately trained specialist.

Although pre-reduction MRI will demonstrate disc herniation in up to half of patients with facet subluxation injuries, the clinical importance of these findings is questionable. Only two case reports exist which document neurological deterioration due to disc herniation following successful closed traction-reduction in awake patients. Both occurred in delayed fashion after closed reduction. In addition, several investigators have demonstrated the lack of correlation between the MRI finding of disc herniation and neurological deterioration in this patient population. The use of pre-reduction MRI has therefore not been shown to improve the safety or efficacy of closed traction-reduction in awake patients. MRI prior to fracture-dislocation reduction may result in unnecessary delays in accomplishing fracture realignment and decompression of the spinal cord. As Class III evidence exists in support of early closed reduction of cervical fracture-dislocation injuries with respect to neurological function, pre-reduction MRI in this setting is not necessary. The ideal timing of reduction is unknown, but many investigators favor reduction as rapidly as possible after injury to maximize the potential for neurological recovery.

Patients who fail attempted closed reduction of cervical fracture injuries have a higher incidence of anatomic obstacles to reduction including facet fractures and discs herniation. Patients who fail closed reduction should undergo more detailed radiographic study prior to attempts at open reduction. The presence of a significant disc herniation in this setting is a relative indication for an anterior decompression procedure, either in lieu of or preceding a posterior procedure.

Patients with cervical fracture dislocation who cannot be examined, due to head injury or intoxication, cannot be assessed for neurologic deterioration during attempted closed traction-reduction. For this reason, an MRI prior to attempted reduction is recommended as a treatment option.

TOPIC 7: MANAGEMENT OF ACUTE SPINAL CORD INURIES IN AN INTENSIVE CARE UNIT OR OTHER MONITORED SETTING

Recommendations

Standards: There is insufficient evidence to support treatment standards.

Guidelines: There is insufficient evidence to support treatment guidelines.

Options:
- Management of patients with acute SCI, particularly patients with severe cervical level injuries, in an intensive care unit or similar monitored setting is recommended.
- Use of cardiac, hemodynamic, and respiratory monitoring devices to detect cardiovascular dysfunction and respiratory insufficiency in patients following acute cervical spinal cord injury is recommended.

Rationale

The intensive care unit (ICU) setting has traditionally been reserved for critically ill patients who require aggressive medical care and exceptional medical attention. Most contemporary medical centers have multiple critical care units; each designed to provide discipline-specific observation and intensive care to patients in need. Select institutions have created Acute Spinal Cord Injury Centers and offer multidisciplinary care including ICU care to patients who have sustained acute spinal cord injuries. Several reports describe improved patient management and lower morbidity and mortality following acute SCI with intensive care unit monitoring and aggressive medical management. Despite this interest in and commitment to more comprehensive care for the patient with acute spinal cord injury (SCI) over the last 30 years by selected individuals and centers, many patients who sustain acute spinal cord injuries are not managed in an ICU setting, nor are they routinely monitored for cardiac or respiratory dysfunction. There exist divergent management strategies for acute SCI patients within regions, communities, even within institutions depending on the training and experiences of the clinicians providing care. Recently completed randomized clinical trials investigating pharmacological agents in the treatment of acute SCI patients did not suggest a specific, common medical management paradigm to guide patient care provided by participating investigators, other than the timing and dosage of the pharmacological agents being tested. These studies included large numbers of seriously injured acute SCI patients managed outside the ICU setting, most without continuous cardiac or respiratory monitoring.

Questions

1. Do patients with acute spinal cord injuries benefit from care in the ICU setting?
2. Is monitoring of cardiac, hemodynamic and pulmonary performance of benefit to patients who have sustained acute SCI?

Summary

Patients with severe acute SCI, particularly cervical level injuries, or patients with multi-system traumatic injury, frequently experience hypotension, hypoxemia, pulmonary dysfunction and many exhibit cardiovascular instability, despite early acceptable cardiac and pulmonary function after initial resuscitation. These occurrences are not limited to acute SCI patients with complete autonomic disruption. Life-threatening cardiovascular instability and respiratory insufficiency may be transient and episodic and may occur in patients who appear to have stable cardiac and respiratory function early in their post-injury course. Patients with the most severe neurological injuries after acute SCI appear to have the greatest risk of these life-threatening events. Monitoring allows the early detection of hemodynamic instability, cardiac rate disturbances, pulmonary dysfunction and hypoxemia. Identification and treatment of these events appears to reduce cardiac and respiratory related morbidity and mortality. Management in an intensive care unit or similar setting with cardiovascular and pulmonary monitoring have an impact on neurological outcome after acute SCI. Patients with acute spinal cord injuries appear to be best managed in the intensive care unit setting for the first seven to fourteen days after injury, the time frame during which they appear most susceptible to significant fluctuations in cardiac and pulmonary performance. This appears to be particularly true for severe cervical SCI patients, specifically acute ASIA grades A and B.

TOPIC 8: BLOOD PRESSURE MANAGEMENT FOLLOWING ACUTE SPINAL CORD INJURY

Recommendations

Standards: There is insufficient evidence to support treatment standards.

Guidelines: There is insufficient evidence to support treatment guidelines.

Options:
- Hypotension (systolic blood pressure <90 mm Hg) should be avoided if possible or corrected as soon as possible following acute SCI.
- Maintenance of mean arterial blood pressure at 85–90 mm Hg for the first seven days following acute SCI to improve spinal cord perfusion is recommended.

Rationale

Acute traumatic spinal cord injury is frequently associated with systemic hypotension. Hypotension may be due to associated traumatic injuries with hypovolemia, direct severe spinal cord trauma itself, or a combination. The occurrence of hypotension has been shown to be associated with worse outcomes after traumatic injury, including severe head injury. While a prospective controlled assessment of the effects of hypotension on acute human SCI has not been performed, laboratory evidence suggests that hypotension contributes to secondary injury after acute SCI by further reducing spinal cord blood flow and perfusion. Hypotension in animal models of spinal cord injury results in worse neurological outcome. Several clinical series of human patients with acute SCI managed in an aggressive fashion with attention to blood pressure, oxygenation and hemodynamic performance report no deleterious effects of therapy and suggest improved neurological outcome. Despite these observations, the majority of patients with acute SCI treated in contemporary practice are not routinely monitored nor treated with blood pressure augmentation following injury. For these reasons the issues of routine blood pressure support and threshold levels of mean arterial pressure maintenance following acute SCI have been raised.

Summary

Hypotension is common after acute traumatic SCI in humans. Hypotension contributes to spinal cord ischemia after injury in animal models and can worsen the initial insult and reduce the potential for neurological recovery. Although unproven by Class I medical evidence studies, it is likely that this occurs in human SCI patients as well. Since the correction of hypotension and maintenance of homeostasis is a basic principle of ethical medical practice in the treatment of patients with traumatic neurological injuries, depriving acute SCI patients of this treatment would be untenable. For this reason, Class I evidence about the effects of hypotension on outcome following acute human SCI will never be obtained. However, correction of hypotension has been shown to reduce morbidity and mortality after acute human traumatic brain injury, and is a guideline level recommendation for the management of TBI. While a similar treatment guideline cannot be supported by the existing spinal cord injury literature, correction of hypotension in the setting of acute human SCI is offered as a strong treatment option. Class III evidence from the literature suggests that maintenance of mean arterial pressure at 85 to 90 mm Hg after acute SCI for a duration of seven days is safe and may improve spinal cord perfusion and ultimately, neurological outcome.

TOPIC 9: PHARMACOLOGICAL THERAPY FOLLOWING ACUTE CERVICAL SPINAL CORD INJURY

Recommendations

STEROIDS

Standards: There is insufficient evidence to support treatment standards.

Guidelines: There is insufficient evidence to support treatment guidelines.

Options: Treatment with methylprednisolone for either 24 or 48 hours is recommended as an option in the treatment of patients with acute spinal cord injuries that should only be undertaken with the knowledge that the evidence suggesting harmful side effects is more consistent than any suggestion of clinical benefit.

GM-1 GANGLIOSIDE

Standards: There is insufficient evidence to support treatment standards.

Guidelines: There is insufficient evidence to support treatment guidelines.

Options: Treatment of patients with acute spinal cord injuries with GM-1 ganglioside is recommended as an option without demonstrated clinical benefit.

Rationale

The hope that administration of a pharmacological agent delivered shortly after acute spinal cord injury might improve neurological function and/or assist neurological recovery has long been held. A variety of promising substances have been tested in animal models of acute spinal cord injury, but few have had potential application to human spinal cord injury patients. Four pharmacological substances have met rigorous criteria in laboratory testing and initial human investigations: two steroids—Methylprednisolone and Tirilazad Mesylate, Naloxone, and GM-1 ganglioside. All four pharmacological agents have been evaluated in controlled, randomized, blinded clinical trials of human patients who have suffered acute spinal cord injuries. Two substances, tirilazad and naloxone, have been studied less extensively and as yet have unclear efficacy in the management of acute human spinal cord injury. The purpose of this medical evidenced-based review is to define the utility of the use of methylprednisolone with or without GM-1 ganglioside in the contemporary management of acute spinal cord injury patients.

Summary

In summary, the available medical evidence does not support a significant clinical benefit from the administration of methylprednisolone in the treatment of patients following acute spinal cord injury for either 24 or 48 hours duration. Three North American, multi-center randomized clinical trials have been completed and several other studies have been accomplished addressing this issue. The neurological recovery benefit of methylprednisolone when administered within eight hours of acute spinal cord injury has been suggested but not convincingly proven. The numerous studies that have attempted to address these issues and from which important conclusions have been drawn do not meet criteria for robust scientific evidence due to significant flaws in study design, trial conduct, statistical analyses, and final presentation of the data. The administration of methylprednisolone for 24 hours has been associated with a significant increase in severe medical complications. This is even more for striking for methylprednisolone administered for 48 hours. In light of the failure of clinical trials to convincingly demonstrate a significant clinical benefit of administration of methylprednisolone, in conjunction with the increased risks of medical complications associated with its use, methylprednisolone in the treatment of acute human spinal cord injuries is recommended as an option that should only be undertaken with the knowledge that the evidence suggesting harmful side effects is more consistent than any suggestion of clinical benefit.

GM-1 GANGLIOSIDE

The available medical evidence does not support a significant clinical benefit from the administration of GM-1 ganglioside in the treatment of patients following acute spinal cord injury. Two North American multi-center, randomized clinical trials have been completed addressing this issue. The neurological recovery benefit of GM-1 ganglioside when administered for 56 days following the administration of methylprednisolone within eight hours of acute spinal cord injury has been suggested but not convincingly proven. At present, GM-1 ganglioside, (a 300mg loading dose followed by 100mg/day for 56 days) when initiated after the administration of methylprednisolone given within eight hours of injury (NASCIS II protocol) is recommended as an option in the treatment of adult patients with acute spinal cord injuries.

TOPIC 10: DEEP VENOUS THROMBOSIS AND THROMBOEMBOLISM IN PATIENTS WITH CERVICAL SPINAL CORD INJURIES

Recommendations

Standards: • Prophylactic treatment of thromboembolism in patients with severe motor deficits due to spinal cord injury is recommended.
• The use of low molecular weight heparins, rotating beds, adjusted dose heparin, or a combination of modalities is recommended as a prophylactic treatment strategy.
• Low dose heparin in combination with pneumatic compression stockings or electrical stimulation is recommended as a prophylactic treatment strategy.

Guidelines: • Low dose heparin therapy alone is not recommended as a prophylactic treatment strategy.
• Oral anticoagulation alone is not recommended as a prophylactic treatment strategy.

Options: • Duplex Doppler ultrasound, impedance plethysmography, and venography are recommended for
use as diagnostic tests for DVT in the spinal cord
injured patient population.
• A 3-month duration of prophylactic treatment for
DVT and PE is recommended.
• Vena cava filters are recommended for patients who
fail anticoagulation or who are not candidates for
anticoagulation and/or mechanical devices.

Rationale

Deep venous thrombosis (DVT) and pulmonary embolism (PE) are
problems frequently encountered in patients who have sustained cervical spinal cord injuries. Several means of prophylaxis and treatment
are available including anticoagulation, pneumatic compression devices, and vena cava filters. The purpose of this evidence-based medicine review is to evaluate the literature on the methods of prevention
and identification of DVT and PE complications in patients following
acute cervical spinal cord injury.

Summary

Thromboembolic disease is a common occurrence in patients who
have sustained a cervical spinal cord injury and is associated with significant morbidity. Class I medical evidence exists demonstrating the
efficacy of several means of prophylaxis for the prevention of thromboembolic events. Therefore, patients with SCI should be treated with
a regimen aimed at prophylaxis.

Although low dose heparin therapy has been reported to be effective as prophylaxis for thromboembolism in several Class III studies,
other Class I, Class II, and Class III medical evidence indicates that
better alternatives than low dose heparin therapy exist. These alternatives include the use of low molecular weight heparin, adjusted dose
heparin, or anticoagulation in conjunction with pneumatic compression devices or electrical stimulation. Oral anticoagulation alone does
not appear to be as effective as these other measures used for prophylaxis.

The incidence of thromboembolic events appears to decrease over
time and the prolonged use of anticoagulant therapy is associated with
a definite incidence of bleeding complications. There are multiple reports of the beneficial effects of the prophylaxis therapy for six to
twelve weeks following spinal cord injury. Very few thromboembolic
events occur beyond three months following injury. For these reasons,
it is recommended that prophylactic therapy be discontinued after
three months unless the patient is at high risk (previous thromboem-

bolic events, obesity, advanced age). It is reasonable to discontinue therapy earlier in patients with retained lower extremity motor function after spinal cord injury, as the incidence of thromboembolic events in these patients is substantially lower than those patients with motor complete injuries.

Caval filters appear to be efficacious for the prevention of PE in SCI patients. The relative efficacy of caval filters versus prophylactic combination therapy with LMWH and pneumatic compression stockings has not been studied. Caval filters are associated with long-term complications in SCI patients, although these complications are relatively rare. Caval filters are recommended for SCI patients who have suffered thromboembolic events despite anticoagulation and for SCI patients with contraindications to anticoagulation and/or the use of pneumatic compression devices.

There are several methods available for the diagnosis of DVT. Venography is considered the "gold standard," but is invasive, not applicable to all patients, and associated with intrinsic morbidity. Duplex Doppler ultrasound and venous occlusion plethysmography have been reported to have sensitivities of approximately 90% and are non-invasive. It is reasonable to use these non-invasive tests for the diagnosis of DVT and to reserve venography for the rare situation when clinical suspicion is high and the results of VOP and ultrasound testing are negative.

TOPIC 11: NUTRITIONAL SUPPORT AFTER SPINAL CORD INJURY

Recommendations

Standards: There is insufficient evidence to support treatment standards.

Guidelines: There is insufficient evidence to support treatment guidelines.

Options: Nutritional support of SCI patients is recommended. Energy expenditure is best determined by indirect calorimetry in these patients as equation estimates of energy expenditure and subsequent caloric need tend to be inaccurate.

Rationale

Hypermetabolism, an accelerated catabolic rate and rampant nitrogen losses are consistent sequelae to major trauma, particularly acute traumatic brain injury and acute spinal cord injury. A well-documented hypermetabolic, catabolic injury cascade is initiated immediately after central nervous system injury which results in depletion of whole body energy stores, loss of lean muscle mass, reduced protein synthesis, and ultimately in loss of gastrointestinal mucosal integrity and compromise of immune competence. Severely injured brain and spinal cord injury patients, therefore, are at risk for prolonged nitrogen losses and advanced malnutrition within two to three weeks following injury with resultant increased susceptibility for infection, impaired wound healing and difficulty weaning from mechanical ventilation. These factors added to the inherent immobility, denervation and muscle atrophy associated with spinal cord injury provide the rationale for nutritional support of spinal cord injured patients following trauma.

Summary

Alterations in metabolism occur after acute SCI, but the marked hypermetabolic response seen after acute traumatic brain injury appears to be blunted in SCI patients, by the flaccidity of denervated musculature after spinal cord transection/injury. As a result, resting energy expenditure (REE) is lower than predicted after acute SCI. Equation estimates of REE in these patients have proven to be inaccurate, therefore indirect calorimetry is the recommended technique to assess energy expenditure in both the acute and chronic settings.

Protein catabolism does occur after acute, severe SCI, and marked losses in lean body mass due to muscle atrophy result in huge nitrogen losses, prolonged negative nitrogen balance and rapid weight loss. Nutritional support of the SCI patient to meet caloric and nitrogen needs, not to achieve nitrogen balance, is safe and may reduce the deleterious effects of the catabolic, nitrogen wasting process that occurs after acute spinal cord injury.

TOPIC 12: MANAGEMENT OF PEDIATRIC CERVICAL SPINE AND SPINAL CORD INJURIES

Recommendations

DIAGNOSTIC

Standards: There is insufficient evidence to support diagnostic standards.

Guidelines: • In children who have experienced trauma and are alert, conversant, have no neurological deficit, no midline cervical tenderness, no painful distracting injury, and are not intoxicated, cervical spine radiographs are unnecessary to exclude cervical spine injury and are not recommended.

- In children who have experienced trauma and who are either not alert or non-conversant, or have neurological deficit, midline cervical tenderness, painful distracting injury, or are intoxicated, it is recommended that A-P and lateral cervical spine radiographs be obtained.

Options:
- In children less than nine years of age who have experienced trauma, and who are non-conversant or have an altered mental status, a neurological deficit, neck pain, a painful distracting injury, are intoxicated, or have unexplained hypotension, it is recommended that AP and lateral cervical spine radiographs be obtained.
- In children nine years of age or older who have experienced trauma, and who are non-conversant or have an altered mental status, a neurological deficit, neck pain, a painful distracting injury, are intoxicated, or have unexplained hypotension it is recommended that AP, lateral, and open-mouth cervical spine radiographs be obtained.
- CT scan with attention to the suspected level of neurological injury to exclude occult fractures, or to evaluate regions not seen adequately on plain radiographs is recommended.
- Flexion and extension cervical radiographs or fluoroscopy may be considered to exclude gross ligamentous instability when there remains a suspicion of cervical spine instability following static radiographs.
- MRI of the cervical spine may be considered to exclude cord or nerve root compression, evaluate ligamentous integrity, or provide information regarding neurological prognosis.

TREATMENT

Standards: There is insufficient evidence to support treatment standards.

Guidelines: There is insufficient evidence to support treatment guidelines.

Options:
- Thoracic elevation or an occipital recess to prevent flexion of the head and neck when restrained supine on an otherwise flat backboard may allow for better neutral alignment and immobilization of the cervical spine in children less than eight years of age

because of the relatively large head in these younger children and is recommended.

- Closed reduction and halo immobilization for injuries of the C2 synchondrosis between the body and odontoid is recommended in children less than seven years of age.
- Consideration of primary operative therapy is recommended for isolated ligamentous injuries of the cervical spine with associated deformity.

Rationale

There are distinct, unique aspects of the management of children with potential injuries of the cervical spinal column and cervical spinal cord compared to adult patients that warrant specific recommendations. The methods of pre-hospital immobilization necessary to approximate "neutral" cervical spinal alignment in a young child differ from those methods commonly employed for adults. The spinal injury patterns among young children differ from those that occur in adults. The diagnostic studies and images necessary to exclude a cervical spine injury in a child may be different than in the adult as well. The interpretation of pediatric radiographic studies must be made with knowledge of age-related development of the osseous and ligamentous anatomy. Methods of reduction, stabilization, and subsequent treatment, surgical and non-surgical, must be customized to each child taking into account the child's degree of physical maturation and his/her specific injury. The purpose of this review is to address the unique aspects of children with real or potential cervical spinal injuries and provide recommendations regarding their management.

Summary

The available medical evidence does not allow the generation of diagnostic or treatment standards for the management of pediatric patients with cervical spine or cervical spinal cord injuries. Only diagnostic guidelines and options, and treatment options are supported by this evidence. The literature suggests that obtaining neutral cervical spine alignment in a child may be difficult when standard backboards are used. The determination that a child does not have a cervical spine injury can be made on clinical grounds alone is supported by Class II and Class III evidence. When the child is alert and communicative and is without neurological deficit, neck tenderness, painful distracting injury, or intoxication, cervical radiographs are not necessary to exclude cervical spinal injury. When cervical spine radiographs are utilized to verify or rule out a cervical spinal injury in children less than nine years of age, only lateral and A-P cervical spine views need be obtained. The traditional three-view x-ray assessment may increase the sensitivity of plain spine radiographs in children nine years of age and older. The vast majority of pediatric cervical spine injuries can be effectively treated non-operatively. The most effective immobilization appears to be accomplished with either halo devices or Minerva jackets. Halo immobilization is associated with acceptable but considerable minor morbidity in children, typically pin site infection and pin loosening. The only specific pediatric cervical spine injury for which medical evidence supports a particular treatment paradigm is an odontoid injury in children less than seven years of age. These children are effectively treated with closed reduction and immobilization. Primarily ligamentous injuries of the cervical spine in children may heal with external immobilization alone, but are associated with a relatively high rate of progressive deformity when treated non-operatively. Pharmacological therapy and intensive care unit management schemes for children with spinal cord injury have not been described in the literature.

TOPIC 13: SPINAL CORD INJURY WITHOUT RADIOGRAPHIC ABNORMALITY (SCIWORA)

Recommendations

DIAGNOSIS

Standards: There is insufficient evidence to support diagnostic standards.

Guidelines: There is insufficient evidence to support diagnostic guidelines.

Options:
- Plain spinal radiographs of the region of injury and CT scan with attention to the suspected level of neurological injury to exclude occult fractures are recommended.
- MR of the region of suspected neurological injury may provide useful diagnostic information.
- Plain radiographs of the entire spinal column may be considered.
- Neither spinal angiography nor myelography is recommended in the evaluation of patients with SCIWORA.

TREATMENT

Standards: There is insufficient evidence to support treatment standards.

Guidelines: There is insufficient evidence to support treatment guidelines.

Options:
- External immobilization is recommended until spinal stability is confirmed flexion and extension radiographs.
- External immobilization of the spinal segment of injury for up to 12 weeks may be considered.
- Avoidance of "high-risk" activities for up to six months following SCIWORA may be considered.

PROGNOSIS

Standards: There is insufficient evidence to support prognostic standards.

Guidelines: There is insufficient evidence to support prognostic guidelines.

Options: MRI of the region of neurological injury may provide useful prognostic information about neurological outcome following SCIWORA.

Rationale

DIAGNOSIS

Pang and Wilberger defined the term SCIWORA (Spinal Cord Injury Without Radiographic Abnormality) in 1982 as "objective signs of myelopathy as a result of trauma" with no evidence of fracture or ligamentous instability on plain spine radiographs and tomography. In their original manuscript they cautioned, "that if the early warning signs of transient symptoms could be recognized and promptly acted upon before the onset of neurological signs, the tragic fate of some of these children might be duly averted". Hamilton and Myles, Osenbach and Menezes, and Pang and Wilberger, have documented the delayed onset of SCIWORA in children as late as four days following injury. Therefore, a concern is whether a child with a normal neurological examination, but with a history of transient neurological symptoms or persisting subjective neurological symptoms referable to traumatic myelopathy should be assigned the diagnosis of SCIWORA and managed accordingly, despite the absence of "objective signs of myelopathy."

Pang and Pollack have recommended obtaining a CT scan focused at the neurological level of injury to exclude an occult fracture in a child with a neurological deficit referable to the spinal cord without abnormalities on plain radiographs of the spine. In addition, dynamic flexion and extension radiographs or fluoroscopy have been advocated to exclude pathological intersegmental motion consistent with ligamentous injury without fracture. If paraspinous muscle spasm, pain, or uncooperation prevents dynamic studies, they recommended external immobilization until the child can flex and extend the spine for dynamic x-ray assessment. The finding of fracture, subluxation, or abnormal intersegmental motion at the level of neurological injury excludes SCIWORA as a diagnosis. In the initial report by Pang and Wilberger, one of 24 children showed pathological motion on initial dynamic radiographs. By their own definition of SCIWORA, this one child would not be diagnosed with SCIWORA because the initial flexion and extension radiographs were abnormal. While concern exists for the development of pathological intersegmental motion in children with SCIWORA following normal flexion and extension studies, there has not been documentation of such instability ever developing.

Magnetic resonance (MR) imaging findings in children with SCIWORA have spanned the spectrum from normal to complete cord disruption, along with evidence of ligamentous and disc injury in some. Possible roles for MR of children with SCIWORA include: 1) exclude compressive lesions of the cord or roots or ligamentous disruption that might warrant surgical intervention, 2) guide treatment regarding length of external immobilization, and/or 3) determine when to allow patients to return to full activity.

TREATMENT

Because there exists no subluxation or malalignment in SCIWORA the mainstay of treatment has been immobilization and avoidance of activity that may lead to either exacerbation of the present injury or increase the potential for recurrent injury. Medical management issues such as blood pressure support and pharmacological therapy are of concern to this population as well, and have been addressed in other guidelines. (Of note, the often-cited prospective studies of pharmacological therapy in the treatment of acute spinal cord injury did not include children younger than 13 years of age).

Pang and Pollack have recommended 12 weeks of external immobilization to allow adequate time for the healing of the presumed ligamentous strain/injury and to prevent exacerbation of the myelopathy. It is unclear however, what role immobilization plays in this population once dynamic radiographs have displayed no instability. The length of and even the need for immobilization remain debatable given the current literature. If the incidence of delayed pathological intersegmental motion in children with SCIWORA who have been proven to have normal dynamic radiographs approaches zero, then the role of spinal immobilization for SCIWORA patients needs to be considered in light of the available literature. If physiological motion (normal) of the spinal column can potentiate spinal cord injury (SCIWORA), in these patients when there is no malalignment, subluxation, or lesion causing cord compression, then immobilization is warranted in these patients.

PROGNOSIS

SCIWORA has been shown to be associated with a high incidence of complete neurological injuries, particularly in children less than nine years of age. Hadley, et al, reported four complete injuries in six children less than ten-years-old with SCIWORA. The regions of complete injury tend to be cervical and upper thoracic. Pang found the presenting neurological examination to relate strongly to outcome. There is some data to suggest that MR abnormalities (or lack of abnormalities) of the cord may be more predictive of outcome than presenting neurological status. Because no child has been documented to develop spinal instability following the diagnosis of SCIWORA, and has by definition, normal flexion and extension radiographs, there has been little impetus to define predictors of instability. On the other hand, children have been documented to suffer recurrent SCIWORA, and predictors of a "high-risk" sub-group of children with SCIWORA for recurrent injury may exist.

Summary

Children presenting with a history of transient neurological signs or symptoms referable to traumatic myelopathy despite the absence of objective evidence of myelopathy and normal radiographs may develop SCIWORA in a delayed fashion.

No child with SCIWORA has developed pathological intersegmental motion with instability after demonstrating normal flexion and extension radiographs.

MRI has not identified any lesion in a child with SCIWORA where the management scheme would be changed by the results of the MRI. Similarly, no child with MRI documented ligamentous injury and SCIWORA has developed evidence of spinal instability.

Hard collar immobilization for patients with cervical level SCIWORA for 12 weeks and avoidance of activities that encourage flexion and extension of the neck for an additional 12 weeks has not been associated with recurrent injury.

The spinal cord findings on MRI imaging provide prognostic information regarding long-term neurological outcome in patients with SCIWORA.

Myelography and angiography have no defined role in the evaluation of children with SCIWORA.

TOPIC 14: DIAGNOSIS AND MANAGEMENT OF TRAUMATIC ATLANTO-OCCIPITAL DISLOCATION INJURIES

Recommendations

DIAGNOSTIC

Standards: There is insufficient evidence to support diagnostic standards.

Guidelines: There is insufficient evidence to support diagnostic guidelines.

Options:
- A lateral cervical radiograph is recommended for the diagnosis of AOD. If a radiological method for measurement is used, the basion-axial interval-basion dental interval (BAI-BDI) method is recommended.
- The presence of upper cervical prevertebral soft tissue swelling on an otherwise non-diagnostic plain radiograph should prompt additional imaging.
- If there is clinical suspicion of AOD, and plain radiographs are non-diagnostic, CT or MR imaging is recommended, particularly for the diagnosis of non-Type II dislocations.

TREATMENT

Standards: There is insufficient evidence to support treatment standards.

Guidelines: There is insufficient evidence to support treatment guidelines.

Options: Treatment with internal fixation and arthrodesis using one of a variety of methods is recommended. Traction may be used in the management of patients with AOD, but is associated with a ten percent risk of neurological deterioration.

Rationale

Although traumatic atlanto-occipital dislocation (AOD) was perceived to be an uncommon injury resulting in frequent death, improvements in emergency management of the patient in the field, rapid transport, and better recognition have resulted in more survivors of AOD in the past two decades. Infrequent observation of patients with AOD and missed diagnoses may impair outcomes of patients with this unusual injury. An assimilation of the reported experiences of clinicians evaluating and managing AOD may facilitate development of diagnostic and treatment options for this traumatic disorder. Specific questions that were evaluated include the sensitivity of plain radiographs, CT, and MR imaging in the diagnosis of AOD, as well as the safety and efficacy of various treatment modalities for AOD, including no treatment, traction, external immobilization, and internal fixation with fusion.

Summary

AOD is an uncommon traumatic injury which is difficult to diagnose and is frequently missed on initial lateral cervical radiographs. Patients who survive often have neurological impairment including lower cranial neuropathies, unilateral or bilateral weakness, or quadriplegia. Yet, nearly 20% of patients with acute traumatic AOD will have a normal neurological examination on presentation. The lack of localizing features may impede diagnosis in the patient with a normal cervical radiograph. A high index of suspicion must be maintained in order to diagnose AOD. Prevertebral soft tissue swelling on a lateral cervical radiograph or craniocervical subarachnoid hemorrhage on axial CT have been associated with AOD and may prompt consideration of the diagnosis. Additional imaging including CT and MR may be required to confirm the diagnosis of AOD if plain radiographs are inadequate. All patients with AOD should be treated. Without treatment, nearly all patients developed neurological worsening, some of whom did not recover. Although treatment with traction and external immobilization has been used successfully in some patients, transient or permanent neurological worsening and late instability have been reported more often in association with these treatments compared to surgical treatment. Consequently, craniocervical fusion with internal fixation is recommended for the treatment of patients with acute traumatic AOD.

TOPIC 15: OCCIPITAL CONDYLE FRACTURES
Recommendations

DIAGNOSTIC

Standards: There is insufficient evidence to support diagnostic standards.

Guidelines: CT imaging is recommended for establishing the diagnosis of occipital condyle fractures. Clinical suspicion should be raised by the presence of one or more of the following criteria: blunt trauma patients sustaining high energy craniocervical injuries, altered consciousness, occipital pain or tenderness, impaired cervical motion, lower cranial nerve paresis, or retropharyngeal soft tissue swelling.

Options: MR imaging is recommended to assess the integrity of the craniocervical ligaments.

TREATMENT

Standards: There is insufficient evidence to support treatment standards.

Guidelines: There is insufficient evidence to support treatment guidelines.

Options: Treatment with external cervical immobilization is recommended.

Rationale

Although traumatic occipital condyle fracture (OCF) was first described by Bell in 1817, more frequent observation of this injury has only been reported during the past two decades. Improvements in computed tomographic (CT) imaging technology and use of CT imaging of the head-injured patient that includes the craniovertebral junction have resulted in more frequent recognition of this injury. However, the overall infrequent occurrence of OCF and missed diagnoses in patients with OCF may result in late neurological deficits in these patients. An analysis of the reported cases of OCF may facilitate development of diagnostic and treatment recommendations for this disorder and are undertaken in this report. Specific questions that were evaluated include: accuracy of plain radiographs and CT imaging in the diagnosis of OCF, as well as the safety and efficacy of various treatment modalities including no treatment, traction, external immobilization, decompression and internal fixation with fusion.

Summary

OCF is an uncommon injury requiring CT imaging for diagnosis. Patients sustaining high energy blunt craniocervical trauma, particularly in the setting of loss of consciousness, impaired consciousness, occipitocervical pain or motion impairment, and lower cranial nerve deficits, should undergo CT imaging of the craniocervical junction. Untreated patients with OCF often develop lower cranial nerve deficits that usually recover or improve with external immobilization. Identification of Type III OCF should prompt external immobilization. Additional treatment may be dictated by the presence of associated cervical fractures or instability.

TOPIC 16: ISOLATED FRACTURES OF THE ATLAS IN ADULTS

Recommendations

Standards: There is insufficient evidence to support treatment standards.

Guidelines: There is insufficient evidence to support treatment guidelines.

Options: Treatment options in the management of isolated fractures of the atlas are based on the specific atlas fracture type. It is recommended that isolated fractures of the atlas with an intact transverse atlantal ligament be treated with cervical immobilization alone. It is recommended that isolated fractures of the atlas with disruption of the transverse atlantal ligament be treated with either cervical immobilization alone or surgical fixation and fusion.

Rationale

The atlas vertebra is subject to a variety of acute fracture injuries and may be associated with other cervical fracture and ligamentous traumatic injuries. While the treatment of atlas fractures in combination with other cervical fracture injuries is most commonly linked to the treatment of the associated injury, isolated fractures of the atlas occur with sufficient frequency to warrant review.

The medical literature addressing the management of fractures of the atlas was examined using evidence-based medicine techniques to determine the optimal treatment for isolated atlas fractures including: Isolated anterior or posterior arch fractures, anterior and posterior arch fractures (burst fractures), lateral mass fractures, comminuted fractures, and transverse process fractures.

Summary

There are no Class I or Class II studies which address the management of patients with isolated atlas fractures. All of the articles reviewed described case series or case reports providing Class III evidence supporting several treatment strategies for patients with acute C1 fracture injuries.

Isolated anterior or posterior atlas arch fractures and fractures of the atlas lateral mass have been effectively treated with external cervical immobilization devices. Rigid collars, SOMI braces and halo ring-vest orthosis have all been utilized for a duration of treatment of

8–12 weeks with good result. No study has provided evidence for using one of these devices over the other.

Combined anterior and posterior arch fractures of the atlas (burst fractures) with an intact transverse atlantal ligament (implying C1-C2 stability) have been effectively managed with use of a rigid collar, a SOMI brace, or a halo orthosis for a duration of 10–12 weeks.

Combined anterior and posterior arch fractures of the atlas (burst fractures) with evidence of transverse atlantal ligament disruption have been effectively treated with either rigid immobilization alone (halo orthosis) for a period of 12 weeks, or surgical stabilization and fusion. The type of C1-C2 internal fixation and fusion procedure performed may influence the need for and duration of post-operative immobilization.

Criteria proposed to determine transverse atlantal ligament injury with associated C1-C2 instability include: Sum of the displacement of the lateral masses of C1 on C2 of greater than 8.1 mm on plain films ("rules of Spence" corrected for magnification), a predental space of greater than 3.0 mm in adults, and magnetic resonance imaging evidence of ligamentous disruption or avulsion.

TOPIC 17: ISOLATED FRACTURES OF THE AXIS IN ADULTS

Recommendations

FRACTURES OF THE ODONTOID

Standards: There is insufficient evidence to support treatment standards.

Guidelines: Type II Odontoid fractures in patients 50 years of age and older should be considered for surgical stabilization and fusion.

Options: Type I, Type II and Type III fractures may be managed initially with external cervical immobilization. Type II and Type III odontoid fractures should be considered for surgical fixation in cases of dens displacement five mm or greater, comminution of the odontoid fracture (Type IIA) and/or inability to achieve or maintain fracture alignment with external immobilization.

TRAUMATIC SPONDYLOLISTHESIS OF THE AXIS
(HANGMAN'S FRACTURE)

Standards: There is insufficient evidence to support treatment standards.

Guidelines: There is insufficient evidence to support treatment guidelines.

Options: Traumatic spondylolisthesis of the axis may be managed initially with external immobilization in the majority of cases. Surgical stabilization should be considered in cases of severe angulation of C2 on C3, (Francis Grade II and IV, Effendi Type II), disruption of the C2-3 disc space, (Francis Grade V, Effendi Type III) or inability to establish or maintain alignment with external immobilization.

FRACTURES OF THE AXIS BODY (MISCELLANEOUS FRACTURES)

Standards: There is insufficient evidence to support treatment standards.

Guidelines: There is insufficient evidence to support treatment standards.

Options: External immobilization is recommended for treatment of isolated fractures of the axis body.

Rationale

Fractures of the axis represent unique cervical vertebral injuries due to the unique anatomy and biomechanics of the C2 vertebra and the stresses applied to the dynamic atlanto-axial complex during trauma. Fractures of the axis may be associated with other cervical fractures or ligamentous injuries. Isolated fractures of the axis are common and warrant independent consideration. Fractures of the axis have been divided into three general subtypes: Fractures of the odontoid process, traumatic spondylolisthesis of the axis (Hangman's fractures), and miscellaneous non-odontoid non-Hangman's fractures of the C2 vertebra. Each of these fracture subtypes has been further subdivided based on the anatomic features and the functional significance of the individual fracture injury. The purpose of this review is to identify evidence-based management strategies for each injury subtype of traumatic fractures of the second cervical vertebra.

Summary

FRACTURES OF THE ODONTOID

There is no Class I medical evidence addressing the issues of management of acute traumatic odontoid fractures. A single Class II evidence paper reviews the management of Type II odontoid fractures in halo immobilization devices. This study demonstrated a 21-fold increase in risk of non-union with halo immobilization in patients over the age of 50 years. All other articles reviewed contain Class III evidence that supports several treatments.

Type II odontoid fractures in patients 50 years of age and older should be considered for surgical stabilization and fusion. Type I, Type II and Type III fractures may be managed initially with external cervical immobilization. Type II and Type III odontoid fractures should be considered for surgical fixation in cases of dens displacement five mm or greater, comminution of the odontoid fracture (Type IIA) and/or inability to achieve or maintain fracture alignment with external immobilization. Isolated Type I and Type III odontoid fractures may be treated with cervical immobilization, resulting in fusion rates of 100% and 84%, respectively. Anterior surgical fixation of Type III fractures has been associated with a 100% fusion rate. Type II odontoid fractures may be treated with external immobilization or surgical fixation and fusion. Halo immobilization and posterior fixation have both been used successfully for these injuries. Anterior odontoid-screw fixation has been reported with up to a 90% fusion success rate, except in older patients. Treatment of Type II odontoid fracture with a cervical collar alone or traction followed by cervical collar immobilization may also be undertaken, but have lower success rates.

TRAUMATIC SPONDYLOLISTHESIS OF THE AXIS

There is no Class I or Class II medical evidence addressing the management of traumatic spondylolisthesis of the axis. All articles reviewed contain Class III evidence that supports a variety of treatments. The majority of Hangman's fractures heal with 12 weeks of cervical immobilization either with a rigid cervical collar or a halo immobilization device. Surgical stabilization is an option in cases of severe angulation (Francis Grade II and IV, Effendi Type II), disruption of the C2-3 disc space (Francis Grade V, Effendi Type III), or the inability to establish or maintain fracture alignment with external immobilization.

FRACTURES OF THE AXIS BODY (MISCELLANEOUS AXIS FRACTURES)

There is no Class I or Class II medical evidence addressing the management of traumatic fractures of the axis body. All articles reviewed contain Class III evidence that supports the use of external immobilization as the initial treatment strategy.

TOPIC 18: MANAGEMENT OF COMBINATION FRACTURES OF THE ATLAS AND AXIS IN ADULTS

Recommendations

Standards: There is insufficient evidence to support treatment standards.

Guidelines: There is insufficient evidence to support treatment guidelines.

Options: Treatment of atlas-axis combination fractures based primarily on the specific characteristics of the axis fracture is recommended. External immobilization of the majority of C1-C2 combination fractures is recommended. C1-Type II odontoid combination fractures with an ADI of five mm or greater and C1-Hangman's combination fractures with C2-C3 angulation of 11 degrees or greater should be considered for surgical stabilization and fusion. In some cases, the surgical technique must modified as a result of the loss of the integrity of the ring of the atlas.

Rationale

Combined fractures of the atlas and axis often present management challenges due to the unique anatomy and biomechanics of the atlantoaxial complex and the untoward stresses applied to the atlantoaxial region during trauma. While the majority of isolated atlas and axis fractures have been managed with cervical immobilization, the occurrence of the two fractures in combination often implies a more significant structural and mechanical injury. Although reports of combination C1-C2 fractures are relatively infrequent, sufficient evidence exists to allow a review of the management of a variety of combinations of atlas and axis fractures. The purpose of this report is to examine the available literature to determine successful treatment strategies for individual C1-C2 combination fracture types.

Summary

Combination fractures involving fractures of both the atlas and axis occur relatively frequently. A higher incidence of neurological deficit is associated with C1-C2 combination fractures compared to either C1 or C2 fractures in isolation. The C1-Type II odontoid combination fracture appears to be the most common combination injury subtype, followed by C1-miscellaneous axis, C1-Type III odontoid and C1-Hangman's combination fractures.

No Class I or Class II evidence addressing the management of patients with combination atlas and axis fractures is available. All of the articles reviewed describe case series or case reports containing Class III evidence supporting a variety of treatment strategies for these unique fracture injuries.

In most circumstances, the specifics of the axis fracture will dictate the most appropriate management of the combination fracture injury.

As reported for isolated atlas and axis fractures, the majority of atlas-axis combination fractures can be effectively treated with rigid external immobilization. Combination atlas-axis fractures with an atlanto-axial interval of five mm or greater or angulation of C2-C3 of 11 degrees or greater may be considered for surgical fixation and fusion. The integrity of the ring of the atlas must often be taken into account when planning a specific surgical strategy utilizing instrumentation and fusion techniques. If the posterior arch of C1 is inadequate, both incorporation of the occiput into the fusion construct (occipitocervical fusion) and posterior C1-C2 transarticular screw fixation and fusion have been successful.

TOPIC 19: OS ODONTOIDEUM

Recommendations

DIAGNOSIS

Standards: There is insufficient evidence to support diagnostic standards.

Guidelines: There is insufficient evidence to support diagnostic guidelines.

Options: Plain radiographs of the cervical spine (A-P, open mouth odontoid, and lateral) and plain dynamic lateral radiographs performed in flexion and extension are recommended. Tomography (computerized or plain) and/or MR of the craniocervical junction may be considered.

MANAGEMENT

Standards: There is insufficient evidence to support treatment standards.

Guidelines: There is insufficient evidence to support treatment guidelines.

Options:
- Patients with os odontoideum, either with or without C1-2 instability, who have neither symptoms nor neurological signs may be managed with clinical and radiographic surveillance.
- Patients with os odontoideum, particularly with neurological symptoms and/or signs, and C1-2 instability may be managed with posterior C1-2 internal fixation and fusion.
- Postoperative halo immobilization as an adjunct to

posterior internal fixation and fusion is recommended unless successful C1-C2 transarticular screw fixation and fusion can be accomplished.
- Occipital-cervical fusion with or without C1 laminectomy may be considered in patients with os odontoideum who have irreducible cervicomedullary compression and/or evidence of associated occipital-atlantal instability.
- Transoral decompression may be considered in patients with os odontoideum who have irreducible ventral cervicomedullary compression.

Rationale

The definition of an os odontoideum (os) is uniform throughout the literature: an ossicle with smooth circumferential cortical margins representing the odontoid process that has no osseous continuity with the body of C2. The etiology of os odontoideum remains debated in the literature with evidence for both acquired and congenital causes. The etiology of os, however, does not play an important role in its diagnosis or subsequent management.

DIAGNOSIS

Os odontoideum can present with a wide range of clinical symptoms and signs, as well as be an incidental finding on imaging. The literature has focused on three groups of patients with os odontoideum, 1) those with occipital-cervical pain alone, 2) those with myelopathy, and 3) those with intracranial symptoms or signs from vertebrobasilar ischemia. Patients with os odontoideum *and* myelopathy have been subcategorized further into those with: 1) transient myelopathy (commonly following trauma), 2) static myelopathy, and 3) progressive myelopathy. Because patients with occipital-cervical pain, myelopathy, or vertebrobasilar ischemia likely will have etiologies other than os, the diagnosis of os odontoideum is not usually considered until imaging is obtained. The presence of an os is usually first suggested after obtaining plain cervical spine radiographs. Most often plain cervical spine radiographs are sufficient to obtain a diagnosis.

Os odontoideum has been classified into two anatomic types, orthotopic and dystopic. Orthotopic defines an ossicle that moves with the anterior arch of C1, while dystopic defines an ossicle that is functionally fused to the basion. The dystopic os may sublux anterior to the arch of C1. Tomograms and computerized tomography have been used to better define the bony anatomy of the os and the odontoid process.

Plain dynamic radiographs in flexion and extension have been used to depict the degree of abnormal motion between C1 and C2. Most often there is anterior instability with the os subluxing forward in relation to the body of C2. However, at times one will see either no discernible instability, or "posterior instability" with the os moving posteriorly into the spinal canal during neck extension.

With respect to diagnosis, the issues regarding the imaging of os odontoideum are two: First, while plain radiographs are often diagnostic for os, the sensitivity and specificity of plain cervical radiographs for os odontoideum have not been reported. The utility of confirmatory studies such as computerized and plain tomography and MR has not been well defined. Second, following the diagnosis of os odontoideum on plain cervical x-rays, instability and osseous anomalies associated with os can influence clinical management. The best methods of further evaluating or excluding these complicating factors deserve definition.

MANAGEMENT

The natural history of untreated os covers a wide spectrum. The literature provides many examples of both asymptomatic and symptomatic patients with known os odontoideum who have never been treated, and who have had no reported new problems in follow-up over many years. Conversely, examples of sudden spinal cord injury in association with os following minor trauma have also been reported. The natural history of os odontoideum is variable, and predictive factors for deterioration, particularly in the asymptomatic patient have not been identified. Indications for surgical stabilization include: simply the existence of an os, os in association with occipital cervical pain alone and/or os in association with neurological deficit. Other factors that may assist in determining the need for stabilization and/or decompression include C1-2 instability, associated deformities, and spinal cord compression. A variety of techniques have been used to stabilize C1 and C2 in patients with os odontoideum. Fusion success rates and complication rates for these various procedures may provide evidence as to whether a preferred method of C1-2 arthrodesis is supported by the literature.

Finally, neural compression is an important consideration in patients with os odontoideum. Neural compression may be anterior from a combination of bone and soft tissue, or posterior from the dorsal arch of C1. Surgical techniques to stabilize and fuse across the craniocervical junction with or without C1 laminectomy, and techniques that provide ventral decompression have been reported in the treatment of os odontoideum with irreducible neural compression. The literature will be examined in light of the risks and benefits these techniques may provide to patients with os odontoideum.

Summary

Plain cervical spine radiographs appear adequate to make a diagnosis of os odontoideum in the vast majority of patients with this disorder. Lateral flexion and extension radiographs can provide useful information regarding C1-2 instability. Tomography (computerized or plain) may be helpful to define the osseous relationships at the skull base, C1 and C2 in patients where the craniovertebral junction is not well visualized on plain radiographs. The degree of C1-C2 instability identified on cervical x-rays does not correlate with the presence of myelopathy. A sagittal diameter of the spinal canal at the C1-2 level of less than 13 millimeters does correlate with myelopathy detected on clinical examination. MR can depict spinal cord compression and signal changes within the cord that correlates with the presence of myelopathy.

Surgical treatment is not required for every patient in whom os odontoideum is identified. Patients who have no neurological deficit and have no instability at C1-2 on flexion and extension studies can be managed without operative intervention. Even patients with documented C1-C2 instability and neurological deficit have been managed non-operatively without clinical consequence during finite follow-up periods. Most investigators of this disorder favor operative stabilization and fusion of C1-C2 instability associated with os odontoideum. The concern exists that patients with os odontoideum with C1-C2 instability have an increased likelihood of future spinal cord injury. While not supported by Class I or Class II evidence from the literature, multiple case series (Class III evidence) suggest that stabilization and fusion of C1-C2 is meritorious in this circumstance. Because a patient with an initially stable os odontoideum has been reported to develop delayed C1-C2 instability, and because there are rare examples of patients with stable os odontoideum who have developed neurological deficits following minor trauma, longitudinal clinical and radiographic surveillance of patients with os odontoideum without instability is recommended.

Posterior C1-2 arthrodesis in the treatment of os odontoideum provides effective stabilization of the atlantoaxial joint in the majority of patients. Posterior wiring and fusion techniques supplemented with postoperative halo immobilization provided successful fusion in 40% to 100% of cases reported. Atlantoaxial transarticular screw fixation and fusion appears to have merit in the treatment of C1-2 instability in association with os odontoideum, and appears to obviate the need for postoperative halo immobilization. Neural compression in association with os odontoideum has been treated with reduction of deformity, dorsal decompression of irreducible deformity, and ventral decompression of irreducible deformity, each in conjunction with C1-C2 or occipital cervical fusion and internal fixation. Each of these combined approaches has provided satisfactory results. Odontoid screw fixation has no role in the treatment of this disorder.

TOPIC 20: TREATMENT OF SUBAXIAL CERVICAL SPINAL INJURIES

Recommendations

SUBAXIAL CERVICAL FACET DISLOCATION INJURIES

Standards: There is insufficient evidence to recommend treatment standards.

Guidelines: There is insufficient evidence to recommend treatment guidelines.

Options:
- Closed or open reduction of subaxial cervical facet dislocation injuries is recommended.
- Treatment of subaxial cervical facet dislocation injuries with rigid external immobilization, anterior arthrodesis with plate fixation, or posterior arthrodesis with plate or rod or interlaminar clamp fixation is recommended.
- Treatment of subaxial cervical facet dislocation injuries with prolonged bedrest in traction is recommended if more contemporary treatment options are not available.

SUBAXIAL CERVICAL INJURIES EXCLUDING FACET DISLOCATION INJURIES

Standards: There is insufficient evidence to recommend treatment standards.

Guidelines: There is insufficient evidence to recommend treatment guidelines.

Options:
- Closed or open reduction of subluxations or displaced subaxial cervical spinal fractures is recommended.
- Treatment of subaxial cervical spinal injuries with external immobilization, anterior arthrodesis with plate fixation, or posterior arthrodesis with plate or rod fixation is recommended.

Rationale

Subaxial cervical vertebral fracture dislocation injuries are common following non-penetrating cervical trauma and are often associated with neurological injury. Prior to the advent of spinal instrumentation, many of these injuries were managed with traction, postural reduction, or external orthoses with frequent success. However, the morbidity and mortality associated with prolonged immobilization for three months or more prompted surgeons to investigate the utility of internal fixation in the management of these injuries. In order to develop treatment recommendations for closed subaxial cervical spinal injuries, an analysis of the articles examining their management is undertaken in this report. In particular, this focused review assessed the utility of closed reduction with or without external immobilization compared to arthrodesis with or without internal fixation.

Summary

In conclusion, closed reduction is successful for most subaxial cervical spinal fracture-dislocation injuries. Failure of closed reduction is more common with facet dislocation injuries. Similarly, treatment with external immobilization is frequently successful in the management of most subaxial cervical spinal injuries, although failure to maintain reduction is more frequent with facet dislocation injuries as well. Virtually all forms of external immobilization have been employed in the treatment of subaxial cervical spinal injuries. More rigid orthoses (halo, Minerva) appear to have better success rates than less rigid orthoses, (collars, traction only) for fracture-dislocation injuries once reduction has been accomplished. Treatment with traction and prolonged bedrest has been associated with increased morbidity and mortality.

Both anterior and posterior cervical fusion procedures are successful in achieving spinal stability for the majority of patients with subaxial cervical spinal injuries. Indications for surgical treatment offered in the literature include failure to achieve anatomic injury reduction (irreducible injury), persistent instability with failure to maintain reduction, ligamentous injury with facet instability, spinal kyphotic deformity greater than 15°, vertebral body fracture compression of 40% or greater, vertebral subluxation of 20% or greater, and irreducible spinal cord compression. Anterior fusion without plate fixation is associated with an increased likelihood of graft displacement and the development of late kyphosis, particularly in patients with distractive flexion injuries. Similarly, late displacement with kyphotic angulation is more common in patients treated for facet dislocation injuries with posterior fusion and wiring compared to those treated with posterior fusion and lateral mass plate or rod or interlaminal clamp fixation. Although patients with persistent or recurrent cervical spinal malalignment often achieve spinal stability with either external immobilization or surgical fusion with or without internal fixation, a greater proportion of these patients have residual cervical pain compared to similarly treated patients in whom anatomic spinal alignment was achieved and maintained.

TOPIC 21: MANAGEMENT OF ACUTE CENTRAL CERVICAL SPINAL CORD INJURIES

Recommendations

Standards: There is insufficient evidence to support treatment standards.

Guidelines: There is insufficient evidence to support treatment standards.

Options:
- Intensive care unit (or other monitored setting) management of patients with acute central cervical spinal cord injuries (ACCSCI), particularly patients with severe neurological deficits, is recommended.
- Medical management including cardiac, hemodynamic and respiratory monitoring, and maintenance of mean arterial blood pressure at 85–90 mm Hg for the first week after injury to improve spinal cord perfusion, is recommended.
- Early reduction of fracture dislocation injuries is recommended.
- Surgical decompression of the compressed spinal cord, particularly if the compression is focal and anterior, is recommended.

Rationale

Central spinal cord injuries are among the most common, well-recognized spinal cord injury patterns identified in neurologically injured patients after acute trauma. Originally described by Richard Schneider in 1954, this pattern of neurologically incomplete spinal cord injury is characterized by "disproportionately more motor impairment of the upper than of the lower extremities, bladder dysfunction and varying degrees of sensory loss below the level of the lesion". It has been associated with hyperextension injuries of the cervical spine, even without apparent damage to the bony spine, but has also been described in association with vertebral body fractures and fracture-dislocation injuries. The natural history of acute central cervical spinal cord injuries indicates gradual recovery of neurological function for most patients, albeit usually incomplete and related to the severity of the original injury and the age of the patient. The role of surgery and its timing for patients with acute central spinal cord injuries without fracture compression or dislocation injuries are the subjects of considerable debate. The optimal management of patients who have sustained acute central cervical spinal cord injuries is the subject of these recommendations.

Summary

The ideal management strategy for patients with acute central cervical spinal cord injuries appears to be multifaceted. As Schneider insisted years ago, a rapid, accurate diagnosis is essential. A detailed clinical examination, cervical spinal radiographs to assess vertebral column injury (see Radiographic Clearance in Symptomatic Patient chapter recommendations) and MRI assessment of the cervical spinal cord for intrinsic injury and/or compression will accomplish this goal. Many of these patients may require management in the ICU setting (see ICU Monitored Setting chapter recommendations) for monitoring and treatment of cardiac, pulmonary and blood pressure disturbances. Blood pressure augmentation to MAP levels of 85 mm Hg to 90 mm Hg may be of benefit (see Blood Pressure Management chapter recommendations). Early reduction of fracture or fracture dislocation injuries should be accomplished (see Closed Reduction and Subaxial Cervical Spinal Injuries chapter recommendations). Administration of pharmacological agents may be of benefit according to specific parameters (see Pharmacological Therapy chapter recommendations). Surgical decompression of the compressed spinal cord, particularly if the compression is focal, anterior and is approached anteriorly, appears to be of benefit in selected patients.

TOPIC 22: MANAGEMENT OF VERTEBRAL ARTERY INJURIES FOLLOWING NON-PENETRATING CERVICAL TRAUMA

Recommendations

DIAGNOSTIC

Standards: There is insufficient evidence to recommend diagnostic standards.

Guidelines: There is insufficient evidence to recommend diagnostic guidelines.

Options: Conventional angiography or magnetic resonance an-
                 giography (MRA) is recommended for the diagnosis of
                 vertebral artery injury (VAI) after nonpenetrating cer-
                 vical trauma in patients who have complete cervical
                 spinal cord injuries, fracture through the foramen
                 transversarium, facet dislocation, and/or vertebral
                 subluxation.

TREATMENT

Standards: There is insufficient evidence to recommend treatment
                 standards.
Guidelines: There is insufficient evidence to recommend treatment
                 guidelines.
Options: • Anticoagulation with intravenous heparin is rec-
                   ommended for patients with vertebral artery injury
                   who have evidence of posterior circulation stroke.
                 • Either observation or treatment with anticoagula-
                   tion in patients with vertebral artery injuries and
                   evidence of posterior circulation ischemia is recom-
                   mended.
                 • Observation in patients with vertebral artery in-
                   juries and no evidence of posterior circulation is-
                   chemia is recommended.

Rationale

The association of cerebrovascular insufficiency and cervical fracture
was first described by Suechting et al in a patient with Wallenburg's
syndrome occurring four days after a C5-C6 fracture-dislocation injury.
Although Schneider et al implicated vertebral artery injury at the site
of cervical fracture dislocation as a cause of posterior circulation cerebral ischemia, Gurdijian et al suggested that unilateral vertebral artery occlusions might be asymptomatic. Subsequent articles described
larger series of patients with asymptomatic vertebral artery injuries
(VAI) after blunt cervical spinal trauma. However, Biffl et al, in the
largest prospective series consisting of 38 patients with VAI diagnosed
by angiography, reported more frequent strokes in patients not treated
initially with intravenous heparin anticoagulation despite an asymptomatic VAI. Fractures through the foramen transversarium, facet fracture-dislocation, or vertebral subluxation are almost always seen in patients with VAI. A cadaveric study demonstrated progressive vertebral
occlusion with greater degrees of flexion-distraction injury, confirming
this clinical observation. In order to develop diagnostic and treatment

recommendations for VAI after blunt cervical trauma, an analysis of the articles examining its management is undertaken in this report. Specific questions that were addressed include: the clinical and radiographic criteria used to prompt diagnostic evaluation, appropriate diagnostic tests for identifying VAI, and the management of VAI (observation versus anticoagulation with heparin).

Summary

The incidence of vertebral artery injury may be as high as 11% after non-penetrating cervical spinal trauma in patients with specific clinical criteria, including facial hemorrhage (bleeding from mouth, nose, ears), cervical bruit in those younger than 50 years of age, expanding cervical hematoma, cerebral infarction by CT, lateralizing neurological deficit, cervical hyper-extension/rotation or hyperflexion injuries, closed head injury with diffuse axonal injury, near hanging, seat belt or other soft tissue injuries to the neck, basilar skull fractures extending into the carotid canal, and cervical vertebral body fractures or distraction injuries. Many patients with VAI have complete spinal cord injuries, fracture through the foramen transversarium, facet dislocation, and/or vertebral subluxation, but many patients with these injuries have normal vertebral arteries when imaged, thus compromising specificity of these injury criteria. Many patients with VAI are asymptomatic, including those with vertebral artery occlusion or dissection. The literature reviewed indicates that patients with posterior circulation stroke and VAI have a better outcome when treated with intravenous heparin compared to those who are not. However, others have reported improvement among patients without anticoagulation. The outcome of patients who develop symptoms of posterior circulation ischemia without stroke treated with intravenous heparin is similar to those patients receiving no treatment. Although the largest prospective study suggested a trend toward less frequent stroke in asymptomatic patients treated with heparin, others have not reported similar observations. Since the risk of significant complications related to anticoagulation is approximately 14% in these studies, there is insufficient evidence to recommend anticoagulation in asymptomatic patients.

AUTHOR'S ADDENUDM, MARCH 2002

Since the presentation of his information in October 2001, the *Guidelines for the Management of Acute Cervical Spine and Spinal Cord Injuries* have been through a rigorous peer review process. They have been formally approved and adopted by the American Association of

Neurological Surgeons and the Congress of Neurological Surgeons. They have been published in their entirety in *Neurosurgery* as a supplement, the full citation for which is: **Neurosurgery** 50(3 Supplement), March 2002, and are available on-line at: www.neurosurgery-online.com.

BIBLIOGRAPHY

1. Acland RH, Anthony A, Inglis G, Walton DI, Xiong X: Methylprednisolone use in acute spinal cord injury. **N Z Med J** 9:99–2001.
2. Aebi M, Zuber K, Marchesi D: Treatment of cervical spine injuries with anterior plating. **Spine** 16:S 38–S 45, 1991.
3. Ahuja A, Glasauer FE, Alker GJ, Klein DM: Radiology in survivors of traumatic atlanto-occipital dislocation. **Surg Neurol** 41:112–118, 1994.
4. Ajani A, Cooper D, Scheinkestel C, Laidlaw J, Tuxen D: Optimal assessment of cervical spine trauma in critically ill patients: A prospective evaluation. **Anaesthesia Intensive Care** 26:487–491, 1998.
5. Aldrich EF, Crow WN: Use of imaging-compatible Halifax interlaminar clamps for posterior cervical fusion. **J Neurosurg** 74:185–189, 1991.
6. Alexander R, Proctor H: Advanced Trauma Life Support Course for Physicians. Chicago: American College of Surgeons, 1993, pp 21–22.
7. Alexander E, Davis C, Forsyth H: Reduction and fusion of fracture dislocation of the cervical spine. **J Neurosurg** 27:588–591, 1967.
8. Allen BL, Ferguson RL, Lehman TR, O'Brien RP: A mechanistic classification of closed indirect fractures and dislocations of the lower cervical spine. **Spine** 7:1–27, 1982.
9. Amar AP, Levy ML: Pathogenesis and pharmacological strategies for mitigating secondary damage in acute spinal cord injury. **Neurosurgery** 44(5):1027–1040, 1999.
10. American Spinal Injury Association: *Standards for Neurological Classification of Spinal Injury Patients.* Chicago, IL: ASIA, 1984.
11. American Spinal Injury Association: *Standards for Neurological Classification of Spinal Injury Patients.* Chicago, IL: ASIA, 1989.
12. Anderson LD, Alonzo RT: Fractures of the odontoid process of the axis. **J Bone Joint Surg Am** 56:1663–1674, 1974.
13. Anderson PA, Montesano PX: Morphology and treatment of occipital condyle fractures. **Spine** 13:731–736, 1988.
14. Anderson PA, Henley MB, Grady MS, Montesano PX, Winn H: Posterior cervical arthrodesis with AO reconstruction plates and bone graft. **Spine** 16:S 72–S 79, 1991.
15. Andersson S, Rodrigues M, Olerud C: Odontoid Fractures: High complication rate associated with anterior screw fixation in the elderly. **Eur Spine J** 9:56–59, 2000.
16. Apfelbaum RI, Lonser RR, Veres R, Casey A: Direct anterior screw fixation for recent and remote odontoid fractures. **J Neurosurg** 93:227–236, 2000.
17. Apostolides PJ, Theodore N, Karahalios DG, et al: Triple anterior screw fixation of an acute combination atlas-axis fracture. **J Neurosurg** 87:96–99, 1997.
18. Argenson C, Lovet J, Sanouiller JL, de Peretti F: Traumatic rotatory displacement of the lower cervical spine. **Spine** 13:767–773, 1988.
19. Armitage JM, Pyne A., et al: Respiratory problems of air travel in patients with spinal cord injuries. **Br Med J** 300(6378):1498–1499, 1990.

20. ASIA/IMSOP: *Standards for Neurological and Functional Classification of Spinal Cord Injury,* Revised 1992. Chicago, IL: ASIA, 1992.
21. ASIA/IMSOP: *International Standards for Neurological and Functional Classification of Spinal Cord Injury,* Revised 1996. Chicago, IL: American Spinal Injury Association, 1996.
22. Augustine J: Spinal Trauma. In *Basic Trauma Life Support: Advanced Pre-Hospital Care.* Englewood Cliffs, NJ: Prentice-Hall, 1998, p 120.
23. Augustine J: Spinal trauma. In *Basic Trauma Life Support for Paramedics and Advanced EMS Providers,* 3rd Edition. Upper Saddle River, NJ: Brady, 1998, p 153.
24. Authority W. *Spinal Injury Assessment and Immobilization, EMS Protocols.* Ann Arbor, MI: University of Michigan Press, 1997.
25. Bachulis B, Long W, Hynes G, Johnson M: Clinical indications for cervical spine radiographs in the traumatized patient. **Am J Surg** 153:473–478, 1987.
26. Balshi JD, Cantelmo NL, Menzoian JO: Complications of caval interruption by Greenfield filter in quadriplegics. **J Vasc Surg** 9:558–562, 1989.
27. Banit D, Grau G, Fisher J: Evaluation of the acute cervical spine: A management algorithm. **J Trauma** 49:450–456, 2000.
28. Banna M, Stevenson GW, Hamilton, Tumiel A: Unilateral atlanto-occipital dislocation complicating an anomaly of the atlas. **J Bone Joint Surg Am** 65A:685–687, 1983.
29. Barboriak JJ, Rooney CB, El Ghatit AZ, et al: Nutrition in spinal cord injury patients. **J Am Paraplegia Soc** 6:32–36, 1983.
30. Barker EG, Jr., Krumpelman J, Long JM: Isolated fracture of the medial portion of the lateral mass of the atlas: A previously undescribed entity. **Am J Roentgenol** 126:1053–1058, 1976.
31. Barney R, Cordell W: Pain associated with immobilization on rigid spine boards (abstract). **Ann Emerg Med** 18:918–1989.
32. Barros TE, Bohlman HH, Capen DA, et al: Traumatic spondylolisthesis of the axis: Analysis of management. **Spinal Cord** 37:166–171, 1999.
33. Bauer D, Kowalski R: Effect of spinal immobilization devices on pulmonary function in the healthy, non-smoking man. **Ann Emerg Med** 17(9):915–918, 1988.
34. Baum JA, Hanley EN, Pullekines J: Comparison of halo complications in adults and children. **Spine** 14:251–252, 1989.
35. Bayless P, Ray V: Incidence of cervical spine injuries in association with blunt head trauma. **Am J Emerg Med** 7:139–142, 1989.
36. Beatson TR: Fractures and dislocation of the cervical spine. **J Bone Joint Surg Br** 45B:21–35, 1963.
37. Becker D, Gonzalez M, Gentili A, Eismont F, Green B: Prevention of deep venous thrombosis in patients with acute spinal cord injuries: Use of rotating treatment tables. **Neurosurgery** 20:675–677, 1987.
38. Bednar DA, Parikh J, Hummel J: Management of type II odontoid process fractures in geriatric patients: A prospective study of sequential cohorts with attention to survivorship. **J Spinal Disord** 8:166–169, 1995.
39. Bednarczyk JH, Sanderson DJ: Comparison of functional and medical assessment in the classification of persons with spinal cord injury. **J Rehabil Research Dev** 30(4):405–411, 1003.
40. Bell C: Surgical observations. **Middlesex Hosp J** 4:469, 1817.
41. Belzberg AJ, Tranmer BI: Stabilization of traumatic atlanto-occipital dislocation. **J Neurosurg** 75:478–482, 1991.
42. Benzel EC, Kesterson L: Posterior cervical interspinous compression wiring and fusion for mid to low cervical spine injuries. **J Neurosurg,**70:893–899, 1989.

43. Benzel EC, Larson SJ: Functional recovery after decompressive spine operation for cervical spine fractures. **Neurosurgery** 20(5):742–746, 1987.
44. Benzel EC, Hadden TA, Saulsbery CM: A comparison of the Minerva and halo jackets for stabilization of the cervical spine. **J Neurosurg** 70:411–414, 1989.
45. Benzel EC, Hart B, Ball P, et al: Fractures of the C2 vertebral body. **J Neurosurg** 81:206–212, 1994.
46. Benzel EC, Hart B, Ball P, Baldwin N, Orrison W, Espinosa M: Magnetic resonance imaging for the evaluation of patients with occult cervical spine injury. **J Neurosurg** 85:824–829, 1996.
47. Berlemann U, Schwarzenbach O: Dens fractures in the elderly. Results of anterior screw fixation in 19 elderly patients. **Acta Orthop Scand** 68:319–324, 1997.
48. Berne J, Velmahos G, El-Tawil Q, Demetriades D, Asensio J, Murray J, Cornwell E, Belzberg H, Berne T: Value of complete cervical helical computed tomographic scanning in identifying cervical spine injury in the unevaluable blunt trauma patient with multiple injuries: A prospective study. **J Trauma** 47:896–903, 1999.
49. Bettini N, Malaguti MC, Sintini M, Monti C: Fractures of the occipital condyles: Report of four cases and review of the literature. **Skeletal Radiol** 2:187–190, 1993.
50. Beyer CA, Cabanela ME, Berquist TH: Unilateral facet dislocations and fracture-dislocations of the cervical spine. **J Bone Joint Surg Br** 73B:977–981, 1991.
51. Biffl WL, Moore EE, Elliot JP, Ray C, Offner PJ, Franciose RJ, Brega KE, Burch JM: The devastating potential of blunt vertebral arterial injuries. **Ann Surg** 231:672–681, 2000.
52. Black CA, Buderer NM: Comparative study of risk factors for skin breakdown with cervical orthotic devices. **J Trauma Nurs** 5(3):62–66, 1998.
53. Blackmore C, Emerson S, Mann F, Koepsell T: Cervical spine imaging in patients with trauma: Determination of fracture risk to optimize use. **Radiology** 211:759–765, 1999.
54. Blackmore C, Ramsey S, Mann F, Deyo R: Cervical spine screening with CT in trauma patients: A cost-effective analysis. **Radiology** 212:117–125, 1999.
55. Blaylock B: Solving the problem of pressure ulcers resulting from cervical collars. **Ostomy Wound Management** 42(4):26–33, 1996.
56. Bloom AI, Neeman Z, Floman Y, Gomori J, Bar-Ziv J: Occipital condyle fracture and ligament injury: Imaging by CT. **Pediatr Radiol** 26:786–790, 1996.
57. Bloom AI, Neeman Z, Slasky BS, Floan Y, Milgrom M, Rivkind A, Bar-Ziv J: Fracture of the occipital condyles and associated craniocervical ligament injury: Incidence, CT imaging and implications. **Clin Radiol** 52:198–202, 1997.
58. Bohay D, Gosselin RA, Contreras DM: The vertical axis fracture: A report on three cases. **J Orthop Trauma** 6:416–419, 1992.
59. Bohler J: An approach to non-union of fractures. **Surg Ann** 14:299–315, 1982.
60. Bohlman HH: Acute fractures and dislocations of the cervical spine: An analysis of three hundred hospitalized patients and review of the literature. **J Bone Joint Surg Am** 61(8):1119–1142, 1979.
61. Bohn D, Armstrong D, Becker L, Humphreys R. Cervical spine injuries in children. J Trauma, 30:463–466, 1990.
62. Bolender N, Cromwell LD, Wendling L: Fracture of the occipital condyle. **Am J Radiology** 131:729–731, 1978.
63. Bools JC, Rose BS: Traumatic atlantooccipital dislocation: Two cases with survival. **Am J Neuroradiol** 7:901–904, 1986.
64. Borckmeyer DL, York JE, Apfelbaum RI: Anatomic suitability of C1-2 transarticular screw placement in pediatric patients. **J Neurosurg** 92(Suppl):7–11, 2000.

65. Borne GM, Bedou GL, Pinaudeau M: Treatment of pedicular fractures of the axis. A clinical study and screw fixation technique. **J Neurosurg** 60:88–93, 1984.

66. Borock E, Gabram S, Jacobs L, Murphy M: A prospective analysis of a two-year experience using computed tomography as an adjunct for cervical spine clearance. **J Trauma** 31:1001–1006, 1991.

67. Bosch A, Stauffer ES, Nickel VL: Incomplete traumatic quadriplegia: A ten-year review. **JAMA** 216(3):473–478, 1971.

68. Bose B, Northrup B, Jewell LO, Cotler J, Ditunno J: Reanalysis of central cervical cord injury management. **Neurosurgery** 15(3):367–372, 1984.

69. Botel U, Glaser E, Niedeggen A: The surgical treatment of acute spinal paralysed patients. **Spinal Cord** 35:420–428, 1997.

70. Botsford DJ, Esses SI: A new scale for the clinical assessment of spinal cord function. **Orthopedics** 15(11):1309–1313, 1992.

71. Boyd CR, Corse KM, et al: Emergency interhospital transport of the major trauma patient: Air versus ground. **J Trauma-Injury Infection Crit Care** 29(6):789–794, 1989.

72. Bozboga M, Unal F, Hepgul K, Izgi N, Turantan I, Tucker K: Fracture of the occipital condyle. Case report. **Spine** 17:1119–1121, 1992.

73. Bracken MB, Holford TR: Effects of timing on methylprednisolone or naloxone administration on recovery of segmental and long-tract neurological function in NASCIS 2. **J Neurosurg** 79:500–507, 1993.

74. Bracken MB, Holford TR: Response: Treatment of spinal cord injury. **J Neurosurg** 80:954–955, 1994.

75. Bracken MB: Response: National acute spinal cord injury study of methylprednisolone or naloxone. **Neurosurgery** 28(4):628–629, 1991.

76. Bracken MB. The use of methylprednisolone. (letter). **J Neurosurg** 93(Spine):340–341, 2000.

77. Bracken MB: Methylprednisolone and spinal cord injury. (Letter). **J Neurosurg** 93(Spine):175–177, 2000.

78. Bracken MB: High dose methylprednisolone must be given for 24 or 48 hours after acute spinal cord injury (Letter). **Br Med J** 322:862–863, 2001.

79. Bracken MB: Pharmacological interventions for acute spinal cord injury (Review). **Cochrane Database Syst Rev** 1:1–32, 2001.

80. Bracken MB, Aldrich EF, Herr DL, Hitchon PW, et al: Clinical measurement, statistical analysis, and risk-benefit: Controversies from trials of spine injury. **J Trauma** 48(3):558–561, 2000.

81. Bracken MB, Collins WF, Freeman DF, Shepard MJ, et al: Efficacy of methylprednisolone in acute spinal cord injury. **JAMA** 251:45–52, 1984.

82. Bracken MB, Shepard MJ, Hellenbrand KG, Collins WF, et al: Methylprednisolone and neurological function 1 year after spinal cord injury. **J Neurosurg** 63:704–713, 1985.

83. Bracken MB, Shepard MJ, Collins WF, Holford TR, et al: A randomized, controlled trial of methylprednisolone or naloxone in the treatment of acute spinal cord injury: Results of the second National Acute Spinal Cord Injury Study (NASCIS II). **N Engl J Med** 322(20):1405–1411, 1990.

84. Bracken MB, Shepard MJ, Collins WF, Holford TR, et al: Methylprednisolone or naloxone treatment after acute spinal cord injury: 1-year follow up data. **J Neurosurg** 76:23–31, 1992.

85. Bracken MB, Shepard MJ, Collins WF, Holford TR, et al: Response: Methylprednisolone for spinal cord injury. **J Neurosurg** 77:325–327, 1992.

86. Bracken MB, Shepard MJ, Holford TR, Leo-Summers L, et al: Administration of

methylprednisolone for 24 or 48 hours or tirilazad mesylate for 48 hours in the treatment of acute spinal cord injury. **JAMA** 277:1597–1604, 1997.

87. Bracken MB, Shepard MJ, Holford TR, Leo-Summers L, et al: Methylprednisolone or tirilazad mesylate administration after acute spinal cord injury: 1-year follow-up results of NASCIS 3. **J Neurosurg** 89:699–706, 1998.

88. Bracken MB, Webb SB, Jr., Wagner FC: Classification of the severity of acute spinal cord injury: Implications for management. **Paraplegia** 15:319–326, 1977.

89. Brady W, Moghtader J, Cutcher D, Exline C, Young J: ED use of flexion-extension cervical spine radiography in the evaluation of blunt trauma. **Am J Emerg Med** 17:504–508, 1999.

90. Brashear R, Venters G, Preston ET: Fractures of the neural arch of the axis. A report of twenty-nine cases. **J Bone Joint Surg Am** 57:879–878, 1975.

91. Bridgman SA, McNab W: Traumatic occipital condyle fracture, multiple cranial nerve palsies, and torticollis: A case report and review of the literature. **Surg Neurol** 38:152–156, 1992.

92. Bridle MJ, Lynch KB, Quesenberry CM: Long-term function following the central cord syndrome. **Paraplegia** 28:178–185, 1990.

93. Brodkey JS, Miller CF, Jr., Harmody RM: The syndrome of acute central cervical spinal cord injury revisited. **Surg Neurol** 14:251–257, 1980.

94. Brohi K, Wilson-Macdonald J: Evaluation of unstable cervical spine injury: A six-year experience. **J Trauma** 49:76–80, 2000.

95. Brooks AL, Jenkins EB: Atlanto-axial arthrodesis by the wedge compression method. **J Bone Joint Surg Am** 60-A:279–284, 1978.

96. Brown LH, Gough JE, et al: Can EMS providers adequately assess trauma patients for cervical spinal injury? **Pre-Hospital Emergency Care** 2(1):33–36, 1989.

97. Bruce D: Comment. **Pediatr Neurosci 15**:175–1989.

98. Brunette D, Rockswold G: Neurologic recovery following rapid spinal realignment for complete cervical spinal cord injury. **J Trauma** 27:445–447, 1987.

99. Bucci MN, Dauser RC, Maynard FA, Hoff JT: Management of post-traumatic cervical spine instability: Operative fusion versus halo vest immobilization. Analysis of 49 cases. **J Trauma** 28:1001–1006, 1988.

100. Bucholz RW, Cheung K: Halo vest versus spinal fusion for cervical injury. **J Neurosurg** 70:884–892, 1989.

101. Bucholz RW: Unstable hangman's fractures. **Clin Orthop** 119–124, 1981.

102. Buhs C, Cullen M, Klein M, Farmer D: The pediatric trauma c-spine: Is the 'odontoid' view necessary? **J Pediatr Surg** 35:994–997, 2000.

103. Bulas DI, Fitz CR, Johnson DL: Traumatic atlanto-occipital dislocation in children. **Radiology** 188:155–158, 1993.

104. Bundschuh CV, Alley JB, Ross M, Porter IS, Gudeman SK: Magnetic resonance imaging of suspected atlanto-occipital dislocation. Two case reports. **Spine** 17:245–248, 1992.

105. Burke D, Berryman D: The place of closed manipulation in the management of flexion-rotation dislocations of the cervical spine. **J Bone Joint Surg Br** 53(B):165–182, 1971.

106. Burke DC, Tiong TS: Stability of the cervical spine after conservative treatment. **Paraplegia** 13:191–202, 1975.

107. Burke JT: Acute injuries of the axis vertebra. **Skeletal Radiol** 18:335–346, 1989.

108. Burney RE, Waggoner R, et al: Stabilization of spinal injury for early transfer. **J Trauma-Injury Infection Crit Care** 29:1497–1499, 1989.

109. Burns GA, Cohn SM, Frumento RJ, Degutis LC, Hammers L: Prospective ultra-

sound evaluation of venous thrombosis in high-risk trauma patients. **J Trauma-Injury Infection Crit Care** 35:405–408, 1993.

110. Butman A, Vomacka R: Part 1: Spine immobilization. **Emergency** 23:48–51, 1991.

111. Cabanela ME, Ebersold MJ: Anterior plate stabilization for bursting teardrop fractures of the cervical spine. **Spine** 13:888–891, 1988.

112. Cahill DW, Bellegarrigue R, Ducker TB: Bilateral facet to spinous process fusion: A new technique for posterior spinal fusion after trauma. **Neurosurgery** 13:1–4, 1983.

113. Cakmpanelli M, Kattner KA, Stroink A, et al: Posterior C1-C2 transarticular screw fixation in the treatment of displaced type II odontoid fractures in the geriatric population—Review of seven cases. **Surg Neurol** 51:600–601, 1999.

114. Capaul M, Zollinger H, Satz N, Dietz V, Lehmann D, Schurch B: Analyses of 94 consecutive spinal cord injury patients using ASIA definition and modified Frankel score classification. **Paraplegia** 32:583–587, 1994.

115. Carey ME, Nance FC, Kirgis HD, et al: Pancreatitis following spinal cord injury. **J Neurosurg** 47:917–922, 1997.

116. Carter VM, Fasen JA, et al: The effect of a soft collar, used as normally recommended or reversed, on three planes of cervical range of motion. **J Orthop Sports Physical Ther** 23(3):209–215, 1996.

117. Casas E, Sanchez M, Arias C, Masip J: Prophylaxis of venous thrombosis and pulmonary embolism in patients with acute traumatic spinal cord lesions. **Paraplegia** 15:209–214, 1978.

118. Castillo M, Mjkherji SK: Vertical fractures of the dens. **Am J Neuroradiol** 17:1627–1630, 1996.

119. Castling B, Hicks K: Traumatic isolated unilateral hypoglossal nerve palsy—Case report and review of the literature. **Br J Oral Maxillofacial Surg** 33:171–173, 1995.

120. Cattell HS, Filtzer DL: Pseudosubluxation and other normal variations in the cervical spine in children. A study of one hundred and sixty children. **J Bone Joint Surg Am** 47-A:1295–1309, 1965.

121. Catz A, Itzkovich M, Agranov E, Ring H, Tamir A: SCIM—Spinal cord independence measure: A new disability scale for patients with spinal cord lesions. **Spinal Cord** 35:850–856, 1997.

122. Chan D, Goldberg R, et al: The effect of spinal immobilization on healthy volunteers. **Ann Emerg Med** 23(1):48–51, 1994.

123. Chan D, Goldberg R, et al: Backboard versus mattress splint immobilization: a comparison of symptoms generated. **J Emerg Med** 14(3):293–298, 1996.

124. Chan RC, Schweigel JF, Thompson GB: Halo-thoracic brace immobilization in 188 patients with acute cervical injuries. **J Neurosurg** 58:508–515, 1983.

125. Chandler DR, Nemejc C, et al: Emergency cervical-spine immobilization. **Ann Emerg Med** 21(10):1185–1188, 1992.

126. Chee S: Review of the role of magnetic resonance imaging in acute cervical spine injuries. **Ann Acad Med** 22:757–761, 1993.

127. Chehrazi B, Wagner FC, Jr., Collins WF, Freeman DF, Jr: A scale for evaluation of spinal cord injury. **J Neurosurg** 54:310–315, 1981.

128. Chen TY, Dickman C, Eleraky MA, Sonntag VKH: The role of decompression for acute incomplete cervical spinal cord injury in cervical spondylosis. **Spine** 23(22):2398–2403, 1998.

129. Chen TY, Lee ST, Lui TN, Wong CW, et al: Efficacy of surgical treatment in traumatic central cord syndrome. **Surg Neurol** 48:435–441, 1997.

130. Cheshire DJE: The stability of the cervical spine following the conservative treatment of fractures and fracture-dislocations. **Paraplegia** 7:193–203, 1969.

131. Cheshire DJE: A classification of the functional end-results of injury to the cervical spinal cord. **Paraplegia** 8:70–73, 1970.
132. Chestnut RM, Marshall LF, Klauber MR, et al: The role of secondary brain injury in determining outcome from severe head injury. **J Trauma** 34:216–222, 1993.
133. Chiba K, Fujimura Y, Toyama Y, et al: Treatment protocol for fractures of the odontoid process. **J Spinal Disord** 9:267–276, 1996.
134. Chu D, Ahn J, Ragnarsson K, Helt J, Folcarelli P, Ramierz A: Deep venous thrombosis: Diagnosis in spinal cord injured patients. **Arch Phys Med Rehabil** 66:365–368, 1985.
135. Clancy M: Clearing the cervical spine of adult victims of trauma. **J Accid Emerg Med** 16:208–214, 1999.
136. Clark CR, White AA: Fractures of the dens. A multicenter study. **J Bone Joint Surg Am** 67:1340–1348, 1985.
137. Clarke KS: Caloric costs of activity in paraplegic persons. **Arch Phys Med Rehabil** 47:427–435, 1966.
138. Clements WD, Mezue W, Matthew B: OS Odontoideum-congenital or acquired? That's not the question. **Injury** 26:640–642, 1995.
139. Cline JR, Scheidel E, et al: A comparison of methods of cervical immobilization used in patient extrication and transport. **J Trauma** 25:649–653, 1985.
140. Cloward R: Reduction of traumatic dislocation of the cervical spine with locked facets. Technical note. **J Neurosurg** 38:527–531, 1973.
141. Cohen ME, Sheehan TP, Herbison GJ: Content validity and reliability of the International Standards for Neurological and Functional Classification of Spinal Cord Injury. **Top Spinal Cord Inj Rehabil** 1:15–31, 1996.
142. Cohen A, Bosshard R, et al: A new device for the care of acute spinal injuries: The Russell Extrication Device (RED). **Paraplegia** 28:151–157, 1990.
143. Cohen ME, Ditunno JF, Jr., Donovan WH, Maynard FM, Jr: A test of the 1992 International Standards for Neurological and Functional Classification of Spinal Cord Injury. **Spinal Cord** 36:554–560, 1998.
144. Cohn S, Lyle W, Linden C, Lancey R: Exclusion of cervical spine injury: A prospective study. **J Trauma** 31:570–574, 1991.
145. Coleman WP, Benzel EC, Cahill DW, Ducker T, et al: A critical appraisal of the reporting of the National Acute Spinal Cord Injury Studies (II and III) of methylprednisolone in acute spinal cord injury. **J Spinal Disord** 13(3):185–199, 2000.
146. Collato PM, DeMuth WW, Schwentker P, Boal D: Traumatic atlanto-occipital dislocation. **J Bone Joint Surg Am** 68A:1106–1109, 1986.
147. Colnet G, Chabannes J, Commun C, Rigal MC, Alassaf M: Luxation occipito-atloidienne et syringomyelie deux complications rares de la tramatologie cervicale. Incidences diagnostiques et therapeutiques. A propros d'un cas. **Neurochirurgie** 35:58–63, 1989.
148. Committee on Injuries: *Emergency Care and Transportation of the Sick and Injured.* Chicago, IL: American Academy of Orthopedic Surgeons, 1971, pp 111– 115.
149. Cone DC, Wydro GC, et al: Current practice in clinical cervical spinal clearance: Implication for EMS. **Pre-Hospital Emergency Care** 3(1):42–46, 1999.
150. Contostavlos DL: Massive subarachnoid hemorrhage due to laceration of the vertebral artery associated with fracture of the transverse process of the atlas. **J Forensic Sci** 16:40–56, 1971.
151. Cooke M: Spinal boards (letter, comment). **J Accid Emerg Med** 13(6):433–1996.
152. Cooper PR, Maravilla KR, Sklar F, Moody SF, Clark WK: Halo immobilization of cervical spine fractures. Indications and results. **J Neurosurg** 50:603–610, 1979.
153. Corric D, Wilson JA, Kelly DL: Treatment of traumatic spondylolisthesis of the

axis with nonrigid immobilization: A review of 64 cases. **J Neurosurg** 85:550–554, 1996.
154. Cotler HB, Cotler JB, Alden ME, Sparks G, Biggs CA: The medical and economic impact of closed cervical dislocations. **Spine** 15:448–452, 1990.
155. Cotler J, Herbison J, Nasuti J, Ditunno J, An H, Wolff B: Closed reduction of traumatic cervical spine dislocation using traction weights up to 140 pounds. **Spine** 18:386–390, 1993.
156. Cotler H, Miller L, Delucia F, Cotler J, Dayne S: Closed reduction of cervical spine dislocations. **Clin Orthop Related Res** 214:185–199, 1987.
157. Cottalorda J, Allard D, Dutour N: Case report: Fracture of the occipital condyle. **J Pediatr Orthop** 5:161–163, 1996.
158. Cox SAR, Weiss SM, Posuniak EA, et al: Energy expenditure after spinal cord injury: An evaluation of stable rehabilitating patients. **J Trauma** 25:419–423, 1985.
159. Coyne TJ, Fehlings M, Wallace MC, Bernstein M, Tator CH: C1-C2 posterior cervical fusion: Long-term evaluation of results and efficacy. **Neurosurgery** 37:688–693, 1995.
160. Craig JB, Hodgson BF: Superior facet fractures of the axis vertebra. **Spine** 16:875–877, 1991.
161. Cruse JM, Lewis RE, Roe DL, et al: Facilitation of immune function, healing of pressure ulcers, and nutritional status in spinal cord injury patients. **Exp Mol Pathol** 68:38–54, 2000.
162. Cruse JM, Lewis RE, Dilioglou S, et al: Review of immune function, healing of pressure ulcers, and nutritional status in patients with spinal cord injury. **J Spinal Cord Med** 23(2):129–135, 2000.
163. Crutchfield W: Skeletal traction in treatment of injuries to the cervical spine. **JAMA** 155:29–1954.
164. Curran C, Dietrich AM, et al: Pediatric cervical-spine immobilization: Achieving neutral position? **J Trauma-Injury Infection Crit Care** 39(4):729–732, 1995.
165. Curri D, Cervellin P, Zanusso M, Benedetti A: Isolated fracture of the occipital condyle. Case report. **J Neurosurg Sci** 32:157–159, 1988.
166. Cybulski GR, Douglas RA, Meyer PR, Rovin RA: Complications in three-column cervical spine injuries requiring anterior-posterior stabilization. **Spine** 17:253–256, 1992.
167. Dai L, Lianshun J: Central cord injury complicating acute cervical disc herniation in trauma. **Spine** 25(3):331–336, 2000.
168. Dai LY, Yuan W, Ni B, et al: Surgical treatment of nonunited fractures of the odontoid process, with special reference to occipitocervical fusion for un-reducible atlantoaxial subluxation or instability. **Eur Spine J** 9:118–122, 2000.
169. Dail L, Yuan W, Ni B, Jai L: OS odontoideum: Etiology, diagnosis, and management. **Surg Neurol** 53:106–109, 2000.
170. D'Alise M, Benzel EC, Hart B: Magnetic resonance imaging evaluation of the cervical spine in the comotose or obtunded trauma patient. **J Neurosurg** 91(Spine 1):54–59, 1999.
171. Davies G, Deakin C, et al. The effect of a rigid collar on intracranial pressure. **Injury** 27(9):647–649, 1996.
172. Davis D, Bohlman HH, Walker E, et al. The pathological findings in fatal craniospinal injuries. **J Neurosurg** 34:603–613, 1971.
173. Davis J, Parks S, Detlefs C, Williams G, Williams J, Smith R: Clearing the cervical spine in obtunded patients: The use of dynamic fluoroscopy. **J Trauma** 39:435–438, 1995.

174. Davis J, Phreaner D, Hoyt D, Mackersie R: The etiology of missed cervical spine injuries. **J Trauma** 34:342–346, 1993.
175. Davis PC, Reisner A, Hudgins PA, Davis WE, O'Brien MS: Spinal injuries in children: Role of MR. **AJNR** 14:607–617, 1993.
176. Davis LA, Warren SA, Reid DC, Oberle K, Saboe LA, Grace MG: Incomplete neural deficits in thoracolumbar and lumbar spine fractures. Reliability of Frankel and Sunnybrook scales. **Spine** 18(2):257–263, 1993.
177. De Lorenzo RA: A review of spinal immobilization techniques. **J Emerg Med** 14(5):603–613, 1996.
178. De Lorenzo RA, Olson JE, et al. Optimal positioning for cervical immobilization (comments). **Ann Emerg Med** 28(3):301–308, 1996.
179. Deeb ZL, Rothfus WE, Goldberg AL, Dafner RH: Occult occipital condyle fractures presenting as tumors. **J Computed Tomography** 12:261–263, 1988.
180. Della Torre F, Rinonapoli E: Halo-cast treatment of fractures and dislocations of the cervical spine. **Int Orthop** 16:227–231, 1992.
181. Demisch S, Linder A, Beck R, Zierz S: Case report. The forgotten condyle: Delayed hypoglossal nerve palsy caused by fracture of the occipital condyle. **Clin Neurol Neurosurg** 100:44–45, 1998.
182. Desai SS, Coumas JM, Danylevich A, Hayes E, Dunn EJ: Fracture of the occipital condyle: Case report and review of the literature. **J Trauma** 30:240–241, 1990.
183. DeSmet L, Vercauteren M, Verdonk R, Claessens H: Severe acute cervical spine injuries. Conservative treatment. **Acta Orthopaedica Belgica** 50:512–520, 1984.
184. DeVivo MJ, Kartus PL, Stover SL, Rutt RD, Fine PR: Cause of death for patients with spinal cord injuries. **Arch Intern Med** 149:1761–1766, 1989.
185. Dibenedetto T, Lee CK: Traumatic atlanto-occipital instability. **Spine** 595–597, 1990.
186. Dick T, Land R: Spinal immobilization devices. Part 1: Cervical extrication collars. **J Emerg Med Serv** 7:26–32, 1982.
187. Dick T, Land R: Full spinal immobilizers. **J Emerg Med Serv** 8:34–36, 1983.
188. Dick T: Comparing the short-board technique (letter). **Ann Emerg Med** 18(1):115–116, 1989.
189. Dickman C, Sonntag VKH: Surgical management of atlantoaxial nonunions. **J Neurosurg** 83:248–253, 1995.
190. Dickman C, Sonntag VKH: Injuries involving the transverse atlantal ligament: Classification and treatment guidelines based upon experience with 39 injuries (Letter). **Neurosurgery** 40:886–887, 1997.
191. Dickman C, Sonntag VKH: Posterior C1-2 transarticular screw fixation for atlantoaxial arthrodesis. **Neurosurgery** 41:275–281, 1998.
192. Dickman C, Greene KA, Sonntag VKH: Injuries involving the transverse atlantal ligament: Classification and treatment guidelines based upon experience with 39 injuries. (Comments). **Neurosurgery** 38:44–50, 1996.
193. Dickman C, Hadley MN, Browner C, et al: Neurosurgical management of acute atlas-axis combination fractures. A review of 25 cases. **J Neurosurg** 70:45–49, 1989.
194. Dickman C, Papadopoulos S, Sonntag VKH, Spetzler RF, Rekate HL: Traumatic occipitoatlantal dislocations. **J Spinal Disord** 6:300–313, 1993.
195. Dickman C, Rekate HL, Sonntag VKH, Zabramski JM: Pediatric spinal trauma: Vertebral column and spinal cord injuries in children. **Pediatr Neurosci** 15:237–256, 1989.
196. Dickman C, Sonntag VKH, Papadopoulos S, Hadley MN: The interspinous method of posterior atlantoaxial arthrodesis. **J Neurosurg** 74:190–198, 1991.

197. Ditunno JF, Jr: New spinal cord injury standards, 1992. **Paraplegia** 30:90–91, 1992.
198. Ditunno JF, Jr: Functional assessment measures in CNS trauma. **J Neurotrauma** 9 (S 1):S 301–S 305, 1992.
199. Ditunno JF, Jr: American spinal injury standards for neurological and functional classification of spinal cord injury: Past, present and future. **J Am Paraplegia Soc** 17:7–11, 1994.
200. Ditunno JF, Jr., Ditunno PL, Graziani V, Scivoletto G, Bernardi M, Castellano V, Marchetti M, Barbeau H, Frankel HL, D'Andrea Greve JM, Ko H-Y, Marshall R, Nance P: Walking index for spinal cord injury (WISCI): An international multicenter validity and reliability study. **Spinal Cord** 38 :234–243, 2000.
201. Ditunno JF, Jr., Young W, Donovan WH, Creasey G: The International Standards Booklet for neurological and functional classification of spinal cord injury. **Paraplegia** 32:70–80, 1994.
202. Dodd F, Simon E, McKeown D, Patrick M: The effect of a cervical collar on the tidal volume of anesthatised adult patients. **Anaesthesia** 50:961–963, 1995.
203. Dodds TA, Martin DP, Stolov WC, Deyo RA: A validation of the functional independence measurement and its performance among rehabilitation inpatients. **Arch Phys Med Rehabil** 74:531–536, 1993.
204. Dolan EJ, Tator CH: The effect of blood transfusion, dopamine, and gamma hydroxybutyrate on post-traumatic ischemia of the spinal cord. **J Neurosurg** 56:350–358, 1982.
205. Domeier RM: Indications for pre-hospital spinal immobilization. **Pre-Hospital Emergency Care** 3(3):251–253, 1999.
206. Domeier RM, Evans RW, Swor R, Rivera-Rivera E, Fredriksen S: High-risk criteria for performing pre-hospital spinal immobilization in trauma. **Ann Emerg Med** 25:142–1995.
207. Domeier RM, Evans RW, et al: Pre-hospital clinical findings associated with spinal injury. **Pre-Hospital Emergency Care** 1(1):11–15, 1997.
208. Domeier RM, Evans RW, et al: Prospective validation of out-of-hospital spinal clearance criteria: A preliminary report (letter). **Acad Emerg Med** 4(6):643–646, 1997.
209. Domeier RM, Evans RW, et al: The reliability of pre-hospital clinical evaluation for potential spinal injury is not affected by the mechanism of injury. **Pre-Hospital Emergency Care** 3(4):332–337, 1999.
210. Donahue DJ, Muhlbauer MS, Kaufman RA, Warner WC, Sanford RA: Childhood survival of atlanto-occipital dislocation: Underdiagnosis, recognition, treatment and review of the literature. **Pediatr Neurosurg** 21:150–111, 1994.
211. Donovan WH, Kopaniky D, Stoltzmann E, Carter RE: The neurological and skeletal outcome in patients with closed cervical spinal cord injury. **J Neurosurg** 66:690–694, 1987.
212. Doran S, Papadopoulos S, Ducker T, Lillehei K: Magnetic resonance imaging documentation of coexistent traumatic locked facets of the cervical spine and disc herniation. **J Neurosurg** 79:341–345, 1993.
213. Dormans JP, Criscitiello AA, Drummond DS, Davidson RS: Complications in children managed with immobilization in a halo vest. **J Bone Joint Surg Am** 77-A:1370–1373, 1995.
214. Dorr LD, Harvey JP, Nickel VL: Clinical review of the early stability of spine injuries. **Spine** 7:545–550, 1982.
215. Dublin AB, Marks WM, Weinstock D, Newton TH: Traumatic dislocation of the atlanto-occipital dislocation articulation (AOA) with short-term survival. **J Neurosurg** 52:541–546, 1980.

216. Ducker T, Zeidman SM: Spinal Cord Injury: Role of steroid therapy. **Spine** 19(20):2281–2287, 1994.
217. Ducker TB, Kindt GW, Kempe LG: Pathological findings in acute experimental spinal cord trauma. **J Neurosurg** 35:700–708, 1971.
218. Duh MS, Shepard MJ, Wilberger J, Bracken MB: The effectiveness of surgery on the treatment of acute spinal cord injury and its relation to pharmacological treatment. **Neurosurgery** 35(2):240–249, 1994.
219. Dunn ME, Seljeskog EL: Experience in the management of odontoid process injuries: An analysis of 128 cases. **Neurosurgery** 18:306–310, 1986.
220. Dyck P: OS odontoideum in children: Neurological manifestations and surgical management. **Neurosurgery** 2:93–99, 1978.
221. Effendi B, Roy D, Cornish B, et al: Fractures of the ring of the axis. A classification based on the analysis of 131 cases. **J Bone Joint Surg Br** 319–327, 1981.
222. Eismont F, Bohlman HH: Posterior atlanto-occipital dislocation with fractures of the atlas and odontoid process. **J Bone Joint Surg Am** 60A:397–399, 1978.
223. Eismont F, Arena M, Green B: Extrusion of an intervertebral disc associated with traumatic subluxation or dislocation of cervical facets. **J Bone Joint Surg Am** 73-A:1555–1560, 1991.
224. Ekong CE, Schwartz MI, Tator CH: Odontoid fracture: Management with early mobilization using the halo device. **Neurosurgery** 9:631–637, 1981.
225. El Masry WS, Silver J: Prophylactic anticoagulant therapy in patients with spinal cord injury. **Paraplegia** 19:334–342, 1981.
226. El Masry WS, Tsubo M, Katoh S, El Miligui YHS: Validation of the American Spinal Injury Association (ASIA) motor score and the National Acute Spinal Cord Injury Study (NASCIS) motor score. **Spine** 21(5):614–619, 1996.
227. Eleraky MA, Theodore N, Adams M, Rekate HL, Sonntag VKH: Pediatric cervical spine injuries: Report of 102 cases and review of the literature. **J Neurosurg** 92(Spine):12–17, 2000.
228. El-Khoury GY, Clark CR, Gravett AW: Acute traumatic rotatory atlanto-axial dislocation in children. **J Bone Joint Surg Am** 66-A:774–777, 1984.
229. Elliott JM, Roers LF, Wissinger JP, et al: The hangman's fracture. Fractures of the neural arch of the axis. **Radiology** 104:303–307, 1972.
230. Emery S, Pathria M, Wilber T, Masaryk T, Bohlman H: Magnetic resonance imaging of post-traumatic spinal ligament injury. **J Spinal Disord** 2:229–233, 1989.
231. Emery E, Saillant G, Ismail M, Fohamo D, Roy-Camille R: Fracture of the occipital condyle: Case report and review of the literature. **Eur Spine J** 4:191–193, 1995.
232. Ersmark H, Kalen R: A consecutive series of 64 halo-vest treated cervical spine injuries. **Acta Orthop Trauma Surg** 105:243–246, 1986.
233. Ersmark H, Lowenhielm P: Factors influencing the outcome of cervical spine injuries. **J Trauma** 28:407–410, 1988.
234. Esses SI, Bednar DA: Screw-fixation of odontoid fractures and non-unions. **Spine** 16:S 483–S 485, 1991.
235. Evans DL, Bethem D: Cervical spine injuries in children. **J Bone Joint Surg Am** 59-A:37–44, 1977.
236. Evans D: Reduction of cervical dislocations. **J Bone Joint Surg Br** 43-B:552–555, 1961.
237. Evarts CM: Traumatic occipitoatlantal dislocation. Report of a case with survival. **J Bone Joint Surg Am** 52A:1653–1660, 1970.
238. Farley FA, Graziano GP, Hensinger RN: Traumatic atlanto-occipital dislocation in a child. **Spine** 17:1539–1541, 1992.

239. Farmer J, Vaccaro A, Albert T, Malone S, Balderston R, Cotler J: Neurologic deterioration after spinal cord injury. **J Spinal Disord** 11:192–196, 1998.
240. Farrington JD: Death in a ditch. **Bull Am Coll Surg** 52:121–130, 1967.
241. Farrington JD: Extrication of victims—surgical principles. **J Trauma** 8:492–1968.
242. Farthing JW: Atlantooccipital dislocation with survival. A case report. **North Carolina Med J** 9:34–36, 1948.
243. Fehlings M, Tator CH: An evidence-based review of decompressive surgery in acute spinal cord injury: Rationale, indications, and timing based on experimental and clinical studies. **J Neurosurg** 91 (S):1–11, 1999.
244. Fehlings MG, Cooper PR, Errico TJ: Posterior plates in the management of cervical instability: Long-term results in 44 patients. **J Neurosurg** 81:341–349, 1994.
245. Fehlings M, Rao S, Tator CH, Skaf G, Arnold P, Benzel EC, Dickman C, Cuddy B, Green B, Hitchon P, Northrup B, Sonntag VKH, Wagner F, Wilberger J: The optimal method for assessing spinal canal compromise and cord compression in patients with cervical spinal cord injury. **Spine** 24:605–613, 1999.
246. Fenstermaker RA: Acute neurologic management of the patient with spinal cord injury. **Urol Clin North Am** 20(3):413–421, 1993.
247. Ferrera PC, Bartfield JM: Traumatic atlanto-occipital dislocation: A potentially survivable injury. **Am J Emerg Med** 14:291–296, 1996.
248. Field-Fote EC, Fluet GG, Schafer SD, Schneider EM, Smith R, Downey PA, Ruhl CD: The spinal cord injury functional ambulation inventory (SCI-FAI). **J Rehabil Med** 33:177–181, 2001.
249. Fielding JW, Hawkins RJ: Atlanto-axial rotary fixation. **J Bone Joint Surg Am** 59A:37–44, 1977.
250. Fielding JW, Cochran GVB, Lawsing JF, et al: Tears of the transverse ligament of the atlas: A clinical and biomechanical study. **J Bone Joint Surg Am** 56A:1683–1691, 1974.
251. Fielding JW, Francis WR, Hawkins RJ, et al: Traumatic spondylolisthesis of the axis. **Clin Orthop** 47–52, 1989.
252. Fielding JW, Hensinger RN, Hawkins RJ. OS Odontoideum: **J Bone Joint Surg Am** 62-A:376–383, 1980.
253. Finch GD, Barnes MJ: Major cervical spine injuries in children and adolescents. **J Pediatr Orthop** 18:811–814, 1998.
254. Flanders A, Schaefer D, Doan H, Mishkin M, Gonzales C, Northrup B: Acute cervical spine trauma: Correlation of MR imaging findings with degree of neurologic deficit. **Radiology** 177:25–33, 1990.
255. Flohr H, Poll W, Brock M: Regulation of spinal cord blood flow. In Russell RWR (ed): *Brain and Blood Flow.* London: Pitman Medical and Scientific Publishing, 1971, pp 406–409.
256. Forhna WJ: Emergency department evaluation and treatment of the neck and cervical spine injuries. **Emerg Med Clin North Am** 17(4):739–791, 1999.
257. Fotter R, Sorantin E, Schneider U, Ranner G, Fast C, Schober P: Ultrasound diagnosis of birth-related spinal cord trauma: Neonatal diagnosis and follow-up and correlation with MRI. **Pediatr Radiol** 24:241–244, 1994.
258. Fowler JL, Sandhu A, Fraser RD: A review of fractures of the atlas vertebra. **J Spinal Disord** 3:19–24, 1990.
259. Francis WR, Fielding JW, Hawkins RJ, et al: Traumatic spondylolisthesis of the axis. **J Bone Joint Surg Br** 313–318, 1981.
260. Frankel HL, Hancock DO, Hyslop G, Melzak J, Michaelis LS, Ungar GH, Vernon JDS, Walsh JJ: The value of postural reduction in the initial management of closed injuries of the spine with paraplegia and tetraplegia. **Paraplegia** 7:179–192, 1969.

261. Frankel H, Michaelis L, Paeslack V, Ungar G, Walsh JJ: Closed injuries of the cervical spine and spinal cord: Results of conservative treatment of vertical compression of the cervical spine. **Proc Vet Admin Spinal Cord Injury Conf** 19:28–32, 1973.

262. Frankenfield DC, Smith JS, Cooney RN: Accelerated nitrogen loss after traumatic injury is not attenuated by achievement of energy balance. **J Parenteral Enteral Nutrition** 21(6):324–329, 1997.

263. Freemyer B, Knopp R, Piche J, Wales L, Williams J: Comparison of five-view and three-view cervical spine series in the evaluation of patients with cervical trauma. **Ann Emerg Med** 18:818–821, 1989.

264. French HJ, Burke SW, Roberts JM, Johnston CEI, Whitecloud T, Edmunds JO: Upper cervical ossicles in Down syndrome. **J Pediatr Orthop** 7:69–71, 1987.

265. Friedman D, Flanders A, Thomas C, Millar W: Vertebral artery injury after acute cervical spine trauma: Rate of occurrence as detected by MR angiography and assessment of clinical consequences. **Am J Roentgen** 164:443–447, 1995.

266. Frisbie JH, Sasahara AA. Low dose heparin prophylaxis for deep venous thrombosis in acute spinal cord injury patients: A controlled study. Paraplegia, 19:343–346, 1981.

267. Frisbie JH, Sharma GV. Pulmonary embolism manifesting as acute disturbances of behavior in patients with spinal cord injury. Paraplegia, 32:570–572, 1994.

268. Fruin AH, Pirotte TP. Traumatic atlanto-occipital dislocation. A case report. J Neurosurg, 46:663–665, 1977.

269. Fujii E, Kobayashi K, Hirabayashi K. Treatment in fractures of the odontoid process. Spine, 13:604–609, 1988.

270. Fujimura Y, Nishi Y, Chiba K, et al: Prognosis of neurological deficits associated with upper cervical spine injuries. **Paraplegia** 33:195–202, 1995.

271. Fujimura Y, Nishi Y, Kobayashi K: Classification and treatment of axis body fractures. **J Orthop Trauma** 10:536–540, 1996.

272. Gabrielsen TO, Maxwell JA: Traumatic atlanto-occipital dislocation with case report of a patient who survived. **Am J Roentgenol** 97:624–629, 1966.

273. Galandiuk S, Raque G, Appel S, Polk HC, Jr: The two-edged sword of large-dose steroids for spinal cord trauma. **Ann Surg** 218(4):419–427, 1993.

274. Garber J: Abnormalities of the atlas and axis vertebrae—Congenital and traumatic. **J Bone Joint Surg Am** 46-A:1782–1791, 1964.

275. Garfin SR, Shackford SR, et al: Care of the multiply injured patient with cervical spine injury. **Clin Orthop Rel Res** 239:19–29, 1989.

276. Garth G: Proposal for the establishment of minimum performance specifications for cervical extrication collars. ASTM Skeletal Support Committee: 14th Annual Meeting, 1988.

277. Gaskill SJ, Marlin AE: Custom fitted thermoplastic Minerva jackets in the treatment of cervical spine instability in preschool age children. **Pediatr Neurosurg** 16:35–39, 1990.

278. Gaufin LM, Goodman SJ: Cervical spine injuries in infants. **J Neurosurg** 42:179–185, 1975.

279. Geerts WH, Code KI, Jay RM, Chen E, Szalai JP: A prospective study of venous thromboembolism after major trauma. **N Engl J Med** 331:1601–1606, 1994.

280. Geisler FH: Commentary. **J Spinal Disord** 5(1):132–133, 1992.

281. Geisler FH: GM-1 ganglioside and motor recovery following human spinal cord injury. **J Emerg Med** 11:49–55, 1993.

282. Geisler FH, Dorsey FC, Coleman WP: Recovery of motor function after spinal cord

injury: A randomized placebo-controlled trial with GM-1 ganglioside. **N Engl J Med** 324:1829–1838, 1991.

283. Geisler FH, Dorsey FC, Coleman WP: Correction: Recovery of motor function after spinal cord injury—A randomized, placebo-controlled trial with GM-1 ganglioside. **N Engl J Med** 325(23):1659–1660, 1991.

284. Geisler FH, Dorsey FC, Coleman WP: GM-1 ganglioside in human spinal cord injury. **J Neurotrauma** 9(S 2):S 517–S 530, 1992.

285. Geisler FH, Dorsey FC, Coleman WP: Response: GM-1 Ganglioside for spinal cord injury. **N Engl J Med** 326(7):494–1992.

286. Geisler FH, Grieco G, Dorsey FC, Poonian D: The GM-1 ganglioside multi-center acute spinal cord injury study. **Spine** (December) 2001.

287. Geisler W, Wynne-Jones M, et al: Early management of the patient with trauma to the spinal cord. **Med Serv J Can** 22:512–523, 1966.

288. George ER, Scholten DJ, Buechler CM, Jordan-Tibbs J, et al: Failure of methylprednisolone to improve the outcome of spinal cord injuries. **Am Surg** 61:659–664, 1995.

289. Georgopolous G, Pizzutillo L, Lee MS: Occipitoatlantal instability in children. A report of five cases and review of the literature. **J Bone Joint Surg Am** 69A:429–436, 1987.

290. Gerhart KA, Johnson RL, Menconi J, Hoffman RE, et al: Utilization and effectiveness of methylprednisolone in a population-based sample of spinal cord injured persons. **Paraplegia** 33:316–321, 1995.

291. Gerndt SJ, Rodriguez JL, Pawlik JW, Taheri PA, et al: Consequences of high-dose steroid therapy for acute spinal cord injury. **J Trauma** 42(2):279–284, 1997.

292. Gerrelts B, Peterson E, Mabry J, Peterson S: Delayed diagnosis of cervical spine injuries. **J Trauma** 31:1622–1626, 1991.

293. Giacobetti FB, Vaccaro A, Bos-Giacobetti MA, Deeley DM, Albert TJ, Farmer JC, Cotler JM: Vertebral artery occlusion associated with cervical spine trauma. A prospective analysis. **Spine** 22:188–192, 1997.

294. Givens TG, Polley KA, Smith GF, Hardin WD, Jr: Pediatric cervical spine injury: A three-year experience. **J Trauma** 41:310–314, 1996.

295. Glaser JA, Whitehill R, Stamp WG, Jane JA: Complications associated with halovest. A review of 245 cases. **J Neurosurg** 65:762–769, 1986.

296. Gleizes V, Jacquot FP, Signoret F, et al: Combined injuries in the upper cervical spine: Clinical and epidemiological data over a 14-year period. **Eur Sine J** 9:386–392, 2000.

297. Godard J, Hadji M, Raul JS: Odontoid fractures in the child with neurological injury. **Child Nerv Sys** 13:105–107, 1997.

298. Goffin J, Plets C, Van den Bergh R: Anterior cervical fusion and osteosynthetic stabilization according to Caspar: A prospective study of 41 patients with fractures and/or dislocation of the cervical spine. **Neurosurgery** 25:865–871, 1989.

299. Goldstein SJ, Woodring JH, Young AB: Occipital condyle fracture associated with cervical spine injury. **Surg Neurol** 17:350–352, 1982.

300. Gonzales R, Fried P, Bukhalo M, Holevar M., Falimirski M: Role of clinical examination in screening for blunt injury. **J Am Coll Surg** 189:152–157, 1999.

301. Goth P: *Spinal Injury: Clinical Criteria for Assessment and Management.* Augusta, ME: Medical Care Development Publishing, 1994.

302. Govender S, Charles RW: Traumatic spondylolisthesis of the axis. **Injury** 18:333–335, 1987.

303. Govender S, Grootboom M: Fractures of the dens—The results of non-rigid immobilization. **Injury** 19:165–167, 1988.

304. Grabb PA, Pang D: Magnetic resonance imaging in the evaluation of spinal cord injury without radiographic abnormality in children. **Neurosurgery** 35:406–414, 1994.
305. Grabb BC, Frye TA, Hedlund GL, Vaid YN, Grabb PA, Royal SA: MRI diagnosis of suspected atlanto-occipital dislocation in childhood. **Pediatr Radiol** 29:275–281, 1999.
306. Grady MS, Howard MA, Jane JA, et al: Use of the Philadelphia collar as an alternative to the halo vest in patients with C2, C3 fractures. **Neurosurgery** 18:151–156, 1986.
307. Grahm TW, Zadrozny DB, Harrington T: Benefits of early jejunal hyperalimentation in the head injured patient. **Neurosurgery** 25:729–735, 1989.
308. Grant G, Mirza S, Chapman J, Winn H, Newell D, Jones D, Grady M: Risk of early closed reduction in cervical spine subluxation injuries. **J Neurosurg** 90 (Spine):13–18, 1999.
309. Graziano AF, Scheidel EA, et al: A radiographic comparison of pre-hospital cervical immobilization methods. **Ann Emerg Med** 16:1127–1131, 1987.
310. Green D, Biddle A, Fahey V, et al: Prevention of thromboembolism in spinal cord injury. **Spinal Cord Med** 20:259–283, 1997.
311. Green D, Chen D, Chmiel JS, et al: Prevention of thromboembolism in spinal cord injury: Role of low molecular weight heparin. **Arch Phys Med Rehabil** 75:290–292, 1994.
312. Green B, Eismont F, et al: Spinal cord injury—a systems approach: Prevention, emergency medical services and emergency room management. **Crit Care Clin** 3:471–493, 1987.
313. Green D, Lee MY, Ito VY, et al: Fixed vs. adjusted-dose heparin in the prophylaxis of thromboembolism in spinal cord injury. **JAMA** 260:1255–1258, 1988.
314. Green D, Lee MY, Lim AC, et al: Comments: Prevention of thromboembolism after spinal cord injury using low-molecular-weight heparin. **Ann Intern Med** 113:571–574, 1990.
315. Greene KA, Dickman C, Marciano FF, et al: Transverse atlantal ligament disruption associated with odontoid fractures. **Spine** 19:2307–2314, 1994.
316. Greene KA, Dickman C, Marciano FF, et al: Acute axis fractures. Analysis of management and outcome in 340 consecutive cases. **Spine** 22:1843–1852, 1997.
317. Greenfield LJ: Does cervical spinal cord injury induce a higher incidence of complications after prophylactic Greenfield filter usage? (Letter). **J Vasc Interv Radiol** 8:719–720, 1997.
318. Gresham GE, Labi MLC, Dittmar SS, Hicks JT, Joyce SZ, Stehlik MAP: The Quadriplegia Index of Function (QIF): Sensitivity and reliability demonstrated in a study of thirty quadriplegic patients. **Paraplegia** 24:38–44, 1986.
319. Griffiths SC: Fracture of the odontoid process in children. **J Pediatr Surg** 7:680–683, 1972.
320. Grisolia A, Bell RL, Peltier LF: Fractures and dislocations of the spine complicating ankylosing spondylitis. A report of 6 cases. **J Bone Joint Surg Am** 49A:339–344, 1967.
321. Griswold DM, Albright JA, Schiffman E, Johnson R, Southwick WO: Atlanto-axial fusion for instability. **J Bone Joint Surg Am** 60A:285–292, 1978.
322. Grogaard B, Dullerud R, Magnaes B: Acute torticollis in children due to atlanto-axial rotary fixation. **Arch Orthop Trauma Surg** 112:185–188, 1993.
323. Grossman M, Reilly P, Gillett T, Gillett D: National survey of the incidence of cervical spine injury and approach to cervical spine clearance in US trauma centers. **J Trauma** 47:684–690, 1999.

324. Gschaedler R, Dollfus P, Mole JP, Mole L, Loeb JP: Reflections on the intensive care of acute cervical spinal cord injuries in a general traumatology centre. **Paraplegia** 17:58–61, 1979.
325. Guigui P, Milaire M, Morvan G, Lassale B, Deburge A: Traumatic atlanto-occipital dislocation with survival: Case report and review of the literature. **Eur Spine J** 4:242–247, 1995.
326. Guiot B, Fessler RG: Complex atlantoaxial fractures. **J Neurosurg** 91:139–143, 1999.
327. Gunby P: New focus on spinal cord injury, medical news. **JAMA** 245:1201–1981.
328. Gunduz S, Ogur E, Mohur H, Somuncu I, Acjksoz E, Ustunsoz B: Deep vein thrombosis in spinal cord injured patients. **Paraplegia** 31:606–610, 1993.
329. Gunn B, Eizenberg N, et al: How should an unconscious person with a suspected neck injury be positioned? **Pre-Hospital Disaster Medicine** 10:239–244, 1995.
330. Gurdjian ES, Hardy WG, Lindner DW, Thomas LM: Closed cervical trauma associated with involvement of carotid and vertebral arteries. **J Neurosurg** 20:418–427, 1963.
331. Guttman L: Initial treatment of traumatic paraplegia and tetraplegia. In *Spinal Injuries.* Edinburgh, Scotland: The Royal College of Surgeons, 1966.
332. Hachen HJ: Anticoagulant therapy in patients with spinal cord injury. **Paraplegia** 12:176–187, 1974.
333. Hachen H: Emergency transportation in the event of acute spinal cord lesion. **Paraplegia** 12:33–37, 1974.
334. Hachen H: Idealized care of the acute injured spinal cord in Switzerland. **J Trauma** 17(12):931–936, 1977.
335. Hadley MN, Argires PJ: The acute/emergent management of vertebral column fracture dislocation injuries. In *Neurological Emergencies.* Park Ridge, IL: American Association of Neurological Surgeons, 1994, pp 249–262.
336. Hadley MN: Hypermetabolism after CNS trauma: Arresting the "injury cascade". **Nutrition** 5(2):143–1989.
337. Hadley MN: Hypermetabolism following head trauma: Nutritional considerations. In Barrow DL (ed): *Complications and Sequelae of Head Injury (Neurosurgical Topics).* Park Ridge, IL: American Association of Neurological Surgeons, 1992, pp 161–168.
338. Hadley MN, Browner C, Sonntag VKH: Axis fractures: A comprehensive reivew of management and treatment in 107 cases. **Neurosurgery** 17:281–290, 1985.
339. Hadley MN, Browner C, Liu SS, et al: New subtype of acute odontoid fractures (Type IIA). **Neurosurgery** 22:67–71, 1988.
340. Hadley MN, Dickman C, Browner C, et al: Acute traumatic atlas fractures: Management and long term outcome. **Neurosurgery** 23:31–35, 1988.
341. Hadley MN, Dickman C, Browner C, et al: Acute axis fractures: A review of 229 cases. **J Neurosurg** 71:642–647, 1989.
342. Hadley MN, Fitzpatrick B, Sonntag VKH, Browner C: Facet fracture-dislocation injuries of the cervical spine. Neurosurgery 30:661–666, 1992.
343. Hadley MN, Grahm TW, Harrington T, et al: Nutritional support and neurotrauma: A critical review of early nutrition in forty-five acute head injury patients. **Neurosurgery** 19:367–373, 1986.
344. Hadley MN, Zabramski JM, Browner C, Rekate HL, Sonntag VKH: Pediatric spinal trauma. **J Neurosurg** 68:18–24, 1988.
345. Hall ED, Wolf DL: A pharmacological analysis of the pathophysiological mechanisms of post-traumatic spinal cord ischemia. **J Neurosurg** 64:951–961, 1986.
346. Hall A, Wagle V, Raycrof J, Goldman R, Butler A: Magnetic resonance imaging in cervical spine trauma. **J Trauma** 34:21–26, 1993.

347. Halliday AL, Henderson BR, Hart BL, Benzel EC: The management of unilateral lateral mass/facet fractures of the subaxial cervical spine: The use of magnetic resonance imaging to predict instability. **Spine** 22:2614–2621, 1997.
348. Hamilton MG, Myles ST: Pediatric spinal injury: Review of 174 hospital admissions. **J Neurosurg** 77:700–704, 1992.
349. Hamilton BB, Granger CV, Sherwin FS, Zielezny M, Tashman JS: A uniform national data system for medical rehabilitation. In *Rehabilitation Outcomes: Analysis and Measurement.* Baltimore: Brookes Publishing, 1987, pp 137–147.
350. Hamilton BB, Laughlin JA, Granger CV, Kayton RM: Interrater agreement of the seven-level functional independece measure (FIM). **Arch Phys Med Rehabil** 72:790–1991.
351. Hamilton BB, Laughlin JA, Fiedler RC, Granger CV: Interrater reliability of the 7-level functional independence measure (FIM). **Scand J Rehabil Med** 26(3):115–119, 1994.
352. Hamilton RS, Pons PT, et al: The efficacy and comfort of full-body vacuum splints for cervical-spine immobilization. **J Emerg Med** 14(5):553–559, 1996.
353. Han SY, Witten DM, Mussleman JP: Jefferson fracture of the atlas. Report of six cases. **J Neurosurg** 44:368–371, 1976.
354. Hanigan WC, Powell FC, Elwood PW, et al: Odontoid fractures in elderly patients. **J Neurosurg** 78:32–35, 1993.
355. Hannigan WC, Anderson RJ: Commentary on NASCIS 2. **J Spinal Disord** 5(1):125–131, 1992.
356. Hanson J, Blackmore C, Mann F, Wilson A: Cervical spine injury: A clinical decision rule to identify high risk patients for helical CT screening. **Am J Roentgenol** 174:713–717, 2000.
357. Hanssen AD, Cabanela ME: Fractures of the dens in adult patients. **J Trauma** 27:928–934, 1987.
358. Harding-Smith J, MacIntosh PK, Sherbon KJ: Fracture of the occipital condyle: A case report and review of the literature. **J Bone Joint Surg Am** 63A:1170–1171, 1981.
359. Harmanlis O, Koyfman Y: Traumatic atlanto-occipital dislocation with survival: Case report and review of the literature. **Surg Neurol** 39:324–330, 1993.
360. Harrington J, Likavec M, Smith A: Disc herniation in cervical fracture subluxation. **Neurosurgery** 29:374–379, 1991.
361. Harris JH, Carson GC, Wagner LK: Radiologic diagnosis of traumatic occipitovertebral dissociation: 1. Normal occipitovertebral relationships on lateral radiographs of supine subjects. **Am J Radiol** 162:881–886, 1994.
362. Harris JH, Carson GC, Wagner F, Kerr N: Radiologic diagnosis of traumatic occipitovertebral dissociation: 2. Comparison of three methods of detecting occipitovertebral relationships on lateral radiographs of supine subjects. **Am J Radiol** 162:887–892, 1994.
363. Harris S, Chen D, Green D: Enoxaparin for thromboembolism prophylaxis in spinal injury. **Am J Phys Med Rehabil** 75:326–327, 1996.
364. Hashimoto T, Watanabe O, Takase M, Koniyama J, Kobota M: Collet-Sicard syndrome after minor head trauma. **Neurosurgery** 23:367–370, 1998.
365. Hauswald M, Ong G, et al: Out-of-hospital spinal immobilization: Its effect on neurologic injury (comments). **Acad Emerg Med** 5(3):214–219, 1998.
366. Hays MB, Alker GJ, Jr: Fractures of the atlas vertebra. The two-part burst fracture of Jefferson. **Spine** 13:601–603, 1988.
367. Hays MB, Bernhang AM: Fractures of the atlas vertebra. A three-part fracture not previously classified. **Spine** 17:240–242, 1992.

368. Heary RF, Hunt DC, Kriger AJ, Antonio C, Livingston DH. Acute stabilization of the cervical spine by halo/vest application facilitates evaluation and treatment of multiple trauma patients. **J Trauma** 33:445–451, 1992.

369. Heller JG, Viroslav S, Hudson T: Jefferson fractures: The role of magnification artifact in assessing transverse ligament integrity. **J Spinal Disord** 6:392–396, 1993.

370. Henry AD, Bohly J, Grosse A: Fixation of odontoid fractures by an anterior screw. **J Bone Joint Surg Br** 81:472–477, 1999.

371. Herr C, Ball P, Sargent S, Quinton H: Sensitivity of prevertebral soft tissue measurement at C3 for detection of cervical spine fractures and dislocations. **Am J Emerg Med** 16:346–349, 1998.

372. Herzenberg JE, Hensinger RN, Dedrick DK, et al: Emergency transport and positioning of young children who have an injury of the cervical spine: The standard backboard may be dangerous. **J Bone Joint Surg Am** 71A:1–1989.

373. Highland TR, Salciccioli GG: Is immobilization adequate treatment of unstable burst fractures of the atlas? A case report with long-term follow-up evaluation. **Clin Orthop** 196–200, 1985.

374. Hladky JP, Lejeune JP, Leclercq F, Dhellemmes P, Christiaens JL: La dislocation occipito-atlodienne traumatique. **Neurochirurgie** 37:312–317, 1991.

375. Hoffman J, Mower W, Wolfson A, Todd K, Zucker M: Validity of a set of clinical criteria to rule out injury to the cervical spine in patients with blunt trauma. **N Engl J Med** 343:94–99, 2000.

376. Hoffman J, Schriger DL, Mower W, Luo J, Zucker M: Low-risk criteria for cervical spine radiography in blunt trauma: A prospective study. **Ann Emerg Med** 21:1454–1460, 1992.

377. Hoffman J, Wolfson A, Todd K, Mower W: Selective cervical spine radiography in blunt trauma: Methodology of the national emergency x-radiography utilization study (NEXUS). **Ann Emerg Med** 32:461–469, 1998.

378. Holliman C, Mayer J, Cook R, Smith J: Is the anteroposterior cervical spine radiograph necessary in initial trauma screening? **Am J Emerg Med** 9:421–425, 1991.

379. Hosono N, Yonenobu K, Ebara S, Ono K: Cineradiographic motion analysis of atlantoaxial instability in os odontoideum. **Spine** 16:S 480–S 482, 1991.

380. Hosono N, Yonenobu K, Kawagoe K, Hirayama N, Ono K: Traumatic anterior atlanto-occipital dislocation. A case report with survival. **Spine** 18:786–790, 1992.

381. Huerta CR, Girffith R, Joyce SM: Cervical spine stabilization in pediatric patients: Evaluation of current techniques. **Ann Emerg Med** 16:1121–1126, 1987.

382. Hulsewe K.W.E., van Acker BACvMMF, Soeters PB: Nutritional depletion and dietary manipulation: Effects on the immune response. **World J Surg** 23:536–544, 1999.

383. Hummel A, Plaue R: Diagnostik und behandlung atlantokzipitaler rupturen. **Unfallchirurgie** 14:311–319, 1988.

384. Hurlbert RJ: Response: The use of methylprednisolone. **J Neurosurg** 93(Spine):340–341, 2000.

385. Hurlbert RJ: Methylprednisolone for acute spinal cord injury: An inappropriate standard of care. **J Neurosurg** 93(Spine 1):1–7, 2000.

386. Ide C, Nisolle JF, Misson N, Trigaux JP, Gustin T, DeCoene B, Gilliard C: Unusual occipitoatlantal fracture dissociation with no neurological impairment. Case report. **J Neurosurg** 88:773–776, 1998.

387. Iida H, Tachibana S, Horiike S, Ohwada T, Fujii K: Association of head trauma with cervical spine injury, spinal cord injury, or both. **J Trauma** 46:450–452, 1999.

478 CLINICAL NEUROSURGERY

388. Ireland A, Britton A, Forrester A: Do supine oblique views provide better imaging of the cervicothoracic junction than swimmer's views? **J Accid Emerg Med** 15:151–154, 1998.
389. Jacobs L, Schwartz R: Prospective analysis of acute cervical spine injury: A methodology to predict injury. **Ann Emerg Med** 15:44–49, 2001.
390. Jacoby CG: Fracture of the occipital condyle. **Am J Radiol** 132:500–1979.
391. Jakim I, Sweet MB: Transverse fracture through the body of the axis. **J Bone Joint Surg Br** 70:728–729, 1988.
392. Jakim I, Sweet MB, Wisniewski T: Isolated avulsion fracture of the anterior tubercle of the atlas. **Arch Orthop Trauma Surg** 108:377–379, 1989.
393. Jarrell BE, Posuniak E, Roberts J, Osterholm JL, Cotler J, Ditunno J: A new method of management using the Kim-Ray Greenfield filter for deep venous thrombosis and pulmonary embolism in spinal cord injury. **Surg Gynecol Obstet** 157:316–320, 1983.
394. Jeanneret B, Magerl F: Primary posterior fusion C1-2 in odontoid fractures: Indications, technique, and results of transarticular screw fixation. **J Spinal Disord** 5:464–475, 1992.
395. Jeanneret B, Magerl F, et al: Over distraction: A hazard of skull traction in the management of acute injuries of the cervical spine. **Arch Orthop Trauma Surg** 110(5):242–245, 1991.
396. Jefferson G: Fractures of the atlas vertebra: Report of four cases and a review of those previously reported. **Br J Surg** 7:407–422, 1920.
397. Jenkins JD, Corric D, Branch CL: A clinical comparison of one- and two-screw odontoid fixation. **J Neurosurg** 89:366–370, 1998.
398. Jevitch V: Traumatic lateral atlanto-occipital dislocation with spontaneous bony fusion. A case report. **Spine** 14:123–124, 1989.
399. Johnson DR, Hauswald M, et al: Comparison of a vacuum splint device to a rigid backboard for spinal immobilization. **Am J Emerg Med** 14(4):369–372, 1996.
400. Jones SL: Spine trauma board. **Phys Ther** 57(8):921–922, 1977.
401. Jones DN, Knox AM, Sage MR: Traumatic avulsion fracture of the occipital condyles and clivus with associated unilateral atlantooccipital distraction. **Am J Neuroradiol** 11:1181–1183, 1990.
402. Jonsson M, Tollback A, Gonzalez H, Borg J: Inter-rater reliability of the 1992 international standards for neurological and functional classification of incomplete spinal cord injury. **Spinal Cord** 38:675–679, 2000.
403. Julien T, Frankel B, Traynelis VC, et al: Evidence-based analysis of odontoid fracture management. **Neurosurg Focus** 8:Article 1-2000.
404. Kalfas I, Wilberger J, Goldberg AL, Prostko ER: Magnetic resonance imaging in acute spinal cord trauma. **Neurosurgery** 23(3):295–299, 1988.
405. Kalff R, Kocks W, Grote W, Scmit-Neuerburg KP: Operative spondylodesis in injuries of the lower cervical spine. **Neurosurg Rev** 16:211–220, 1993.
406. Kaneriya P, Schwetizer M, Spettell C, Cohen M, Karasick D: The cost effectiveness of oblique radiography in the exclusion of C7-T1 injury in trauma patients. **Am J Radiology** 171:959–962, 1998.
407. Katzberg R, Benedetti P, Drake C, Ivanovic M, Levine R, Beatty C, Nemzek W, McFall R, Ontell F, Bishop D, Poirier V, Chong B: Acute cervical spine injuries: Prospective MR imaging assessment at a level-one trauma center. **Radiology** 213:203–212, 1999.
408. Kaufman RA, Dunbar JS, Botsford JA, McLaurin RL: Traumatic longitudinal atlanto-occipital distraction injuries in children. **Am J Neuroradiol** 3:415–419, 1982.

409. Kaufman HH, Rowlands BJ, Stein DK, Kopaniky DR, et al: General metabolism in patients with acute paraplegia and quadriplegia. **Neurosurgery** 16(3):309–313, 1985.
410. Kaups K, Davis J: Patients with gunshot wounds to the head do not require cervical spine immobilization and evaluation. **J Trauma** 44:865–867, 1998.
411. Kawabe N, Hirotani H, Tanaka O: Pathomechanism of atlanto-axial rotary fixation in children. J **Pediatr Orthop** 9:569–574, 1989.
412. Kearns PJ, Thompson JD, Werner PC, et al: Nutritional and metabolic response to acute spinal cord injury. **J Parenteral Enteral Nutrition** 16(1):11–15, 1992.
413. Keiper MD, Zimmerman RA, Bilaniuk LT: MRI in the assessment of the supportive soft tissues of the cervical spine in acute trauma in children. **Neuroradiology** 40:359–363, 1998.
414. Kesterson L, Benzel EC, Orrison W, et al: Evaluation and treatment of atlas burst fractures (Jefferson fractures). **J Neurosurg** 75:213–220, 1991.
415. Key A: Cervical spine dislocations with unilateral facet interlocking. **Paraplegia** 13:208–215, 1975.
416. Khansarinia S, Dennis JW, Veldenz HC, Butcher JL, Hartland L: Prophylactic Greenfield filter placement in selected high-risk trauma patients. **J Vasc Surg** 22:231–235, 1995.
417. Kilburn MPB, Smith DP, Hadley MN: The initial evaluation and treatment of the patient with spinal trauma. In Batjer HH, Loftus CL (eds): *Textbook of Neurological Surgery.* Philadelphia: Lippincott Williams & Wilkins, 2001.
418. Kindt GW, Ducker TB, Huddlestone J: Regulation of spinal cord blood flow. In Russell RWR (ed.): *Brain and Blood Flow.* London: Pitman Medical and Scientific Publishing, 1971, pp 401–405.
419. King BS, Gupta R, Narayan RK: The early assessment and intensive care unit management of patients with severe traumatic brain and spinal cord injuries. **Surg Clin North Am** 80(3):855–870, 2000.
420. Kinney TB, Rose SC, Valji K, Oglevie SB, Roberts AC: Comments: Does cervical spinal cord injury induce a higher incidence of complications after prophylactic Greenfield inferior vena cava filter usage? **J Vasc Interv Radiol** 7:907–915, 1996.
421. Kiwerski JE: Early anterior decompression and fusion for crush fractures of cervical vertebrae. **Int Orthop** 17:166–168, 1993.
422. Klein G, Vaccaro A, Albert T, Schwetizer M, Deely D, Karasick D, Cotler J: Efficacy of magnetic resonance imaging in the evaluation of posterior cervical spine fractures. **Spine** 24:771–774, 1999.
423. Kleyn P: Dislocations of the cervical spine: Closed reduction under anaesthesia. **Paraplegia** 22:271–281, 1984.
424. Klose KJ, Green BA, Smith RS, Adkins RH, MacDonald AM: University of Miami Neuro-Spinal Index (UMNI): A quantitative method for determining spinal cord function. **Paraplegia** 18:331–336, 1980.
425. Kobrine AI, Doyle TF, Martins AN: Autoregulation of spinal cord blood flow. In Wilkins RH (ed.): *Clinical Neurosurgery,* Baltimore, MD: Williams & Wilkins (Congress of Neurological Surgeons), 573–581, 1974.
426. Kobrine AI, Doyle TF, Rizzoli HV: Spinal cord blood flow as affected by changes in systemic arterial blood pressure. **J Neurosurg** 44:12–15, 1976.
427. Kolb JC, Summers RL, et al: Cervical collar-induced changes in intracranial pressure. **Am J Emerg Med** 17(2):135–137, 1999.
428. Koop SE, Winter RB, Lonstein JE: The surgical treatment of instability of the upper part of the cervical spine in children and adolescents. **J Bone Joint Surg Am** 66A:403–411, 1987.

429. Kornberg M: Atypical unstable burst fracture of the atlas. Treated by primary atlantoaxial fusion. **Orthop Rev** 15:727–729, 1986.
430. Korres DS, Zoubos AB, Kavadias K, et al: The "tear drop" (or avulsed) fracture of the anterior inferior angle of the axis. **Eur Spine J** 3:151–154, 1994.
431. Koskinen EVS, Nieminen R: Fractures and dislocations of the cervical spine. Treatment and results of 159 cases. **Int Surg** 47:472–485, 1967.
432. Kossuth LC: Removal of injured personnel from wrecked vehicles. **J Trauma** 5:704–705, 1965.
433. Kossuth LC: The initial movement of the injured. **Mil Med** 132(1):18–21, 1967.
434. Kowalski HM, Cohen WA, Cooper P, Wisoff J.H. Pitfalls in the CT diagnosis of atlanto-axial rotary subluxation. **AJR** 149:595–600, 1987.
435. Kreipke D, Gillespie K, McCarthy M, Mail J, Lappas J, Broadie T: Reliability of indications for cervical spine films in trauma patients. **J Trauma** 29:1438–1439, 1989.
436. Kucukdeveci AA, Yazuver G, Tennant A, Suldur N, Sonel B, Arasil T: Adaptation of the modified Barthel index for use in physical medicine and rehabilitation in Turkey. **Scand J Rehabil Med** 32:87–92, 2000.
437. Kuhns LR, Loder RT, Farley FA, Hensinger RN: Nuchal cord changes in children with os odontoideum: Evidence for associated trauma. **J Pediatr Orthop** 18:815–819, 1998.
438. Kulkarni JR, Burt AA, Tromans AT, Constable PD: Prophylactic low dose heparin anticoagulant therapy in patients with spinal cord injuries: A retrospective study. **Paraplegia** 30:169–172, 1992.
439. Laham JL, Cotcamp CH, Gibbons PA, Kahana MD, Crone KR: Isolated head injuries versus multiple trauma in pediatric patients: do the same indications for cervical spine evaluation apply? **Pediatric Neurosurg** 21:221–226, 1994.
440. Lam CH, Stratford J: Bilateral hypoglossal nerve injury with occipital condyle fracture. **Can J Neurol Sci** 23:145–148, 1996.
441. Lamb GC, Tomski MA, Kaufman J, Maiman D: Is chronic spinal cord injury associated with increased risk of venous thromboembolism? **J Am Paraplegia Soc** 16:153–156, 1993.
442. Landells CD, Van Peteghem PK: Fractures of the atlas: Classification, treatment and morbidity. **Spine** 13:450–452, 1988.
443. Landi G, Ciccone A: GM-1 ganglioside for spinal cord injury (Letter). **N Engl J Med** 326(7):493–1992.
444. Lazar RB, Yarkony GM, Ortolano D, Heinemann A, Perlow E, Lovell L, Meyer P: Prediction of functional outcome by motor capability after spinal cord injury. **Arch Phys Med Rehabil** 70(12):819–822, 1989.
445. Ledsome JR, Sharp JM: Pulmonary function in acute cervical cord injury. **Am Rev Respir Dis** 124:41–44, 1981.
446. Lee C, Woodring J: Unstable Jefferson variant atlas fractures: An unrecognized cervical injury. **Am J Neuroradiol** 12:1105–1110, 1991.
447. Lee TT, Green BA, Petrin DR: Treatment of stable burst fracture of the atlas (Jefferson fractures) with rigid cervical collar. **Spine** 23:1963–1967, 1998.
448. Lee A, Maclean J, Newton D: Rapid traction for reduction of cervical spine dislocations. **J Bone Joint Surg Br** 76-B:352–356, 1994.
449. Lee C, Woodring JH, Goldstein SJ, Daniel TL, Young AB, Tibbs PA: Evaluation of traumatic atlanto-occipital dislocations. **Am J Neuroradiol** 8:19–26, 1987.
450. Lee C, Woodring JH, Walsh JW: Carotid and vertebral injury in survivors of atlanto-occipital dislocations: Case reports and literature review. **J Trauma** 31:401–407, 1991.

451. Legros B, Fournier P, Chiaroni P, Ritz O, Fusciardi J: Basal fracture of the skull and lower (IX, X, XI, XII) cranial nerves palsy: Four case reports including two fractures of the occipital condyle—A literature review. **J Trauma** 48:342–348, 2000.
452. Lehmann KG, Lane JG, Piepmeier JM, Batsford WP: Cardiovascular abnormalities accompanying acute spinal cord injury in humans: Incidence, time course and severity. **J Am Coll Cardiol** 10(1):46–52, 1987.
453. Lemons VR, Wagner FC: Stabilization of subaxial cervical spinal injuries. **Surg Neurol** 39:511–518, 1993.
454. Lennarson PJ, Mostafavi H, Traynelis VC, et al: Management of Type II dens fractures: A case-control study. **Spine** 25:1234–1237, 2000.
455. Leone A, Cerase A, Colosimo C, Lauro L, Puca A, Marano P: Occipital condylar fractures: A review. **Radiology** 216:635–644, 2000.
456. Lerner E.B., Billittier AJT, et al: The effects of neutral positioning with and without padding on spinal immoibilization of healthy subjects. **Pre-Hospital Emergency Care** 2(2):112–116, 1998.
457. Leventhal MR, Boydston WR, Sebes JI, Pinstein ML, Watridge CB, Lowery R: The diagnosis and treatment of fractures of the occipital condyle. **Orthopaedics** 15:944–947, 1992.
458. Levi L, Wolf A, Rigamonti D, Ragheb J, Mirvis S, Robinson WL: Anterior decompression in cervical spine trauma: Does the timing of surgery affect the outcome? **Neurosurgery** 29(2):216–222, 1991.
459. Levi L, Wolf A, Belzberg H: Hemodynamic parameters in patients with acute cervical cord trauma: Description, intervention, and prediction of outcome. **Neurosurgery** 33(6):1007–1017, 1993.
460. Levine AM, Edwards CC: The management of traumatic spondylolisthesis of the axis. **J Bone Joint Surg Am** 67:217–226, 1985.
461. Levine AM, Edwards CC: Treatment of injuries in the C1-C2 complex. **Orthop Clin North Am** 17:31–44, 1986.
462. Levine AM, Edwards CC: Fractures of the atlas. **J Bone Joint Surg Am** 73:680–691, 1991.
463. Levine AM, Mazel C, Roy-Camille R: Management of fracture separations of the articular mass using posterior cervical plating. **Spine** 17:S 447–S454, 1992.
464. Levine AM, Nash MS, Green BA, et al: An examination of dietary intakes and nutritional status of chronic healthy spinal cord injured individuals. **Paraplegia** 30:880–889, 1992.
465. Lewelt W, Jenkins LW, Miller JD: Autoregulation of cerebral blood flow after experimental fluid percussion injury of the brain. **J Neurosurg** 53:500–511, 1980.
466. Lewis L, Docherty M, Ruoff B, Fortney J, Keltner R, Britton P: Flexion-extension views in the evaluation of cervical spinal injuries. **Ann Emerg Med** 20:117–121, 1991.
467. Lieberman IH, Webb JK: Cervical spine injuries in the elderly. **J Bone Joint Surg Br** 76B:877–881, 1994.
468. Liew S, Hill D: Complications of hard cervical collars in multi-trauma patients. **Aust N Z J Surg** 64:139–140, 1994.
469. Lifeso RM, Colucci MA: Anterior fusion for rotationally unstable cervical spine fractures. **Spine** 25:2028–2034, 2000.
470. Linares HA, Mawson AR, et al: Association between pressure sores and immobilization in the immediate post-injury period. **Orthopedics** 10(4):571–573, 1987.
471. Lind B, Nordwall A, Sihlbom H: Odontoid fractures treated with halo-vest. **Spine** 12:173–177, 1987.

472. Lind B, Sihlbom H, Nordwall A: Halo-vest treatment of unstable traumatic cervical spine injuries. **Spine** 13:425–432, 1988.
473. Lindsey R, Diliberti T, Doherty B, Watson A: Efficacy of radiographic evaluation of the cervical spine in emergency situations. **Southern Med J** 86:1253–1255, 1993.
474. Link TM, Schuierer G, Hufendiek A, Horch C, Peters PE: Substantial head trauma: Value of routine CT examination of the cervicocranium. **Radiology** 196:741–745, 1995.
475. Lipson SJ: Fractures of the atlas associated with fractures of the odontoid process and transverse ligament ruptures. **J Bone Joint Surg Am** 59:940–943, 1977.
476. Lockey A, Handley R, Willett K: Clearance of cervical spine injury in the obtunded patient. **Injury** 29:493–497, 1998.
477. Louw JA, Mafoyane NA, Small B, Neser CP: Occlusion of the vertebral artery in cervical spine dislocations. **J Bone Joint Surg Br** 72 B:679–681, 1990.
478. Lowry DW, Pollack IF, Clyde B, Albright AL, Adelson PD: Upper cervical spine fusion in the pediatric population. **J Neurosurg** 87:671–676, 1997.
479. Lu K, Lee T, Chen H: Closed reduction of bilateral locked facets of the cervical spine under gneeral anaesthesia. **Acta Neurochir** 40:1055–1061, 1998.
480. Lu K, Lee TC, Liang CL, Chen HJ: Delayed apnea in patients with mid- to lower cervical spinal cord injury. **Spine** 25(11):1332–1338, 2000.
481. Lucas JT, Ducker TB: Motor classification of spinal cord injuries with mobility, morbidity and recovery indices. **Am Surg** 45:151–158, 1979.
482. Ludwig S, Vaccaro A, Balderston R, Cotler J: Immediate quadriparesis after manipulation for bilateral cervical facet subluxation. **J Bone Joint Surg Am** 79-A:587–590, 1997.
483. Lui TN, Lee ST, Wong CW, Yeh YS, Tzaan WC, Chen TY, Hung SY: C1-C2 fracture dislocations in children and adolescents. **J Trauma** 40:408–411, 1996.
484. Lukhele M: Fractures of the vertebral lamina associated with unifacet and bi-facet cervical spine dislocations. **S African J Surg** 32:112–114, 1994.
485. Lyons MK, Partington MD, Meyer FB: A randomized, controlled trial of methylprednisolone or naloxone in the treatment of acute spinal-cord injury (Letter). **N Engl J Med** 323(17):1207–1208, 1990.
486. Macdonald R, et al: Diagnosis of cervical spine injury in motor vehicle crash victims: How many x-rays are enough? **J Trauma** 30:392–397, 1990.
487. Mace S: Emergency evaluation of cervical spine injuries: CT versus plain radiographs. **Ann Emerg Med** 14:973–975, 1985.
488. Mace S: Unstable occult cervical spine fracture. **Ann Emerg Med** 20:1373–1375, 1991.
489. MacKinnon JA, Perlman M, Kirpalani H, Rehan V, Sauve R, Kovacs L: Spinal cord injury at birth: Diagnostic and prognostic data in twenty-two patients. **J Pediatr** 122:431–437, 1993.
490. Mahadevan S, Mower W, Hoffman J, Peeples W, Goldberg W, Sonner R: Interrater reliability of cervical spine injury criteria in patients with blunt trauma. **Ann Emerg Med** 31:197–201, 1998.
491. Mahale Y, Silver J: Progressive paralysis after bilateral facet dislocation of the cervical spine. **J Bone Joint Surg Br** 74-B:219–223, 1992.
492. Mahale Y, Silver J, Henderson N: Neurological complications of the reduction of cervical spine dislocations. **J Bone Joint Surg Br** 75-B:403–409, 1993.
493. Mahoney FI, Barthel DW: Functional evaluation: The Barthel Index. **Maryland Med J** 14:61–65, 1965.
494. Maiman DJ, Larson SJ: Management of odontoid fractures. **Neurosurgery** 11:820–1982.

495. Maiman D, Barolat G, Larson S: Management of bilateral locked facets of the cervical spine. **Neurosurgery** 18:542–547, 1986.
496. Mandabach M, Ruge JR, Hahn YS, McLone DG: Pediatric axis fractures: Early halo immobilization, management and outcome. **Pediatric Neurosurg** 19:225–232, 1993.
497. Mann FA, Coheen W: Occipital condyle fracture: Significance in the assessment of occipitoatlantal stability. **Am J Radiol** 163:193–194, 1994.
498. Mansel JK, Norman JR: Respiratory complications and management of spinal cord injuries. **Chest** 97(6):1446–1452, 1990.
499. Marar BC, Tay CK: Fracture of the odontoid process. **Aust N Z J Surg** 46:231–236, 1976.
500. Mariani PJ: Occipital condyle fracture presenting as a retropharyngeal hematoma. **Ann Emerg Med** 19:1447–1449, 1990.
501. Marino RJ, Huang M, Knight P, Herbison GJ, Ditunno JF Jr, Segal M: Assessing selfcare status in quadriplegia: Comparison of the quadriplegia index of function (QIF) and the functional independence measure (FIM). **Paraplegia** 31(4):225–233, 1993.
502. Marino RJ, Rider-Foster D, Maissel G, Ditunno JF: Superiority of motor level over single neurological level in categorizing tetraplegia. **Paraplegia** 33:510–513, 1995.
503. Markenson D, Foltin G, et al: The Kendrick extrication device used for pediatric spinal immobilization. **Pre-Hospital Emergency Care** 3(1):66–69, 1999.
504. Marks DS, Roberts P, Wilton PJ, Burns LA, Thompson AG: A halo jacket for stabilization of the paediatric cervical spine. **Arch Orthop Trauma Surg** 112:134–135, 1993.
505. Maroon JC: "Burning Hands" in football spinal cord injuries. **JAMA** 238(19):2049–2051, 1977.
506. Marshall LF, Knowlton S, et al: Deterioration following spinal cord injury. A multicenter study. **J Neurosurg** 66(3):400–404, 1987.
507. Massaro F, Lanotte M: Case reports. Fracture of the occipital condyle. **Injury** 24:419–420, 1993.
508. Matava MJ, Whitesides TE, Davis PC: Traumatic atlanto-occipital dislocations with survival. Serial computerized tomography as an aid to diagnosis and reduction: A report of three cases. **Spine** 18:1897–1903, 1993.
509. Matsui H, Imada K, Tsuji H: Radiographic classification of Os odontoideum and its clinical significance. **Spine** 22:1706–1709, 1997.
510. Matsumoto T, Tamaki T, Kawakami M, Yoshida M: Early complications of high-dose methylprednisolone sodium succinate treatment in the follow-up of acute cervical spinal cord injuyr. **Spine** 26(4):426–430, 2001.
511. Maves CK, Souza A, Prenger EC, Kirks DR: Traumatic atlanto-occipital disruption in children. **Pediatr Radiol** 21:504–507, 1991.
512. Mawson AR, Biundo JJ, Jr., et al: Risk factors for early occurring pressure ulcers following spinal cord injury. **Am J Phys Med Rehabil** 67(3):123–127, 1988.
513. Maynard FM, Bracken MB, Creasey G, Ditunno JF, Jr., Donovan WH, Ducker TB, Garber SL, Marino RJ, Stover SL, Tator CH, Waters RL, Wilberger JE, Young W: International standards for neurological and functional classification of spinal cord injury. **Spinal Cord** 35:266–274, 1997.
514. Maynard FM, Reynolds GG, Fountain S, Wilmot C, Hamilton R: Neurological prognosis after traumatic quadriplegia. Three-year experience of California Regional Spinal Cord Injury Care System. **J Neurosurg** 50(May):611–616, 1979.
515. Mazolewski PMTH: The effectiveness of strapping techniques in spinal immobilization. **Ann Emerg Med** 23(6):1290–1295, 1994.

516. McCabe JB, Nolan DJ: Comparison of the effectiveness of different cervical immobilization collars. **Ann Emerg Med** 15:50–53, 1986.
517. McGuire RA, Harkey HL: Primary treatment of unstable Jefferson's fractures. **J Spinal Disorders** 8:233–236, 1995.
518. McGuire RA Jr: Protection of the unstable spine during transport and early hospitalization. **J Miss State Med Assoc** 32(8):305–308, 1991.
519. McGuire RA, Degnan G, et al: Evaluation of current extrication orthoses in immobilization of the unstable cervical spine. **Spine** 15(10):1064–1067, 1990.
520. McGuire RA, Neville S, et al: Spinal instability and the log-rolling maneuver. **J Trauma-Injury Infection Crit Care** 27(5):525–531, 1987.
521. McHugh TP, Taylor JP: Unnecessary out-of-hospital use of full spinal immobilization (letter). **Acad Emerg Med** 5(3):278–280, 1998.
522. McKinley WO, Jackson AB, Cardenas DD, DeVivo MJ: Long-term medical complications after traumatic spinal cord injury: A regional model systems analysis. **Arch Phys Med Rehabil** 80:1402–1410, 1999.
523. McLaurin RL, Vernal R, Salmon JH: Treatment of fractures of the atlas and axis by wiring without fusion. **J Neurosurg** 36:773–780, 1972.
524. McMichan JC, Michel L, Westbrook PR: Pulmonary dysfunction following traumatic quadriplegia. **JAMA** 243(6):528–531, 1980.
525. McNamara R, Heine E, Esposito B: Cervical spine injury and radiography in alert, high risk patients. **J Emerg Med** 8:177–182, 1990.
526. McSwain N: Spine management skills. In *Pre-Hospital Trauma Life Support* (2nd Edition), Akron, OH: Educational Direction, Inc., 225–256, 1990.
527. McSwain N: Proper c-spine immobilization. **Emerg Med** 27:120–121, 1995.
528. Meldon SW, Brant TA, et al: Out-of-hospital cervical spine clearance: Agreement between EMTs and Emergency Physicians. **J Trauma-Injury Infection Crit Care** 45(6):1058–1061, 1998.
529. Menezes AH, Ryken TC: Craniovertebral abnormalities in Down's Syndrome. **Pediatric Neurosurg** 18:24–33, 1992.
530. Menticoglou SM, Perlman M, Manning FA: High cervical spinal cord injury in neonates delivered with forceps: A report of 15 cases. **Obstet Gynecol** 86:589–594, 1995.
531. Merianos P, Tsekouras G, Koskinas A: An unusual fractures of the atlas. **Injury** 22:489–490, 1991.
532. Merli G, Crabbe S, Doyle L, Ditunno J, Herbison G: Mechanical plus pharmacological prophylaxis for deep vein thrombosis in acute spinal cord injury. **Paraplegia** 30:558–562, 1992.
533. Merli G, Herbison G, Ditunno J, et al: Deep vein thrombosis: Prophylaxis in acute spinal cord injured patients. **Arch Phys Med Rehabil** 69:661–665, 1988.
534. Merriam WF, Taylor TKF, Ruff SJ, McPhail MJ: A reappraisal of acute traumatic central cord syndrome. **J Bone Joint Surg Br** 65B:708–713, 1986.
535. Mestdagh H, Letendart J, Sensey JJ, et al: (Treatment of fractures of the posterior axial arch. Results of 41 cases). **Rev Chir Orthop Reparatrice Appar Mot** 70:21–28, 1984.
536. Mirvis S, Diaconis J, Chirico P, Reiner B, Joslyn J, Militello P: Protocol driven radiologic evaluation of suspected cervical spine injury: Efficacy study. **Radiology** 170:831–834, 1989.
537. Mirvis SE, Geisler FH, Jelinek JJ, Joslyn J, et al: Acute cervical spine trauma: Evaluation with 1.5-T MR imaging. **Radiology** 166:807–816, 1988.
538. Mirvis S, Young J, Lim AC, et al: Hangman's fracture: Radiologic assessment in 27 cases. **Radiology** 163:713–717, 1987.

539. Mody BS, Morris EW: Fracture of the occipital condyle: Case report and review of the world literature. **Injury** 23:350–352, 1992.
540. Mollan RA, Watt PC: Hangman's fracture. **Injury** 14:265–267, 1982.
541. Montane I, Eismont F, Green BA: Traumatic occipitoatlantal dislocation. **Spine** 16:112–116, 1991.
542. Montesano PX, Anderson PA, Schlehr F, et al: Odontoid fractures treated by anterior odontoid screw fixation. **Spine** 16(S): 33–S 37, 1991.
543. Morandi X, Hanna A, Hamlat A, et al: Anterior screw fixation of odontoid fractures. **Surg Neurol** 51:236–240, 1999.
544. Morgan MK, Onofrio BM, Bender CE: Familial os odontoideum. Case report. **Neurosurgery** 70:636–639, 1989.
545. Moylan JA: Trauma Injuries. Triage and stabilization for safe transfer. **Postgrad Med** 78(5):166–177, 1985.
546. Mubarak SJ, Camp JF, Vuletich W, Wenger DR, Garfin SR: Halo application in the infant. **J Pediatr Orthop** 9:612–614, 1989.
547. Muhr MD, Seabrook DL, et al: Paramedic use of a spinal injury clearance algorithm reduces spinal immobilization in the out-of-hospital setting. **Pre-Hospital Emergency Care** 3(1):1–6, 1999.
548. Muller EJ, Wick M, Russe O, et al: Management of odontoid fractures in the elderly. **Eur Spine J** 8:360–365, 1999.
549. Muller EJ, Wick M, Muhr G: Traumatic spondylolisthesis of the axis: Treatment rationale based on the stability of the different fracture types. **Eur Spine J** 9:123–128, 2000.
550. Myllynen P, Kammonen M, Rokkanen P, Bostman O, Lalla M, Laasonen E: Deep venous thrombosis and pulmonary embolism in patients with acute spinal cord injury: A comparison with non-paralyzed patients immobilized due to spinal fractures. **J Trauma-Injury Infection Crit Care** 25:541–543, 1985.
551. Naso F: Pulmonary embolism in acute spinal cord injury. **Arch Phys Med Rehabil** 55:275–278, 1974.
552. Naso WB, Cure J, Cuddy BG: Retropharyngeal pseudomeningocele after atlanto-occipital dislocation: Report of two cases. **Neurosurgery** 40:1288–1291, 1997.
553. Nazarian SM, Louis RP: Posterior internal fixation with screw plates in traumatic lesions of the cervical spine. **Spine** 16:S 64–S 71, 1991.
554. Neifeld G, Keene J, Hevesy G, Leikin J, Proust A, Thisted R: Cervical injury in head trauma. **J Emerg Med** 6:203–207, 1988.
555. Nesathurai S: Steroids and spinal cord injury: Revisiting the NASCIS 2 and NASCIS 3 trials. **J Trauma** 45(6):1088–1093, 1998.
556. Neville S, Watts C: Management of the unstable cervical spine in transport: A reevaluation. **Aeromed J** 32:1987.
557. Newey ML, Sen PK, Fraser RD: The long-term outcome after central cord syndrome. **J Bone Joint Surg Br** 82B:851–855, 2000.
558. Nischal K, Chumas P, Sparrow O: Prolonged survival after atlanto-occipital dislocation: Two case reports and review. **Br J Neurosurg** 7:677–682, 1993.
559. Noble ER, Smoker WRK: The forgotten condyle: The appearance, morphology, and classification of occipital condyle fractures. **Am J Neuroradiol** 17:507–513, 1996.
560. Nunez D, Quencer R: The role of helical CT in the assessment of cervical spine injuries. **Am J Radiology** 171:951–957, 1998.
561. Nypaver M, Treloar D: Neutral cervical spine positioning in children. **Ann Emerg Med** 23(2):208–211, 1994.
562. Oda T, Panjabi MM, Crisco JJD, et al: Experimental study of atlas injuries. II. Relevance to clinical diagnosis and treatment. **Spine** 16 S:S 466–S 473, 1991.

563. Oda T, Panjabi MM, Crisco JJD: Multidirectional instabilities of experimental burst fractures of the atlas. **Spine** 17:1285–1290, 1992.
564. Odent T, Langlais J, Glorion C, Kassis B, Bataille J, Pouliquen JC: Fractures of the odontoid process: A report of 15 cases in children younger than 6 years. **J Pediatr Orthop** 19:51–54, 1999.
565. Olerud C: Compression of the cervical spinal cord after reduction of fracture dislocations. Report of 2 cases. **Acta Orthop Scand** 62:1991.
566. Olson CM, Jastremski MS, et al: Stabilization of patients prior to interhospital transfer. **Am J Emerg Med** 5(1):33–39, 1987.
567. Olsson R, Kunz R: Fracture of the occipital condyle as an incidental finding during CT—Evaluation of a maxillary fracture. **Acta Radiologica** 35(1):90–91, 1994.
568. Orbay T, Aykol S, Seckin Z, Ergun R: Late hypoglossal nerve palsy following fracture of the occipital condyle. **Surg Neurol** 31:402–404, 1989.
569. Ordonez BJ, Benzel EC, Naderi S, Weller SJ: Cervical facet dislocation: Techniques for ventral reduction and stabilization. **J Neurosurg** 92(Spine 1):18–23, 2000.
570. Orledge JD, Pepe PE: Out-of-hospital spinal immobilization: Is it really necessary? **Acad Emerg Med** 5(3):203–204, 1998.
571. Osenbach RK, Menezes AH: Spinal cord injury without radiographic abnormality in children. **Pediatr Neurosci** 15:168–175, 1989.
572. Osenbach RK, Menezes AH: Pediatric spinal cord and vertebral column injury. **Neurosurgery** 30:385–390, 1992.
573. Osterholm JL: The pathophysiological response to spinal cord injury: The current status of related research. **J Neurosurg** 40:5–33, 1974.
574. Osti O, Fraser R, Griffiths E: Reduction and stabilisation of cervical dislocations. **J Bone Joint Surg Br** 71-B:275–282, 1989.
575. Ota T, Akaboshi K, Nagata M, Sonoda S, Domen K, Seki M, Chino N: Functional assessment of patients with spinal cord injury: Measured by the motor score and the Functional Independence Measure. **Spinal Cord** 34:531–535, 1996.
576. Paeslack V, Frankel H, Michaelis L: Closed injuries of the cervical spine and spinal cord: Results of conservative treatment of flexion fractures and flexion fracture dislocation of the cervical spine with tetraplegia. **Proc Vet Admin Spinal Cord Injury Conf** 19:39–42, 1973.
577. Page CP, Story JL, Wissinger JP, Branch CL: Traumatic atlanto-occipital dislocation. Case report. **J Neurosurg** 39:394–397, 1973.
578. Paley MD, Wood GA: Traumatic bilateral hyperglossal nerve palsy. **Br J Oral Maxillofacial Surg** 33:239–241, 1995.
579. Palmer MT, Turney SZ: Tracheal rupture and atlanto-occipital dislocation: Case report. **J Trauma-Injury Infection Crit Care** 37:314–317, 1994.
580. Pang D, Hanley EN: Special problems of spinal stabilization in children. In Cooper PR (ed): *Management of Posttraumatic Spinal Instability*. Park Ridge, IL: AANS, 1990, pp 181–206.
581. Pang D, Pollack IF: Spinal cord injury without radiographic abnormality in children—The SCIWORA syndrome. **J Trauma** 29:654–664, 1989.
582. Pang D, Wilberger J: Traumatic atlanto-occipital dislocation with survival: Case report and review. **Neurosurgery** 7:503–508, 1980.
583. Pang D, Wilberger J: Spinal cord injury without radiographic abnormalities in children. **J Neurosurg** 57:114–129, 1982.
584. Panjabi MM, Oda T, Crisco JJD, et al: Experimental study of atlas injuries. I. Biomechanical analysis of their mechanisms and fracture patterns. **Spine** 16 S:S 460–S 465, 1991.

585. Papadopoulos S, Dickman C, Sonntag VKH, Rekate HL, Spetzler RF: Traumatic atlanto-occipital dislocation with survival. **Neurosurgery** 28:574–579, 1991.
586. Paramore CG, Dickman C, Sonntag VKH: The anatomical suitability of the C1-2 complex for transarticular screw fixation. **J Neurosurg** 85:221–224, 1996.
587. Pasciak M, Doniec J: Results of conservative treatment of unilateral cervical spine dislocations. **Arch Orthop Trauma Surg** 112:226–227, 1993.
588. Pasquale M, Fabian T, ATEAH Committee: The East Ad Hoc Committee on Practice Management Guidelines for Trauma from the Eastern Association for the Surgery of Trauma. **J Trauma** 44:945–946, 1998.
589. Patton J, Kralovich K, Cuschieri J, Gasparri M: Clearing the cervical spine in victims of blunt assault to the head and neck: What is necessary? **Am Surg** 66:326–330, 2000.
590. Pedersen AK, Kostuik JP: Complete fracture-dislocation of the atlantoaxial complex: Case report and recommendations for a new classification of dens fractures. **J Spinal Disord** 7:350–355, 1994.
591. Peiffer SC, Blust P, Leyson JFJ: Nutritional assessment of the spinal cord injured patient. **J Am Diet Assoc** 78:501–505, 1981.
592. Pennecot GF, Leonard P, Peyrot des Gachons S, Hardy JR, Pouliquen JC: Traumatic ligamentous instability of the cervical spine in children. **J Ped Orthop** 4:339–345, 1984.
593. Pepin JW, Hawkins RJ: Traumatic spondylolisthesis of the axis: Hangman's fracture. **Clin Orthop** 133–138, 1981.
594. Pepin JW, Bourne RB, Hawkins RJ: Odontoid fractures, with special reference to the elderly patient. **Clin Orthop** 178–183, 1985.
595. Perkash A, Prakash V, Perkash I: Experience with the management of thromboembolism in patients with spinal cord injury: Part I. Incidence, diagnosis, and role of some risk factors. **Paraplegia** 16:322–331, 1978.
596. Perry SD, McLellan B, et al: The efficacy of head immobilization techniques during simluated vehicle motion. **Spine** 24(17):1839–1844, 1999.
597. Phillips WA, Hensinger RN: The management of rotatory atlanto-axial subluxation in children. **J Bone Joint Surg Am** 71A:664–668, 1989.
598. Piepmeier JM, Lehmann K.B., Lane JG: Cardiovascular instability following acute cervical spinal cord trauma. **Central Nervous System Trauma** 2(3):153–160, 1985.
599. Pitzen T, Caspar W, Steudel WI, et al: [Dens fracture in elderly patients and surgical management]. **Aktuelle Traumatol** 24:56–59, 1994.
600. Plaiser B, Gabram S, Schwartz R, Jacobs L: Prospective evaluation of craniofacial pressure in four different cervical orthoses. **J Trauma-Injury Infection Crit Care** 37:714–720, 1994.
601. Podolsky S, Baraff LJ, et al: Efficacy of cervical spine immobilization methods. **J Trauma-Injury Infection Crit Care** 23(6):461–465, 1983.
602. Podolsky S, Hoffman JR, et al: Neurologic complications following immobilization of cervical spine fracture in a patient with ankylosing spondylitis. **Ann Emerg Med** 12(9):578–580, 1983.
603. Pointillart V, Petitjean ME, Wiart L, Vital JM, et al: Pharmacological therapy of spinal cord injury during the acute phase. **Spinal Cord** 38:71–76, 2000.
604. Polin RS, Szabo T, Bogaev CA, et al: Nonoperative management of Types II and III odontoid fractures: The Philadelphia collar versus the halo vest. **Neurosurgery** 38:450–457, 1996.
605. Pollack IF, Pang D, Sclabassi R: Recurrent spinal cord injury without radiographic abnormalities in children. **J Neurosurg** 69:177–182, 1988.

606. Powell M, Kirschblum S, O'Connor K: Duplex ultrasound screening for deep vein thrombosis in spinal cord injured patients at rehabilitation admission. **Arch Phys Med Rehabil** 80:1044–1046, 1999.
607. Powers B, Miller MD, Kramer RS, Martinez S, Gehweiler JA: Traumatic anterior atlanto-occipital dislocation. **Neurosurgery** 4:12–17, 1979.
608. Poynton AR, O'Farrell DA, Shannon F, Murray P, et al: An evaluation of the factors affecting neurological recovery following spinal cord injury. **Injury** 28(8): 545–548, 1997.
609. Prabhu V, Kizer J, Pail A, Hellbusch L, Taylon C, Leibrock L: Vertebrobasilar thrombosis associated with nonpenetrating cervical spine trauma. **J Trauma** 40:130–137, 1996.
610. Prasad VS, Schwartz A, et al: Characteristics of injuries to the cervical spine and spinal cord in polytrauma patient population: Experience from a regional trauma unit. **Spinal Cord** 37(8):560–568, 1999.
611. Priebe MM, Waring WP: The interobserver reliability of the revised American Spinal Injury Association standards for neurological classification of spinal injury patients. **Am J Phys Med Rehabil** 70(5):268–270, 1991.
612. Przybylski GJ, Clyde BL, Fitz CR: Craniocervical subarachnoid hemorrhage associated with atlanto-occipital dislocation. **Spine** 21:1761–1768, 1996.
613. Putnam WE, Stratton FT, Rohr RJ, Stitzell W, Roat G: Traumatic atlanto-occipital dislocations: Value of the Power's ratio in diagnosis. **J Am Osteopath Assoc** 86:798–804, 1986.
614. Quencer RM, Bunge RP, Egnor M, Green BA, et al: Acute traumatic central cord syndrome: MRI-pathological correlations. **Neuroradiology** 34:85–94, 1992.
615. Quirke TE, Ritota PC, Swan KG: Inferior vena caval filter use in US trauma centers: A practitioner survey. **J Trauma-Injury Infection Crit Care** 43:333–337, 1997.
616. Raila FA, Aitken AT, Vivkers GN: Computed tomography and three-dimensional reconstruction in the evaluation of occipital condyle fracture. **Skeletal Radiol** 22:269–271, 1993.
617. Ralston ME, Chung K, Barnes PD, Emans JB, Schutzman SA: Role of flexion-extension radiographs in blunt pediatric cervical spine injury. **Academic Emerg Med** 8:237–245, 2001.
618. Ramon S, Dominguez R, Ramierez A, Paraira M, Olona M, Castello T, Garcia-Fernandez L: Clinical and magnetic resonance imaging correlation in acute spinal cord injury. **Spinal Cord** 35:664–673, 1997.
619. Ramsay AH, Waxman BP, O'Brien JF: A case of traumatic atlanto-occipital dislocation with survival. **Injury** 17(6):412–413, 1986.
620. Raphael J, Chotai R: Effects of the cervical collar on cerebrospinal fluid pressure. **Anaesthesia** 49:437–439, 1994.
621. Rapp RP, Young B, Twymann D, et al: The favorable effect of early parenteral feeding on survival in head injured patients. **J Neurosurg** 58:906–912, 1983.
622. Rathbone D, Johnson G, Letts M: Spinal cord concussion in pediatric athletes. **J Ped Ortho** 12:616–620, 1992.
623. Reid D, Henderson R, Saboe L, Miller J: Etiology and clinical course of missed spine fractures. **J Trauma** 27:980–986, 1987.
624. Reines HD, Harris RC: Pulmonary complications of acute spinal cord injuries. **Neurosurgery** 21(2):193–196, 1987.
625. Reinges MHT, Mayfrank L, Rohde V, Spetzger U, Gilsbach JM: Surgically treated traumatic synchondrotic disruption of the odontoid process in a 15-month-old girl. **Childs Nervous System** 14(1–2):85–87, 1998.

626. Riley KO, May AK, Hadley MN: Neurological injury and nutritional support. In Batjer HH, Loftus CL (eds): *Textbook of Neurological Surgery.* Philadelphia: Lippincott Williams & Wilkins, 2001.
627. Rimel RW, Jane JA, et al: An educational training program for the care at the site of injury of trauma to the central nervous system. **Resuscitation** 9:23–28, 1981.
628. Ripa DR, Kowall MG, Meyer PR, Rusin JJ: Series of ninety-two traumatic cervical spine injuries stabilized with anterior ASIF plate fusion technique. **Spine** 16:S 46–S 55, 1991.
629. Rizzolo S, Vaccaro A, Cotler J: Intervertebral disc injury complicating cervical spine trauma. **Spine** 16(6 Suppl):S187–189, 1991.
630. Roberge R, Wears R, Kelly M, Evans T, Kenny M, Daffner R, Kremen R, Murray K, Cottington E: Selective application of cervical spine radiography in alert victims of blunt trauma: A prospective study. **J Trauma** 28:784–788, 1988.
631. Robertson P, Ryan M: Neurological deterioration after reduction of cervical subluxation. **J Bone Joint Surg Br** 74-B:224–227, 1992.
632. Rockswold GL, Seljeskog EL: Traumatic atlantocranial dislocation with survival. **Minnesota Med** 62:151–152, 1979.
633. Rockswold G, Bergman TA, Ford SE: Halo immobilization and surgical fusion: Relative indications and effectiveness in the treatment of 140 cervical spine injuries. **J Trauma** 30:893–898, 1990.
634. Rodgers JA, Rodgers WB: Marginal mandibular nerve palsy due to compression by a cervical hard collar. **J Orthopaedic Trauma** 9(2):177–179, 1995.
635. Rodriguez DJ, Benzel EC: Nutritional support. In Benzel EC (ed): *Spine Surgery: Techniques, Complication Avoidance, and Management.* New York: Churchill Livingstone, 1999, pp 1321–1331.
636. Rodriguez DJ, Benzel EC, Clevenger FW: The metabolic response to spinal cord injury. **Spinal Cord** 35:599–604, 1997.
637. Roozmon P, Gracovetsky SA, et al: Examining motion in the cervical spine. I: Imaging systems and measurement techniques. **J Biomed Eng** 15:5–12, 1993.
638. Rorabeck CH, Rock MG, Hawkins RJ, Bourne RB: Unilateral facet dislocation of the cervical spine. An analysis of the results of treatment in 26 patients. **Spine** 12:23–27, 1987.
639. Rose L: Thoracolumbar spinal instability during variations of the log-roll maneuver (comment). **Pre-Hospital Disaster Med** 7:138–1992.
640. Rosen PB: Comparison of two new immobilization collars. **Ann Emerg Med** 21(10):1189–1195, 1992.
641. Rosenfeld J, Vaccaro A, Albert T, Klein G, Cotler J: The benefits of early decompression in cervical spinal cord injury. **Am J Orthopedics** 27:23–28, 1998.
642. Rosner MJ: National acute spinal cord injury study of methylprednisolone or naloxone (Correspondence). **Neurosurgery** 28(4):628–1991.
643. Rosner MJ: Methylprednisolone for spinal cord injury. **J Neurosurg** 77:324–325, 1992.
644. Rosner MJ: Treatment of spinal cord injury. **J Neurosurg** 80:954–1994.
645. Ross S, O'Malley K, DeLong W, Born C, Schwab C: Clinical predictors of unstable cervical spine injury in multiply injured patients. **Injury** 23:317–319, 1992.
646. Rossitch E, Oakes WJ: Perinatal spinal cord injury. **Pediatric Neurosurg** 18:149–152, 1992.
647. Roth EJ, Lawler MH, Yarkony GM: Traumatic central cord syndrome: Clinical features and functional outcomes. **Arch Phys Med Rehabil** 71:18–23, 1990.
648. Roth B, Martin R, Foley PBP, Kennedy P: Roentgenographic evaluation of the cervical spine. **Arch Surg** 129:643–645, 1994.

649. Roussi J, Bentolila S, Boudaoud L, et al: Contribution of D-Dimer determination in the exclusion of deep venous thrombosis in spinal cord injury patients. **Spinal Cord** 37:548–552, 1999.
650. Roy-Camille R, Benazet JP, Saillant G, Henry P, Mamoudy P, Leonard PH: Luxation traumatique occipito-atloidienne. Interet de nouveaux signes radiologiques (A propro de deux cas). **Revue de Chirurgie Orthopedique** 72:303–309, 1986.
651. Roy-Camille R, Saillant G, Laville C, Benazet JP: Treatment of lower cervical spinal injuries—C3 to C7. **Spine** 17:S 442–S 446, 1992.
652. Ruge JR, Sinson GP, McLone DG, Cerullo LJ: Pediatric spinal injury: The very young. **J Neurosurg** 68:25–30, 1988.
653. Rutledge G, Sumchai A, et al: A safe method for transportation of patients with cervical spine injuries. **Aeromed J** 33:1987.
654. Ryan MD, Henderson JJ: The epidemiology of fractures and fracture-dislocations of the cervical spine. **Injury** 23:38–40, 1992.
655. Ryan MD, Taylor TK: Odontoid Fractures. A rational approach to treatment. **J Bone Joint Surg Br** 64:416–421, 1982.
656. Ryan M, Taylor T: Odontoid fractures in the elderly. **J Spinal Disorders** 6:397–401, 1993.
657. Sabiston C, Wing P, Schweigel J, Peteghem P, Yu W: Closed reduction of dislocations of the lower cervical spine. **J Trauma** 28:832–835, 1988.
658. Salmon JH: Fractures of the second vertebra: Internal fixation by interlaminar wiring. **Neurosurgery** 1:125–127, 1977.
659. San Mateo County C. EMS System Policy Memorandum #F–3A. 1991.
660. Sandler AN, Tator CH: Effect of acute spinal cord compression injury on regional spinal cord blood flow in primates. **J Neurosurg** 45:660–676, 1976.
661. Sandler AN, Tator CH: Review of the effect of spinal cord trauma on the vessels and blood flow in the spinal cord. **J Neurosurg** 45:638–646, 1976.
662. Savini R, Parisini P, Cervellati S: The surgical treatment of late instability of flexion-rotation injuries in the lower cervical spine. **Spine** 12:178–182, 1987.
663. Savolaine ER, Ebraheim NA, Jackson WT, Rusin JJ. Case report. Three-dimensional computed tomography in the evaluation of occipital condyle fracture. **J Orthop Trauma**, 3:71–75, 1989.
664. Scarrow A, Levy E, Resnick D, Adelosn P, Sclabassi R: Cervical spine evaluation in obtunded or comatose pediatric trauma patients: A pilot study. **Pediatric Neurosurg** 30:169–175, 1999.
665. Schaefer DM, Flanders A, Northrup BE, Doan HT, Osterholm JL: Magnetic resonance imaging of acute cervical spine trauma. **Spine** 14(10):1090–1095, 1989.
666. Schellinger PD, Schwab S, Krieger D, Fiebach JB, Steiner T, Hund EF, Hacke W, Meinck HM: Masking of vertebral artery dissection by severe trauma to the cervical spine. **Spine** 26:314–319, 2001.
667. Schleehauf K, Ross SE, Civil ID, Schwab CW: Computed tomography in the initial evaluation of the cervical spine. **Ann Emerg Med** 18:815–817, 1989.
668. Schlicke LH, Callahan RA: A rational approach to burst fractures of the atlas. **Clin Orthop** 18–21, 1981.
669. Schneider RC: A syndrome in acute cervical spine injuries for which early operation is indicated. **J Neurosurg** 8:360–367, 1951.
670. Schneider R: "Hangman's fracture" of the cervical spine. **J Neurosurg** 22:141–154, 1965.
671. Schneider RC, Cherry G, Pantek H: The syndrome of acute central cervical spinal cord injury. **J Neurosurg** 546–577, 1954.
672. Schneider RC, Crosby EC, Russo RH, Gosch HK: Traumatic spinal cord syndromes and their management. **Clin Neurosurg** 20:424–492, 1973.

673. Schneider RC, Thompson JC, Bebin J: The syndrome of acute central cervical spinal cord injury. J **Neurol Neurosurg Psychiat** 21:216–227, 1958.
674. Schonhofer PS: GM-1 Ganglioside for spinal cord injury (Letter). **N Engl J Med** 326(7):493–1992.
675. Schriger DL: Immobilizing the cervical spine in trauma; Should we seek an optimal position or an adequate one? (editorial comment). **Ann Emerg Med** 28(3):351–353, 1996.
676. Schriger DL, Larmon B, et al: Spinal immobilization on a flat backboard: Does it result in neutral position of the cervical spine? **Ann Emerg Med** 20(8):878–881, 1991.
677. Schwarz N: The fate of missed atlanto-axial rotatory subluxation in children. **Arch Ortho Trauma Surg** 117:288–289, 1998.
678. Schwarz N, Buchinger W, Gaudernak T, Russe F, Zechner W: Injuries to the cervical spine causing vertebral artery trauma: Case reports. **J Trauma** 31:127–133, 1991.
679. Schwarz N, Genelin F, Schwarz AF: Post-traumatic cervical kyphosis in children cannot be prevented by non-operative methods. **Injury** 25:173–175, 1994.
680. Sears W, Fazl M: Prediction of stability of cervical spine fracture managed in the halo vest and indications for surgical intervention. **J Neurosurg** 72:426–432, 1990.
681. Sedlock DA, Laventure SJ: Body composition and resting energy expenditure in long term spinal cord injury. **Paraplegia** 28:448–454, 1990.
682. Sees D, Cruz LR, Flaherty S, Coceri D: The use of bedside fluoroscopy to evaluate the cervical spine of obtunded patients. **J Trauma** 45:768–771, 1998.
683. Segal LS, Grimm JO, Stauffer ES: Non-union of fractures of the atlas. **J Bone Joint Surg Am** 69:1423–1434, 1987.
684. Seljeskog EL, Chou SN: Spectrum of the hangman's fracture. **J Neurosurg** 45:3–8, 1976.
685. Seljeskog EL: Non-operative management of acute upper cervical injuries. **Acta Neurochir** 41:87–100, 1978.
686. Senter HJ, Venes JL: Loss of autoregulation and post-traumatic ischemia following experimental spinal cord trauma. **J Neurosurg** 50:198–206, 1979.
687. Seybold EA, Bayley JC: Functional outcome of surgically and conservatively managed dens fractures. **Spine** 23:1837–1846, 1998.
688. Shacked I, Ram Z, Hadani M: The anterior cervical approach for traumatic injuries to the cervical spine in children. **Clin Orthop Rel Res** 292:144–150, 1993.
689. Shafermeyer RW, Ribbeck BM, Gaskins J, Thomason S, Harlan M, Attkisson A: Respiratory effects of spinal immobilization in children. **Ann Emerg Med** 20:1017–1019, 1991.
690. Shaffer M, Doris P: Limitation of the cross table lateral view in detecting cervical spine injuries: A prospective analysis. **Ann Emerg Med** 10:508–513, 1981.
691. Shah S, Vanclay F, Cooper B: Improving the sensitivity of the Barthel Index for stroke rehabilitation. **J Clin Epidemiol** 42(8):703–709, 1989.
692. Shapiro S: Methylprednisolone for spinal cord injury. **J Neurosurg** 77:324–1992.
693. Shapiro S: Management of unilateral locked facet of the cervical spine. **Neurosurgery** 33:832–837, 1993.
694. Shapiro S, Snyder W, Kaufman K, Abel T: Outcome of 51 cases of unilateral locked cervical facets: Interspinous braided cable for lateral mass plate fusion compared with interspinous wire and facet wiring with iliac crest. **J Neurosurg** 91(Spine 1):19–24, 1999.
695. Sharma BS, Mahajan S, Khosla VK: Collet-Sicard syndrome after closed head injury. **Clin Neurol Neurosurg** 96:197–198, 1994.

492   CLINICAL NEUROSURGERY

696. Shaw M, Burnett H, Wilson A, Chan O: Pseudosubluxation of C2 on C3 in poly-traumatized children: Prevalence and significance. **Clin Radiol** 54:377–380, 1999.
697. Sherk HH, Nicholson JT: Fractures of the atlas. **J Bone Joint Surg Am** 52:1017–1024, 1970.
698. Sherk HH, Nicholson JT, Chung SMK: Fractures of the odontoid process in young children. **J Bone Joint Surg Am** 60:921–924, 1978.
699. Shirasaki N, Okada K, Oka S, Hosono N, Yonenobu K, Ono K: Os odontoideum with posterior atlantoaxial instability. **Spine** 16:706–715, 1991.
700. Short DJ: Use of steroids for acute spinal cord injury must be reassessed. **Br Med J** 321:1224–2000.
701. Short DJ, El Masry WS, Jones PW: High dose methylprednisolone in the management of acute spinal cord injury—a systematic review from a clinical perspective. **Spinal Cord** 38:273–286, 2000.
702. Shoung H, Lee L: Anterior metal plate fixation in the treatment of unstable lower cervical spine injuries. **Acta Neurochir** 98:55–59, 1989.
703. Shrosbee R: Neurological sequelae of reduction of fracture dislocations of the cervical spine. **Paraplegia** 17:212–221, 1979.
704. Shrosbree RD: Acute central cervical spinal cord syndrome—Aetiology, age incidence, and relationship to orthopaedic injury. **Paraplegia** 14:251–258, 1977.
705. Sim E, Schwarz N, Biowski-Fasching I, Biowski P: Color-coded duplex sonography of vertebral arteries. **Acta Orthop Scand** 64:133–137, 1993.
706. Sim E, Vaccaro A, Berzlanovich A, Pienar S: The effects of staged static cervical flexion-distraction deformities on the patency of the vertebral arterial vasculature. **Spine** 25:2180–2186, 2000.
707. Smith M, Bourn S, et al: Ties that bind: Immobilizing the injured spine. **J Emerg Med Services** 14:28–35, 1989.
708. Smith MD, Phillips WA, Hensinger RN: Fusion of the upper cervical spine in children and adolescents. **Spine** 16:695–701, 1991.
709. Song WS, Chiang YH, Chen CY, Lin SZ, Liu MY: A simple method for diagnosing traumatic occlusion of the vertebral artery at the craniovertebral junction. **Spine** 19:837–839, 1994.
710. Sonntag VKH: Management of bilateral locked facets of the cervical spine. **Neurosurgery** 8:150–152, 1981.
711. Spence KF, Jr., Decker S, Sell KW: Bursting atlantal fracture associated with rupture of the transverse ligament. **J Bone Joint Surg Am** 52:543–549, 1970.
712. Spencer JA, Yeakley JW, Kaufman HH: Fracture of the occipital condyle. **Neurosurgery** 15:101–103, 1984.
713. Spierings EL, Braakman R. The management of os odontoideum. Analysis of 37 cases. **J Bone Joint Surg Br** 64-B:422–428, 1982.
714. Sponseller PD, Cass JR: Atlanto-occipital fusion for dislocation in children with neurological preservation. A case report. **Spine** 22:344–347, 1997.
715. Starr JK, Eismont FJ: Atypical hangman's fractures. **Spine** 18:1954–1957, 1993.
716. Starr A, Jones A, Cotler J, Balderston R, Sinha R: Immediate closed reduction of cervical spine dislocations using traction. **Spine** 15:1068–1072, 1990.
717. Stauffer ES, Kelly EG: Fracture-dislocation of the cervical spine. Instability and recurrent deformity following treatment by anterior interbody fusion. **J Bone Joint Surg Am** 59A:45–48, 1977.
718. Stauffer ES: Orthotics for spinal cord injuries. **Clin Orthopaedics Related Res** 102:92–99, 1974.
719. Stevens JM, Chong WK, Barber C, Kendall BE, Crockard HA: A new appraisal of

abnormalities of the odontoid process associated with atlantoaxial subluxation and neurological disability. **Brain** 117:133–148, 1994.

720. Stineman MG, Marino RJ, Deutsch A, Granger CV, Maislin G: A functional strategy for classifying patients after traumatic spinal cord injury. **Spinal Cord** 37:717–725, 1999.

721. Stover S, Fine PR. Spinal cord injury. In *The Facts and Figures*. Birmingham, AL: The University of Alabama at Birmingham, 1986, p 45.

722. Stroobants J, Fidlers L, Storms JL, Klaes R, Dua G, Van Hoye M: High cervical pain and impairment of skull mobility as the only symptom of an occipital condyle fracture. **J Neurosurg** 81:137–138, 1994.

723. Strrobants J, Seynaeve P, Fidlers L, Klaes R, Brabants K, Van Hoye M: Occipital condyle fracture must be considered in the pediatric population: Case report. **J Trauma** 36:440–441, 1994.

724. Subach BR, McLaughlin MR, Albright AL, Pollack IF: Current management of pediatric atlanto-axial rotatory subluxation. **Spine** 23:2174–2179, 1998.

725. Subach BR, Morone MA, Haid RW, et al: Management of acute odontoid fractures with single-screw anterior fixation. **Neurosurgery** 45:812–820, 1999.

726. Suechting RL, French LA: Posterior inferior cerebellar artery syndrome following a fracture of the cervical vertebra. **J Neurosurg** 12:187–189, 1955.

727. Sun PP, Poffenbarger GJ, Durham S, Zimmerman RA: Spectrum of occipitoatlantoaxial injury in young children. **J Neurosurg** 93(Spine 1):28–39, 2000.

728. Suter R, Tighe T, et al: Thoracolumbar spinal instability during variations of the log-roll maneuver. **Pre-Hospital Disaster Medicine** 7:133–138, 1992.

729. Swain A, Dove J, et al: ABCs of major trauma. Trauma of the spine and spinal cord—I. **Br Med J** 301(6742):34–38, 1990.

730. Sweeney J, Rosemurgy A, Gill S, Albrink M: Is the cervical spine clear? Undetected cervical fractures diagnosed only at autopsy. **Ann Emerg Med** 21:1288–1290, 1992.

731. Swischuk LE, John SD, Hendrick EP: Is the open-mouth odontoid view necessary in children under 5 years? **Pediatr Radiol** 30:186–189, 2000.

732. Taggard DA, Menezes AH, Ryken TC: Treatment of Down syndrome-associated craniovertebral abnormalities. **J Neurosurg** 93:205–213, 2000.

733. Tan ES, Balachandran N: Hangman's fracture in Singapore (1975–1988). **Paraplegia** 30:160–164, 1992.

734. Tan E, Schwetizer M, Vaccaro A, Spettell C: Is computed tomography of nonvisualized C7-T1 cost effective? **J Spinal Disorders** 12:472–476, 1999.

735. Tator CH, Fehlings M: Review of the secondary injury theory of acute spinal cord trauma with emphasis on vascular mechanisms. **J Neurosurg** 75:15–26, 1991.

736. Tator CH: Vascular effects and blood flow in acute spinal cord injuries. **J Neurosurg Sci** 28(3–4):115–119, 1984.

737. Tator CH: Hemodynamic issues and vascular factors in acute experimental spinal cord injury. **J Neurotrauma** 9(2):139–141, 1992.

738. Tator CH: Ischemia as a secondary neural injury. In Salzman SK, Faden AL (eds): *Neurobiology of Central Nervous System Trauma*. New York: Oxford University Press, 1994, 209–215.

739. Tator CH: Experimental and clinical studies of the pathophysiology and management of acute spinal cord injury. **J Spinal Cord Med** 19(4):206–214, 1996.

740. Tator CH: Biology of neurological recovery and functional restoration after spinal cord injury. **Neurosurgery** 42:696–708, 1998.

741. Tator CH, Duncan EG, Edmonds VE, Andrews DF: Comparison of surgical and medical management in 208 patients with acute spinal cord injury. **Can J Neurol Sci** 14:60–69, 1987.

742. Tator CH, Duncan EG, Edmonds VE, Lapczak LI, Andrews DF: Changes in epidemiology of acute spinal cord injury from 1947 to 1981. **Surgical Neurology** 40:207–215, 1993.

743. Tator CH, Rowed DW, Schwartz MI: Sunnybrook Cord Injury Scales for assessing neurological injury and neurologic recovery. In Tator CH (ed): *Early Management of Acute Spinal Cord Injury.* New York: Raven Press, 1982, pp 17–24.

744. Tator CH, Rowed DW, et al: Management of acute spinal cord injuries. **Can J Surg** 27(3):289–294, 1984.

745. Tehranzadeh J, Bonk R, Ansari A, Mesgarzadeh M: Efficacy of limited CT for nonvisualized lower cervical spine in patients with blunt trauma. **Skeletal Radiology** 23:349–352, 1994.

746. Thibodeaux LC, Hearn AT, Peschiera JL, Deshmukh RM, Kerlakian GM, Welling RE, Nyswonger GD: Extracranial vertebral artery dissection after trauma: A five-year review. **Br J Surg** 84:94–1997.

747. Todd JW, Frisbie JH, Rossier AB, et al: Deep venous thrombosis in acute spinal cord injury: A comparison of 1251 fibrinogen leg scanning, impedance plethysmography and venography. **Paraplegia** 14:50–57, 1976.

748. Toh E, Arima T, Mochida J, Omata M, Matsui S: Functional evaluation using motor scores after cervical spinal cord injuries. **Spinal Cord** 36:491–496, 1998.

749. Tola JC, Holtzman R, Lottenberg L: Bedside placement of inferior vena cava filters in the intensive care unit. **Am Surg** 65:833–837, 1999.

750. Torreman M: Long-term prognosis of the hangman's fracture. **Ned Tijdschr Geneeskd** 134:1173–1176, 1990.

751. Toscano J: Prevention of neurological deterioration before admission to a spinal cord injury unit. **Paraplegia** 26(3):143–150, 1988.

752. Totten VY, Sugarman DB: Respiratory effects of spinal immobilization. **Pre-Hospital Emergency Care** 3(4):347–352, 1999.

753. Tracy P, Wright R, Hanigan W: Magnetic resonance imaging of spinal injury. **Spine** 14:292–301, 1989.

754. Trauma CO: Advanced trauma life support. In *Advanced Trauma Life Support.* Chicago: American College of Surgeons, 1993, pp 214–218.

755. Trauma CO: Advanced trauma life support. In *Advanced Trauma Life Support.* Chicago: American College of Surgeons, 1993, p 201.

756. Trauma CO: Spine and spinal cord trauma. In *Advanced Trauma Life Support for Doctors, Student Course Manual,* 6th ed. Chicago: American College of Surgeons, 1997, pp 215–242.

757. Traynelis VC: Evidence-based management of Type II odontoid fractures. **Clin Neurosurg** 44:841–929, 1997.

758. Traynelis VC, Marano GD, Dunker RO, Kaufman HH: Traumatic atlanto-occipital dislocation. Case report. **J Neurosurg** 65:863–870, 1986.

759. Treloar DJ, Nypaver M: Angulation of the pediatric cervical spine with and without cervical collar. **Pediatric Emergency Care** 13(1):5–8, 1997.

760. Tuite GF, Veres R, et al: Use of an adjustable, transportable, radiolucent spinal immobilization device in the comprehensive management of cervical spine instability. Technical note. **J Neurosurg** 85(6):1177–1180, 1996.

761. Tuli S, Tator CH, Fehlings M, Mackay M: Occipital condyle fractures. **Neurosurgery** 41:368–377, 1997.

762. Tulyapronchote R, Selhorst JB, Malkoff MD, Gomez CR: Delayed sequelae of vertebral artery dissection and occult cervical fractures. **Neurology** 44:1397–1399, 1994.

763. Turgut M, Akpmar G, Akalan N, Ozcan OE: Spinal injuries in the pediatric age group. **Eur Spine J** 5:148–152, 1996.

764. Turnbull IM: Microvasculature of the human spinal cord. **J Neurosurg** 35:141–147, 1971.
765. Turnbull IM: Blood supply of the spinal cord: Normal and pathological considerations. In Wilkins RH (ed): *Clinical Neurosurgery.* Baltimore: Williams & Wilkins (Congress of Neurological Surgeons), 1973, pp 56–84.
766. Turnbull IM, Brieg A, Hassler O: Blood supply of cervical spinal cord in man. A microangiographic cadaver study. **J Neurosurg** 24:951–965, 1966.
767. Urculo E, Arrazola M, Riu I, Moyua A: Delayed glossopharyngeal and vagus nerve paralysis following occipital condyle fracture. Case report. **J Neurosurg** 84:522–525, 1996.
768. Vaccaro A, An H, Lin S, Sun S, Balderston R, Cotler J: Non-contiguous injuries of the spine. **J Spinal Disorders** 5:320–329, 1992.
769. Vaccaro A, Falatyn A, Flanders R, Balderston R, Northrup B, Cotler J: Magnetic resonance evaluation of the intervertebral disc, spinal ligaments, and spinal cord before and after closed traction-reduction of cervical spine dislocations. **Spine** 24:1210–1217, 1999.
770. Vaccaro A, Klein GR, Flanders AE, Albert TJ, Balderston R, Cotler JM: Long-term evaluation of vertebral artery injuries following cervical spine trauma using magnetic resonance angiography. **Spine** 23:789–795, 1998.
771. Valaskatzis EP, Hammer AJ: Fracture of the occipital condyle. A case report. **S African Med J** 77:47–48, 1990.
772. Vale FL, Burns J, Jackson AB, Hadley MN: Combined medical and surgical treatment after acute spinal cord injury: Results of a prospective pilot study to assess the merits of aggressive medical resuscitation and blood pressure management. **J Neurosurg** 87:239–246, 1997.
773. Verbeist H: Anterolateral operations for fractures and dislocations in the middle and lower parts of the cervical spine. **J Bone Joint Surg Am** 51A:1489–1530, 1969.
774. Verheggen R, Jansen J: Hangman's fracture: Arguments in favor of surgical therapy for Type II and III according to Edwards and Levine. **Surg Neurol** 49:253–262, 1998.
775. Verska JM, Anderson PA: Os odontoideum. A case report of one identical twin. **Spine** 22:706–709, 1997.
776. Viccellio P, Simon H, Pressman BD, Shah MN, Mower W, Hoffman J: A prospective multi-center study of cervical spine injury in children. **Pediatrics** 108:1–6, 2001.
777. Vital J, Gille O, Senegas J, Pointillart V: Reduction technique for uni- and biarticular dislocations of the cervical spine. **Spine** 23:949–955, 1998.
778. Vogel LC: Unique management needs of pediatric spinal cord injury patients: Etiology and Pathophysiology. **J Spinal Cord Med** 20:10–13, 1997.
779. Waddell J, Reardon G: Atlantoaxial arthrodesis to treat odontoid fractures. **Can J Surg** 26:255–258, 1983.
780. Wagner FC, Jr., Johnson RM: Cervical bracing after trauma. **Medical Instrumentation** 16(6):287–288, 1982.
781. Wallace MC, Tator CH: Successful improvement of blood pressure, cardiac output, and spinal cord blood flow after experimental spinal cord injury. **Neurosurgery** 20(5):710–715, 1987.
782. Walsh M, Grant T, et al: Lung function compromised by spinal immobilization (letter). **Ann Emerg Med** 19(5):615–616, 1990.
783. Walters B: Clinical practice parameter development in neurosurgery. In Bean J (ed): *Neurosurgery in Transition.* Baltimore: Williams & Wilkins, 1998, pp 99–111.
784. Walton G: A new method of reducing dislocation of cervical vertebrae. **J Nervous Mental Disorders** 20:609–1893.

785. Walton R, DeSalvo JF, et al: Padded vs. unpadded spine board for cervical spine immobilization. **Academic Emerg Med** 2(8):725–728, 1995.
786. Wang GJ, Mabie KN: The nonsurgical management of odontoid fracture in adults. **Spine** 9:229–230, 1984.
787. Wang J, Vokshoor A, Kim S, Elton S, Kosnik E, Bartkowski H: Pediatric atlanto-axial instability: Management with screw fixation. **Pediatric Neurosurg** 30:707–708, 1999.
788. Wani MA, Tandon PN, Banerji AK, Bhatia R: Collet-Sicard syndrome resulting from closed head injury: Case report. **J Trauma** 31:1437–1439, 1991.
789. Waring WP, Karunas RS: Acute spinal cord injuries and the incidence of clinically occurring thromboembolic disease. **Paraplegia** 29:8–16, 1991.
790. Wasserberg J, Bartlett RJV: Occipital condyle fractures diagnosed by high-definition CT and coronal reconstruction. **Neuroradiology** 37:370–373, 1995.
791. Watanabe M, Toyama Y, Fujimura Y: Atlantoaxial instability in os odontoideum with myelopathy. **Spine** 21:1435–1439, 1996.
792. Waters RL, Adkins RH, Yakura JS: Definition of complete spinal cord injury. **Paraplegia** 9:573–581, 1991.
793. Waters RL, Adkins R, Yakura J, Vigil D: Prediction of ambulatory performance based on motor scores derived from standards of the American Spinal Injury Association. **Arch Phys Med Rehabil** 75(July):756–760, 1994.
794. Waters RL, Meyer PR, Jr., et al: Emergency, acute, and surgical management of spine trauma. **Arch Phys Med Rehabil** 80(11):1383–1390, 1999.
795. Watridge CB, Orrison WW, Arnold H, Woods GA: Lateral atlanto-occipital dislocation: A case report. **Neurosurgery** 17:345–347, 1985.
796. Watson N: Venous thrombosis and pulmonary embolism in spinal cord injury. **Paraplegia** 6:113–121, 1968.
797. Watson N: Anti-coagulant therapy in the prevention of venous thrombosis and pulmonary embolism in the spinal cord injury. **Paraplegia** 16:265–269, 1978.
798. Weinstein PR, Karpman RR, Gall EP, Pitt M: Spinal cord injury, spinal fracture, and spinal stenosis in ankylosing spondylitis. **J Neurosurg** 57:609–616, 1982.
799. Weller SJ, Rossitch E, Malek AM: Detection of vertebral artery injury after cervical spine trauma using magnetic resonance angiography. **J Trauma** 46:660–666, 1999.
800. Wells JD, Nicosia S: Scoring acute spinal cord injury: A study of the utility and limitations of five different grading systems. **J Spinal Cord Med** 18:33–41, 1995.
801. Wessels LS: Fracture of the occipital condyle: A report of 3 cases. **S African Med J** 28:155–156, 1990.
802. White AJ, Panajabi M: *Biomechanics of the Spine.* Philadelphia: J.B. Lippincott, 1990.
803. White P, Seymour R, Powell N: MRI assessment of the pre-vertebral soft tissues in acute cervical spine trauma. **Br J Radiology** 818–823, 1999.
804. Wholey MH, Bruwer AJ, Baker HL: The lateral roentgenogram of the neck (with comments on the atlanto-odontoid-basion relationship). **Radiology** 71:350–356, 1958.
805. Wilberger J: Immobilization and traction. In Tator CH, Benzel EC (eds): *Contemporary Management of Spinal Cord Injury: From Impact to Rehabilitation.* 2000, pp 91–98.
806. Williams TG: Hangman's fracture. **J Bone Joint Surg Br** 57:82–88, 1975.
807. Willis BK, Greiner F, Orrison W, Benzel EC: The incidence of vertebral artery injury after midcervical spine fracture or subluxation. **Neurosurgery** 34:435–442, 1994.

808. Wilson JT, Rogers FB, Wald SL, Shackford SR, Ricci MA: Prophylactic vena cava filter insertion in patients with traumatic spinal cord injury: Preliminary results. **Neurosurgery** 35:234–239, 1994.
809. Winemiller MH, Stolp-Smith KA, Silverstein MD, Therneau TM: Prevention of venous thromboembolism in patients with spinal cord injury: Effects of sequential pneumatic compression and heparin. **J Spinal Cord Med** 22:182–191, 1999.
810. Wing PC, Nance P, Connell DG, Gagnon F: Risk of avascular necrosis following short term megadose methylprednisolone treatment. **Spinal Cord** 36:633–636, 1998.
811. Wolf A, Levi L, Mirvis S, Ragheb J, Huhn S, Rigamonti D, Robinson WL: Operative management of bilateral facet dislocation. **J Neurosurg** 75:883–890, 1991.
812. Wood-Jones F: The ideal lesion produced by judicial hanging. **Lancet** 1:53–1913.
813. Woodring J, Lee C: Limitations of cervical radiography in the evaluation of acute cervical trauma. **J Trauma** 34:32–39, 1993.
814. Woodring JH, Lee C, Duncan V: Transverse process fractures of the cervical vertebrae: Are they insignificant? **J Trauma** 34:797–802, 1993.
815. Woodring JH, Selke AC, Duff DE: Traumatic atlanto-occipital dislocation with survival. **Am J Radiology** 137:21–24, 1981.
816. Worsing RA, Jr: Principles of pre-hospital care of musculoskeletal injuries. **Emerg Med Clin North Am** 2(2):205–217, 1984.
817. Xiong X, Bean A, Anthony A, Inglis G, Waltom D: Manipulation for cervical spinal dislocation under general anaesthesia: Seriel review for 4 years. **Spinal Cord** 36:21–24, 1998.
818. Yamaguchi N, Ikeda K, Ishise J, Yamashita J: Traumatic atlanto-occipital dislocation with long-term survival. **Neurol Med Chir** 36:36–39, 1996.
819. Yamashita Y, Takahashi M, Sakamoto Y, Kojima R: Atlantoaxial subluxation. Radiography and magnetic resonance imaging correlated to myelopathy. **Radiologica** 30:135–140, 1989.
820. Yarkony GM, Roth E, Lovell L, Heinemann A, Katz RT, Wu Y: Rehabilitation outcomes in complete C5 quadriplegia. **Am J Phys Med Rehabil** 69:73–76, 1988.
821. Yashon D, Tyson G, Vise W: Rapid closed reduction of the cervical fracture dislocation. **Surgical Neurology** 4:513–514, 1975.
822. Yavuz N, Tezyurek M, Akyuz M: A comparison of two functional tests in quadriplegia: The quadriplegia index of function and the functional independence measure. **Spinal Cord** 36:832–837, 1998.
823. Yelnik A, Dizien O, Bussel B, et al: Systemic lower limb phlebography in acute spinal cord injury in 147 patients. **Paraplegia** 29:253–260, 1991.
824. Young W, Bracken MB: The Second National Acute Spinal Cord Injury Study (NASCIS 2). **J Neurotrauma** 9(S 1):S 397–S 405, 1992.
825. Young B, Ott L, Twymann D, et al: The effect of nutritional support on outcome from severe head injury. **J Neurosurg** 67:668–676, 1987.
826. Young B, Ott L, Rapp RP, Norton J: The patient with critical neurological disease. **Crit Care Clin** 3(1):217–233, 1987.
827. Young WF, Rosenwasser RH, Getch C, Jallo J: Diagnosis and management of occipital condyle fractures. **Neurosurgery** 34:257–261, 1994.
828. Zach GA, Seiler W., Dollfus P: Treatment results of spinal cord injury in the Swiss Paraplegic Centre. **Paraplegia** 14(1):58–65, 1976.
829. Zampella EJ, Duvall ER, Langford KH: Computed tomography and magnetic resonance imaging in traumatic locked-in syndrome. **Neurosurgery** 22:591–593, 1988.
830. Zavanone M, Guerra P, Rampini P, et al: Traumatic fractures of the craniovertebral junction. Management of 23 cases. **J Neurosurg Sci** 35:17–22, 1991.

831. Zeidman SM, Ling GSF, Ducker TB, Ellenbogen RG: Clinical applications of pharmacologic therapies for spinal cord injury. **J Spinal Disorders** 9(5):367–380, 1996.
832. Zigler JE, Waters RL, Nelson RW, Capen DA, Perry J: Occipito-cervico-thoracic spine fusion in a patient with occipito-cervical dislocation and survival. **Spine** 11:645–646, 1986.
833. Zimmerman E, Grant J, Vise WM, et al: Treatment of Jefferson fracture with a halo apparatus. Report of two cases. **J Neurosurg** 44:372–375, 1976.

21

Advances in Minimally Invasive Spine Surgery

KEVIN T. FOLEY, M.D., AND MICHAEL A. LEFKOWITZ, M.D.

INTRODUCTION

When spinal surgery is deemed necessary for optimal patient management, consideration must be given to minimizing surgical morbidity. A portion of this morbidity is attributable to tissue trauma related to the surgical approach. Approach-related morbidity increases postoperative pain, diminishes spinal function, and can lengthen the patient's recovery time. For all patients, but particularly for athletes, maximizing postoperative function and hastening return to full activity are important surgical goals. Thus, surgical procedures that lessen tissue trauma are desirable.

This chapter will describe how advances in surgical technique and technology have enabled the "reinvention" of several commonly performed spinal procedures through the adoption of minimally invasive approaches. A wide spectrum of procedures has benefited from these advances, including microdiscectomy, interbody fusion, and pedicle screw/rod fixation. Importantly, while these spinal procedures are minimally invasive, they are not minimally effective. In fact, reinvention of these operations has resulted in improvements in several important clinical parameters, such as incision size, surgical blood loss, length of hospitalization, and return to activity.

MINIMALLY INVASIVE SPINE SURGERY

Definition

Minimally invasive surgery refers to a variety of techniques for which one of the primary objectives is the minimization of trauma to surrounding anatomic structures during the approach to a surgical site. The notion of minimally invasive surgery is relative; it is characterized in terms of the context in which it is performed. The nature of a specific minimally invasive surgical procedure is determined by many factors: the disease process to be treated, the goals of the surgery, and the anatomy of the target organ and its surrounding structures.

Benefits

There are a number of benefits to minimally invasive spine surgery. Smaller incisions and less invasive surgical approaches result in less tissue disruption; therefore, blood loss and pain are reduced and cosmesis is improved. Postoperative recovery is shortened, both in terms of the length of hospitalization and the length of outpatient convalescence prior to a return to normal activity levels.

The notion of reduced dissection of surrounding tissues merits further discussion. For certain intracranial procedures (e.g., skull base surgeries), more extensive resection of surrounding bony structures has allowed neurosurgeons to minimize brain retraction and limit neurologic morbidity. Of course, preservation of neural elements is of paramount importance in any neurosurgical procedure. In the spine, however, it must be noted that the vertebrae, intervertebral discs, facet joints, paraspinous muscles, and various spinal ligaments form a dynamic biomechanical construct, the performance of which is critical to overall spinal function. Surgical resection or disturbance of one or more of these non-neural structures can have adverse effects on both short- and long-term outcomes.

Increasing evidence suggests that iatrogenic muscle injury during spinal surgery initiates biochemical reactions and morphological alterations that have clinically significant implications in terms of reduction in muscle strength, decreased endurance and increased pain. Kawaguchi (1, 2) has monitored the effects of retractor pressure on muscle during lumbar spine surgery. He has demonstrated that muscle injury, as indicated by the release of certain isoenzymes, is dependent upon retraction pressure and duration. He has also found that morphological damage to muscle may be evident as long as 10 months after surgery. Styf (3) has demonstrated that retractor blades used during dorsal lumbar spine surgery may increase intramuscular pressure in paravertebral muscles to levels that induce ischemia within these muscles. Rantanen and associates (4) have found that patients with poor outcomes after lumbar spine surgery are more likely to have persistent selective type 2 muscle fiber atrophy and pathological structural changes in the paraspinous muscles. Sihvonen (5) has demonstrated that local denervation atrophy due to damage of dorsal rami after lumbar spine surgery is associated with an increased incidence of failed back syndrome.

Results of these studies suggest that, in contrast to intracranial procedures, a different balance must be struck between preservation of neural and neural-supporting elements in the spine. In all procedures involving the nervous system, neural elements must be preserved to the greatest extent possible. However, the functional responsibilities of neural-supporting elements in the spine dictate that they must also be accorded a high degree of respect. This is the rationale for minimally invasive surgery of the spine.

Limitations

Minimally invasive spine surgery is not without its drawbacks. As with all new surgical procedures, a learning curve is encountered during the process of attaining technical proficiency. These operations are likely to be more technically demanding than their open surgical counterparts, and, at least initially, the complication rate may be higher. Frequently, the procedures are longer in duration than conventional surgeries, even after considerable experience. Minimally invasive procedures often require the use of intraoperative imaging or image-guidance. As a result, rather than performing a surgery under direct visualization, a surgeon is operating while looking at a live or virtual fluoroscopic image on a monitor or at a three-dimensional reconstruction of the surgical anatomy on a frameless stereotactic system. This can be disorienting for surgeons who have less experience in recognizing their three-dimensional position using two-dimensional images or who have had limited exposure to image-guided surgery systems. It should also come as no surprise to practitioners that minimally invasive surgery can be both capital- and labor-intensive. The aforementioned image-guidance systems, as well as the specialized surgical sets, are expensive. Their use requires the availability of experienced surgical technicians and surgical device representatives. Finally, the long-term efficacy of many minimally invasive procedures has not been proven. In fact, some minimally invasive spinal procedures have indeed been shown to be minimally effective (6).

METRX TUBULAR RETRACTOR SYSTEM

The METRx (**M**inimal **E**xposure **T**ubular **R**etractor) tubular retractor system is a tool that facilitates minimally invasive spinal exposure. The system consists of a series of concentric dilators and thin-walled retraction tubes of varying lengths. The advantage of this system is that it provides access to bony elements of the spine using muscle-splitting, rather than muscle-dissecting, techniques. The tubular retractor minimizes the stripping of muscle from the spine, producing less tissue trauma than standard exposures. In addition, it is thin-walled (0.9 mm) and displaces muscle circumferentially. Thus, a 16-mm-diameter METRx tube (through which lumbar discectomy is performed) displaces muscle no more than 8 mm in any direction, minimizing muscle retraction.

The tubular retractor system was developed in 1994 and was studied in the laboratory for two years prior to clinical use (7, 8). Initially developed in conjunction with endoscopic visualization of the spinal anatomy (and thus termed "microendoscopic discectomy," or "MED"), it was later adapted for use with the operating microscope or with surgical loupes. Although it may be used in many situations where there is a desire for minimally invasive access to the spine, the system has been used primarily for lumbar microdiscectomies and fusions, as well as cervical and lumbar laminotomies and foraminotomies. Since April 1996, the system has been used in over 6,000 cases at over 550 institutions worldwide.

Lumbar Discectomy Using METRx

The standard lumbar discectomy was first described by Mixter and Barr in 1933 (9). The procedure was performed through a laminotomy at the level of the lesion. Even at this early stage, Mixter and Barr recognized the importance of preservation of the bony and ligamentous elements during the procedure, "for we believe that a ruptured disc is a weakened disc and the strength of the spine should be preserved as much as possible." This belief did not, however, extend to the treatment of the paraspinous muscles. In conventional descriptions of the procedure, no attempts were made to localize the appropriate spinal level radiographically (10). For herniated discs at the L4-5 or L5-S1 levels, a 10-cm midline skin incision was made at the rostral tip of the L4 spinous process and was extended down to the sacrum. In 1971, Simeone (11) first described the use of magnification in the form of operative loupes for lumbar discectomy. He performed his procedures through 4-cm incisions; the L4-5 and L5-S1 levels were confirmed visually in relation to the sacrum. In 1978, Williams (12) first reported on the microscopic lumbar discectomy. His procedure was devised in response to a patient population that demanded optimization of cosmesis and spine function after discectomy—the Las Vegas showgirl. Although it met with some initial skepticism, his technique was eventually widely accepted and resulted in reductions in length of hospitalization and return to work intervals (13, 14). *Figure 21.1* and *Table 21.1* demonstrate these improvements in length of hospitalization and return to work intervals with change in operative technique. *Figure 21.2* and *Table 21.2* demonstrate the relationship between incision length, hospital stay and the era for lumbar discectomy.

Lumbar microdiscectomy using the METRx system employs operative techniques similar to those of conventional microdiscectomy; however, the tubular retractor allows for a smaller incision and less mus-

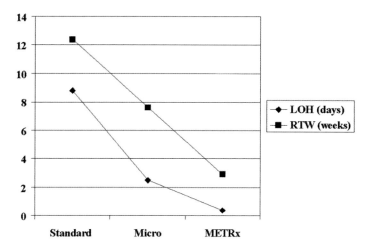

F<small>IG.</small> 21.1 Comparison of parameters for standard discectomy, open microdiscectomy, and METRx discectomy.

cle disruption. *Figure 21.3* illustrates a 16-mm-diameter METRx tube in place during microdiscectomy. *Figure 21.4* shows the sutured skin incision after completion of the microdiscectomy.

One hundred patients who underwent lumbar microdiscectomy using the METRx system were studied prospectively in an effort to determine the benefits of this technique in terms of operative utility and clinical outcome. There were 66 males and 34 females with an average age of 44 years (range: 18–76 years). Mean follow-up was 43 months (range: 35–50 months). Nine patients were involved in Workers' Compensation claims.

Preoperatively, 100% of the patients had radicular leg pain, 56% percent had motor deficits, and 69% had sensory deficits. The distribution of disc level pathology was as follows: L5-S1: 58%; L4-5: 33%; L3-4: 7%; L2-3: 2%. Eleven percent of the patients had far lateral herniated discs.

T<small>ABLE</small> 21.1
A comparison of parameters for standard discectomy, standard microdiscectomy, and microdiscectomy using METRx

Parameter	Standard Discectomy*	Standard Microdiscectomy	METRx Microdiscectomy
Postoperative hospital stay (days)	8.75 ± 0.59	2.47 ± 0.16	0.40
Return to work interval (weeks)	12.43 ± 2.48	7.59 ± 0.93	2.86

*Reference: Andrews and Lavyne[13]

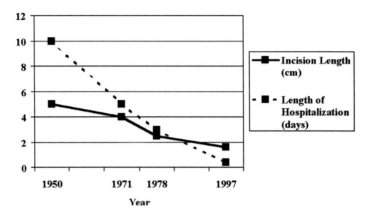

FIG. 21.2 Relationship of incision length and length of hospitalization to surgical era for lumbar discectomies.

At surgery, 52% of the patients were found to have contained disc herniations, 48% had non-contained disc herniations, and 16% had concomitant lateral recess stenosis. Mean operative time was 110 minutes for the first 30 cases, 75 minutes for the last 30 cases. There were two intraoperative complications: one dural laceration, which was identified and repaired intraoperatively, and one delayed pseudomeningocele. Mean length of hospitalization was 9.5 hours (range: 2–23 hours).

Postoperatively, 90% of the patients had resolution of their radicular pain and 10% noted improvement. Using the modified Macnab criteria for outcome after lumbar spine surgery *(Fig. 21.5)*, 85% of the results were characterized as excellent, 19% as good, 1% as fair, and 3% as poor (all three of these patients required reoperation—one for pseudomeningocele and two for recurrent disc herniation). The average time required to return to work was 20 days. This compared with 44 days for a matched cohort of patients who underwent open microdiscectomy.

TABLE 21.2
The relationship between incision length and length of
hospitalization to surgical era for lumbar discectomies

Author	Year	Incision Length	Length of Hospitalization
Semmes[10]	1950s	5 cm	10 days
Simeone[11]	1971	4 cm	5 days
Williams[12]	1978	2.5 cm	3 days
Foley[7]	1997	1.6 cm	0.40 days

Zappulla[41] reported an average length of stay of 10 days for standard lumbar laminectomy and 5 days for lumbar microdiscectomy.

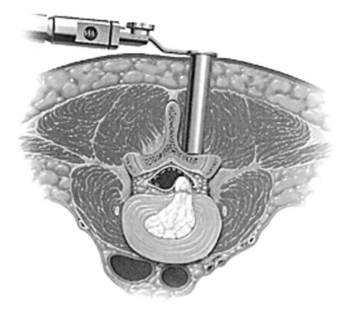

FIG. 21.3 Illustration of a 16-mm-diameter METRx tubular retractor in place during lumbar microdiscectomy.

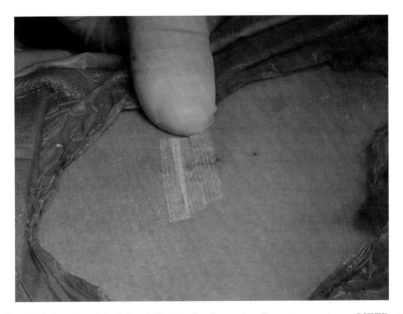

FIG. 21.4 A sutured incision following lumbar microdiscectomy using a METRx tubular retractor.

Modified Macnab Criteria

Excellent	•Free of pain •No restriction of mobility •Able to return to normal work & activities
Good	•Occasional non-radicular pain •Relief of presenting symptoms •Able to return to modified work
Fair	•Some improved functional capacity •Still handicapped and/or unemployed
Poor	•Continued objective symptoms of root involvement •Additional operative intervention needed at the index level, irrespective of repeat or length of postoperative follow-up

FIG. 21.5 Modified Macnab criteria for lumbar discectomy outcomes.

The Oswestry Low Back Pain Questionnaire was employed to assess pre- and postoperative back and leg pain (15). For this scale, a score of zero indicates no pain and a score of 100 indicates that pain medications have no impact on pain. For complaints of back pain, the average preoperative score was 57. At 6 weeks and 6 months postoperatively, the average scores had decreased to 25 and 20, respectively. For complaints of leg pain, the average preoperative score was 64. At 6 weeks and 6 months postoperatively, the average score was 25 and 6, respectively. The SF-36 was also administered to patients preoperatively and postoperatively at 6 months (16, 17). With regard to physical functioning, the average score improved from 28 preoperatively to 85 six months after surgery; social functioning improved from 34 to 88; mental health perception improved from 57 to 82; bodily pain improved from 22 to 74.

An assessment of procedural costs was performed to compare inpatient and outpatient METRx procedures with inpatient microdiscectomy. The inpatient METRx procedure was slightly less expensive than inpatient microdiscectomy—$11,800 versus $13,000. The outpatient METRx procedure was the least expensive—$4,000.

PERCUTANEOUS PEDICLE SCREW AND ROD INSERTION USING SEXTANT

History of Pedicle Screw and Rod Insertion

Lumbar spinal fusion was first performed in the early 1900s by Albee (18) and Hibbs (19). This technique was originally used for treatment of deformities arising from Pott's disease, although the indications were later expanded to include scoliosis and fractures. The concept of internal fixation using a cantilever-beam construct was introduced in the 1940s by King (20). The pedicle screw was first employed by Boucher (21), and the first use of a pedicle screw in association with a dorsal plate was reported by Roy-Camille in 1963 (22). These techniques were largely effective, but the extensive exposures needed to perform them resulted in significant iatrogenic morbidity.

In 1982, Magerl (23) first used percutaneous pedicle screws in association with an external fixator. The limitations of this technology included the risk of infection and patient discomfort associated with external instrumentation. In 1995, Matthews (24) described the use of percutaneous pedicle screws in association with subcutaneous, suprafascial fixators. This technique reduced patient discomfort and the incidence of infection, but the mechanical construct was inefficient because the long moment arm led to suboptimal fixation.

Rationale for Percutaneous Pedicle Screw/Rod Fixation

A system for percutaneous pedicle screw/rod insertion has been developed to address the limitations of existing dorsal thoracolumbar fixation systems (25). As previously discussed, an expanding body of literature has demonstrated that the extensive tissue dissection performed during open posterior lumbar approaches results in histologic and biochemical disruptions in paraspinous muscle that can lead to significant long-term morbidity. The design criteria included the ability to percutaneously insert a biomechanically sound pedicle screw and rod construct into a standard anatomic position.

The Sextant system (Medtronic Sofamor Danek, Memphis, TN) is a percutaneous pedicle screw and rod insertion system consisting of several components (polyaxial pedicle screws, screw extenders, rod inserter, and pre-contoured rods) with design characteristics that are essential to the overall function of the device (25). The pedicle screws used in this system are a modified version of those used for conventional pedicle fixation. They are cannulated, with polyaxial heads that allow for multiple degrees of freedom during screw head alignment (*Fig. 21.6*). The screw extenders, which connect to the pedicle screws prior to insertion, allow the screw heads to be percutaneously aligned so that they can accept a percutaneously-inserted rod. The screw extenders also hold lock plugs that affix the rod to the pedicle screw heads. *Figure 21.7* shows a screw with an attached extender. The rod inserter attaches to the screw extenders in such a fashion that the rod is geometrically constrained to pass along an arc intersecting the screw heads, like a thread through the eye of a needle. The rod inserter allows percutaneous passage of the pre-contoured rods through the pedi-

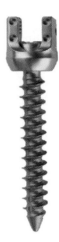

FIG. 21.6 The polyaxial head pedicle screw used for percutaneous pedicle screw/rod insertion.

cle screw heads without the need for direct visualization and with minimal disturbance of the paraspinous muscles. *Figure 21.8* depicts the rod inserter attached to the screw extenders, prior to rod insertion. The screw extender and rod inserter combine to allow the remote place-

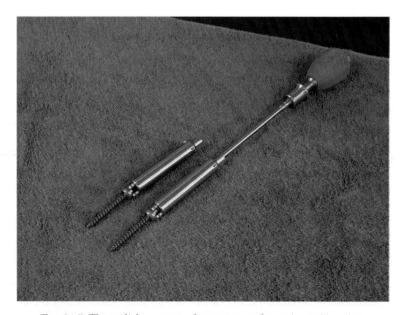

FIG. 21.7 The pedicle screw and screw extender, prior to insertion.

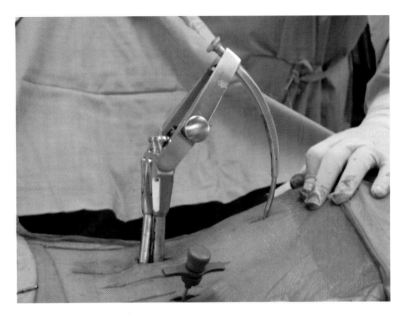

Fig. 21.8 The rod inserter, or "Sextant" device, attached to the screw extenders. A pre-contoured rod is in place and is ready for percutaneous insertion.

ment of instrumentation in a biomechanically sound, anatomically ideal fashion. The design of this system allows the insertion of the pedicle screws through 12-mm skin incisions. In the case of screw/rod fixation at the L5-S1 level, the lordosis of the spine permits placement of both screws through a single 24-mm incision.

Results

Twenty-two patients underwent percutaneous pedicle screw and rod insertion at our institution between March 2000 and September 2001. Twelve of these patients have been followed for at least 9 months and are the subjects of this report. Six patients were male, six were female; mean age was 47 years (range: 23–68 years). Eleven patients had spondylolisthesis as a component of their pathology; seven patients had a grade I slip, three had a grade II slip, and one had a grade III slip. One patient with degenerative disc disease was treated for nonunion of a prior stand-alone interbody fusion. Ten patients had one-level disease: six at L5-S1; three at L4-5; and one at L2-3. Two patients had two-level disease: one at L3-4 and L4-5, the other at L4-5 and L5-S1. Ten patients had mechanical back pain and radiculopathy; two patients had mechanical back pain only. Eleven patients underwent concomitant anterior or posterior lumbar interbody fusion

(ALIF or PLIF) procedures; one patient had a percutaneous postero-lateral onlay fusion at L5-S1.

Eleven patients underwent placement of bilateral percutaneous pedicle screws and rods and one had unilateral screw/rod placement. Two patients had two-level screw/rod placements. Average blood loss for the percutaneous pedicle screw/rod procedures was 65 cc. Average length of hospitalization was 2.1 days.

Mean length of follow-up was 12.8 months (range: 9–18 months). All patients improved clinically and developed solid fusions by radiographic criteria. One patient required replacement of a loose lock plug one month postoperatively. The patient did well clinically and the event was asymptomatic. Reoperation to replace the lock plug was carried out on an outpatient basis. This event occurred early in our clinical experience and led to a redesign of the lock plug. No other device-related problems have been experienced.

POSTERIOR LUMBAR INTERBODY FUSION USING METRX

Posterior lumbar interbody fusion (PLIF) is a technique indicated for restoring spinal stability in the presence of degenerative disc disease or spondylolisthesis when spinal canal or neural foraminal compromise is present. The procedure was originally performed by Cloward in 1940, although he did not report his results until a number of years later (26, 27). PLIF was performed without posterolateral stabilization until Steffee proposed supplementation with pedicle screw fixation in the 1980s (28, 29). Historically, the approach for this procedure has been one of the most invasive in the spinal armamentarium, due to its disruption of the paraspinous musculature, the posterior interspinous and interlaminar (ligamentum flavum) ligaments, and the posterior bony elements (spinous process, lamina, and facets). As a result, this procedure is an excellent candidate for the development of a minimally invasive alternative.

In an attempt to minimize the approach-related morbidity of the PLIF procedure, a minimally invasive surgery has been conceived whereby PLIF is performed through bilateral 22-mm METRx tubular retractors and pedicle screws and rods are placed percutaneously using the Sextant system. The pedicle screws are inserted through the same incisions used for the tubular retractors, after the retractors have been removed.

To date, seven patients (three male, four female; mean age: 62 years) have undergone this procedure. Five patients had L4-5 involvement; two had L5-S1 involvement. One patient had degenerative disc disease only, five patients had grade I spondylolisthesis and one had grade II spondy-lolisthesis. One patient had neurogenic claudication only, one had mechanical back pain only, four had mechanical back pain and unilateral radiculopathy, and one had mechanical back pain and bilateral radiculopathy. The average duration of symptoms was 26 months.

Minimally invasive PLIF was performed successfully in all seven patients. Bilateral pedicle screws were placed in six patients and unilateral pedicle screws were placed in one patient. *Figure 21.9* illustrates the incisions resulting from a minimally invasive PLIF with percutaneous pedicle screw and rod insertion. *Figure 21.10* shows the anteroposterior and lateral lumbar spine plain films following a minimally invasive PLIF and percutaneous instrumentation. Average total operative time and blood loss were 6 hours, 18 minutes and 314 cc, respectively. Average length of hospitalization was 2.4 days. All patients showed improvement in clinical symptoms.

Brantigan, et al. (30) reported on open PLIF using carbon fiber interbody cages and posterolateral pedicle screw and rod fixation with the Steffee plate. They reported a mean intraoperative blood loss of 1066 ml, an average operative time of 261 minutes, and a mean length of hospitalization of 6.4 days. *Table 21.3* compares the results for open and minimally invasive PLIF procedures. Although the results are pre-

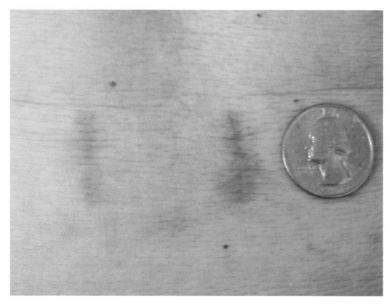

FIG. 21.9 The skin incisions following minimally invasive PLIF and percutaneous pedicle screw and rod insertion.

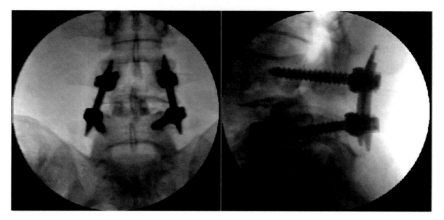

FIG. 21.10 Anteroposterior (left) and lateral (right) lumbar spine plain films following minimally invasive PLIF and percutaneous pedicle screw and rod insertion.

liminary and the number of patients is quite small, minimally invasive PLIF is associated with less blood loss and a significantly shorter hospital stay.

ANTERIOR LUMBAR INTERBODY FUSION

Anterior lumbar interbody fusion (ALIF) has been used for spinal degenerative disorders since 1932, when Carpenter first described the technique for treatment of spondylolisthesis (31). The procedure is now commonly used for a variety of spinal conditions. It offers several potential benefits, such as preservation of posterior spinal elements, reduction of risk to neural elements, and avoidance of epidural scarring. A number of implants have been used for ALIF, including femoral ring allografts, cylindrical bone dowels, cylindrical (32) and tapered threaded metallic cages, and carbon fiber cages (33). In all cases, the

TABLE 21.3

Comparison of EBL, length of surgery, and length of hospitalization for open PLIF and minimally invasive PLIF with instrumentation

Parameter	Open PLIF (Brantigan[30])	Minimally Invasive PLIF (Foley)
Estimated blood loss	1,066 ml	314 ml
Operative time	261 minutes	378 minutes
Length of hospitalization	6.4 days	2.4 days

ultimate strength and stability of the ALIF depends on the achievement of a solid bony fusion.

ALIF was originally performed through an open retroperitoneal approach. In the mid-1980s, reports were published which described a simultaneous combined anterior and posterior approach for spinal fusion (34). The procedure was characterized by a 25-cm incision extending from the midline to the lateral border of the rectus abdominus, 400–600 cc of intraoperative blood loss, a surgical duration of 3.25 hours and hospitalizations typically lasting 10–14 days (34, 35). In the mid-1990s, mini-open retroperitoneal (36, 37), mini-open transperitoneal (36), laparoscopic transperitoneal (38, 39), and laparoscopic retroperitoneal (40) approaches were developed for ALIF. Many of these procedures were performed in a "stand-alone" manner (i.e., without adjunctive posterior stabilization). For these approaches, emphasis was placed on minimization of tissue disruption during the exposure. Incision length was reduced to a single 5-cm incision for the mini-open approach and four 1- to 2-cm incisions for the laparoscopic approach. Operative blood loss was reduced to 150–300 cc for each approach (36, 37) and length of hospitalization was reduced to 3.3–4.0 days (37). Operative time was not significantly reduced by these approaches. It is unclear whether these approaches have had any impact upon the long-term efficacy of ALIF.

Concerns about the success of fusion with stand-alone ALIF have been raised, particularly with regard to situations involving true spinal instability, patients with "tall" discs, and spondylolisthesis. However, the addition of supplemental pedicle fixation has typically involved an open dorsal spinal exposure with its attendant approach-related morbidity. In an effort to optimize treatment of patients with symptomatic spondylolisthesis in a minimally invasive manner, a protocol has been developed for a 360° repair employing a laparoscopic insertion of cortical bone dowels followed by percutaneous pedicle screw and rod insertion. The laparoscopic procedure is performed through three or four 1- to 2-cm incisions, depending on the amount of bowel retraction required. Percutaneous screws are placed through 12-mm skin incisions. *Figure 21.11* shows the lateral lumbar spine plain films before and after this procedure.

Fourteen patients (13 males, 1 female; mean age: 45 years) underwent laparoscopic ALIF and percutaneous insertion of pedicle screws using the Sextant system between May 2000 and September 2001. Thirteen patients had L5-S1 spondylolisthesis and one had L4-5 spondylolisthesis. Seven patients had grade I spondylolisthesis and seven had grade II spondylolisthesis. Seven patients had mechanical back pain and radiculopathy, four had mechanical back pain only, and three had radiculopathy only. Average duration of symptoms was 47 months.

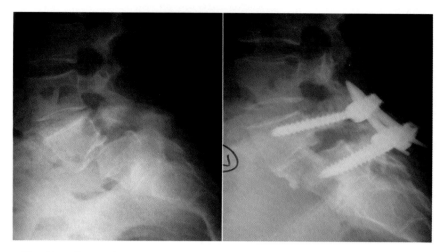

Fig. 21.11 Lateral lumbar spine plain films before (left) and after (right) laparoscopic ALIF and percutaneous pedicle screw and rod insertion for L5-S1 spondylolisthesis.

Laparoscopic ALIF with bilateral pedicle screw placement was performed in twelve patients and unilateral pedicle screw placement was performed in two patients. Average total operative time and blood loss were 6.25 hours and 213 cc, respectively, for the combined anterior and posterior procedure. Mean length of hospitalization was 2.7 days. Average clinical and radiographic follow-up was 8 months. All patients showed significant improvement in symptoms and had excellent fusion by radiographic criteria. There were two surgical complications: one patient sustained a bladder tear during the ALIF that was repaired intraoperatively and a second patient experienced transient retrograde ejaculation postoperatively.

Minimally invasive ALIF with percutaneous pedicle screw insertion was found to be a safe and effective treatment for symptomatic spondylolisthesis. *Table 21.4* summarizes the comparison between intraop-

TABLE 21.4
Comparison of incision length, EBL, length of surgery (LOS), and hospital stay (LOH) for open versus minimally invasive ALIF with posterior fixation

Author	Incision	EBL (cc)	LOS (min)	LOH (days)
O'Brien[34] (open, including posterior fusion)	Anterior: 25 cm	600	195	10–14
Foley (laparoscopic, including percutaneous pedicle screw placement)	Anterior: 4 × 1–2 cm	211	375	2.7

erative blood loss, length of hospitalization, and incision length for an open ALIF with open posterior fixation versus minimally invasive ALIF with percutaneous posterior fixation. The minimally invasive procedure, while taking longer to perform, is associated with less blood loss and a significantly shorter hospital stay.

FUTURE CHALLENGES AND OPPORTUNITIES

Minimally invasive spinal surgery is in its infancy. Despite the recent progress documented in this chapter, more work remains to be done and great promise lies ahead. Most importantly, outcome studies are needed to validate the efficacy of minimally invasive spinal surgical procedures in comparison to time-tested approaches to spinal surgery. That being said, it is clear that new technologies are providing the tools to allow surgeons to perform effective spinal surgery in a fashion that minimizes trauma to surrounding structures, yet follows the same principles and accomplishes the same goals as conventional open surgeries. Recent biomedical advances, including image-guided surgery and genetically-engineered products such as bone morphogenetic proteins, should expand our abilities to surgically treat the spine in a percutaneous, less invasive fashion.

BIBLIOGRAPHY

1. Kawaguchi Y, Matsui H, Tsuji H: Back muscle injury after posterior lumbar spine surgery. A histologic and enzymatic analysis. **Spine** 21(8):941–944, 1996.
2. Kawaguchi Y, Matsui H, Tsuji H: Back muscle injury after posterior lumbar spine surgery. Part 2: Histologic and histochemical analyses in humans. **Spine** 19(22): 2598–2602, 1994.
3. Styf JR, Willen J: The effects of external compression by three different retractors on pressure in the erector spine muscles during and after posterior lumbar spine surgery in humans. **Spine** 23(3):354–358, 1998.
4. Rantanen J, Hurme M, Falck B, Alaranta H, Nykvist F, Lehto M, Einola S, Kalimo H: The lumbar multifidus muscle five years after surgery for a lumbar intervertebral disc herniation. **Spine** 18(5):568–574, 1993.
5. Sihvonen T, Herno A, Paljiarvi L, Airaksinen O, Partanen J, Tapaninaho A: Local denervation atrophy of paraspinal muscles in postoperative failed back syndrome. **Spine** 18(5):575–581, 1993.
6. Kahanovitz N, Viola K, Goldstein T, Dawson E: A multicenter analysis of percutaneous discectomy. **Spine** 15(7):713–715, 1990.
7. Foley KT, Smith MM: Microendoscopic discectomy. **Tech Neurosurg** 3(4):301–307, 1997.
8. Foley KT, Smith MM, Rampersaud YR: Microendoscopic discectomy. In Schmidek HH (ed): *Operative Neurosurgical Techniques: Indications, Methods, and Results,* 4th ed. Philadelphia: WB Saunders, 2000.
9. Mixter WJ, Barr JS: Rupture of the intervertebral disc with involvement of the spinal canal. **New Engl J Med** 211:210–214, 1933.

10. Semmes RE: *Ruptures of the Lumbar Intervertebral Disc.* Springfield, IL: Charles C Thomas. 1984, pp 30–34.
11. Simeone FA: The neurologic approach to lumbar disc disease. **Orthop Clin North Am** 2:499–506, 1971.
12. Williams RW: Microlumbar discectomy: A conservative surgical approach to the virgin herniated lumbar disc. **Spine** 3:175–182, 1978.
13. Andrews DW, Lavyne MH: Retrospective analysis of microsurgical and standard lumbar discectomy. **Spine** 15(4):329–335, 1990.
14. Wilson DH, Harbaugh R: Microsurgical and standard removal of the protruded lumbar disc: a comparative study. **Neurosurgery** 8(2):422–425, 1979.
15. Fairbank JC, Couper J, Davies JB, O'Brien JP: The Oswestry low back pain questionnaire. **Physiotherapy** 66(8):271–273, 1980.
16. Ware JE Jr, Sherbourne CD: The MOS 36-item short-form health survey (SF-36). I. Conceptual framework and item selection. **Med Care** 30(6):473–483, 1992.
17. McHorney A, Ware JE Jr, Raczek AE: The MOS 36-item short-form health survey (SF-36): II. Psychometric clinical tests of validity in measuring physical and mental health constructs. **Med Care** 31(3):247–263, 1993.
18. Albee FH: Transplantation of a portion of the tibia into the spine for Pott's disease. **JAMA** 57:885–886, 1911.
19. Hibbs RA: An operation for progressive spinal deformities. **NY Med J** 93:1013–1016, 1911.
20. King D: Internal fixation for lumbosacral fusion. **J Bone Joint Surg** 30A:560–565, 1948.
21. Boucher HH: A method of spinal fusion. **J Bone Joint Surg** 41-B:248–259, 1959.
22. Roy-Camille R, Saillant G, Mazel C: Internal fixation of the lumbar spine with pedicle screw plating. **Clin Orthop** 203:7–17, 1986.
23. Magerl FP: External skeletal fixation of the lower thoracic and the lumbar spine. In Uhthoff HK, Stahl E (eds): *Current Concepts of External Fixation of Fractures.* New York: Springer-Verlag, 1982, pp 353–366.
24. Matthews HH, Long BH: Endoscopy assisted percutaneous anterior interbody fusion with subcutaneous suprafascial internal fixation: evolution of technique and surgical considerations. **Orthop Int Ed** 3:496–500, 1995.
25. Foley KT, Gupta SK, Justis JR, Sherman MC: Percutaneous pedicle screw fixation of the lumbar spine. **Neurosurg Focus** 10(4):1–8, 2001.
26. Cloward RB: New treatment for ruptured intervertebral disc. Annual Meeting of Hawaii Territorial Medical Association, May 1945.
27. Cloward RB: The treatment of ruptured intervertebral discs by vertebral body fusion. Indications, operative technique, after care. **J Neurosurg** 10:154–168, 1953.
28. Steffee AD, Sitkowski DJ: Posterior lumbar interbody fusion and plates. **Clin Orthop** 227:99–102, 1988.
29. Steffee AD: The variable screw placement system with posterior lumbar interbody fusion. In Lin PM, Gill K (eds): *Lumbar Interbody Fusion.* Rockville, MD, Aspen Publishers, 1989, pp 81–93.
30. Brantigan JW, Steffee AD, Lewis ML, Quinn LM, Persenaire JM: Lumbar interbody fusion using the Brantigan I/F Cage for posterior lumbar interbody fusion and the variable pedicle screw placement system. **Spine** 25(11):1437–1446, 2000.
31. Carpenter N: Spondylolisthesis. **Br J Surg** 19:374–386, 1932.
32. Bagby G: Arthrodesis by the distraction—compression methods using a stainless steel implant. **Orthopedics** 11:931–934, 1988.
33. Brantigan JW, Steffee AD: A carbon fiber implant to aid interbody lumbar fusion: Two-year clinical results in the first 26 patients. **Spine** 18:2106–2117, 1993.

34. O'Brien JP, Dawson MHO, Heard CW, Momberger G, Speck G, Weatherly CR: Simultaneous combined anterior and posterior fusion: A surgical solution for failed spinal surgery with a brief review of the first 150 patients. **Clin Orthop Rel Res** 203:191–195, 1986.
35. Crock HV: Anterior lumbar interbody fusion: Indications for its use and notes on surgical technique. **Clin Orthop Rel Res** 165:157–163, 1982.
36. Mayer HM: A new microsurgical technique for minimally invasive anterior lumbar interbody fusion. **Spine** 22:691–700, 1997.
37. Regan JJ, Yuan H, McAfee PC: Laparoscopic fusion of the lumbar spine: Minimally invasive spine surgery. **Spine** 24:402–411, 1999.
38. Zucherman JF, Zdeblick TA, Bailey SA, Mahvi D, Hsu KY, Kohrs D: Instrumented laparoscopic spinal fusion. **Spine** 20:2029–2035, 1995.
39. Zdeblick TA: Laparoscopic spinal fusion. **Orthop Clin North Am** 29(4):635–645, 1998.
40. McAfee PC, Regan JJ, Geis WP, Fedder IL: Minimally invasive anterior retroperitoneal approach to the lumbar spine. Emphasis on the lateral BAK: **Spine** 23: 1476–1484, 1998.
41. Zappulla RA, Hollis PH: The microsurgical approach to the herniated lumbar disc. In Camins M, O'Leary P (eds): *The Lumbar Spine*. Raven Press: New York, 1987, pp 143–148.

22

Fractures, Stenosis, and Sports: Guidance for Participation

BRIAN R. SUBACH, M.D., REGIS W. HAID, JR., M.D.,
GERALD E. RODTS, JR., M.D.AMORY FIORE, M.D.,
PRAVEEN MUMMANENI, M.D, AND CARMEN A. PETRAGLIA, B.S.

INTRODUCTION

Each of us has had the pleasure of diagnosing and treating spinal and spinal cord injuries in an athlete at some point in our career. While many athletes are young, healthy, and motivated individuals, participating at a very high levels of organized competition, there are just as many aging individuals who play competitive recreational sports such as tennis, running, skiing, and golf. Although the frequency of involvement in contact sports tends to decrease as the age of the athlete increases, the desire to return to play often burns just as brightly in the aging athlete. It is this same desire to return to active sport participation that often causes the most significant problems in the recovering athlete.

It seems that one of our roles as spinal surgeons has evolved. Not only are we responsible for managing the initial injury, but we also must develop a rehabilitation schedule, marked by graduated increases in activity, with the endpoint being a return to full participation in the sport. The simple decision to ban further play is a difficult one to make. On one hand we wish to successfully return our patients to their prior level of functioning and play. On the other hand, we realize that their spine and spinal cord may not be able to endure the likely stresses placed upon them. Banning further play in a professional athlete may alienate the physician from the patient and may also have mental and financial repercussions which impact well beyond the athlete himself *(Fig. 22.1)*. Conversely, counseling a high school athlete and his family about the likelihood of a future disabling spinal cord injury may be rewarding.

Factors which must be considered by both the surgeon and the athlete in determining the appropriate course of action after injury include the inherent risk of the sport itself based upon degree of contact and likelihood of future injury, the level of participation in the sport, ranging from grade school player to professional athlete or competitive recre-

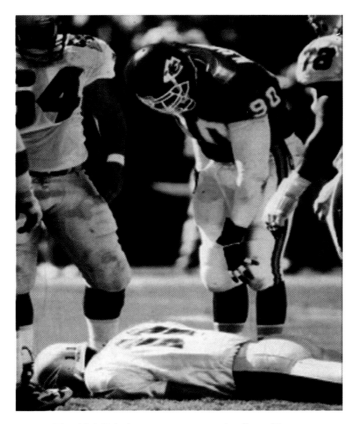

FIG. 22.1 Injuries may occur even in elite athletes.

ational athlete, the presence of prior injury, the degree of muscular, spinal, and ligamentous injury, and the extent of neurological deficit, whether temporary or permanent. Despite a clear and careful analysis of the individual factors leading to your decision, it will be a difficult one to make. Sport is more than just a game to an athlete. It may be as important and intrinsic to them as eating and breathing. The athlete may define himself as a person based on his batting average, his nickname, or even the number on his jersey. Realize the importance of your decisions, think carefully, discuss frankly, and you will not err.

DEFINING CERVICAL SPINAL STENOSIS: THE TORG RATIO

Numerous attempts have been made to radiographically define cervical spinal stenosis, particularly as it relates to the competitive athlete. Since there is obviously no absolute number based on the various body types and structures, Torg et al. described a ratio of the anteroposterior diameter of the spinal canal divided by the anteroposterior diameter of the adjacent vertebral body. The Torg ratio, as it has come to be called, is obtained from dimensions taken from plain lateral radiographs and is commonly used to define congenital spinal stenosis (12). A ratio of less than or equal to 0.8 has been found to be 93% sensitive in describing clinically significant stenosis in a symptomatic athlete. It has been found to be less effective as a screening method prior to participation given a relatively low positive predictive value (0.2%). Since the size of the vertebral bodies in athletes may be considerably larger than in non-athletes, but the spinal canal is similar in size, use of the Torg ratio may falsely identify spinal stenosis. In such cases, the absolute canal diameter, typically greater than 12 mm should be considered as well, prior to making the determination. Although less than ideal, this ratio lends an important perspective to dealing with symptomatic cervical stenosis. An examination with a better predictive value is yet to be found.

THE STINGER OR BURNER SYNDROME

The syndrome which has come to be known as the "stinger" or "burner" among athletes, is typically viewed as a trivial or inconsequential injury. The injury typically occurs among athletes participating in contact sports such as football, hockey, and lacrosse, but has been described in non-contact sports by athletes striking the ground or another immobile object. The primary symptoms include transient, burning, radicular pain and paresthesias in the arm. It is typically a unilateral syndrome, involving one arm only, and may be associated with weakness and neck pain which is exacerbated by extension (Fig. 22.2). Estimated to occur in more than 50% of collegiate athletes participating in contact sports, the extent of such injuries is often underestimated. When the initial injury occurs, the athlete will usually leave the playing field while supporting the affected extremity. When questioned by the trainer, he will describe a painful, burning, or tingling sensation which runs from the back of the neck to the fingertips. The pain may last only a short time, however, the associated motor and sensory findings may persist for days or weeks (7).

The burner most commonly affects either the C5 or C6 dermatomes. The muscles involved are usually the deltoid (C5), the biceps (C5, C6), the supraspinatus (C5, C6), and the infraspinatus (C5, C6). Physicians

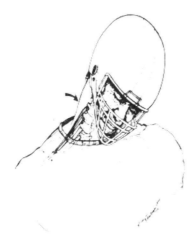

FIG. 22.2 One of the postulated mechanisms for a "burner": ipsilateral shoulder depression with contralateral head tilt causing brachial plexus stretch injury.

and athletic trainers have attributed the frequency of involvement of these nerve roots to their proximity to the clavicle and the significant degree of lateral neck bending which occurs at the mid-cervical spine. Three mechanisms have been postulated as possible causes for burners. One possibility is simply a stretch or traction injury to the brachial plexus, caused by depression of the ipsilateral shoulder with a head tilt toward the contralateral side of the body. A second proposed mechanism is cervical hyperextension with concomitant axial loading. This could lead to transient foraminal compression of the exiting nerve roots. Finally, it is also possible to deliver a blow directly to the brachial plexus, specifically near Erb's point, where the upper trunk of the plexus is tethered to the transverse processes of the cervical spine.

Irrespective of the precise causative mechanism, the syndrome likely represents a neuropraxic injury. With repetitive trauma, the typically transient signs and symptoms may become chronic. Often by modification of the player's habits and equipment, such chronic changes may be avoided. It remains critical to differentiate the signs and symptoms of nerve root or brachial plexus involvement from the more serious spinal cord involvement.

TRANSIENT QUADRIPARESIS

The stingers and burners, sustained by both recreational and competitive athletes, clearly represent the majority of sport-related cervical syndromes. Similar to the neuropraxic injuries to the roots, the spinal cord itself, may sustain a traumatic neuropraxia. Such injuries to the cord are often grouped under the heading of syndromes called transient quadriparetic injuries. Transient quadriparesis may occur as a result of an impact, with either the ground or another athlete. It is typically described as proximal weakness involving both upper and lower extremities causing the athlete to remain on the ground after the impact. Initial evaluations by trainers and physicians will focus upon both the head and cervical spine. The athlete usually remains conscious throughout the entire episode, but may need assistance to roll into a recovery position. Occasionally, a mild respiratory distress syndrome may accompany the presentation. Although the subjective weakness may resolve in a matter of seconds, the athlete often notices dysesthetic, burning paresthesias involving both upper extremities which typically last 10–15 minutes, but may persist up to 48 hours. Since the initial inciting episode and transient weakness may go unnoticed by coaching and medical personnel, it is critical to carefully examine any athlete complaining of bilateral, dysesthetic sensations.

The incidence of dysesthesias and transient quadriparesis related to this syndrome has been reported to be 7.3 per 10,000 athletes. It is believed to occur more frequently in higher levels of competition where the athletes are faster and the collision impact forces are greater. It may be less frequently reported at the level of elite intercollegiate and professional athletes, since an athlete may not verbalize health concerns, which may alter his play status or have financial implications.

The proposed mechanism of injury appears to be axial compression with some degree of hyperextension or hyperflexion. Often, there may be coexisting congenital cervical stenosis, loss of cervical lordosis, kyphosis, congenital fusion of interspaces (Klippel-Feil abnormality), degenerative disc disease (Speartackler's spine), or segmental instability. The extent of the compressive force often determines the degree of spinal cord injury and the severity and duration of symptoms. Sensory abnormalities range from paresthesias or burning pain to complete loss of sensation in more than one dermatome. The multiple nerve distributions and bilaterality will help to differentiate this syndrome from a burner. Typically, the extent of motor involvement is less severe than the sensory disturbance, however, transient quadriplegia has been reported particularly in cases with preexisting disease.

Various attempts have been made to correlate canal diameter with the occurrence of transient quadriparesis. Torg et al. applied the ratio of anteroposterior diameter of canal to cervical vertebrae to athletes sustaining a single neuropraxic event. Of the 110 athletes studied, Torg made two interesting observations. First, athletes sustaining a single episode of transient quadriparesis have a 56% chance of a recurrence if play continues. Second, there was no greater risk of permanent neurological injury in athletes experiencing a single event.

RETURN-TO-PLAY CRITERIA

The decision to remove an athlete from competition is not an easy one. Although he may have the player's best medical interests in mind, the team physician is seldom applauded by coaches, trainers, and the athletes themselves, even in cases of temporary restriction of play. Social

TABLE 22.1

Guidelines for Return to Play Based Upon Cervical Spinal Abnormalities

Absolute Contraindications
1. Atlantoaxial instability or subluxation.
2. Atlanto-occipital fusion.
3. Abnormalities of the odontoid process.
4. Complex congenital spinal fusion (Type I and Type III Klippel-Feil abnormalities).
5. Radiographic evidence of Speartackler's spine (congenital cervical stenosis with loss of normal lordosis).
6. Evidence of subaxial cervical instability on dynamic radiographs (>3.5 mm translation or >11° angulation between adjacent vertebrae[16]).
7. Acute fracture of the vertebrae or posterior elements.
8. Healed subaxial fractures with residual canal compromise or malalignment.
9. Healed cervical fusion in the presence of congenital stenosis.
10. Abnormal neurological examination, abnormal range of motion, or persistent pain in the presence of a healed cervical fracture.
11. Cervical disc herniation (acute or chronic) with pain, motor or sensory deficits, or abnormal cervical range of motion.

Relative Contraindications
1. Presence of a healed fracture of the atlas or axis with a normal range of motion, without pain or neurological deficit.
2. Healed, minimally displaced, vertebral compression fracture with normal alignment.
3. Healed fracture of the posterior elements (excluding spinous process fractures).
4. Radiographic evidence of facet joint instability with concomitant disc disease.
5. Healed multi-level cervical fusion.

No Contraindications
1. Congenital cervical fusion, one or two levels (Type II Klippel-Feil anomaly), without significant stenosis, instability, or disc disease.
2. Spina bifida occulta.
3. Healed, minimally displaced, vertebral compression fracture with normal alignment.
4. Asymptomatic cervical disc herniation.
5. Healed single level cervical fusion without pain or neurologic deficit.

From Torg/Ramsey-Emrheim (13).

and financial pressures often complicate decisions and may sway the physician to take a less conservative course of action. Maroon and Bailes found themselves faced with such decisions in dealing with the Pittsburgh Steelers. They developed a three-tiered classification system (Types I–III), in an attempt to generate guidelines for return to play after cervical spinal cord injury. Type I injuries consisted of athletes with clinical evidence of permanent spinal cord damage. Ranging from complete cord injuries to the many incomplete cord syndromes (anterior, central, etc.). Type I injuries were considered absolute contraindications to play. Type II injuries typically included transient spinal cord syndromes, such as transient quadriparesis, spinal cord contusions, and the burning hands syndrome. As relative contraindi-

TABLE 22.2

Guidelines for Return to Play Based Upon Cervical Spinal Abnormalities

Absolute Contraindications

Cervical Injury
• More than two episodes of transient quadriparesis / neuropraxia.
• Clinical evidence of cervical myelopathy.
• Persistent neck pain, limited range of motion, or neurological deficit after previous cervical injury.

Postsurgical Conditions
• Healed C1-C2 fusion.
• Healed cervical laminectomy.
• Healed multilevel (>3) cervical fusion.

Soft-Tissue Abnormalities
• Ligamentous laxity (>3.5 mm translation or >11° angulation between adjacent vertebrae[16]).
• Radiographic evidence of C1-C2 hypermobility with the atlantodental interval of >3.5 mm (adult) or >4.0 mm (child).
• Radiographic evidence of a distraction/extension cervical injury.
• Symptomatic cervical disc herniation.

Isolated Radiographic Findings
• Plain Radiographs
  ○ Speartackler's spine.
  ○ Multi-level Klippel-Feil abnormality.
  ○ Ankylosing spondylosis or diffuse idiopathic skeletal hyperostosis.
• Magnetic Resonance Imaging
  ○ Arnold-Chiari malformation
  ○ Healed subaxial cervical fracture with residual stenosis.
  ○ Any spinal cord abnormality.
  ○ Evidence of basilar invagination.
• Computed Tomography
  ○ Fixed atlantoaxial rotatory abnormality
  ○ Occipital-C1 assimilation.

From Vaccaro/Watson (15).

cations, these injuries would mandate restriction of play while symptoms were present, followed by a complete examination and thorough discussion with the athlete, prior to a return-to-play status. Repetitive Type II injuries or persistent neurological dysfunction following such an injury should warrant serious discussion with both the athlete and coaching staff, as to possible permanent restriction from play. Type III injuries basically encompassed radiographic abnormalities such as spinal stenosis, fractures, degenerative disc disease, or ligamentous instability. Maroon and Bailes recommended close evaluation of the individual athlete in such cases.

In 1997, Torg and Ramsey-Emrhein developed a second set of guidelines, similar to Maroon and Bailes' guidelines, which outlined absolute contraindications, relative contraindications, and non-contraindications to return to play *(Table 22.1)*. The guidelines were

TABLE 22.3
Guidelines for Return to Play Based Upon Cervical Spinal Abnormalities

Relative Contraindications
Cervical Injury
- Two episodes of transient quadriparesis / neuropraxia without pain, neurologic deficit, or abnormal cervical range of motion.
- Three or more previous episodes stingers/burners without pain, neurologic deficit, or abnormal cervical range of motion.
- Prolonged stinger/burner or transient quadriparesis lasting >24 hours.

Postsurgical Conditions
- Following a healed two-level anterior cervical fusion
- Healed single level posterior cervical fusion.

No Contraindications
Cervical Injury
- Healed C1 or C2 fracture with normal cervical range of motion.
- Healed subaxial fracture without sagittal plane deformity.
- Asymptomatic spinous process fracture.
- Prior episode (<3) of a stinger/burner lasting <24 hours without abnormal cervical range of motion or neurologic deficit.
- Single episode of transient quadriparesis with a full range of cervical motion, no evidence of neurologic deficit, and no radiographic evidence of cervical instability or disc herniation.

Degenerative / Postsurgical Conditions
- Cervical disc disease treated conservatively, without neurological deficit.
- Healed cervical laminoforaminotomy (single or multiple levels).
- Healed sinlgle-level cervical fusion.

Congenital Abnormalities
- Single level Klippel-Feil anomaly not involving the C0/C1 articulation.
- Spina bifida occulta.
- Asymptomatic Torg ratio

From Vaccaro/Watson (15).

much more detailed and specific, thereby enhancing the strength of the criteria (13).

In July 2001, Vaccaro and Watkins reviewed the available guidelines set forth by Maroon, Torg, Cantu, and others (15). In attempting to identify a single, logical classification system, they adapted the absolute-relative-non-contraindication format, which had been previously utilized *(Tables 22.2 and 22.3)*. Prior to employing the guidelines, the initial management of all injured athletes is the same. The principles of immobilization and prevention of on-field injury exacerbation are critical. Restriction from play until all symptoms have resolved and a complete physical and radiographic evaluation can be carried out, is mandatory. These maneuvers are well described in other forums.

REFERENCES

1. Clarke KS: Epidemiology of athletic neck injury. **Clin Sports Med** 17:83–97, 1998.
2. Cantu RC: Stingers, transient quadriplegia, and cervical spinal stenosis: return to play criteria. **Med Sci Sports Exerc** 29:S233–S235, !997.
3. Cantu RC, Bailes JE, Wilberger JE: Guidelines for return to contact or collision sport after cervical spine injury. **Clin Sports Med** 17:137–146, 1998.
4. Clancy WG, Brand RL, Bergfield JA: Upper trunk brachial plexus injuries in contact sports. **Am J Sports Med** 5:209–216, 1977.
5. Levitz CL, Reilly PJ, Torg JS: The pathomechanics of chronic, recurrent cervical nerve root neuropraxia. **Am J Sports Med** 25:73–76, 1997.
6. Markey KL, Di Benedetto M, Curl WW: Upper trunk brachial plexopathy: the stinger syndrome. Am J Sports Med 21:650–655, 1993.
7. Maroon JC, Bailes JE: Athletes with cervical spine injury. **Spine** 21:2294–2299, 1996.
8. Meyer SA, Schulte KR, Callaghan JJ: Cervical spinal stenosis and stingers in collegiate football players. **Am J Sports Med** 22:158–166, 1994.
9. Morganti C, Sweeney CA, Albanese SA, Hosea T, Burnk C, Connolly PJ: Return to play after cervical spine injuy. **Spine** 26:1131–1136, 2001.
10. Torg JS, Corcoran TA, Thibault LE: Cervical cord neuropraxia: classification, pathomechanics, morbidity, and management guidelines. **J Neurosurg** 87:843–850, 1997.
11. Torg JS, Naranja RJ, Pavlov H, Galinat BJ, Warren R, Stine RA: The relationship of developmental narrowing of the cervical spinal canal to reversible and irreversible injury of the cervical spinal cord in football players. **J Bone Joint Surg Am** 78:1308–1314, 1996.
12. Torg JS, Pavlov H, Genuario SE: Neurapraxia of the cervical spinal cord with transient quadriplegia. **J Bone Joint Surg Am** 68:1354–1370, 1986.
13. Torg JS, Ramsey-Emrhein JA: Suggested management guidelines for participation in collision activities with congenital, developmental, or post-injury lesions involving the cervical spine. **Med Sci Sports Exerc** 29:S256–S272, 1997.
14. Torg JS, Sennett B, Pavlov H, Leventhal MR, Glasgow SG: Spear tackler's spine. An entity precluding participation in tackle football and collision activities that expose the spine to axial energy inputs. **Am J Sports Med** 21:640–649, 1993.

15. Vaccaro AR, Watkins R, Albert TJ, Pfaff WL, Klein GR, Silber JS: Cervical spine injuries in athletes: current return to play criteria. **Orthopedics** 24(7):699–703, 2001.
16. Weinstein SM: Assessment and rehabilitation of an athlete with a "stinger". A model for the management of noncatastrophic athletic cervical spine injury. **Clin Sports Med** 17:127–135, 1998.
17. White AA, Johnson RM, Panjabi MM, Southwick WO: Biomechanical analysis of clinical stability in the cervical spine. **Clin Orthop** 109:85–96, 1975.
18. Wilberger JE: Athletic spinal cord and spine injuries: guidelines for initial management. **Clin Sports Med** 17:111–120, 1998.

23

Spondylolysis and Spondylolisthesis in the Athlete

DAVID A. LUNDIN, M.D., DIANA B.WISEMAN, M.D.,
AND CHRISTOPHER I. SHAFFREY, M.D.

INTRODUCTION

Episodes of minor lower back pain (LBP) are a fairly common occurrence in recreational and competitive adolescent athletes (1). Most episodes of pain are brief, self-limited, and medical evaluation is infrequently obtained. While spondylolysis and spondylolisthesis are usually asymptomatic in the adult population, they are frequent causes of disabling LBP in young athletes. Spondylolysis and spondylolisthesis are responsible in less than 5% of all cases of adult low back pain but cause 15% of the LBP in competitive athletes in the second and third decades and almost 50% in adolescent athletes. In athletes greater than 40 years of age degenerative changes of the spine are the most likely causes of LBP. Degenerative spondylolisthesis can rarely be the source of LBP in the older athlete. Many different treatment regimens have been suggested with varying degrees of success for these conditions. This article represents a review of treatment options and gives suggested algorithms for treating spondylolysis and spondylolisthesis in the athlete.

EPIDEMIOLOGY AND CLASSIFICATION

The incidence of spondylolysis is reported to be between 3–7% (2–4). On review of 4200 cadaver spines, Roche and Rowe found that the incidence varies with race and gender. Caucasian males and females have a rate of 6.4% and 2.3% respectively while African-American males and females have a rate of 2.8% and 1.1% respectively. In general males are effected 2 to 3 times more commonly than females. Age beyond childhood does not appear to change the rate of occurrence (4). When spondylolysis is radiographically visible, there is an associated spondylolisthesis approximately 25% of the time. In one radiographic study of 500 newborns, no cases of spondylolysis were found (3). Rosenburg evaluated 143 adult patients who had been non-ambulatory their entire life and found no cases of pars defects (5). Among 500 6-year-olds, an overall incidence of 4.4% was found which increased to 6% by adulthood in the same population (3). Most cases likely develop during childhood and are associated with activity.

The higher incidence in the athletic population lends support to activity as a cause of the spondylolysis. Jackson studied 100 young female gymnasts and found an 11% rate, which is significantly higher than expected in population based studies previously performed (6). Rossi in a review of 1430 adolescent athletes noted a 15% incidence of spondylolysis, with wrestlers, gymnasts, divers and weight lifters representing a larger majority affected within this group (7). Soler evaluated 3152 athletes and found an overall incidence of 8.02%. Among the athletes, throwing sports (discus, shot put) had an incidence of 26.7%, gymnastics 16.9%, rowing 16.9% and swimming 10.2% (8). Jones reviewed pre-participation radiographs of Division 1 college football players and compared them to controls. He found comparable rates among athletes and controls. The rate of spondylolysis was 4.8% in athletes and 6% in controls, while the rate of spondylolisthesis was 3.8% in athletes and 3.6% in controls (9) Other studies have reported 10.1–50% spondylolysis rates for down-lineman. Micheli and Wood evaluated adolescents presenting for low back pain (LBP) to a sports medicine clinic compared to a control population of adults with LBP and found 47% of the adolescents had spondylolysis in comparison to 5% of adults (10). Shaffer reviewed questionnaires completed by NFL and 25 top NCAA team physicians. The known prevalence of spondylolisthesis was 1%. Of patients with symptomatic spondylolisthesis who underwent fusion 50% returned to participate (11).

The majority of spondylitic defects occur at the L5 level, 85–95%, while the next most common level is L4, 5–15% (12). Wiltse in 1976 classified spondylolysis and spondylolisthesis into one of five types.

- Type I: dysplastic–due to congenital defects of L5 and/or the upper sacrum.
- Type II: isthmic–3 subtypes exist: (a) lytic lesion–fatigue fracture of the pars, (b) elongated intact pars, (c) acute fracture. Type II lesions represent the majority of the pathology involved in clinically symptomatic spondylolysis of adolescents.
- Type III: degenerative.
- Type IV: traumatic–an acute fracture elsewhere in the neural arch other than the pars.
- Type V: pathological–for example metastatic disease (13).

PRESENTATION AND DIAGNOSIS

The majority of spondylolysis cases are asymptomatic. When clinically symptomatic, patients often describe low back pain that may radiate into the buttock or proximal lower extremities. Physical exam findings include hyperlordotic posture with tight hamstrings. Hyperextension and rotation may aggravate symptoms as may standing on one leg while leaning backwards.

Radiographic evaluation begins with plain radiographs. AP, lateral and bilateral oblique radiographs make up the basic set of evaluation films. On plain oblique films the pars lesion is described as a collar on the "Scotty dog." Amato found that a spot lateral view of the lumbosacral junction was the most sensitive view in his series of radiographs, disclosing the defect 84% of the time (2). Bone scan is often positive in new lesions but negative in long-term lesions. Bone scan may be helpful identifying symptomatic pars lesions by increased activity at the defect. CT scan is more sensitive than plain films or nuclear medicine studies on identifying pars lesions, but is not considered 100 % sensitive or specific. SPECT (single photon emission computed tomography) has advantages over bone scan and plain ra-

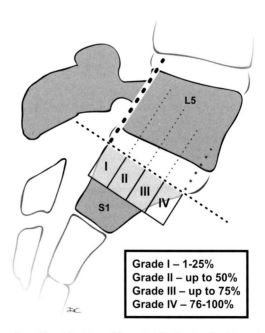

Grade I – 1-25%
Grade II – up to 50%
Grade III – up to 75%
Grade IV – 76-100%

FIG. 23.1 Meyerding Classification of Spondylolisthesis. Grading of spondylolisthesis is measured as a percentage anterior slippage relative to the antero-posterior diameter of the sacrum.

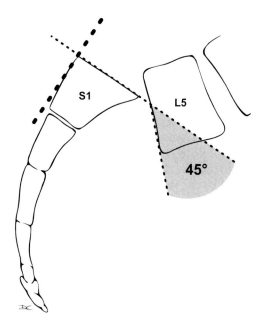

FIG. 23.2 Slip Angle. Measured as the intersection of a line drawn parallel to the L5 superior endplate and one drawn perpendicular to a line along the posterior cortex of the S1 and S2 bodies.

diographs. Unfortunately SPECT has greater sensitivity than specificity for demonstrating a pars defect. MRI has a less defined role in imaging pars lesions, but helps evaluate other possible pathology such as disc herniation, disc degeneration, annular disruption or the presence of infection or tumor.

When spondylolisthesis is present, the Meyerding classification is used to grade it. On viewing lateral plain radiographs the anterior-posterior diameter of the superior surface of the vertebra is divided into quarters. A grade of I to IV is assigned based on slippage of 1 to 4 quarters of the A-P diameter *(Fig. 23.1)*. Slip angle, a measure of the kyphosis caused by the spondylolisthesis is also measured and described. The angle is the intersection of a line drawn parallel to the L5 superior endplate and one drawn perpendicular to a line along the posterior cortex of the S1 and S2 bodies *(Fig. 23.2)*.

RISK OF PROGRESSION

The risk of progression of spondylolisthesis depends on a number of factors. Younger age (decreased skeletal maturity), slip of greater than

50%, slip angle greater than 40 to 50 degrees (0–10 degrees is normal), female, dome shaped sacrum and dysplastic vs. isthmic spondylosis. Multiple studies have looked at factors associated with risk of progression. Bladburne noted than no patient with a slip less than 30% progressed to beyond 30%. Progressive slippage that did occur was predominantly noted during puberty and had an association with spina bifida occulta (14). Saraste, in a study of 255 patients followed for minimum 20 years, noted a mean slip progression of 4 mm with 11% of adolescents and 5% of adults progressing to more than 10 mm (15). Muschik reported on 86 young athletes, 6–20 years old, with spondylolysis or listhesis. 12% of patients showed a slip progression of more than 10 % over a period of 4.8 years. Progression of greater than 20% occurred in 1 of 86 patients. The mean initial degree of slip was 10.1%. 47% of patients had no progression, 44% had slip progression and 9% improved. An increased risk of progression was found during puberty and with an increased slip angle and sacral inclination. No increased risk was associated with spina bifida occulta or continued activity (16).

TREATMENT

Although the majority of the cases of spondylolysis are asymptomatic, and require no treatment, occasionally these lesions can be associated with significant low back pain. This is often the case with adolescent and young adult athletes who ultimately present to spine surgeons with complaints of severe focal low back pain that can be debilitating and prevents participation in sporting activities. The pain is often exacerbated with activities involving lumbar extension and rotation, and occasionally can extend into the buttock or proximal lower extremities, though true radiculopathy is less common (17). True radicular symptoms require evaluation for disc herniation, foraminal stenosis or significant instability and radiographic evaluation including dynamic radiographs and a MRI should be considered. The presence of decreased flexibility and tight hamstrings often leads to more frequent muscle strains (12, 18). The combination of these findings often limits physical function and optimal performance in athletic programs. Therefore, all treatment options aim to relieve pain, optimize physical function, and promote bony healing of the underlying defect of the pars interarticularis.

We propose a treatment protocol based on a review of the literature and our clinical experience in treating athletes with symptomatic spondylolysis with or without spondylolisthesis. Reviews of the literature on standard treatment of spondylolysis and spondylolisthesis can be confusing because the natural history of symptoms in the athlete is not clearly defined. Considerable debate exists over the indications for non-operative treatment including the indications for bracing, the type of brace that is best tolerated and best relieves symptoms, the value of physical therapy, the timing of return to athletic training and the time period required to define a failure of non-operative therapy.

A variety of treatment options have been effectively demonstrated in the literature and clear superiority of a specific treatment regimen has not been defined. Finally the medical literature is often confounded with clinical reviews which have involved diverse groups of patient that often mix groups containing children, adolescents and adults, as well as a variety in the types and degrees of the spondylolisthesis treated. Despite this, we have determined an effective and thoughtful model on how the athlete with a symptomatic pars defect should be approached. As outlined, the treatment of children and adolescents differs from young adults *(Figs. 23.3 and 23.4)*.

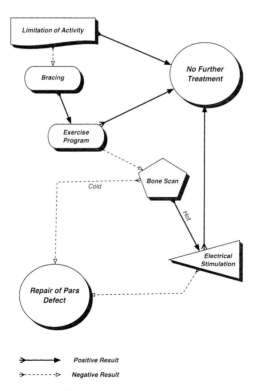

FIG. 23.3 Spondylolysis in Children and Adolescents. Typical flow chart describes steps in work-up and treatment of children and adolescents with symptomatic spondylolysis and/or spondylolisthesis. Solid arrows denote positive or effective results while broken arrows represent negative or failed results unless otherwise specified.

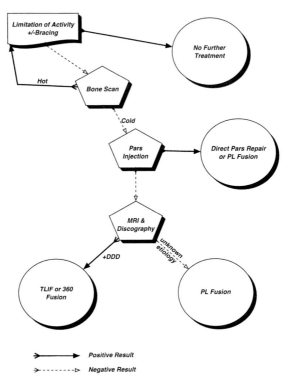

FIG. 23.4 Spondylolysis in Young Adults. Typical flow chart describes steps in work-up and treatment of young adults with symptomatic spondylolysis and/or spondylolis-thesis. Solid arrows denote positive or effective results while broken arrows represent negative or failed results unless otherwise specified.

Initial treatment options focus on non-operative management, with surgical intervention being reserved for definite failure of those treated with limitation of activity, bracing and a rehabilitation program as defined below. Initial treatment plans encompass some degree of activity restriction, which is usually defined as restriction from current sporting activities. Specific restriction of activities resulting in repetitive flexion, extension and rotation of the lumbar spine are specifically restricted in the early treatment phase. Thoracolumbosacral bracing and abdominal strengthening exercises often supplements these programs.

Steiner and Micheli reported on 67 patients with spondylolysis or low grade spondylolisthesis whom they treated in a modified Boston brace for 6 months followed by a 6-month weaning period in which physical therapy and gradual return to athletics was allowed (19).

They noted an 18% rate of bony healing, though 78% of patients had good to excellent clinical results including full return to activity.

Blanda and colleagues reported their experience treating young athletes with pars defects (20). Initially all patients were managed with activity restriction and bracing for 2 to 6 months followed by a gradual exercise and stretching program. Radiographic union of these defects was noted in 37% of patients. However, only 15% of patients failed non-operative management after greater than 6 months without relief, and therefore required surgical intervention. Notably, 96% of all patients had a good or excellent result as determined by return to normal activity and either no lumbago or minimal symptoms with strenuous activity.

In a study of 185 adolescent athletes with spondylolysis, Morita and associates further classified pars defects with plain radiographs and CT as early, progressive, or terminal stage (21). Patients were then restricted from sporting activity and braced with a conventional lumbar corset for 3 to 6 months, followed by rehabilitation and bracing with an extension limiting corset. They confirmed bony fusion with follow up imaging in 37.9% of all patients. They noted however, that 73% of early stage defects, 38.5% of progressive stage, and 0% of terminal stage defects healed. They concluded that pars defects diagnosed in early stages could be effectively treated using conservative measures.

Our preference is a Boston brace that is generally the most commonly used brace used today for this condition (18). It is molded to a $0°$ lordosis to help reduce the load on the posterior elements and is usually worn 23 hours a day for at least 4 months, though 6–9 months of bracing may be required in some cases (10, 19).

In children, patients who have significant or complete resolution of symptoms after such conservative measures, a gradual reconditioning program in initiated prior to the return to routine sporting activities. A physical therapy program focusing on stretching the lumbodorsal fascia, strengthening the paraspinous and abdominal musculature without hyperextension of the spine is performed. Following reconditioning, the asymptomatic patient is allowed a gradual return to full athletic activity. However, for those patients who fail such treatment or develop a recurrence of symptoms after resumption of athletic activity, further evaluation is warranted.

We recommend a bone scan as the first level of investigation. Bone scans and single photon emission computed tomography (SPECT) can detect early stress fractures of the pars interarticularis, and determine whether the injury is acute or chronic in nature. An acute spondylolysis has greater potential for healing than with chronic processes. In our younger patients (<21 years old), a positive bone scan after failure of bracing and recondition is followed by a second course of activity restriction and bracing in combination with electrical stimulation.

The addition of external electrical stimulation in promoting healing of pars defects has gained attention in recent years. The first indication that this technology might be successful in promoting healing of a pars defect was its effect on improving healing after other types of spinal fusion. Mooney tested the effect pulsed electromagnetic fields had on interbody lumbar fusions in 195 patients operated for various diagnosis, including spondylolisthesis (22). In patients who had actively used the electromagnetic device in addition to standard bracing, he observed a 92.2% fusion rate in comparison to the control groups, which had a 67.9% fusion rate. These encouraging results lead us to use electrical stimulation in combination with bracing to treat spondylolysis in adolescent athletes. Pettine and colleagues treated an adolescent athlete with acute spondylolysis with intermittent bracing and daily external electric stimulation, noting progressive bony healing within 3 months of starting electrical treatments (23). In a similar study, Fellander-Tsai and Micheli treated two patients successfully with bracing and electric stimulation who had previously failed conservative treatment without such stimulation (24). Though further studies are needed to clearly evaluate the overall efficacy of electrical stimulation to promote bony healing of pars defects, we often find it to be of clinical utility and without significant drawbacks. In young adults however, electrical stimulation has not been clearly defined and therefore, only continual bracing and activity restriction is recommended.

The vast majority of patients with spondylolysis and many patients with spondylolisthesis can be managed non-operatively. The reported incidence of cases that ultimately require surgery has varied from 9–53%. (12, 17, 19, 20, 25).Traditionally, intertransverse fusion procedures have been performed in children, adolescent, and adults who have failed non-operative treatment. Indications for surgery include: uncontrolled pain or major symptoms despite activity modification and bracing, slip greater than 50% or progressive slip from 25-50%, high slip angle greater than 30% with significant growth remaining, presence of sciatic scoliosis, or progressive neurological deficit (16).

Non-operative management of spondylolysis and spondylolisthesis generally has a greater likelihood of returning the athlete to their previous level of performance. Some studies appear to indicate that there is a selection process that occurs in elite level athletes where incidence of spondylolysis and spondylolisthesis is reduced when higher levels of performance is required. Shaffer and colleagues studied the prevalence of spondylolisthesis in the top 25 NCAA Division I college football teams and all 28 NFL teams through questionnaires submitted to team physicians. Although many authors have reported a high prevalence of spondylolysis and spondylolisthesis among football players, Shaffer found that only 0.9% of college athletes and 1.5% of NFL players had a known deformity. Furthermore, 96% of NFL team physicians stated that they downgraded players with known spondylolisthesis during the annual draft, suggesting these players are eliminated from participation prior to entering the professional arena (11). It appears there are few professional athletes who have had spinal surgery for correction of a spondylolysis or spondylolisthesis. In his study, Shaffer found six college players who had had surgery for spondylolisthesis and only two NFL players with prior surgery. Of these eight patients, only 50% of them were able to return to participate at the same level. Given these facts, surgical correction should be the last resort and performed only after all other treatment options are exhausted.

In selected cases, less invasive surgical approaches, such as decompression alone or direct pars interarticularis repair can be an effective alternative to traditional spinal fusion and can maintain the integrity of the motion segment. The use of decompression alone has been advocated some authors especially if an isolated radiculopathy alone exists. Lapras used simple decompression in 45 patients with grade I and II spondylolisthesis and obtained 68% good and excellent results. However, this technique has a high risk of progressive slippage in children, and is therefore not generally advocated. In fact, 44 of the patients operated on by Lapras and colleagues were adults (26). We will occasionally perform a partial hemilaminectomy and foraminotomy in adult patients with spondylolysis or grade I spondylolisthesis with no motion on dynamic radiographs that have radiculopathy without significant back pain.

Selected young patients (<25 years old) with spondylolysis or grade I spondylolisthesis who fail nonoperative management are considered for repair the pars defects primarily. Several studies have demonstrated the efficacy of direct repair of pars defects in this patient population (27–29). Buck originally described repair of defects in the pars interarticularis in 1970 (30). The advantage of such procedures is that it preserves the anatomic integrity and motion of the affected segment. In a recent study, Dai and associates examined the efficacy of direct pars repair in 46 patients with lumbar spondylolysis or mild (Meyerding grade I or II) isthmic spondylolisthesis (27). They attained an excellent or good functional outcome in 93.4% of all patients. No significant improvement was found with the addition of facet fusion. They, however, noted that the success of such a procedure was highly dependent on the presence of normal adjacent disks as assessed by

MRI. This is based on the notion that in the presence of significant disk degeneration, the segment with the spondylolysis or spondylolisthesis is predisposed to instability, and bony fusion is impaired. Szypryt stated that given the increased degree of disk degeneration of the affected spinal segment with age, segmental fusion is recommended in patients over the age of 25 years old with spondylolysis or spondylolisthesis (31). Kakiuchi described results in patients with spondylolysis and spondylolisthesis using a variable angle screw in the pedicle and a laminar hook compressing across the pars defect (29). The authors have frequently employed a similar technique with great success *(Figs. 23.5 and 23.6)*. Use of direct repair of the pars interarticularis in cases of multilevel pars defects has been reported (32). Although this technique is very effective in the general adolescent and young adult population, there is no literature describing its effectiveness in competitive athletes.

Early disk degeneration in athletes with spondylolysis and spondylolisthesis is commonly seen. The authors order a MRI scan in all pa-

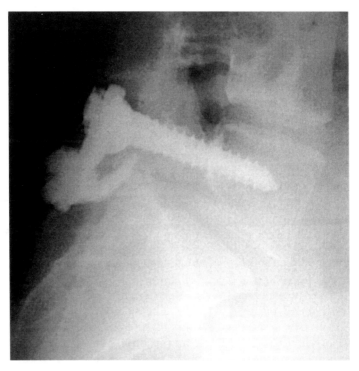

FIG. 23.5 Postoperative Lateral Radiograph of Direct Pars Repair. Pedicle screws and a laminar hook are used to compress across the pars defect.

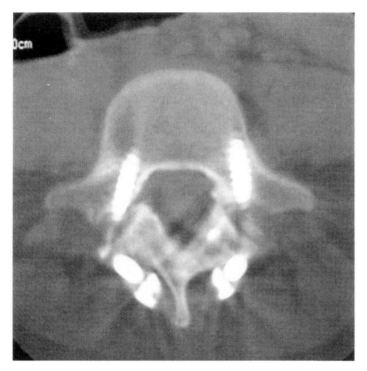

FIG. 23.6 Postoperative Axial CT Scan of Direct Pars Repair. Construct shows complete reduction of pars defect.

tients considered for a pars interarticularis repair to assess the hydration and integrity of the discs at the level of the pars defect and the adjacent segments. If any question exists about the disc as a pain source, we routinely perform direct pars injection with local anesthetic in the course of our surgical evaluation. Wu and colleagues showed that patients with a positive pars injection were highly likely to have a good or excellent outcome with operative repair. In their evaluation of 100 patents that had positive pars injections, as defined by reproduction of the patient's similar pain with needle insertion, and at least 70% pain relief for more than six hours, 85 patients (91.3%) had good or excellent outcomes after an average of 30.4 months (25). In patients without relief of symptoms with a pars injection, other sources of pain such as intervertebral disc disruption or facet joint arthropathy must be considered. Further investigation such as discography might be warranted. In cases of substantial disc degeneration or segmental instability posterolateral fusion with or without instrumentation is the procedure of choice.

Non-instrumented (*in situ*) posterolateral fusion is also effective option is some cases of spondylolysis and spondylolisthesis especially in younger patients (children and adolescents). This procedure has been shown to reduce symptoms in 70–100% of cases, though overall fusion rates are slightly lower and can range from 40–100% (33–38). Fusion rates are lower in patients with higher-grade spondylolisthesis especially with an increased slip angle. Traditionally non-instrumented procedures were managed with pantaloon spica casting until the fusion consolidated. There has been an increasing trend to the use of a thoracolumbar or thoracolumbosacral with thigh extension orthosis in this patient population. Although an effective modality of treatment most cases of spondylolisthesis, it frequently does not improve slip angle found in cases of higher-grade spondylolisthesis. We usually reduce the slip angle by preoperative traction and/or with the use of transpedicular instrumentation in this patient population. Though non-instrumented fusion can be accompanied with decompression, there remains a higher risk of slip progression and non-union. This is especially true for patients with a slip angle greater than 25 degrees, grade III and IV spondylolisthesis, presence of a trapezoidal L5 segment or dome shaped sacrum, or hyperlordotic (>50%) lumbar spine (35, 36, 38–44).

The advent and success of instrumented fusions for other spinal disorders has led to several authors advocating various combinations of such procedures for spondylolisthesis. Posterior segmental instrumentation and fusion can be performed with or without reduction and has the benefit over non-instrumented fusion in that it permits correction of the slip angle which improves body posture and mechanics. Instrumentation increases fusion rate in higher-grade spondylolisthesis while allowing full neural decompression. Molinari noted that non-instrumented arthrodesis had a higher nonunion rate compared with patients with posterior segmental instrumentation or after circumferential procedures in high-grade spondylolisthesis patient (45). In adults with grade I or II isthmic spondylolisthesis, the advantages of instrumentation are less clear-cut. In a recent prospective randomized study, Moller and Hedlund compared the role of instrumented versus non-instrumented posterolateral fusion in 77 patients with isthmic spondylolisthesis and greater than 1 year for low back pain or sciatica (46). They included patients 18 to 55 years of age and those with grades I, II, and III spondylolisthesis. Counterintuitively, radiographic fusion was higher (78%) in the non-instrumented patients vs. those instrumented groups (65%). Although pain and disability indices were significantly improved in both groups, there were no significant differences between groups. Further, blood loss and operating time was longer in instrumented patients and two patients (5.4%) had pedicle screw related nerve root injuries. Despite the lack of clear-cut evidence, the authors utilize transpedicular instrumentation in cases of grade III or greater spondylolisthesis, in cases where the slip angle is greater than 30 degrees and in most patients requiring an inter-transverse fusion greater than 18 years of age.

In cases of high-grade spondylolisthesis the chances of returning to high performance athletics is low. Treatment of high-grade spondylolisthesis may require the use of anterior or combined anterior/posterior procedures to relieve symptoms and obtain a solid arthrodesis (45) *(Figs. 23.7 and 23.8)*. The addition of anterior procedures allows the fusion to heal under compression, and is frequently used as a salvage procedure for failed posterior fusions. Theoretically, additional complications, such as retrograde ejaculation can occur, though the overall incidence has not been quantified. Muschik retrospectively evaluated the use of anterior in situ fusion versus anterior spondylodesis with posterior transpedicular instrumentation and reduction

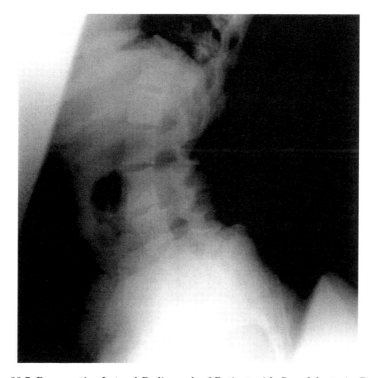

FIG. 23.7 Preoperative Lateral Radiograph of Patient with Spondyloptosis. Demonstrates greater than 100% slip with a slip angle of approximately 72 degrees.

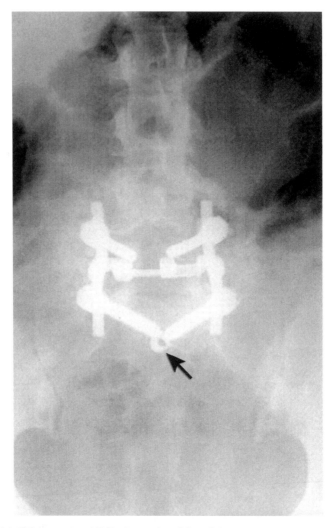

FIG. 23.8 Postoperative A/P Radiographs of Spondyloptosis Repair. Demonstrate correction of slip angle and partial reduction of spondyloptosis. Arrow demonstrates fibular allograft placed through sacrum into the instrumented L5 vertebral body.

and found significantly lower rates of pseudarthrosis, reduced degree of slip, reduced lumbosacral kyphosis, and decreased fusion time in patients with transpedicular instrumentation. Although there was a trend toward improved clinical outcome in combined approaches, with 87% patients symptom free at follow-up versus 69% using anterior approaches only, this difference was not statistically significant.

THE OLDER ATHLETE

Lower back pain in the older athlete (>45 years old) is frequently related to degenerative changes of the functional spinal unit and may have components of disc degeneration, facet joint arthropathy, spinal stenosis or degenerative spondylolisthesis. There is even less literature regarding the optimal treatment of athletes in this population group. In patients with spondylolisthesis a major consideration is the presence or absence of a neurological deficit. As is the case for younger patients, non-operative management gives the greatest chance of return to vigorous athletics. A description of the non-operative management of the various degenerative conditions affecting the lumbar spine in the older athlete is beyond the scope of this review. Surgery is usually reserved for patients with a radiculopathy, neurogenic claudication and/or a neurological deficit. Our surgical management of degenerative spondylolisthesis in the older athlete parallels the operative management described by Watkins (47). Decompression, but not fusion, is performed in fixed (no motion of dynamic radiographs) grade I lesions. An instrumented arthrosis is performed in grade I lesions if there is >3.5 mm of slippage or greater than 10 degrees of angulation on dynamic radiographs and in all grade II lesions.

REHABILITATION AFTER SPINE SURGERY

One goal of surgery is to allow patients the potential to return to the sporting activities they desire. The question as to when the athlete can return to sports after spinal surgery is dependent on a number of different factors. These include the patient's diagnosis, age, and general medical condition, type of surgery performed, and ultimately, the type of sporting activity desired (47). Given this multifactorial approach, it is difficult to prescribe a set protocol for all patients. However, as a rule of thumb, we typically restrict activity to those required for routine tasks for a period of 6 weeks, allowing lifting of no more than 5 pounds. For more complex spinal fusion procedures, we occasionally extend this period to 3 months. After this initial period of activity restriction, the post-operative rehabilitation program begins with neutral positioning and isometric strengthening. The goal is to regain proper muscle control and strength to the trunk. Once this is obtained, we slowly progress though range of motion activities that mimic those required in the sport of choice. This is done under the auspices of our physical therapist and rehabilitation medicine colleagues. If the patient demonstrates adequate strength and mobility in these exercises, they can then safely return to a gradual return to sports.

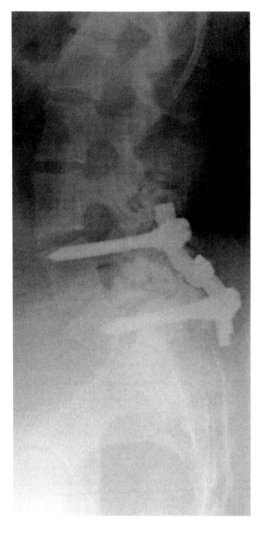

FIG. 23.9 Postoperative Lateral Radiographs of Spondyloptosis Repair. Demonstrate correction of slip angle and partial reduction of spondyloptosis. Arrow demonstrates fibular allograft placed through sacrum into the instrumented L5 vertebral body.

CONCLUSION

In summary, the majority of cases of spondylolysis or isthmic spondylolisthesis in athletes is asymptomatic and requires no treatment. The childhood, adolescent, or young adult athletes are at higher risk for development of symptoms than the general population and these conditions can impair optimal performance in sporting events. Usually, nonoperative measures that include activity restriction and bracing are all that are needed to eliminate symptoms. It is unusual to have younger athletes present with significant radicular pair or a neurological deficit and further investigation including an MRI should be considered in these cases. Surgical intervention is reserved for a clear failure of nonoperative management. The range of such procedures is dependent on the age of the patient, the presence of neurological deficit and the specific type of lesion present. If treated appropriately, most patients do well from a clinical perspective and should be able to return to athletics.

REFERENCES

1. Balague F, Dutoit G, Waldburger M: Low back pain in schoolchildren. An epidemiological study. **Scand J Rehabil Med** 20(4):175–179, 1988.
2. Amato M, Totty WG, Gilula LA: Spondylolysis of the lumbar spine: demonstration of defects and laminal fragmentation. **Radiology** 153(3): 627–629, 1984.
3. Fredrickson BE, et al: The natural history of spondylolysis and spondylolisthesis. **J Bone Joint Surg Am** 66(5):699–707, 1984.
4. Roche MA, et al: The incidence of separate neural arch and coincident bone variations: a survey of 4,200 skeletons. **Anat Rec** 109:233–252, 1951.
5. Rosenberg NJ, Bargar WL, Friedman B: The incidence of spondylolysis and spondylolisthesis in nonambulatory patients. **Spine** 6(1):35–38, 1981.
6. Jackson DW, Wiltse LL, Cirincoine RJ: Spondylolysis in the female gymnast. **Clin Orthop** 117:68–73, 1976.
7. Rossi F: Spondylolysis, spondylolisthesis and sports. **J Sports Med Phys Fitness** 18(4):317–340, 1978.
8. Soler T, Calderon C: The prevalence of spondylolysis in the Spanish elite athlete. **Am J Sports Med** 28(1):57–62, 2000.
9. Jones DM, et al: Radiographic abnormalities of the lumbar spine in college football players. A comparative analysis. **Am J Sports Med** 27(3):335–338, 1999.
10. Micheli LJ, Wood R: Back pain in young athletes. Significant differences from adults in causes and patterns. **Arch Pediatr Adolesc Med** 149(1):15–18, 1995.
11. Shaffer B, Wiesel S, Lauerman W: Spondylolisthesis in the elite football player: an epidemiologic study in the NCAA and NFL. **J Spinal Disord** 10(5):365–370, 1997.
12. Standaert CJ, Herring SA: Spondylolysis: a critical review. **Br J Sports Med** 34(6):415–422, 2000.
13. Wiltse LL, Newman PH, Macnab I: Classification of spondylolisis and spondylolisthesis. **Clin Orthop** 117:23–29, 1976.
14. Blackburne JS, Velikas EP: Spondylolisthesis in children and adolescents. **J Bone Joint Surg Br** 59-B(4):490–494, 1977.
15. Saraste H: Long-term clinical and radiological follow-up of spondylolysis and spondylolisthesis. **J Pediatr Orthop** 7(6):631–638, 1987.
16. Muschik M, et al: Competitive sports and the progression of spondylolisthesis. **J Pediatr Orthop** 16(3):364–369, 1996.
17. Standaert CJ, et al: Spondylolysis. **Phys Med Rehabil Clin North Am** 11(4):785–803, 2000.
18. Omey ML, Micheli LJ, Gerbino PG 2nd: Idiopathic scoliosis and spondylolysis in the female athlete. Tips for treatment. **Clin Orthop** 372:74–84, 2000.
19. Steiner ME, Micheli LJ: Treatment of symptomatic spondylolysis and spondylolisthesis with the modified Boston brace. **Spine** 10(10):937–943, 1985.
20. Blanda J, et al: Defects of pars interarticularis in athletes: a protocol for nonoperative treatment. **J Spinal Disord** 6(5):406–411, 1993.

21. Morita T, et al: Lumbar spondylolysis in children and adolescents. **J Bone Joint Surg Br** 77(4):620–625, 1995.
22. Mooney V: A randomized double-blind prospective study of the efficacy of pulsed electromagnetic fields for interbody lumbar fusions. **Spine** 15(7):708–712, 1990.
23. Pettine KA, Salib RM, Walker SG: External electrical stimulation and bracing for treatment of spondylolysis. A case report. **Spine** 18(4):436–439, 1993.
24. Fellander-Tsai L, Micheli LJ: Treatment of spondylolysis with external electrical stimulation and bracing in adolescent athletes: a report of two cases. **Clin J Sport Med** 8(3):232–234, 1998.
25. Wu SS, Lee CH, Chen PQ: Operative repair of symptomatic spondylolysis following a positive response to diagnostic pars injection. **J Spinal Disord** 12(1):10–16, 1999.
26. Lapras C, et al: [Treatment of spondylolisthesis (stage I-II) by neurosurgical decompression without either osteosynthesis or reduction]. **Neurochirurgie** 30(3):147–152, 1984.
27. Dai LY, et al: Direct repair of defect in lumbar spondylolysis and mild isthmic spondylolisthesis by bone grafting, with or without facet joint fusion. **Eur Spine J** 10(1):78–83, 2001.
28. Gillet P, Petit M: Direct repair of spondylolysis without spondylolisthesis, using a rod-screw construct and bone grafting of the pars defect. **Spine** 24(12):1252–1256, 1999.
29. Kakiuchi M: Repair of the defect in spondylolysis. Durable fixation with pedicle screws and laminar hooks. **J Bone Joint Surg Am** 79(6):818–825, 1997.
30. Buck JE: Direct repair of the defect in spondylolisthesis. Preliminary report. **J Bone Joint Surg Br** 52(3):432–437, 1970.
31. Szypryt EP, et al: The prevalence of disc degeneration associated with neural arch defects of the lumbar spine assessed by magnetic resonance imaging. **Spine** 14(9):977–981, 1989.
32. Eingorn D, Pizzutillo PD: Pars interarticularis fusion of multiple levels of lumbar spondylolysis. A case report. **Spine** 10(3):250–252, 1985.
33. Harris IE, Weinstein SL: Long-term follow-up of patients with grade-III and IV spondylolisthesis. Treatment with and without posterior fusion. **J Bone Joint Surg Am** 69(7):960–969, 1987.
34. Freeman BL 3rd, Donati NL: Spinal arthrodesis for severe spondylolisthesis in children and adolescents. A long-term follow-up study. **J Bone Joint Surg Am** 71(4):594–598, 1989.
35. Johnson JR, Kirwan EO: The long-term results of fusion in situ for severe spondylolisthesis. **J Bone Joint Surg Br** 65(1):43–46, 1983.
36. Laurent LE, Osterman K: Operative treatment of spondylolisthesis in young patients. **Clin Orthop** 117:85–91, 1976.
37. Hensinger RN, Langm JR, MacEwen GD: Surgical management of spondylolisthesis in children and adolescents. **Spine** 1(4):206–216, 1976.
38. Burkus JK, et al: Long-term evaluation of adolescents treated operatively for spondylolisthesis. A comparison of in situ arthrodesis only with in situ arthrodesis and reduction followed by immobilization in a cast. **J Bone Joint Surg Am** 74(5):693–704, 1992.
39. Dimar JR, Hoffman G: Grade 4 spondylolisthesis. Two-stage therapeutic approach of anterior vertebrectomy and anterior-posterior fusion. **Orthop Rev** 15(8):504–509, 1986.
40. Carragee EJ: Single-level posterolateral arthrodesis, with or without posterior decompression, for the treatment of isthmic spondylolisthesis in adults. A prospective, randomized study. **J Bone Joint Surg Am** 79(8):1175–1180, 1997

41. Matthiass HH, Heine J: The surgical reduction of spondylolisthesis. **Clin Orthop** 203:34–44, 1986.
42. Schnee CL, Freese A, Ansell LV: Outcome analysis for adults with spondylolisthesis treated with posterolateral fusion and transpedicular screw fixation. **J Neurosurg** 86(1):56–63, 1997.
43. Bassewitz H, Herkowitz H: Lumbar stenosis with spondylolisthesis: current concepts of surgical treatment. **Clin Orthop** 384:54–60, 2001.
44. Fischgrund JS, et al: 1997 Volvo Award winner in clinical studies. Degenerative lumbar spondylolisthesis with spinal stenosis: a prospective, randomized study comparing decompressive laminectomy and arthrodesis with and without spinal instrumentation. **Spine** 22(24):2807–2812, 1997.
45. Molinari RW, et al: Complications in the surgical treatment of pediatric high-grade, isthmic dysplastic spondylolisthesis. A comparison of three surgical approaches. Spine 24(16):1701–1711, 1999.
46. Moller H, Hedlund R:Instrumented and noninstrumented posterolateral fusion in adult spondylolisthesis—a prospective randomized study: part 2. Spine 25(13):1716–1721, 2000.
47. Watkins RG, Campbell DR: The older athlete after lumbar spine surgery. Clin Sports Med 10(2):391–399, 1991.

CHAPTER

24

Energy Sources in the Posterior Fossa: The Role of Radiosurgery

DOUGLAS KONDZIOLKA, M.D., JOHN C. FLICKINGER, M.D., AND L. DADE LUNSFORD, M.D.

INTRODUCTION

Stereotactic radiosurgery can be used to treat a variety of disorders that occur within the posterior fossa of the brain. Over the last 30 years, radiosurgery has proven effective for patients with selective vascular malformations, benign or malignant tumors, and some functional disorders such as trigeminal neuralgia. In the posterior fossa, the role of radiosurgery is defined by a number of factors. These include lesion diagnosis, other available therapies, the risks and benefits of different management strategies, brain location, or relationship to specific cranial nerves, volume of brain stem parenchyma involved, extension outside the posterior fossa contents, and patient goals and expectations. We will discuss the role of radiosurgery for different disorders in the context of all of these clinical issues. At the University of Pittsburgh, stereotactic radiosurgery has been used since August 1987 in over 4,500 patients. A listing of those disorders in the posterior fossa is shown in *Table 24.1*. The technique of radiosurgery has evolved over time but the lessons learned regarding the radiation tolerance of different brain structures remains consistent.

ARTERIOVENOUS MALFORMATIONS

Arteriovenous malformations (AVM) that involve the parenchyma of the brain stem or cerebellum may be suitable candidates for radiosurgery particularly when the lesion volume is relatively small. For AVMs within the brainstem parenchyma, surgical resection may be associated with such high risk that it is not a desired treatment approach. The proximity of small perforating arteries and the variable blood supply to the brainstem may make endovascular embolization problematic and often not associated with cure. Thus, radiosurgery is

TABLE 24.1
Posterior Fossa Radiosurgery at the
University of Pittsburgh (n = 1925)

Diagnosis	Number of Patients
AVM	107
Cavernous malformation	53
Vestibular schwannoma	700
Other schwannoma	51
Meningioma	329
Brain metastasis	139
Glial neoplasms	68
Hemangioblastoma	24
Chordoma/chondrosarcoma	34
Glomus tumor	10
Trigeminal neuralgia	410

an attractive treatment for brainstem AVMs and is a valuable alternative for selected patients with cerebellar AVMs (1–10).

In a recent analysis, we reviewed brainstem AVMs from several centers (47). These include AVMs in the midbrain ($n = 52$), pons ($n = 22$), middle cerebellar peduncle ($n = 7$), and medulla oblongata ($n = 6$). Forty-six patients had at least 2 years imaging follow-up. Complete obliteration was found in 29 patients (63%), and subtotal obliteration in 16 (35%). Evaluations were made with angiography or MRI. Three patients had a hemorrhage after radiosurgery, and two recovered fully. One patient with a hemorrhage died. The lower obliteration rate when compared to non-brainstem AVMs is a reflection of the modest dose reduction necessary in this brain location.

We performed radiosurgery in 65 patients with cerebellar arteriovenous malformations. These lesions varied widely in size, and included some patients with large malformations who had undergone prior embolization or resection. Dose selection is more consistent with supratentorial malformations, and is not so limited as with brainstem AVMs, unless the anterior margin of the AVM involves the brainstem parenchyma. The highest obliteration rates are found after radiosurgery for the smaller AVMs, where a margin dose of at least 20 Gy can be administered safely.

CAVERNOUS MALFORMATIONS

At our center, radiosurgery is used for symptomatic patients with hemorrhagic cavernous malformations who have usually sustained two or more symptomatic hemorrhages (11). The vast majority of our patients have had cavernous malformations in the brainstem because surgical resection was found to be associated with high risk. Most of these malformations have been of relatively small volume. Initial flexion of the radiosurgical dose was based upon little prior available information. In early experience, the dose of the margin of the malformation varied from 16 to 20 Gy. At present, this dose varies from 13 to 16 Gy for most patients (12). A decrease in the delivered dose has not been associated with an increase in the hemorrhage rate, but has been associated with a decrease in complications. The brainstem cavernous malformation radiosurgery can be difficult since the target vol-

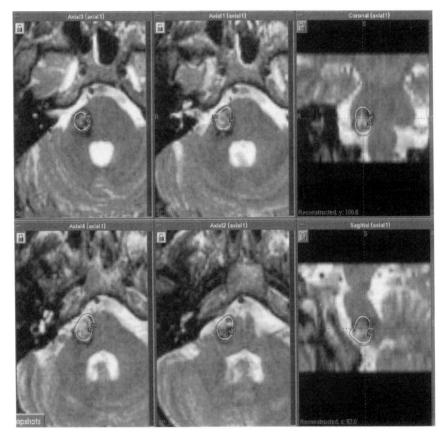

Fig. 24.1 MR images at radiosurgery using long relaxation time sequences. This 45-year-old woman with a cavernous malformation of the pons had a history of multiple symptomatic hemorrhages. The 50% peripheral isodose line was kept inside the hemosiderin rim to deliver a dose of 15 Gy.

ume is not seen on angiography and poorly demonstrated by CT scan. Stereotactic magnetic resonance imaging (MRI) is necessary to identify the core of the malformation *(Fig. 24.1)*. Usually, the peripheral radiation isodose is kept within the hemosiderin ring that surrounds the malformation. Any small blood clots that may be eccentric to the malformation are usually not irradiated.

We reviewed pre and post Gamma knife radiosurgery data on 82 patients managed between 1987 and 2000. Most patients had multiple hemorrhages from brainstem or diencephalic cavernous malformations. Follow-up data was examined to identify hemorrhages and an overall hemorrhage rate was calculated. Observation prior to treatment averaged 4.33 years (range 0.17–18 years) for a total of 354 patient years. During this period, 202 hemorrhages were observed for an annual hemorrhage rate of 33.9%, excluding the first hemorrhage. Temporal clustering of hemorrhages was not significant. After radiosurgery, patient follow-up averaged 5 years (range, 0.42–12.08 years), for a total of 401 patient years. During this period, 18 hemorrhages were identified, 16 in the first 2 years post treatment and two after 2 years. The annual hemorrhage rate was 11.6% per year for the first 2 years after radiosurgery, followed by 0.76% per year from years 2–12. Twelve patients had new neurological symptoms without hemorrhage after radiosurgery (14.6%). The symptoms in nine of these patients were minor and five were temporary. Radiosurgery confers a dramatic reduction in the risk of hemorrhage for high-risk cavernous malformations. Risk reduction, while in evidence during initial follow up, is most pronounced after 2 years.

POSTERIOR FOSSA SCHWANNOMAS

The most common intracranial schwannoma is a vestibular schwannoma, which has made up the vast majority of benign tumors irradiated at our center. Since more patients undergo neuroimaging studies with earlier onset symptoms, smaller tumors are being identified. Increasing numbers of patients are choosing radiosurgery over resection or observation. We have treated patients with trigeminal schwannomas, and jugular foramen region schwannomas within the posterior fossa that provide evidence of different cranial nerve tolerances (42).

At our center we have treated 700 patients with vestibular schwannomas (12–19). The results of radiosurgery have been consistent with a tumor control rate (no need for further treatment) in the range of 97–98% over the last 14 years. With judicious dose selection and highly conformal radiosurgical dose planning *(Fig. 24.2)*, the current risk of facial neuropathy is less than 1%, trigeminal neuropathy less than 2%

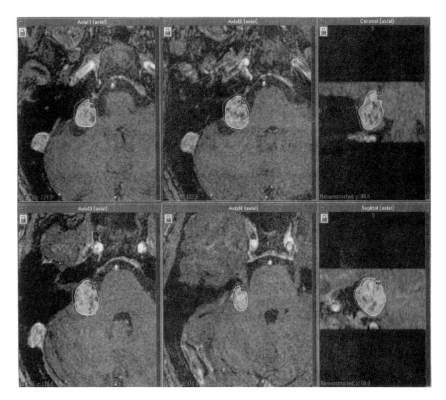

Fig. 24.2 MR images at radiosurgery in a patient with a right vestibular schwannoma. A conformal radiosurgical volume was created with multiple 8- and 4-mm isocenters to deliver a tumor margin dose of 13 Gy.

(depending on volume), and hearing preservation in the range of 60–90%, also depending on tumor size. Such dose planning cannot be achieved in fractionated radiotherapy, nor is any attempt made to tailor the radiation dose precisely to the tumor margin. It appears that the facial nerve is tolerant to a radiosurgery dose of 13 Gy and that high rates of hearing preservation similarly can be achieved at that dose. The reason for trigeminal symptoms in patients with larger tumors remains unclear. Initially it was believed that the dose received by the trigeminal nerve may have been responsible for the decrease in sensation, but we also suspect that it may be irradiation of the trigeminal nucleus within the brainstem itself. When the trigeminal nerve receives much higher doses (i.e., 80 Gy, as in trigeminal neuralgia radiosurgery), the risk for trigeminal sensory loss still remains low.

For patients with vestibular schwannomas large enough to compress the middle cerebellar peduncle, the tumor margin dose between 12–16 Gy rarely causes brain stem effects. In our early experience, rare patients had the appearance of MR signal changes indicative of transient edema in the peduncle but such changes have not been seen for many years. Again it appears that the brain stem tissue is very tolerant to doses less than 13 Gy (19). Similarly we have not seen late infarctions that might be due to occlusion of irradiated perforating arteries in this site or at any other location of the skull base.

Other schwannomas include those related to the trigeminal nerve ($n = 25$), jugular foramen region ($n = 22$), or facial nerve ($n = 1$). Other cranial nerves can also form schwannomas and we have managed patients with hypoglossal or abducens nerve tumors. Many of these patients have undergone partial resection before radiosurgery. The hourglass shape of trigeminal schwannomas can be quite typical, and primary radiosurgery can be effective for patients with smaller tumors.

MENINGIOMAS

Radiosurgery has been used to treat meningiomas at many dural locations in the posterior fossa (20–24). These range from the cavernous sinus and petroclival area superiorly to the foramen magnum inferiorly and the cerebellar convexity posteriorly. The role of radiosurgery is based upon tumor size, patient symptoms, and degree of brain stem compression. For those patients with significant brainstem compression causing a pronounced neurologic deficit, we recommend microsurgical resection (either total or partial) to relieve pressure on the brain as quickly as possible. Radiosurgery is used as adjuvant treatment to halt the growth of a new residual tumor should it remain. The long-term success rate of meningioma radiosurgery has been above 95% for patients who have had radiosurgery as primary treatment and above 90% for those where radiosurgery has had an adjuvant role. A similar margin dose to schwannomas, (12–16 Gy) is often used for posterior fossa meningiomas. This has been associated with a very low chance for brainstem symptoms or cranial neuropathy. One early patient with a petroclival meningioma had a margin dose of 20 Gy that was also received by the superior pons. One year later she developed a transient leg weakness and abducens deficit that resolved completely. Transient enhancement of the adjacent brainstem was seen. Such high doses are no longer used in the posterior fossa for meningiomas and such complications have not been seen for over 11 years.

BRAIN METASTASES

The most common intracranial tumor treated by radiosurgery is the brain metastasis (25–34). Symptoms with brainstem metastasis often harbor a dismal prognosis and little has been written about this entity.

In fact there are no surgical resection series specifically on brainstem metastases to our knowledge and most patients have undergone conventional fractionated radiation therapy. The expected survival with that treatment usually is 3 to 4 months. We have been aggressive with the use of radiosurgery for patients with good performance status and brainstem tumors. The presence of active extracranial disease has not limited the role of radiosurgery at our center. A recent review of patients with brainstem metastasis showed a high rate of long-term tumor control and a median survival of 9 months *(Fig. 24.3)* (28). We recommend that tumor dose selection is in the range of 15 to 18 Gy depending on volume. Since this disease is so invasive and destroys the brainstem parenchyma,

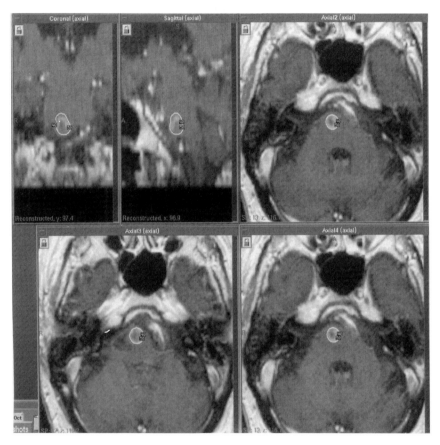

FIG. 24.3 Stereotactic radiosurgery in a patient with metastatic lung cancer to the pons. He presented with diplopia and received whole brain radiotherapy prior to radiosurgery. He also had a small right temporal lobe metastasis. Using two 8-mm isocenters, a margin dose of 16 Gy was delivered.

we usually accept a higher risk with radiosurgery in this setting than with a benign tumor where a longer survival would be expected.

Radiosurgery has changed the surgical management of patients with cerebellar metastasis. Surgeons have long managed patients with cerebellar tumors with some urgency, particularly when surrounding edema or fourth ventricular compression was identified. It is clear that most patients have adequate relief of symptoms with corticosteroid therapy alone, and they can be treated effectively with radiation therapy and radiosurgery, or radiosurgery alone should the metastasis be solitary. At our center, resection of a cerebellar metastasis infrequently performed and not often necessary. For patients with large tumors (above 3 cm in diameter with significant edema) we continue to advocate surgery. However in an era of frequent staging imaging scans and earlier diagnosis, this is becoming a less and less frequent occurrence.

The effects of radiosurgery can be stratified by tumor type. The median survival seen at our center for lung cancer, renal cancer, melanoma, breast cancer, and cancer of unknown origin have been 11 months, 11 months, 7 months, 13 months, and 15 months respectively.

BRAINSTEM ASTROCYTOMA

Patients with glial neoplasms of the brainstem or cerebellum may be suitable for radiosurgery (35–37). At our center, the most common patient in this category is a child with a residual or recurrent pilocytic astrocytoma. Radiosurgery for this tumor can be followed by marked tumor regression on imaging, with good long-term rates of tumor arrest. Malignant glial tumors also may be suitable for boost radiosurgery. Ependymomas or anaplastic ependymomas, also often in children, can be effectively treated with radiosurgery (37). These patients unfortunately remain at risk for the development of new tumors outside the radiosurgical treatment volume.

OTHER TUMORS

Radiosurgery has been used for other tumors in the posterior fossa. Hemangioblastomas, with or without von Hippel Lindau disease can be effectively managed (41). Selected extracranial tumors of the nasopharynx can involve the adjacent posterior fossa and can be boosted with radiosurgery in addition to radiotherapy (38, 40). Chordomas and chondrosarcomas of the petrous bone and clivus are also suitable for primary or adjuvant radiosurgery (39). Jugular foramen region and petrous bone glomus tumors are appropriate for radiosurgery if the tumor does not extend inferiorly into the neck *(Fig 24.4.)*

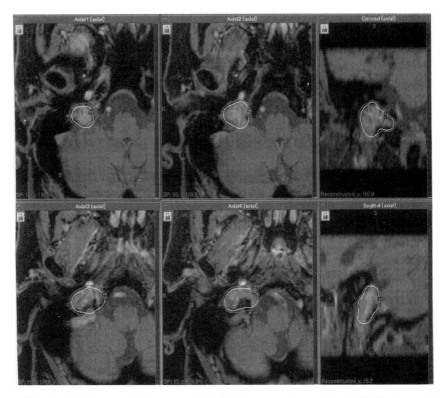

FIG. 24.4 MR images (fat suppression) at radiosurgery in a patient with tinnitus and right hearing dysfunction from a glomus tumor in the jugular foramen. Radiosurgery was performed with multiple 8-mm isocenters to deliver a margin dose of 14 Gy.

TRIGEMINAL NEURALGIA

Although performed sporadically over the last decades, trigeminal neuralgia radiosurgery began in earnest in 1992 (43–46). Many patients fail or cannot tolerate medical therapy, and eventually require surgical intervention. In the past, surgery typically involved either microvascular decompression or one of several percutaneous ablative procedures. Although often associated with initial pain relief, all surgical procedures have variable but definite rates of recurrence and morbidity. Gamma knife radiosurgery has been advocated as a minimally invasive alternative surgical approach for trigeminal neuralgia.

At present we have treated 410 patients with trigeminal neuralgia. Dr. Ronald Young also has a large patient series, and other centers have large experiences in excess of 100 patients. Our last review of 264 consecutive Gamma knife radiosurgery procedures for trigeminal neuralgia performed between 1992 and 1998 was published recently (46). Two hundred and twenty patients had trigeminal neuralgia that was idiopathic, long-standing, and refractory to medication therapy such as carbamazepine, phenytoin, baclofen, or gabapentin as well as a variety of analgesic medications.

Prior surgery was performed in 135 patients (61.4%), including microvascular decompression, glycerol rhizotomy, radiofrequency rhizotomy, balloon microcompression, peripheral neurectomy, or ethanol injections. In these 135 patients, 86 (39.1%) had one, 39 (17.7%) had two, and 10 (4.5%) had three or more procedures prior to radiosurgery. Thus, the majority of patients represented both medical and surgical failures.

MR imaging was performed using contrast-enhanced, short repetition time (TR) sequences and axial volume acquisitions of 512×216 matrices divided into 1-mm slices *(Fig. 24.5)*. A single 4-mm isocenter

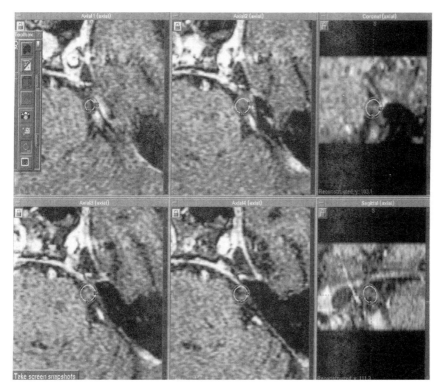

FIG. 24.5 Gamma knife radiosurgery in an 88-year-old man with left trigeminal neuralgia, refractory to medical therapy. A single 4-mm isocenter was targeted to the trigeminal nerve to deliver a maximum dose of 80 Gy.

was used in 192 patients (87.3%) and two 4-mm isocenters were used in 28 patients (12.7%). With a single isocenter, the target was 2 to 4 mm anterior from the junction of the trigeminal nerve and pons. The isocenter was usually located so that brainstem surface was irradiated at the 30% isodose line. We administered maximum doses of 60 Gy (2.7%), 70 Gy (24.1%), 75 Gy (21.8%), 80 Gy (48.6%), 85 Gy (1.8%) and 90 Gy (0.9%).

The outcome of the intervention was graded into four categories: excellent, good, fair, and poor. Complete pain relief without the use of any medication was defined as an *excellent* outcome. We recommended all patients with complete pain relief to taper off their medications, and some patients were in the process of tapering at the time of evaluation (or refused to taper off because of the fear of a recurrence). Those patients with complete pain relief but who were still using some medication were considered as *good* outcomes. Patients with partial pain relief (more than 50% pain relief) were considered to have a *fair* outcome. No pain relief or less than 50% pain relief were considered as *poor*. Thus, though outcomes in 220 patients were calculated using actuarial statistics over a 6.5-year period, the median follow-up duration was 2 years (median, 22 months; range, 6–78).

Most of the patients responded to radiosurgery within 6 months of the procedure (median, 2 months). At the initial follow-up assessment, excellent results were obtained in 105 patients (47.7%), and excellent plus good results were found in 139 patients (63.2 %). More than 50% pain relief (excellent, good, or fair) was noted in 181 patients (82.3%). At the last follow-up evaluation, 88 patients (40%) had excellent outcomes, 121 patients (55.9%) had excellent plus good outcomes, and 152 were fair or better (69.1%). Thirty patients (13.6%) had recurrence of pain after the initial achievement of pain relief (25 patients after complete relief, 5 patients after more than 50% relief) between 2 and 58 months after radiosurgery. Recurrences occurred at a mean of 15.4 months from irradiation.

More than 50% pain relief (excellent, good or fair) was achieved and maintained in 75.8 ± 2.9% of patients at 1 year, 71.3 ± 3.3% of patients at 2 years, and 67.2 ± 3.9% of patients at 3 years. Complete pain relief (excellent or good) was achieved and maintained in 63.6 ± 3.3% of patients at 1 year, and 59.2 ± 3.5% of patients at 2 years, results similar to other series with a high proportion of patients who had failed prior surgery. No patient sustained an early complication after any radiosurgery procedure. Seventeen patients (7.7%) developed increased facial paresthesiae and/or facial numbness that lasted more than 6 months. No patient developed a mastication deficit after radiosurgery or noted problems in facial motor function. The median time to developing paresthesiae was 8 months (range, 1–19 months). After 19 months, no patient developed any new sensory symptoms. In our study, preoperative paresthesia and prior surgery were factors associated with duration of pain relief. Prior surgery may have injured the trigeminal nerve and caused a sensory disturbance. Seventy percent of patients without any prior surgery ($n = 85$) maintained complete pain relief at 9 months and also at 5 years. We did not identify a recurrence in this group past 9 months (46). With this result, it is possible that primary radiosurgery could provide a high rate of long-term pain control, as is found after microvascular decompression. This will require further longer-term follow up.

REFERENCES

1. Lunsford LD, Kondziolka D, Flickinger J, et al: Stereotactic radiosurgery for arteriovenous malformations of the brain. **J Neurosurg** 75:512–524, 1991.
2. Pollock BE, Kondziolka D, Lunsford LD, Bissonette D, Flickinger JC: Repeat stereotactic radiosurgery of arteriovenous malformations: Factors associated with incomplete obliteration. **Neurosurgery** 38:318–324, 1996.
3. Yamamoto M, Jimbo M, Kobayashi M, et al: Long-term results of radiosurgery for arteriovenous malformation: Neurodiagnostic imaging and histological studies of angiographically confirmed nidus obliteration. **Surg Neurol** 37:219–230, 1992.
4. Hadjipanayis C, Levy E, Niranjan A, Firlik A, Kondziolka D, Flickinger J, Lunsford LD: Stereotactic radiosurgery for motor cortex region arteriovenous malformations. **Neurosurgery** 48:70–77, 2001.
5. Mathis J, Barr J, Horton J, et al: The efficacy of particulate embolization combined with stereotactic radiosurgery for treatment of large arteriovenous malformations of the brain. **AJNR** 16:299–306, 1995.
6. Kondziolka D, Lunsford LD, Kanal E, et al: Stereotactic magnetic resonance angiography for targeting in arteriovenous malformation radiosurgery. **Neurosurgery** 35:585–591, 1994.
7. Maesawa S, Flickinger JC, Kondziolka D, Lunsford LD: Repeated radiosurgery for incompletely obliterated arteriovenous malformations. **J Neurosurg** 92:961–970, 2000.
8. Levy E, Niranjan A, Thompson T, Scarrow A, Kondziolka D, Flickinger JC, Lunsford LD: Radiosurgery for childhood intracranial arteriovenous malformations. **Neurosurgery** 47:834–842, 2000.
9. Flickinger JC: An integrated logistic formula for prediction of complications from radiosurgery. **Int J Radiat Oncol Biol Phys** 17:879–885, 1989.
10. Flickinger JC, Kondziolka D, Pollock BE, Maitz A, Lunsford LD: Complications from arteriovenous malformation radiosurgery: Multivariate analysis and risk modeling. **Int J Radiat Oncol Biol Phys** 38:485–490, 1997
11. Kondziolka D, Lunsford LD, Coffey R, et al: Stereotactic radiosurgery of angiographically occult vascular malformations: Indications and preliminary experience. **Neurosurgery** 27:892–900, 1990.
12. Kondziolka D, Lunsford LD, Flickinger JC, et al: Reduction of hemorrhage risk after stereotactic radiosurgery for cavernous malformations. **J Neurosurg** 83:825–831, 1995.
13. Pollock B, Lunsford LD, Flickinger J, Clyde B, Kondziolka D: Vestibular schwan-

noma management. Part I. Failed microsurgery and the role of delayed stereotactic radiosurgery. **J Neurosurg** 89:944–948, 1998.
14. Pollock B, Lunsford LD, Kondziolka D, Sekula R, Subach B, Foote RL, Flickinger J: Vestibular schwannoma management. Part II. Failed radiosurgery and the role of delayed microsurgery. **J Neurosurg** 89:949–955, 1998.
15. Kondziolka D, Lunsford LD, McLaughlin M, Flickinger JC: Long-term outcomes after radiosurgery for acoustic neuromas. **N Engl J Med** 339:1426–1433, 1998.
16. Subach B, Kondziolka D, Lunsford LD, Bissonette D, Flickinger JC, Maitz A: Stereotactic radiosurgery in the management of acoustic neuromas associated with neurofibromatosis-type II. **J Neurosurg** 90:815–822, 1999.
17. Niranjan A, Lunsford LD, Flickinger J, Maitz A, Kondziolka D: Dose reduction improves hearing preservation rates after intracanalicular acoustic tumor radiosurgery. **Neurosurgery** 45:753–765, 1999.
18. Pollock BE, Lunsford LD, Kondziolka D, et al: Outcome analysis of acoustic neuroma management: A comparison of microsurgery and stereotactic radiosurgery. **Neurosurgery** 36:215–229, 1995.
19. Flickinger JC, Kondziolka D, Niranjan A, Lunsford LD: Results of acoustic neuroma radiosurgery: An analysis of 5 years' experience using current methods. **J Neurosurg** 94:1–6, 2001
20. Kondziolka D, Lunsford LD, Coffey RJ, et al: Stereotactic radiosurgery of meningiomas. **J Neurosurg** 74:552–559, 1991.
21. Subach B, Lunsford LD, Kondziolka D, Maitz A, Flickinger JC, et al: Management of petroclival meningiomas by stereotactic radiosurgery. **Neurosurgery** 42:437–445, 1998.
22. Kondziolka D, Flickinger JC, Perez B: Judicious resection and/or radiosurgery for parasagittal meningiomas: Outcomes from the Gamma knife meningioma study group. **Neurosurgery** 43:405–414, 1998.
23. Duma CM, Lunsford LD, Kondziolka D, et al: Stereotactic radiosurgery of cavernous sinus meningiomas as an addition or alternative to microsurgery. **Neurosurgery** 32:699–705, 1993.
24. Kondziolka D, Levy E, Niranjan A, Flickinger J, Lunsford LD: Long-term outcomes after meningioma radiosurgery: physicians and patients perspective. **J Neurosurg** 91:44–50, 1999.
25. Kim Y, Kondziolka D, Flickinger JC, Lunsford LD: Stereotactic radiosurgery for patients with non-small cell lung cancer metastatic to the brain. **Cancer** 80:2075–2083, 1997.
26. Mori Y, Kondziolka D, Lunsford LD, Logan T, Flickinger J: Stereotactic radiosurgery for brain metastases from renal cell carcinoma. **Cancer** 83:344–353, 1998.
27. Mori Y, Kondziolka D, Flickinger J, Kirkwood JM, Agarwala S, Lunsford LD: Stereotactic radiosurgery for cerebral metastatic melanoma: Factors affecting local disease control and survival. **Int J Radiat Oncol Biol Phys** 42:581–589, 1998.
28. Huang CF, Kondziolka D, Flickinger JC, Lunsford LD: Stereotactic radiosurgery for brainstem metastases. **J Neurosurg** 91:563–568, 1999.
29. Firlik K, Kondziolka D, Flickinger J, Lunsford LD: Stereotactic radiosurgery for brain metastases from breast cancer. **Ann Surg Oncol** 7:333–338, 2000.
30. Maesawa S, Kondziolka D, Thompson T, Flickinger J, Lunsford LD: Brain metastases in patients with no known primary tumor: The role of stereotactic radiosurgery. **Cancer** 89:1095–1101, 2000.
31. Loeffler JS, Kooy H, Wen P, et al: The treatment of recurrent brain metastases with stereotactic radiosurgery. **J Clin Oncol** 8:576–582, 1990.
32. Flickinger JC, Kondziolka D, Lunsford LD, et al: A multi-institutional experience

with stereotactic radiosurgery for solitary brain metastases. **Int J Radiat Oncol Biol Phys** 28:797–802, 1994.

33. Kondziolka D, Patel A, Lunsford LD, Kassam A, Flickinger JC: Stereotactic radiosurgery plus whole brain radiotherapy versus radiotherapy alone for patients with multiple brain metastases. **Int J Radiat Oncol Biol Phys** 45:427–434, 1999

34. Rutigliano M, Lunsford LD, Kondziolka D, et al: The cost effectiveness of stereotactic radiosurgery versus surgical resection in the treatment of solitary metastatic brain tumors. **Neurosurgery** 37:445–455, 1995.

35. Kondziolka D, Flickinger JC, Bissonette DJ, Bozik M, Lunsford LD: Survival benefit of stereotactic radiosurgery for patients with malignant glial neoplasms. **Neurosurgery** 41:776–785, 1997.

36. Shrieve D, Alexander E, Wen P, et al: Comparison of stereotactic radiosurgery and brachytherapy in the treatment of recurrent glioblastoma multiforme. **Neurosurgery** 36:275–284, 1995.

37. Jawahar A, Kondziolka D, Lunsford LD, Flickinger JC: Stereotactic radiosurgery for anaplastic ependymomas in children and adults. **Stereotact Funct Neurosurg** 73:23–30, 1999.

38. Kondziolka D, Lunsford LD: Stereotactic radiosurgery for squamous cell carcinoma of the nasopharynx. **Laryngoscope** 101:519–522, 1991.

39. Muthukumar N, Kondziolka D, Lunsford LD, Flickinger J.et al: Stereotactic radiosurgery for chordoma and chondrosarcoma: Further experiences. **Int J Radiat Oncol Biol Phys** 41:387–393, 1998.

40. Firlik KS, Kondziolka D, Lunsford LD, Janecka IP, Flickinger JC: Radiosurgery for recurrent cranial base cancer arising from the head and neck. **Head Neck** 18:160–166, 1996.

41. Jawahar A, Kondziolka D, Garces Y, Pollock B, Flickinger J, Lunsford LD: Stereotactic radiosurgery for hemangioblastomas of the brain. **Acta Neurochir** 142:641–645, 2000.

42. Muthukumar N, Kondziolka D, Lunsford LD, Flickinger J: Stereotactic radiosurgery for jugular foramen schwannomas. **Surg Neurol** 52:172–179, 1999.

43. Leksell L: Stereotaxic radiosurgery and trigeminal neuralgia. **Acta Chir Scand** 137:311–314, 1971.

44. Kondziolka D: Functional radiosurgery. **Neurosurgery** 44:12–22, 1999.

45. Kondziolka D, Flickinger JC, Lunsford LD, et al: Stereotactic radiosurgery for trigeminal neuralgia: A multi-institution study using the gamma unit. **J Neurosurg** 84:940–945, 1996.

46. Maesawa S, Salame C, Pirris S, Flickinger JC, Kondziolka D, Lunsford LD: Clinical outcomes after stereotactic radiosurgery for idiopathic trigeminal neuralgia. **J Neurosurg** 94:14–20, 2001.

47. Massager N, Regis J, Kondziolka D, Njee T, Levivier M: Gamma knife radiosurgery for brainstem arteriovenous malformations: preliminary results. **J Neurosurg** (suppl 3) 93:102–103, 2000.

CHAPTER

25

Reaching for Utopia[*] and Slouching Towards Gomorrah[†]
2000 Congress of Neurological Surgeons: Presidential Address

Daniel L. Barrow, M.D.

It is a unique privilege to address the 50th annual meeting of the Congress of Neurological Surgeons during this first year of a new century and millennium. I owe recognition and thanks to many people for their overwhelming support. I would like to thank my parents, Dr. and Mrs. Warren Barrow, and my grandmother, Mrs. Emma Pessina, who are here in the audience, for providing me with a nurturing environment, an education, and encouragement to pursue my career and life goals. I owe a great debt to my many mentors, particularly Drs. George Tindall, John Jane, Thor Sundt, David Piepgras, and Robert Spetzler, who all offered sound advice and numerous opportunities during my career. I thank all the members of the dozen Executive Committees, with whom I have had the privilege to work, and past CNS Presidents Mike McWhorter, Mike Salcman, and Bill Chandler for taking a chance and entrusting me with the most important jobs in the CNS. I want to personally thank my partners in the Department of Neurosurgery at Emory for their collegial support and tolerance during this past year. Most importantly, I want to express my heartfelt thanks, admiration, and love for my wife and best friend, Mollie, and our three children, Emily, Jack, and Tom. Your patience and support throughout has been uncompromising and greatly appreciated.

A golden anniversary, the end of a century or the beginning of a new millennium are tricks of the calendar, arbitrary calls to reflect upon our past accomplishments and failures and to predict our future courses. Fifty years is a short interval in the context of recorded history. Consider that there have been only 85 generations since the time of Jesus, only 18 since Gutenberg invented the printing press, a mere seven sets of grandparents since the American Revolution and fewer than three from Kitty Hawk to space walks. Centuries of change now occur in one lifetime. The past 50

*From "Utopia" by Sir Thomas More (10)
†From "Slouching Towards Gomorrah" by R.H. Bork (3)

years has witnessed some of the most astounding advances in science of any previous period of similar length. Our specialty has benefited immensely from this scientific renaissance and has been transformed from a fledgling subspecialty of general surgery into a complex and rewarding discipline that neurosurgeons of 1951 would have difficulty recognizing.

One of the primary endeavors of civilized man has been the pursuit of utopia, a state of an impossible ideal (1). Plato was the first to systematically analyze the concept of utopia in *The Republic* (25) and greatly influenced Sir Thomas More, who published *Utopia* and coined the term in 1516 (18). This extraordinary work introduced the promise of "science as liberator and universal benefactor," a view also championed by Francis Bacon in his *New Atlantis* in 1627 (2). While envisioning landmark scientific advances, Bacon postulated that, through skillful research and subsequent discovery, society would have the means to harness nature, achieving both panacea and ultimate liberation. The staggering scientific progress achieved over the past half century has supported the belief that we can accomplish everything in this generation, particularly if we are able to apply the proper technology. Indeed, medical research and discovery during the past 50 years have made the age-old dream of a disease-free world no longer seem foolish and unattainable (29). Within the next 50 years, aging itself may prove to be simply another disease to be treated. Some experts believe that the human life span should not encounter any theoretical natural limits before 120 years, and with continuing advances in molecular biology and a growing understanding of the aging process, that limit could rise to 130 years or more (32). There has already been an explosion in the population of centenarians, with the result that survival to the age of 100 is no longer the newsworthy feat it was when my great-grandmother turned 100 *(Fig. 25.1)*. There were approximately 40,000 centenarians in the United States when she died in 1997 at the age of 110.

Unfortunately, the marvelous accomplishments in science over the past half century that have provided a surge towards a medical utopia contrast with a simultaneous decline in our national character and a crisis of our cultural values. The past 50 years has been characterized by a collapse of our popular culture, a weakening of the intellect, the growth of an intrusive government guided by irrational incentives and a transformation of the federal courts into cultural institutions promoting a politically correct agenda. Robert H. Bork has described this culture in decline in his book, *Slouching Towards Gomorrah,* a reference to the biblical city burned to the ground for the sinfulness of its people (5). He attributes our decline to the "rise of modern liberalism, which stresses the dual forces of radical egalitarianism (the equality of outcome rather than the equality of opportunity) and radical individualism (the drastic reduction of limits to per-

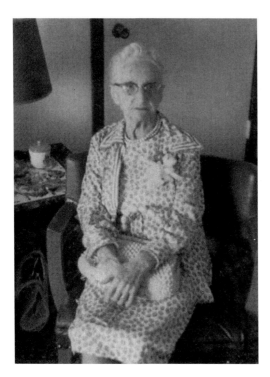

FIG. 25.1 Elvira Arnado (Mama Vera), my 110-year-old great grandmother.

sonal gratification)" (5). Let us explore the changes that have occurred in our society over the past half-century and compare and contrast those changes with the transfiguration of medicine over the past half-century. In doing so, I would submit that, as we have been reaching for Utopia in science and medicine, we are slouching towards Gomorrah in our cultural values and national character.

Much in this country and in the world was different 50 years ago. In 1951, the population of the United States was 155 million, an increase of more than 3 million from 1950. This was the peak year in population growth after World War II, giving rise to the term "baby boom" (33). The presidency of Harry Truman was nearing its conclusion and Dwight Eisenhower would begin his administration in 1952. Politics was characterized by the Cold War and the containment of communism. Fifty years ago this past June, North Korean troops invaded South Korea, marking the beginning of a 3-year war that left nearly 37 thousand Americans dead and thousands more captured or missing in an effort to stand up against communist expansion. In 1951, The United States economy consisted of 48 billion dollars in receipts and 44 billion dollars in expenditures (10). The average per capita income was $1,436.00. Prime television shows in

1951 included *Your Show of Shows* starring Sid Caesar and Imogene Coca, and *You Bet Your Life* starring Groucho Marx. *The Roy Rogers Show* debuted in 1951. Major films in the year of the first meeting of the CNS included *An American in Paris* with Gene Kelly, *A Streetcar Named Desire* with Marlon Brando and Vivian Leigh, and Walt Disney's *Alice in Wonderland*. Popular books in 1951 included *The Kane Mutiny* by Herman Wouk, *From Here to Eternity* by James Jones, and *The Sea Around Us* by Rachel Carson. Joe DiMaggio retired from baseball in 1951 and Ben Hogan won the Masters. 1951 was the first year comic strip kid, "Dennis the Menace," began annoying Mr. Wilson. In the 1951 music scene, Pete Seeger released "On Top of Old Smokey" and Cleveland disc jockey, Allen Freed, coined the term "rock and roll." In the area of science and technology, 1951 saw the explosion of the first hydrogen bomb, the introduction of power steering by Chrysler and the availability of "Super Glue." The world's first electronic digital computer for commercial use was unveiled in 1951. The Universal Automatic Computer, or UNIVAC, weighed 8 tons, consumed 100 kilowatts of power, and performed 2000 calculations per second.

In 1951, health care costs were relatively low because there was little doctors could do for a large percentage of patients. A physical examination, simple blood tests, and X-rays of the chest, bowel and bone, could identify a few treatable disorders; however, many afflictions that are readily controlled by modern medicine led to incapacitation and early mortality in those days (29). "Patients with severe congestive heart failure spent their days in padded chairs designed to keep the edema from settling in their lungs. Patients with medically refractory angina pectoris were effectively disabled. Those with malignant hypertension suffered severe headaches, loss of vision and anticipated kidney failure and stroke in their futures" (29).

Much was different in neurosurgery in 1951. The specialty was guided by indirect and often inaccurate imaging studies, lack of magnification and good illumination in the operating room, marginal neuroanesthetic techniques, and a more primitive understanding of neuropathology. The field was fraught with excessive morbidity and poor outcomes, thus attracting a special breed of physicians.

In 1951 there were approximately 400 neurosurgeons practicing in the United States, 1 for every 387,000 people (10). The majority of neurosurgeons were clustered in major metropolitan areas, most in close proximity to a medical school. The average physician income in 1949 was $11,053, led by neurosurgeons with an average of $28,628. In California in the early 1950s, the annual premium for $10,000 of malpractice coverage was $50 (10).

In 1951, the evaluation of a patient suspected to have an intracranial mass would include a medical history, physical, neurological and funduscopic examinations, x-ray films of the skull and chest and perimetry. Pneumoencephalography and ventriculography were the principle procedures used to confirm or rule out mass lesions, although angiography was being introduced in large medical centers. All contrast studies were done by neurosurgeons and they accounted for about 50% of the neurosurgeon's work and income (36). Other common procedures in 1951 included sympathectomy for hypertension, discectomy, exploratory craniotomy, and tracheostomy, since common endotracheal intubation was still 5 years away.

For decades, neurosurgeons had depended on local anesthesia with the airway kept clear for spontaneous breathing. Devices for head fixation were not in general use in 1951 and combinations of straps and adhesive tape were used to stabilize the head. Neurosurgeons scrubbed their hands with bar soap timed by a 10-minute hourglass. The forearms were then immersed in cylinders of alcohol, followed by immersion in bichloride of mercury which turned the fingernails brown. The hands were then dusted with a packet of talc and were gloved.

Osteoplastic craniotomy was performed with hand-operated instruments—burrs, the Gigli saw and guide and the Stille double-action rongeur. Adequate illumination in a deep exposure was as much a problem in 1951 as it had been in 1907 when Herman Schloffer described how he moved an operating table to a window so that his mirror could direct reflected light into the cavity leading to the patient's sella (28).

Hemostasis was obtained with cotton pledgets, bits of crushed temporal muscle, gel foam and bone wax. Bipolar coagulation was not available in 1951, although James Greenwood had been experimenting with the technique since 1940.

Management of intracranial hypertension was primitive by today's standards. Medical management with hyperventilation, urea and mannitol came in the decade after 1951, and the reality was stark. A patient was nursed in a ward close to the nurse's station as there were no intensive care units. The hyperosmolar agent in use was 50% dextrose, and ventricular tapping was the principle measure for reducing intracranial pressure. Surgical management of uncal herniation, introduced in the 1930s and still in use in 1951, consisted of resection of the uncus and division of the tentorium.

My mentor and teacher, George Tindall, used to tell "war stories" of neurosurgery in the 1950s at Duke University where he trained under Guy Odom and Barnes Woodhall and took his first academic position. He told of patients becoming so ill from pneumoencephalography that they would routinely be whisked from the pneumo chair directly to surgery. If they had time to reconsider their limited options after pneumoencephalography, many patients would simply refuse further treatment. He told stories of "woodpecker surgery": multiple burr holes placed bilaterally to search for treatable, extra-axial hematomas in trauma patients. As a resident I remember asking Dr. Tindall, "Whatever possessed you and your colleagues to enter a field with such poor outcomes and so little to offer?" He responded, "We all knew it had to get better." And better it got!

The major thrust towards a medical utopia can be traced to the same period of history in which the CNS was established. As the United States emerged victorious from World War II, scientists and government leaders believed that the success of research efforts like the Manhattan Project could be emulated in the area of medical research with aggressive governmental support (29). As a result, the National Institutes of Health (NIH) began its re-invention from a small agency with a budget of $26 million in 1948. By 1950, Congress had provided the NIH with an impressive new building in Bethesda, Maryland, along with expanded resources that transformed it into the Goliath of today with an estimated budget of nearly $18 billion *(Fig. 25.2)* (5).

These leaders could not have anticipated the magnitude of the success of the technological revolution they were about to unleash. Consider that in 1951 it would still be two years before James Watson and Frederick Crick published their seminal report on the molecular structure of DNA *(Fig. 25.3)* (34). This paper, published in *Nature,* contained only 128 lines

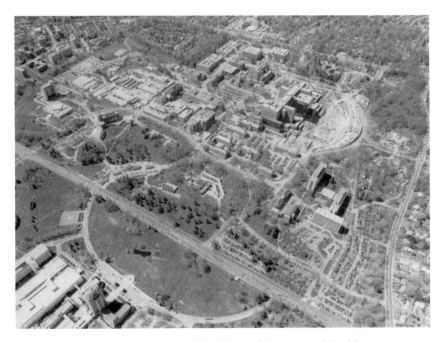

FIG. 25.2 Aerial view of the National Institutes of Health.

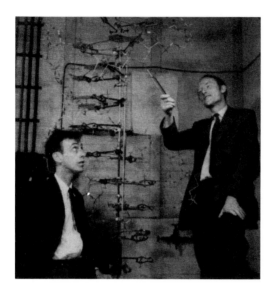

FIG. 25.3 James Watson and Francis Crick with a model of the molecular structure of DNA. (Reprinted with permission from Crick JD: *The Double Helix*. New York: MacMillan.)

but would impact science and medicine as profoundly as Darwin's *On the Origin of Species* or Einstein's *Special Theory of Relativity* (27). Less than 50 years later, the progress that has been made in the field of molecular biology is bewildering. Earlier this year, two independent groups simultaneously announced completion of mapping the human genome—nature's instructions for making and maintaining human beings.

Some important foundations for the current state of neurosurgery had their genesis in this same era in which the CNS was established. Carrea and coworkers performed the first carotid reconstruction in Buenos Aires on October 20, 1951 (8). 1951 was the year Lars Leksell first described and invented the technique for radiosurgery of the brain, and it was the year Hassler and Riechart successfully treated Parkinson's disease with stereotactic lesions in the ventrolateral thalamus (13, 15). Matson introduced ventriculoureterostomy, and Nulsen and Spitz described valve-regulated ventriculo-venous shunting in 1951 (16, 24). This was the same year that first saw the therapeutic use of hypophysectomy for breast and prostate cancer (26). In 1951, Sweet proposed the possible use of neutron-capturing isotopes such as boron-10 in the treatment of brain neoplasms. Sydney Sunderland provided his five-grade classification of peripheral nerve injury (30), and Mulder discussed the causative mechanism for Morton's metatarsalgia in the year of the inaugural CNS meeting (20). In 1951, continuous monitoring of intracranial pressure was first described by Guillaume and Janny and the strain gauge was used experimentally by Eli Goldensohn to establish that hypercarbia raises intracranial pressure (11, 12). These advances were the key to an explosion of laboratory and clinical work during the following decades that changed the field of neurosurgery forever.

Neurosurgeons depending upon pneumoencephalography to peer into the human brain would be astonished by the elegance and accuracy of magnetic resonance imaging (MRI) in detailing the elusive anatomy of the central nervous system. Neurosurgeons of the early 1950s would be shocked by today's routine microsurgical treatment of arteriovenous malformations (AVMs) and aneurysms with little morbidity. Obliteration of deep-seated AVMs by radiosurgical devices or elimination of inoperable aneurysms by electrolytic coils under fluoroscopic guidance would seem unreal. The use of an operating microscope maneuvered by frameless stereotactic MRI guidance would seem like science fiction.

A half-century of unprecedented scientific discovery, however, has not resulted in a social panacea. I believe it is essential to periodically survey and critique the health of our culture and speak out in opposition to trends that may jeopardize our future generations. "This century's battles have, above all, involved ideas, particularly about liberty and equality. Those ideas remain at the center of our debates and anxieties: about globalization, about the balance between governments and markets, the environment, the status of women, the rights of minorities, the fate of the poor, the virtues and vices of capitalism. Liberty and equality are such simple and seemingly virtuous words that it is hard to believe they have caused so much trouble" (31). They have done so for many reasons. One reason is, simply, due to linguistic abuse. Consider the Democratic People's Republic of Korea (aka North Korea) or the People's Republic of China, both founded a half century ago supposedly in the name of freedom and equality. There has also been a long dispute over what liberty actually means and the fact that liberty and equality do not sit happily side-by-side. "Indeed, in many respects they are in conflict. The conflict arises whenever equality is taken to mean equality of outcomes. For to achieve that, it is necessary to take, by force, from some people to give to others. This is also true of the more realistic meaning of equality, namely equality of opportunity. But the sacrifice of liberty required to invest in mass public education or to forbid discrimination in jobs or elsewhere on irrelevant grounds such as race or sex, is one that people, in general, have been willing to make voluntarily. During the past fifty years they have done so with spectacular results. The dispute has been over whether true freedom requires guidance or other intervention from another authority" (31). A rise in contemporary liberalism over the past 50 years has led to a redefinition of liberty and equality, resulting in a crisis in our cultural values, a weakening of our collective intellect and a decline in our national character. Liberty and equality, promoted by traditional liberalism, is what

America is all about. Thomas Jefferson, in drafting the Declaration of Independence, stated, "We hold these truths to be self-evident, that all men are created equal, that they are endowed with certain unalienable Rights, that among these are Life, Liberty and the Pursuit of Happiness." What distinguishes traditional liberalism from contemporary liberalism is not a difference in the central role of liberty and equality, but a difference in the influence of the other forces that modify or constrain radical forms of equality and liberty—the forces of law, religion, family, community and morality. "American conservatism is simply liberalism that accepts the constraints that must necessarily be placed upon the main thrusts of liberalism—liberty and equality. Thomas Jefferson and the signers of the Declaration of Independence understood this. Once they won their independence and got down to the business of running a nation, the Founders were not so lyrical. "Unalienable rights" of the Declaration frequently became alienable. For example, the Fifth Amendment of the Constitution explicitly assumes that a criminal may be punished by depriving him of life or liberty, which has a tendency to interfere with one's pursuit of happiness" (5). Over the past 50 years, the constraints that moderate the drive toward radical egalitarianism and radical liberty are evaporating.

There are many examples of our "slouch towards Gomorrah," including a collapse of popular culture, a decline in our educational system, the atrocious condition of our inner cities, particularly the scourge of illegitimacy, the redefinition of our legal system, and the failure of a social welfare system promulgated by a government with misguided compassion and irrational incentives.

Popular culture provides a reflection of the attitudes and mores of the society. In that arena we have declined precipitously in the past half-century. In 1951, one of the most popular songs in this country was Irving Gordon's "Unforgettable," a beautiful and melodious love song.

In our time, a liberal definition must be applied to the word "music" if it is to describe such modern classics as Nine Inch Nails' "Big Man With a Gun," which resonates with violence and sex.

Michael Bywater writes that "the music industry has somehow reduced humanity's greatest achievement—the near universal language of pure transcendence—into a knuckle-dragging sub-pidgin of grunts and snarls, capable of fully expressing only the more pointless forms of violence and the more brutal forms of sex" (7).

The popular TV show, *I Love Lucy,* debuted in 1951 and provided decent and principled humor and entertainment. Today, television talk shows provide an astonishing example of our ethical and moral deterioration. There are nearly 25 hosts competing for audiences that generate about 100 hours of programs weekly. The question is often asked, "Where do these shows find people willing to appear and reveal their most vulgar intimacies?" A better question might be, "Where do the networks find an estimated audience of 50 million people who want to watch such things as women who marry their rapists or mothers and daughters having affairs with the same man?" "Popular culture is popular because an American public consumes it. The demand for vulgarity and decadence exists without the music, television, and movie industries forcing it upon a reluctant public. This fact, however, does not excuse the industries of fault any more than an addict's demand for heroin excuses the actions of the drug dealer" (5).

The title of a recent book by William Bennett, *The Death of Outrage,* describes our situation (3). "Our culture is attacked by delivering shocks to its moral standards. When that culture keeps revising its standards by accumulating each new outrage, it is necessary to keep upping the ante by being ever more shocking. Large sections of our society, like drug-resistant bacteria, are approaching the state of being unshockable(3)." As Pat Moynihan has stated, "we have, as a society, defined deviancy down" (19). We have argued that if something is prevalent it must be normal, and if it is normal then it must be acceptable.

This decline in our popular cultural can be traced to a modern emphasis on radical individualism or unrestrained personal gratification. To propose a ban on anything that can be called "expression" is an attempt to "take away our constitutional rights." "Such reactions," says Robert Bork, an expert in constitutional law, "reveal a profound ignorance of the history of the First Amendment. Until quite recently, nobody even raised the question of that amendment in prosecutions of pornographers; it was not thought relevant even by the pornographers . . . First Amendment jurisprudence has shifted from the protection of the exposition of ideas towards the protection of self-expression—however lewd, obscene, or profane" (5).

How could I discuss a decline in morality at this time without mentioning our current Commander-in-Chief? In 1951, the stage was set for Dwight Eisenhower, a war hero and virtuous family man, to become the next President of the United States. In contrast, I quote Senator Joe Lieberman, now the Democratic Vice Presidential candidate, on the subject of William Jefferson Clinton's publicly displayed extramarital affair in the vicinity of the Oval Office with an employee half his age: " . . . such behavior is not just inappropriate. It is immoral. And it is harmful, for it sends a message of what is acceptable behavior to the larger American family, particularly to our children, which is as influential as the negative messages communicated by the entertainment culture" (16).

There are other examples of our cultural descent. The past 50 years has witnessed a worrisome decline of intellect and a collapse of our educational system. Today our schools are graduating the first generation in

American history that is less well educated than the prior generation. "Every employer recognizes that it is perfectly possible for an individual to graduate from an American high school and be functionally illiterate—incapable of writing or reading a complicated paragraph" (35). The explanation for this decline is also rooted in behavior and ideas. Richard Hofstadter wrote in 1962, "It has been noticed that intellect in America is resented as a kind of excellence, as a claim to distinction, as a challenge to egalitarianism . . . anti-intellectualism made its way into our politics because it became associated with our passion for equality" (14). Again, the problem can be traced to one of the products of modern liberalism, the promotion of radical egalitarianism, the equality of outcomes rather than opportunities. Egalitarianism was a positive force in gradually extending education to all children and adolescents, but egalitarianism also led to the concept that education must be largely the same for all levels of ability. An egalitarian educational system opposes meritocracy and reward for achievement. Those with greater academic potential were no longer encouraged to achieve as they once were. The result has been declining SAT scores (22), American students falling well behind the students of many other nations on international science and mathematics tests, and even college students frequently lacking basic historical and geographical knowledge.

The National Association of Scholars (NAS) conducted a systematic survey of the evolution of university education in 50 highly selective institutions over a period of 80 years. The result was a scathing report card on American higher education, characterized by the dissolution of structure, the evaporation of content, and the decline of rigor. General education requirements have been abandoned, producing students who have information about small niches of a subject but no conception of the larger context that alone can give the niches meaning. The percentage of institutions with requirements in literature, philosophy, religion, social science, natural science and mathematics has plummeted. The NAS report paints "a discouraging portrait of diminishing rigor at the most prestigious colleges and universities in our land. Thus, by 1993, students graduating from these elite schools not only had fewer assignments to complete but were asked to do considerably less to complete them." In 1914, 98% of the surveyed schools had Saturday classes. By 1993, only 6% had Saturday classes and there was "a widespread impression within academe that even Friday classes are becoming a rarity" (22).

Over the past 50 years it has been assumed that the best predictor of a school's success was the amount of money spent on the school. More recent objective analysis has demonstrated that the best predictor of a school's performance is the quality of the families from which the school children come (9). The most important variables can explain approximately 90% of the difference in school performances: 1) the number of parents in the home; 2) the quantity and quality of reading material in the home; 3) the amount of homework done in the home; and 4) the amount of television watched in the home (35).

The decline in education, therefore, is related to another major concern on the minds of the American public at the beginning of the 21st century, namely the condition of our cities and its underclass and its effect on families. As George Will has stated, "We are evolving in America today a kind of civilization that never existed before and should not exist here—one in which the cities are important not as centers of cultural and commercial vitality but are important, rather, only as burdens. We are experiencing something without precedent in urban history—broad scale social regression in the midst of rising prosperity. The principle correlate of this is family disintegration, the principle consequence is the intergenerational transmission of poverty and the sound effect is gun fire" (35).

Charles Murray, a political scientist, contends that "illegitimacy is the single most important social problem of our time—more important than crime, drugs, poverty, illiteracy, welfare, or homelessness because it drives everything else" (21). In 1965, Pat Moynihan, then a young social scientist in the government, published a famous report on the crisis in the black family. He declared that our country was in the midst of a crisis because 26% of all children born to black mothers were born out of wedlock. At the end of the 20th century, the number was 68% and still rising. Twenty four percent of white children are born out of wedlock today, just 2% below what it was in black America when Moynihan rightly declared a crisis, rising faster in white America than in black America. The frightening fact is that no one truly understands how this happened; the collapse of a timeless, ancient norm. "It was a mark of disgrace, a stigma, to be associated with the cruel and reckless act of bringing a child into the world for whom you had neither the will nor the capacity to properly parent. This revolution in values has occurred, not in a nation ravaged by war, famine and pestilence, but in the United States of America during peace and prosperity" (35).

If a rise in modern liberalism is a driving force behind our decline, a bloated and intrusive federal government, guided by irrational incentives, is the engine behind that rise and the federal courts have become the vehicle for that rise. In 1950, the average American family of four sent 2% of its income to the Federal government. Today it sends 24%, twelve times the amount. Not many Americans are convinced they are getting twelve times better government. It is likely that our liberal social policies of the past 50 years have been fundamentally incorrect. "The politicians responsible for designing and implementing our social welfare state were from a generation influenced by the hardening experience of unemployment in the Depression. This era of politicians believed that social problems and dysfunctional behavior have material bases and, therefore, have material solutions. Our social welfare system has blundered under the assumption that what the poor really need are goods and services that only the government can deliver to them" (35). Most of the social welfare programs instated over the past 50 years began as morally sound ideas but suffer from misguided compassion and irrational incentives. As an example, consider the program for Aid to Dependent Children. This well-intentioned program provided federal funding to unwed mothers to assist in the responsibility of raising their illegitimate children. The program, however, became nothing more than government paid prostitution, as it provided a disincentive to marriage and increased funding for the addition of more children born out of wedlock.

At the end of this last century, the future of our welfare system is in jeopardy due to a paradox articulated by George Will. "The great achievement of 20th century liberalism is the welfare state. That great achievement now makes liberal governance impossible. It makes it impossible because the welfare state has swallowed the federal budget—the great consumers of welfare state transfer payments are the elderly—pension and medical care. And we are an aging population. Demography is destiny and that is the great demographic fact" (35). Medical science has already made the very old the fastest growing segment of our population. Since 1960, the American population has grown 30%, but the American population age group 85 or older has grown 230% and it will continue (32). Currently, 50% of the federal budget is earmarked for entitlement programs. Another 14% is used to pay interest on the national debt, leaving 1/3 of the budget for all domestic discretionary spending and all defense spending.

It is a fact that our medical successes have created some new social challenges. One of the most pressing fiscal issues is the increasing cost of health care and the means to pay for the delivery of the many products of our medical successes. The advances that have occurred in medicine in the past 50 years are taken for granted and the role these advances have played in driving up costs is generally forgotten. There has been a tendency, particularly among politicians, to blame inefficiency and greed in the health care system rather than facing the paramount issue that advancing technology continually opens up new therapeutic and diagnostic opportunities that must be paid for. During the past two decades, new technology has been responsible for approximately half of the 6% (inflation-adjusted) annual rise in expenditures on medical care (29). The rest is due to rising costs of wages and supplies. This issue was notably absent from the debate that surrounded the most recent attempt to expand government control of our economy. That occurred in 1994 when the Democratic Party put forth a health care plan that would be the "social security of the nineties," in an effort to again convince the middle class of the central role of government in our society. Allow me to rehearse that debate in the style of George Will (35). The Clinton administration stated that we were having a health care crisis because we were spending 14 % of GDP on health care and that's too much. Critics asked, "How do you know that's too much?" And they said, "Well, it's more than Austria spends." And the critics asked, "Well, since when did Austria become an American aspiration?" And they said, "Well, it's more than we spent in 1960. In 1960 we spent only 6% of GDP on health care." And the critics said, "Well, good, all in favor of going back to 1960s medicine, say you're in favor of giving up MRIs, lasers and molecular biology." As recently as the mid 1970s there were only 10,000 coronary bypass operations performed in America in a year. This year, there will be about 600,000. Is that too many? About 600,000 Americans think that's exactly the right number. Then they said, "Well, we have a crisis in health care because infant mortality rates are scandalously high." Indeed they are. In some of our central cities they are at third world levels. But that, ladies and gentlemen, is because of children having babies, low birth-weight babies born to young women out of wedlock. That is not an inefficiency in the health care system, it is a crisis of cultural values. They say, "Well, the life expectancy in Japan is longer than here in the United States." Quite right. Of course, we have an AIDS rate 200 times that of Japan and more hand guns in private ownership in this city than in all of the Japanese islands. Not an inefficiency of the health care system, a crisis in cultural values.

Today, the courts view themselves as political and cultural institutions. The Supreme Court, without authorization from the law, is taking out of the hands of the American people the most basic and moral cultural decisions. In his First Inaugural Address, Abraham Lincoln asserted, "The candid citizen must confess that if the policy of the Government upon vital question affecting the whole people is to be irrevocably fixed by decision of the Supreme Court . . . the people will have ceased to be their own rulers, having to that extent practically resigned their Government into the hands of that eminent tribunal." President Lincoln was referring to the Dred Scott decision, the infamous decision that created a constitutional right to own slaves. Lincoln's words were a harbinger of things to come and we have not heeded his warning. Into the hands of the federal judiciary we have resigned ever more vital questions affecting our nation. Modern Supreme Court decisions have repeatedly maximized individual rights at the expense of corporate rights of what sociologists call "intermediate institutions"—families, schools, business organizations, private associations, local and state governments (4, 23).

With a change in the role of the courts from judiciary to political institutions have come the gradual elimination of personal accountability and the extortion of legitimate business. The government has promoted and made lucrative the idea that most Americans are victims of American society. Americans are encouraged to organize into grievance groups and petition the government for entitlements and reparations for the wickedness done to them by American society.

Notwithstanding the concerns I have expressed about our society's slouch, I remain optimistic that we can avoid Gomorrah. Unlike early Eutopian authors who placed their ultimate faith in "science as liberator and universal benefactor," I am optimistic because of my faith in the ability of the American people to achieve and succeed once a challenge is identified and a goal is established. Larger segments of our society are recognizing the decline I speak of. If a consensus cries out for a restoration of our national character and an enhancement of our cultural values, the challenge will be identified. If we devote our inner resources to these social goals today as we did our scientific goals over the past half-century, I am confident we can avoid Gomorrah and benefit from a cultural and ethical renaissance. Ultimately, we are responsible for the world we create and no generation gets a free pass. Right now, we need the willingness and emotional courage to restore ethical and moral behavior into our culture, to bring the Supreme Court back to its constitutional legitimacy, to restore American education to its former level of rigor and substance, and to eliminate the perverted and illogical government incentives that reward deviant and risky behavior. The only impediment is the will of the people. That will begins with people like you and me. Through our positions as professionals, physicians, surgeons, educators, philanthropists, and parents, we have the ability and duty to influence positive change in our culture and national character.

Despite my criticisms of our society and culture, the past 50 years has witnessed many social and cultural triumphs. The staggering progress of the past half-century in science and technology has been created and funded by this society. Great strides have been made in civil rights over the past 5 decades. The cold war was won and the threat of war casts its dark shadow over a smaller proportion of the world's population than before. Fewer people live in constant fear of arbitrary arrest and torture, and political, economic and personal liberty has become a widespread fact for the first time.

As we focus our attention on improving our moral and ethical health, we must not forget that much remains undone in our specialty. In our field, more reliable therapeutic options are needed for the management of cerebral ischemia, chronic pain and neurodegenerative diseases. Spinal cord injury remains a devastating problem and the management of head injury remains suboptimal. *Figure 25.4* is a picture of my younger sister

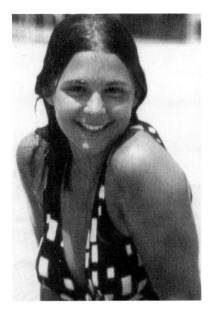 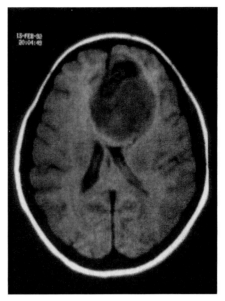

FIG. 25.4 *Left:* Photograph of my younger sister, Kris Barrow. *Right:* Axial MRI demonstrating her glioblastoma.

and an MRI revealing her glioblastoma. At the time of her diagnosis in 1992, her outlook was, for practical purposes, no better than that of a similar patient in 1951. We have much yet to accomplish. We must not only elude Gomorrah but also continue to reach for Utopia.

REFERENCES

1. Apuzzo MLJ: Brave New World: Reaching for Utopia. Editor's Letter. **Neurosurgery** 46:1033, 2000.
2. Bacon F: *New Atlantis.*
3. Bennett WJ: *The Death of Outrage. Bill Clinton and the Assault on American Ideals.* New York: The Free Press, 1998.
4. Berger PL, Neuhaus RJ: *To Empower People: From State to Civil Society,* 2nd edition, Washington, DC: The AEI Press, 1996.
5. Bork RH: *Slouching Towards Gomorrah. Modern Liberalism and American Decline.* New York: Regan Books, HarperCollins, 1996.
6. Bork RH: *The Tempting of America: The Political Seduction of the Law.* New York: The Free Press, 1990.
7. Bywater M: Never mind the width, feel the lack of quality (reviewing the Faber Book of Pop, London, Faber, 1995). **The Spectator,** May 13, 1995, p 44.
8. Carrea RME, Molins M, Murphy G: Surgical treatment of spontaneous thrombosis of the internal carotid artery in the neck, carotid-carotideal anastomosis: Report of a case. **Acta Neurol Lationam** 1:71–78, 1955.

9. Faria MA Jr.: Why the decline in American education (and morals). Editor's Corner. **Medical Sentinel** 2:14–15, 1997.
10. Florin RE: Status of neurosurgery in 1951: A socioeconomic perspective. In Barrow DL, Kondziolka D, Laws ER, Traynelis VC (eds): *Fifty Years of Neurosurgery: The Golden Anniversary of the Congress of Neurological Surgeons.* Baltimore: Lippincott, Williams & Wilkins, 2000.
11. Goldensohn E, Whitehead R, Parry T, Spencer J, Grover R, Dreper W: Effect of diffusion respiration and high concentrations of CO2 on cerebrospinal fluid pressure of anesthetized dogs. **Am J Physiol** 165:334–340, 1951.
12. Guillaume J, Janny P: [Continuous intracranial manometry]. **Rev Neurol** 84:131–142, 1951. (Article in French).
13. Hassler R, Reichert T: Indikationen und Lokalisationsmethode der gezielten Hirnoperationen. **Nervenarzt** 25:441–447, 1954.
14. Hofstadter R: *Anti-intellectualism in American Life.* New York: Vintage Books, 1962, p 51.
15. Leksell L: The stereotaxic method and radiosurgery of the brain. **Acta Chir Scand** 10:316–319, 1951.
16. Lieberman J: Address to the Senate Regarding President Clinton and the Independent Counsel's Investigation. Washington Post, September 3, 1998.
17. Matson DD: Ventriuloureterostomy. **J Neurosurg** 8:398–404, 1951.
18. More T: *Utopia.*
19. Moynihan DP: Defining deviancy down. **The American Scholar,** Winter, 1993, p 17.
20. Mulder JD: The causative mechanism in Morton's metatarsalgia. **J Bone Joint Surg** 33B:94, 1951.
21. Murray C: The Coming White Underclass, *The Wall Street Journal,* October 29, 1993, p A14.
22. National Association of Scholars: *The Dissolution of General Education: 1914–1993.* Princeton: National Association of Scholars, 1996.
23. Nisbit R: *Twilight of Authority.* New York: Oxford University Press, 1975.
24. Nulsen F, Spitz E: Treatment of hydrocephalus by direct shunt from ventricle to jugular vein. **Surg Forum** 2:399–403, 1951.
25. Plato: *The Republic.*
26. Ray BS: Intracranial hypophysectomy. J Neurosurg 28:180–186, 1968.
27. Rutka JT, Taylor M, Mainprize T, Langlois A, Ivanchuk S, Mondal S, Dirks P: Molecular biology and neurosurgery in the third millennium. **Neurosurgery** 46: 1034–1051, 2000.
28. Schloffer H: Erfolgreiche operation eines hypophysen-tumors auf nasalen wege. **Wein Klin Wochenschr** 20:621–624, 1907.
29. Schwartz, WB: *Life Without Disease. The Pursuit of Medical Utopia.* Berkeley and Los Angeles: University of California Press, 1998.
30. Sunderland S: A classification of peripheral nerve injuries producing loss of function. **Brain** 74:491, 1951.
31. **The Economist:** Liberty, Equality, Humility. September 11, 1999.
32. U.S Bureau of the Census: Current population report, special studies: 65+ in the United States. Washington DC: U.S. Government Printing Office, 1996; Social Security Administration, Office of the Actuary. Tables used in support of the 1995 Trustees Report, Alternative 2 Life Expectancy Series.
33. United States Census Bureau: Historical National Population Estimates: July 1900 to July 1998. United States Census Bureau, Washington, DC.

34. Watson JD, Crick FHC: Molecular structure of nucleic acids: A structure for deoxyribose nucleic acid. **Nature** 171:737–738, 1953.
35. Will G: Address to the Annual Meeting of The Society of Actuaries. Boston, Massachusetts, 1995.
36. Wilson CB, Rosegay, H: The status of neurosurgery in 1951: Clinical practice. In Barrow DL, Kondziolka D, Laws ER, Traynelis VC (eds): *Fifty Years of Neurosurgery: The Golden Anniversary of the Congress of Neurological Surgeons.* Baltimore: Lippincott, Williams & Wilkins, 2000.

Author Index

Subject Index